MEDICAL CONSULTATION

The Internist on Surgical, Obstetric, and Psychiatric Services

Second Edition

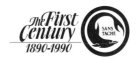

MEDICAL CONSULTATION

The Internist on Surgical, Obstetric, and Psychiatric Services

Second Edition

Co-Editors

William S. Kammerer, M.D.
Associate Professor of Medicine
Department of Medicine
Milton S. Hershey Medical Center
The Pennsylvania State University

Richard J. Gross, M.D.
Assistant Professor of Medicine
The Johns Hopkins University School of Medicine
Department of Medicine
The Johns Hopkins Hospital *and*
the Francis Scott Key Medical Center
Baltimore, Maryland

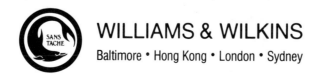

WILLIAMS & WILKINS
Baltimore • Hong Kong • London • Sydney

Editor: Michael G. Fisher
Associate Editor: Carol Eckhart
Project Editor: Teresa A. Tamargo
Designer: Wilma E. Rosenberger
Illustration Planner: Wayne Hubbel
Production Coordinator: Charles E. Zeller

Copyright © 1990
Williams & Wilkins
428 East Preston Street
Baltimore, Maryland 21202, USA

Accurate indications, adverse reactions, and dosage schedules for drugs are provided in this book, but it is possible that they may change. The reader is urged to review the package information data of the manufacturers of the medications mentioned.

Printed in the United States of America

First Edition 1983

Library of Congress Cataloging-in-Publication Data

Medical consultation : the internist on surgical, obstetric, and
  psychiatric services / co-editors, William S. Kammerer, Richard J.
  Gross.—2nd ed.
      p.   cm.
  Includes bibliographical references.
  ISBN 0-683-04506-7
  1. Internal medicine.   2. Medical consultation.   3. Internists.
I. Kammerer, William S.   II. Gross, Richard J. (Richard Joseph),
1948–   .
  [DNLM: 1. Internal Medicine.   2. Referral and Consultation.   W 64
M489]
RC48.M43   1990
616—dc20
DNLM/DLC
for Library of Congress   89-16705
                                                                  CIP

90 91 92 93
1 2 3 4 5 6 7 8 9 10

To Graham H. Jeffries, M.B., Ch.B., D.Phil., Founding Chairman of the Department of Medicine and, for 20 years, Professor of Medicine at the University Hospital of The Pennsylvania State University. Mentor and friend. Pre-eminent consultant. He leads by example.

Foreword to the First Edition

When thou arte callde at anye time,
A patient to see;
And doste perceave the cure too grate,
And ponderous for thee;

See that thou laye disdeyne aside,
And pride of thyne owne skyll;
And thinke no shame counsell to take,
But rather wyth good wyll.

Gette one or two of experte men,
To help thee in that nede;
And make them partakers wyth thee,
In that worke to procede.

—John Halle, M.D. (1529–1566)
From *Goodlye Doctrine and Instruction*

The practicing internist is often called on to provide advice to colleagues. The time devoted to this endeavor during medical residency training varies from program to program but in general is not consonant with the need. A busy general internist may spend up to 40% of practice time providing consultations. The error made in most training programs is the assumption that, if a physician is competent to care for the diabetic on a medicine service, then he or she is competent to manage the diabetic through delivery or a surgical procedure. In fact, to give valuable service the consultant needs to understand the exigencies of anesthesia, the surgical procedure, the dynamics of pregnancy, labor, and delivery, and the disposition of colleagues.

The general internist is often in the best position to understand and work with these multiple variables. By virtue of their usual practice mix, general internists are faced daily with "interface medicine." Multiple medical problems in the same patient are the rule in general internal medicine, and the proper care of such patients requires knowledge of the effects of one disease on another, the hazards of polypharmacy, and the importance of the larger picture of health and disease.

Because these considerations and techniques are not the province of traditionally oriented textbooks, the editors felt the need to present this information in a composite form. Although chaptered and indexed in usual organ or disease entity ways, the information stresses the effects of surgery or pregnancy on a disease process or, conversely, the effects of a disease or pregnancy on the outcome of surgery. Further, the editors and contributors provide specific practical management advice designed to minimize these effects.

Before launching into the specific portions of this text, we would offer some general recommendations regarding the conduct of consultations which experience has taught us are worth bearing in mind as you make your appointed rounds.

KNOW FOR WHOM YOU ARE PROVIDING THE SERVICE. Different services may be looking for different kinds of advice. So, too, some individual physicians may routinely call for specific types of assistance.

KNOW WHY YOU ARE BEING CONSULTED. In general terms the request may be: "Help! What do I do now?"; "Come argue with another consultant"; or "Come see what a nice job I've done." More specifically, try to elicit the exact question being asked.

BE BRIEF—ALLOW FOR SELECTIVE READING OF YOUR NOTE. Long notes are not read. You should title sections of your note so that areas of interest for different readers will be readily identified. If you wish to record information for your own future review or to help a covering consultant, separate it from the rest of your text.

BE SPECIFIC WITH RECOMMENDATIONS. Therapeutic measures should be spelled out with respect to drug, dose, route of administration, desired effect, and toxicity.

SUPPORT YOUR RECOMMENDATIONS AND IMPRESSIONS. Your text should include the data to warrant a diagnosis and the indications for diagnostic and therapeutic recommendations.

TEACH THE READER. You have been asked to provide a special service. This is an admission that the requestor seeks information. Your experience with similar cases and pertinent points from the literature are appropriate.

FOLLOW-UP. It is a rare consultation which should involve one visit. If that is the case, you should indicate that you will not return unless requested.

Your note should include what progress you expect and should provide the opportunity to change your problem list as the data base expands. Flow sheets which you can initiate might be a worthwhile venture. The follow-up visit is your best learning device.

BE CHARITABLE. You do not help the patient when you shame or anger his doctor.

ATTEMPT PERSONAL COMMUNICATION. This is a courtesy which allows you to amplify your note and reinforce your recommendations.

BE HONEST. You have been called in as an expert. Do not suggest diagnoses which are not supported by the data. Get help when you need it or recommend other consultants who can deal adequately with the situation.

The editors and contributors to this volume are from two training programs that endeavor to stress consultation skills as important educational components. All have wide experience in both providing and teaching consultations. Their contributions contain the science of the discipline and the wisdom of having done it many times.

J. W. Burnside

Preface to the Second Edition

Plus ca change, plus c'est la meme chose

The central theme of the second edition remains the same: a well-prepared general internist with a special interest in consultation medicine will best serve the interests of patients with medical problems on nonmedical services. Recent changes in insurance and hospital regulations, philosophy, training programs, and knowledge base are markedly altering medical consultation. Increased emphasis is being placed on elective outpatient evaluation; more than one-half of all evaluations are now being performed on an outpatient basis, a marked change that has occurred in a little more than 5 years. The general internist is ideally qualified to perform outpatient evaluations, but these require even more attention to proper communication and efficiency.

The increased number of surgical patients with multiple problems or in intensive care units is consuming greater proportions of physicians' time, changing the way physicians practice, and altering training programs. The amount of information to be collected and the therapeutic interventions available expand on an almost-daily basis. Under these conditions, it has been the well-trained general internist committed to patient care who has been called upon to care for the "whole patient" again, to coordinate multiple (and, occasionally, conflicting) strategies of subspecialty consultants, and to function effectively and efficiently in the absence of all the data that would ideally be available. For effective consultation, both communication skills and a command of an expanding knowledge base are required.

To meet these changing conditions, this edition has been expanded by the addition of new chapters on general medical evaluation of the preoperative patient, evaluation of the presumably healthy patient, evaluation for outpatient surgery, invasive cardiovascular monitoring, and the oncology patient requiring surgery. Most chapters have been extensively expanded based on new developments.

We welcome several new authors (J. Ballard, J. Field, B. Ford, R. Simons) who have given this edition "new blood." Although we are aware of many new concepts and techniques in various disciplines, we have not included every new idea reported if it is untested or too "subspecialized" (e.g., intraoperative EEG monitoring). We have used the same criteria for adding new references. In an effort to assist the reader, we have highlighted key concepts and information throughout the text.

This text selectively emphasizes information on medical problems of surgical, obstetric, and psychiatric patients that is *different* from that for the usual medical patients. We have not tried to reproduce another textbook of general medicine; this would necessitate the reader plucking what was "different" in the nonmedical patient from a mass of general medical knowledge. The precise focus of this text is to highlight these differences. Likewise, the amount of literature available varies tremendously, from the massive number of articles in cardiology, to relatively few in gastroenterology. This makes uniformity in style difficult. The editors have again decided to allow individual chapter authors wide latitude in order to best present their material. Whereas this decision yields variation in editorial uniformity, we believe it best achieves our goal of presenting the field of medical consultation in a clear, practical manner.

This book was conceived as an equal effort between the two editors and their general internal medicine faculties. They bring to this edition varied and complementary interests, skills, and experience.

There remain many gaps in knowledge in this field and in the bibliography. We hope this text will stimulate our readers to fill these gaps with careful clinical research. As before, we welcome suggestions or corrections from readers for future editions.

Our goal continues to be providing the consulting internist with practical information for the care of our sickest and most complex patients.

William S. Kammerer
Richard J. Gross

Preface to the First Edition

"Operating on someone who has no place else to go."
—Dr. John Kirklen, quoted by Dr. C. B. Mullins, with permission.

What would motivate one to put together a multiauthored text on a subject traditionally learned through years of trial and error at the bedside and hours of labor in the library? We felt that, by bringing together the views of experienced internist consultants and a widely scattered literature, we could provide a nidus for an effective teaching program for residents, as well as a reference for continuing self-education for the practicing internist. Because medical consultations to non-medical services make up a large part of an average working day for practicing internists and medical residents, most training programs now include a rotation on a general medical consultation service. However, teaching on such services is hampered by the lack of reference material and the experience is often haphazard, isolated, and unsupervised. Many medical residents thus come to dread this activity and feel it is irrelevant and unscientific.

By categorizing the lessons learned from personal experience and the thinking of experienced internists, we hope that the prolonged floundering of trial and error learning will thereby be shortened and given direction. Consultation medicine is one of the few remaining areas in a subspecialty world where the venerable concept of the general internist as a master diagnostician of all ills "from the skin in" can come alive and allow the full utilization of all of his/her skills.

Recognizing that even the most complete general internist tends to become more proficient in one area than another, we felt a multiauthored approach, representing several institutions and styles of practice, would best serve the goals of this book. With few exceptions (e.g., anesthesiology, mechanical respiratory support, and dermatology) dictated by special skills and knowledge, all of the contributors are practicing general internists.

Undoubtedly, some subspecialists will find omissions or generalizations in the text which are unacceptable to them. However, rather than attempting an encyclopedic subspecialty reference text, our goal is to provide an approach as practiced by experienced general internists to specific perioperative problems and to medical problems in pregnancy and psychiatry. This approach emphasizes clinical decision making and practical management techniques rather than extended discussions of medical, surgical, and anesthetic pathophysiology. Due to the complex interrelationships at the interface of medical, surgical, and anesthetic problems and to the rapid changes in their relative importance through the pre-, intra-, and postoperative periods, pathophysiologic generalizations are often impossible to apply to the individual patient. Thus, we place the majority of our emphasis on clinical decision-making based on well-designed empirical studies and extensive personal experience. However, in areas where a general understanding of current surgical or anesthetic pathophysiology cannot reasonably be expected of the general internist, it is incorporated in the appropriate clinical discussions. Obviously, this approach assumes a general familiarity with a wide range of medical and surgical problems.

While attempting to keep the general structure and organization of all sections reasonably uniform, the remaining diversity in styles tends to reemphasize the need for versatility and practicality in the approach to medical consultations to surgical and non-medical services.

Discerning readers will note that the

bibliography occasionally appears dated, or even absent, for common consultation problems. Perhaps this observation will provide a stimulus to our readers to fill these gaps.

We hope the book will serve the needs of both medical residents and the consulting general internist and prove practical, educational, and stimulating.

W. S. Kammerer, M.D.
R. J. Gross, M.D.

Acknowledgments

We gratefully acknowledge Kay Cassel for her superior word processing abilities and indispensable secretarial and organizational skills. We also acknowledge the efforts of librarians Jean Shipman and Mary Lee Pabst for locating and copying references.

For their encouragement and support, we thank Donald O. Wood, M.D., Barbara Grosz, Ph.D., Kathleen A. Gross, Brent Petty, L. R. Barker, D. Levine, and Gina Chiloro. For their patience and for comic relief during our labors, we thank our children, Christopher, Stacey, Cal, David, and Jonathan.

We thank also our toughest critics, our senior residents and colleagues, for their constructive criticism of much of this second edition: Drs. Mahmood Ali Kahn, Mark Bates, Deborah Bethards, Barry Clemson, Joseph Converse, Robert Cordes, Claude Fanelli, Colleen Fletcher, Kevin Green, Charles Haile, A. I. Mushlin, Michael Pasquale, David Pawlush, David Roberts, Howard Rudnick, and Thomas Ruth.

The authors and editors, however, take responsibility for the final choice of content and for any errors.

Contributors

JAMES O. BALLARD, M.D.
Associate Professor of Medicine
Division of Hematology
Milton S. Hershey Medical Center
The Pennsylvania State University
Hershey, Pennsylvania

GARY R. BRIEFEL, M.D.
Associate Professor of Medicine
The Johns Hopkins University School of
  Medicine
Director of Dialysis Services
Francis Scott Key Medical Center
Baltimore, Maryland

JOHN W. BURNSIDE, M.D.
Associate Dean for Clinical Affairs
Southwestern Medical School
University of Texas Health Science Center
Dallas, Texas

LOURDES C. CORMAN, M.D.
Associate Professor of Medicine
Division of General Internal Medicine
University of Florida College of Medicine
Gainesville, Florida

JOHN M. FIELD, M.D.
Associate Professor of Medicine and Sur-
  gery
Director, Emergency Medical Services
Milton S. Hershey Medical Center
The Pennsylvania State University
Hershey, Pennsylvania

BARBARA G. FORD, R.D., M.P.H.
Assistant Professor of Medicine and Family
  Medicine
Department of Medicine
Milton S. Hershey Medical Center
The Pennsylvania State University
Hershey, Pennsylvania

ROBERT A. GORDON, M.D.
Clinical Associate Professor of Medicine
Milton S. Hershey Medical Center
The Pennsylvania State University
Hershey, Pennsylvania
Associate Director of Medical Education
Polyclinic Medical Center
Harrisburg, Pennsylvania

RICHARD J. GROSS, M.D., SC.M. (HYG.)
Assistant Professor of Medicine
The Johns Hopkins University School of
  Medicine
Francis Scott Key Medical Center and
The Johns Hopkins Hospital
Baltimore, Maryland

LARRY B. GROSSMAN, M.D.
Clinical Assistant Professor of Anesthe-
  siology
Milton S. Hershey Medical Center
The Pennsylvania State University
Hershey, Pennsylvania
Medical Director/Chief of Outpatient
  Anesthesia
Chestnut Hill Hospital Outpatient Sur-
  gical Center
Philadelphia, Pennsylvania

WILLIAM S. KAMMERER, M.D.
Associate Professor of Medicine
Division of Internal Medicine
Milton S. Hershey Medical Center
The Pennsylvania State University
Hershey, Pennsylvania

DAVID E. KERN, M.D., M.P.H.
Assistant Professor of Medicine
The Johns Hopkins University School of
  Medicine
Co-Director, Division of General Internal
  Medicine
Francis Scott Key Medical Center
Baltimore, Maryland

DONALD P. LOOKINGBILL, M.D.
Professor of Medicine
Chief, Division of Dermatology
Milton S. Hershey Medical Center
The Pennsylvania State University
Hershey, Pennsylvania

THOMAS J. MCGLYNN, JR., M.D.
Associate Professor of Medicine
Division of Internal Medicine
Milton S. Hershey Medical Center
The Pennsylvania State University
Hershey, Pennsylvania

RICHARD J. SIMONS, JR., M.D.
Assistant Professor of Medicine
Division of Internal Medicine
Milton S. Hershey Medical Center
The Pennsylvania State University
Hershey, Pennsylvania

JOHN STUCKEY, M.D.
Assistant Professor of Medicine
George Washington University School of
  Medicine
Chairman, Section of General Internal
  Medicine
Washington Hospital Center
Washington, D.C.

KERMIT R. TANTUM, M.D.
Clinical Professor of Anesthesia
Milton S. Hershey Medical Center
The Pennsylvania State University
Hershey, Pennsylvania
Chairman, Department of Anesthesia
Harrisburg Hospital
Harrisburg, Pennsylvania

JOSEPH J. TRAUTLEIN, M.D.
Associate Professor of Medicine
Division of Internal Medicine
Milton S. Hershey Medical Center
The Pennsylvania State University
Hershey, Pennsylvania

HAROLD TUCKER, M.D.
Assistant Professor of Medicine
The Johns Hopkins University School of
  Medicine
Baltimore, Maryland

PAUL E. TURER, M.D.
Staff Nephrologist, St. Agnes Hospital
Medical Director, Catonsville Dialysis
  Facility
Baltimore, Maryland

JANET WOODCOCK, M.D.
Director
Division of Biological Investigational New
  Drugs, FDA
Office of Biological Product Review
Center for Biologic Evaluation and
  Research
Rockville, Maryland

Contents

1/ General Medical Consultation Service: The Role of the Internist

—Richard J. Gross and William S. Kammerer

2/ Function of a General Internal Medicine Consultation Service

—William S. Kammerer and Richard J. Gross

3/ Evaluation of Medical Risks in the Surgical Patient

—Richard J. Gross

4/ Anesthesia: Organ Effects, Risks, and General Principles

—Kermit R. Tantum

5/ Nutritional Assessment and Support

—William S. Kammerer and Barbara G. Ford

6/ Preoperative Pulmonary Evaluation

—Joseph J. Trautlein

7/ Basic Mechanical Respiratory Support

—Larry B. Grossman

8/ Invasive Physiologic Monitoring
—John M. Field

9/ Thromboembolic Disorders
—Thomas J. McGlynn, Jr.

10/ Cardiovascular Disease and Hypertension
—Richard J. Gross and David E. Kern

11/ Renal, Fluid and Electrolyte, and Acid-Base Disorders
—Paul E. Turer and Gary R. Briefel

12/ Gastroenterology
—Harold Tucker

13/ Endocrine Disorders

—Thomas J. McGlynn, Jr. and Richard J. Simons

14/ Hematology

—Robert A. Gordon and James O. Ballard

15/ Oncology

—Robert A. Gordon

16/ Infectious Disease

—John Stuckey and Richard J. Gross

17/ Dermatology

—Donald P. Lookingbill

18/ Orthopaedics and Rheumatology

—John W. Burnside

19/ Neurologic Conditions in the Perioperative Setting

—Lourdes C. Corman

1

General Medical Consultation Service: The Role of the Internist

Richard J. Gross and William S. Kammerer

Little formal attention has been directed to the role of the internist as a consultant. Most authors have concentrated on a brief list of responsibilities or ethical constraints to prevent patient stealing or fee splitting. A few of the major figures in American medicine in the early 20th century commented briefly on the consultant's role, but none elucidated their philosophy in detail. The purpose of this chapter is to outline the consulting internist's role in relationship to the patient, the problem, and the consulting physician.

The opinions and reports of the Judicial Council of the American Medical Association contain the most comprehensive list of consultant responsibilities (1). The AMA document lists nine ethical principles of consultation:

1. One physician should be in charge of the patient's care;
2. The attending physician has overall responsibility for the treatment of the patient;
3. The consultant should not assume primary care of the patient without the consent of the referring physician;
4. The consultation should be done punctually.
5. Discussions in consultation should be with the referring physician and only with the patient with the prior consent of the referring physician;
6. Conflicts of opinion should be resolved by a second consultation or withdrawal of the consultant; however, the consultant has the right to give his opinion to the patient in the presence of the referring physician.*

A consultation should be differentiated from a referral, although these two terms are often used interchangeably. A consultation is strictly defined as requesting another physician to give his opinion on diagnosis or management. Referral means to request another physician to assume direct responsibility for a portion or all of the patient's care. A referral may be for a specific problem or total care of the patient.

We have conceptualized the role of the consultant as outlined below, based on clinical experience, discussion with other internists, and review of available literature. The performance of a consultation involves the phases of initial contact, completion of the consultation report, and follow-up (Table 1.1).

---

*The other three principles involve responsibilities of the referring physician for obtaining consultations. 1) Consultations are indicated "upon request," in doubtful or difficult cases, or when they enhance the quality of medical care. 2) Consultations are primarily for the patient's benefit. 3) A case summary should be sent to the consulting physician unless a verbal description of the case has been given.

1

INITIAL CONTACT

The Consultation Request (Statement of the Problem)

Commonly, consultations are submitted without a clear statement of the question(s) to be answered by the consultant. A consultation request stating the problem as "angina" might be submitted in the following greatly different situations: a patient with atypical chest pain where the referring physician wants confirmation of a noncardiac etiology; a patient with refractory angina referred for cardiac catheterization prior to noncardiac surgery; a patient with stable angina where the surgeon desires to know if further therapy is necessary; a patient with new chest pain and gallbladder disease where the physician desires to know the etiology of the pain; or the patient with symptomatic gallstones where the referring physician desires to know if the patient can withstand surgery. **A precise understanding of the reason(s) for a consultation** is imperative for the consultant to provide optimal service to the referring physician and to the patient. Poorly defined reasons for consultation often lead to duplication of effort, increased costs to the patient, and suboptimal care.

In addition, it is important for the consultant to know what procedure is planned, what alternatives the referring surgeon will or will not consider, what benefits the procedure or alternatives offer the patient, and the extent of involvement in patient care and follow-up desired by the referring physician. Speaking with the referring surgeon for a few minutes before seeing the patient to clarify the reason for consultation will save time and result in more specific suggestions. The consultant should remember that he was called to help and not to be another burden with peripheral questions and suggestions that are not pertinent to the problem at hand.

The Referring Physician

Conflicts over patient management between referring physicians and consultants are among the most difficult areas of interprofessional relationships. Contributing factors to these disagreements are differences in expertise between physicians as training becomes more specialized; differences in the approach to common problems between internists, anesthesiologists, and surgeons; and differences in philosophy between internists and surgeons about how closely the patient needs to be followed or the urgency for surgery. In academic institutions, the departmental structure can foster conflicts between different services.

It serves no purpose to criticize the referring physician because of differences in knowledge or in philosophy of patient care. This serves only to increase the resistance to recommendations or to decrease appropriate consultation in the future, both of which depend on some goodwill. In our experience, the best way to prevent conflicts is communication prior to the consultation as described above, and verbal, as well as written, transmission of recommendations, especially when some controversy is anticipated. Restricting recommendations to those that will have an impact on diagnosis and therapy is appreciated by many surgeons and patients.

Methods of resolving conflicts vary in academic and community practice situations. In academic settings, a case conference including residents, consultants, and attending physicians is useful, especially if guided by a senior attending physician. Communication between senior attending physicians can often resolve problems that begin on the resident or fellow level. In either training or private practice settings, utilizing persuasion by other consultants or obtaining a second formal consultation can be helpful.

The Patient

The following information should be explained to the patient at the beginning of the consultant's visit: (1) your name, (2) that you are a consultant requested by his/her physician, (3) the service that you represent, and (4) the reason for the consultation. If more than one person from the consulting service will see the patient (e.g., medical student, fellow), this should be explained along with each person's role.

It is regarded by many physicians as discourteous, if not "unethical," for a consultant to discuss diagnostic and therapeutic recommendations with the patient before obtaining the specific approval of the referring physician. The consultant must work out any differences of opinion with the referring physician before relating these to the patient. If important, irreconcilable differences of opinion exist, they should be cited specifically in the chart with a request for another opinion to help resolve the dilemma. If all else fails, the consultant should indicate to the patient his intention to withdraw from the case because of disagreement with the patient's physician on a diagnosis or a management plan, and explain that it is the patient's right to request that his physician seek another opinion.

COMPLETION OF THE CONSULTATION REPORT

The Existing Data Base (Chart)

A careful review of the patient's chart is necessary for a complete consultation. This review should include obtaining out-side office or hospital records, unreturned laboratory data (especially those tests sent to bacteriology, serology, or out-of-hospital laboratories), and a personal review of electrocardiograms, x-rays, and gram-stained smears.

The Consultation Report

A consultation to a nonmedical service should include a very brief summary of the history and hospital course. The aspects of the physical examination important to the problems for which the consultation was obtained should be detailed, particularly any differences from those recorded by the primary physician. Only pertinent laboratory data should be listed, preferably in a flow sheet form. Most emphasis should be placed on the consultant's impressions and recommendations including a brief discussion of:

1. How the conclusions were reached;
2. The reasons for suggestions listed in the recommendations.

We have found the following format useful for recording consultations: Impressions; Recommendations; Discussion; References (see Figs. 2.1, 2.2, pp. 12–15). The impression, discussion, and recommendations should specifically address the central question asked by the referring physician, as well as more general problems.

Consultations on medical services will, in most instances, be somewhat longer and more detailed. References supporting recommendations are often appreciated, especially on academic services. These are generally interpreted as indicators of the enthusiasm of the consultant and often help to forestall disagreements based upon opinions rather than on fact.

A complete recording of a comprehensive history and physical examination for a hospitalized patient should not be necessary. This is the responsibility of the primary service. The consultant's report should be confined to the major and pertinent problems identified and to any differences in observations from those recorded by the primary physician.

Recommendations should be as specific as possible because the referring physician may not be familiar with the performance of certain tests or the use of unfamiliar drugs. For example, one should not write to "digitalize the patient," but to give "digoxin 0.25 mg orally now, again in 6 hours, and then once a day." Large numbers of recommendations are less likely to be carried out on surgical services. There should be some balance between the desire to comprehensively cover all problems no matter how unrelated or minor, and what can be practically achieved. Some non-acute recommendations may need to be deferred to later follow-up notes in complex patients, to increase the likelihood that suggestions will be carried out. Critical or stat recommendations should be listed first and clearly labeled as urgent (1–8). It is useful to discuss specific impressions and recommendations with the referring service; this is mandatory if recommendations are urgent or many.

The consultant should provide the surgeon with: (1) a clear, concise evaluation of medical risks; (2) measures to improve or stabilize the patient preoperatively; (3) postoperative medical considerations; and (4) the role he/she will assume in the overall care of the patient (9, 10).

Timeliness

Consultations are often asked for in a rushed manner, whether because of the patient's critical state or for the convenience of the referring physician. There is some truth to the saying, "consultations requested today were urgently needed yesterday, and should have been requested one week ago." Such "urgent" consultations should be seen promptly, regardless of whether mandated by the patient's condition or the physician's request. Elective consultations for surgery should be done so as not to postpone surgery, even if the request was received late. Patients will appreciate this courtesy as it may often prevent prolonging costly hospitalization. In cases of repeated unnecessary requests for urgent consultation, a gentle reminder of the inconvenience is usually sufficient. Regardless, all consultations should be seen for at least a brief triage assessment on the day they are received. The problem of unrecognized severity is just as important and common as the situation where the severity is known to the referring surgeon. If the consultation cannot be completed on the day received, the anticipated delay must be immediately and directly communicated to the referring physician.

Relationship to Other Consultants

The general internist is commonly in a position of being one of a number of medical consultants on an individual patient (60% of the time in a study from the University of Chicago) (8). A common mistake is to simply make suggestions for the specific problem(s) relating to one's specialty. Conflicts with the suggestions of other consultants most often arise in this manner. Conflicts may include different advice for the same problem and recommendations for therapy that may adversely affect another problem or interfere with another consultant's recommendations. The consulting internist needs to keep abreast of the suggestions of other consultants and, in many cases, to negotiate with them as indicated. One of the functions of the general internist should be to integrate advice from the subspecialists and to help resolve conflicting suggestions.

FOLLOW-UP

There are no specific data on how often follow-up visits need to be made by the consultant. The consultant's advice is more likely to be taken if follow-up is more frequent and documented with a progress note (6, 11). The need for follow-up visits ranges from 2–3 visits per day for a critically ill patient (e.g., with a myocardial infarction after surgery), 2–3 visits per week for a relatively stable patient (e.g., with a resolving postoperative pneumonia), or one visit per week for a stable patient (e.g., awaiting return of a laboratory value for an elective workup). **The type and frequency of follow-up should be specifically listed** as part of the recommendations/plan in the initial consultation note.

Brief progress notes should usually be made for each consultation visit. Emphasis should be placed on new data, changes in impressions, and suggested changes in tests or therapy. Problem oriented flowsheets attached to the patient's original consultation and updated on each visit are an efficient way of recording data. The frequency of or need for continued follow-up should be questioned if the consultant does not feel that follow-up notes need to be made on more than an occasional visit. Recommendations should be documented in follow-up notes as well as communicated verbally, since the record provides the only means of reviewing the longitudinal course of the patient. Verbal interchange is quite useful for the same reasons as the initial consultation report. **A written note should document when the consultant will no longer follow the patient and that the consultation is complete.** A common and inexcusable practice by many consultants is to just stop seeing the patient with only a vague word to the referring service that follow-up is discontinued. This may mislead the referring physician into thinking that everything is going well with the patient, when in reality the patient is doing poorly and is not being followed.

A final job of the consultant is to assure continuity of the patient's care for medical problems after discharge. It is easily accomplished if the consultant is also the patient's primary physician. Minor problems are often adequately handled by mentioning to the surgeon what information should be communicated to the primary physician, either verbally or in the discharge summary. Contact between the consultant and the patient's primary medical physician is important for serious medical problems or complex patients. In this case, a letter to the primary physician is often indicated, after coordinating one's recommendations with the physician who requested the consultation. The consultant should assist in making arrangements for medical follow-up care when the patient has no primary medical physician.

EFFECTIVENESS OF CONSULTATIONS: AN EVALUATION

Considerable literature has recently become available on the effectiveness of medical consultants on nonmedical services (1–8, 10, 11, 13, 14). Using the principles of consultation listed above, certain aspects of the consultant's role can be identified that have the most influence on his recommendations being carried out by the referring physician (the "best" measure of consultation "quality").

The available literature is limited because only one measure of consultation quality was examined (the referring physician's compliance with carrying out the consultant's advice) and because the data were gathered from mostly academic institutions, where the consulting and referring physicians may be attendings, residents, or medical students. The relevance of this data for the different setting of private practice is not established.

Compliance with the advice of the consultant ranged from 54–77% of recommendations made in academic centers (Table 1.2). A study (3) from a military teaching hospital found that 90% of recommendations made were done, suggesting compliance may be higher in nonacademic settings.

In studies of medical consultation on nonmedical services, the referring and

Table 1.2.   % Compliance with Advice of Medical Consultant

Study	% Compliance*
Klein (1)	54%
Sears (4)	77%
Pupa (3)	90%
Ballard (5)	72%

*% Compliance = number of recommendations carried out/total number of recommendations by consultant.

consulting physicians disagreed in some manner on the major reason for the consultation in about 14–36% of cases (Table 1.3). The reasons for the disagreements varied among studies, including the referring physician never having stated a reason for the consult, the consulting physician's note not answering the major question asked by the referring physician, or both physicians having stated different reasons for the consultation. Obviously, if the consultant does not answer the *"central question"* (2) for the consultation *specifically* in his report, the consultation has not served its intended purpose, no matter how much more important or interesting other problems may be. Several factors have been noted to improve compliance with the consultant's advice in multiple studies, (Table 1.4) (3).

Most of these factors are within the consultant's ability to change, except the severity of illness and type of recommendation (diagnostic vs. therapeutic) (9, 10

Table 1.3.   Referring/Consulting M.D. Disagreement* on Central Reason for Consultation

Study	% Disagreement
Lee (7)	14%
Horowitz (6)	18%
Rudd (8)	36%

*Disagreement was defined variously as different reasons, no stated reason for consult, or consult report not answering question listed by referring physician.

Table 1.4.   Factors Improving Compliance with Medical Consultant's Recommendations

	Ref.
1. Consultation performed within 24 hrs. of request.	6
2. Follow-up (frequent, follow-up notes more than 2 follow-up visits.	6, 11
3. Verbal contact with referring M.D.; positive attitude towards referring service.	3, 7, 8
4. Limited number of recommendations (≤5).	1–4
5. Recommendation related to *"central reason"* for consultation.	2, 4, 7
6. Definitiveness of recommendation.	1, 2, 6–8
7. "Crucial" (vs. routine) recommendation.	3–5
8. Specific details for drug recommendations (dose, duration).	6, 8, 11
9. Medication/treatment (vs. diagnostic) recommendation.	1–5
10. Severely ill patient.	4, 5

in Table 1.4). The way the consultation is performed affects it outcome. Improved compliance was found when the consult was performed promptly (within 24 hours), follow-up was frequent and noted in the chart, and when the consultant discussed his findings with the referring physician. Aspects of the recommendations that improved the consultation included limiting the number of recommendations to five or less, keeping recommendations tied to the central reason for the consultation, making the recommendation definite (i.e., written as "do today" versus "suggested"), and listing specific details, especially for drug recommendations (such as dose and route of administration).

Although, performing the consultation within the points listed (Table 1.4) improves compliance with advice, these points cannot always be followed. Many patients have multiple serious problems requiring recommendations other than the disease for which the consultation was requested. Severely ill patients tend to have more recommendations made by the consultant (3–5); often these cannot be reduced to five or less recommendations. There is a need to document recommendations for unrelated problems affecting the patient's health for medicolegal reasons. An approval to take in handling consultations where the points in Table 1.4 must be violated (e.g., a large number of recommendations), includes personal, verbal discussion with the referring physician (1, 2, 7, 12), often on a repeated basis during the follow-up period. More elective recommendations for peripheral problems can be deferred to follow-up notes once the critical recommendations are carried out. There is a tendency to list every recommendation in the initial consultation report, even if they involve long-term, non-acute problems, which may overwhelm the referring physician caring for an acutely ill patient, and be forgotten later in the course.

Two recent preliminary studies have suggested that the yield (in terms of new problems identified) of perioperative medical consultation are found mostly in high-risk patients (such as over age 50 or ASA Class III–IV) (15, 16).

SUMMARY

Burnside (17), Goldman and Rudd (18) and Merli and Weitz (19) have summarized a philosophy of consultation into the "Ten Commandments of Consultation" (Table 1.5) based on their experience as consultants and on the literature cited above. They serve as a brief (pocket) reminder of the important points of consultation listed above.

The skills and process of consultation are learned through experience and through observing accomplished senior consultants. This analysis is not intended to supplant such experiences, but to complement them by providing an outline for critical observation of patient care. A

Table 1.5. Ten Commandments for Consultations*

1. Determine the question.
2. Establish urgency.
3. Obtain your own primary data.
4. Be brief in your report.
5. Be specific in your recommendations; support your impressions and recommendations. (Be honest.)
6. Provide contingency plans.
7. Respect the referring physician's prerogatives.
8. Teach.
9. Talk with the referring physician.
10. Provide follow-up

*Slightly adapted from ref. 17–19.

number of residency programs have established general medical consultation services with the aim of teaching these consultation skills (see pp. 10–11).

In summary, the ideal consultant as described by Bates (20, 21) is one who, "informs without patronizing, educates without lecturing, directs without ordering, and . . . solves the problem without making the referring physician look stupid." The consultant, then, should try always to support the referring physician, comfort the patient, and be specific.

READINGS

1. Klein LE, Levine DM, Moore RD, et al.: The Preoperative Consultation: Response to Internists' Recommendations. *Arch Intern Med* 143:743–744, 1983.
2. Klein LE, Moore RD, Levine DM, et al.: Effectiveness of Medical Consultations. *J Med Ed* 58:149–151, 1983.
3. Pupa LE, Coventry JA, Hanley JF, et al.: Factors Affecting Compliance for General Medicine Consultations to Non-Internists. *Am J Med* 81:508–514, 1986.
4. Sears CL, Charlson ME: The Effectiveness of a Consultation. *Am J Med* 74:870–876, 1983.
5. Ballard W, Gold JP, Charlson ME: Compliance with the Recommendations of Medical Consultants. *J Gen Intern Med* 1:220–224, 1986.
6. Horwitz RL, Henes CG, Horwitz SM: Developing Strategies for Improving the Diagnostic and Management Efficacy of Medical Consultations. *J Chronic Dis* 36:213–218, 1983.
7. Lee T, Pappius EM, Goldman L: Impact of Inter-Physician Communication on the Effectiveness of Medical Consultations. *Am J Med* 74:106–112, 1983.
8. Rudd P, Siegler M, Byyny RL: Perioperative

Diabetic Consultation: A Plea for Improved Training." *J Med Ed* 53:590–596, 1978.

9. *Opinions and Reports of the Judicial Council.* Chicago, American Medical Association, 1960.

10. Burke GR, Corman LC: The General Medicine Consult Service in a University Teaching Hospital. *Med Clin N Am* 63:1353–1358, 1979.

11. Mackenzie TB, Popkin MK, Callies AL, et al.: The Effectiveness of Cardiology Consultation. *Chest* 79:16–22, 1981.

12. Charlson ME, Cohen RP, Sears CL: General Medical Consultation: Lessons from a Clinical Service. *Am J Med* 75:121–128, 1983.

13. Moore RA, Kammerer WS, McGlynn TJ, et al.: Consultations in Internal Medicine: A Training Program Resource. *J Med Ed* 52:323–327, 1977.

14. Robie PW: The Service and Educational Contributions of a General Internal Medicine Consultation Service. *J Gen Intern Med* 1:225–227, 1986.

15. Gluck R, Munoz E, Wise L: "Preoperative and Postoperative Medical Evaluation of Surgical Patients." *Am J Surg* 155:730–734, 1088.

16. Levinson W: Preoperative Evaluations by an Internist—Are They Worthwhile?" *West J Med* 141:395–398, 1984.

17. Burnside JW: Commandments for Consultants. *Hosp Physician* 7:53–54, 1973.

18. Goldman L, Rudd P. Ten Commandments for Effective Consultations. *Arch Intern Med* 143:1753–1755, 1983.

19. Merli GJ, Weitz HH: The Medical Consultant. *Med Clin N A* 71:353–354, 1987.

20. Bynny RL, Siegler M, Taylor AR: Development of an Academic Section of General Internal Medicine. *Am J Med* 63:493–498, 1977.

21. Bates RC: The Two Sides of Every Successful Consultation. *Med Econ* December 10:173–180, 1979.

22. Golden WE, Lavender RC: Preoperative Cardiac Consultations in a Teaching Hospital. *S Med J* 82:292–295, 1989.

2

Function of a General Internal Medicine Consultation Service

William S. Kammerer and Richard J. Gross

The reappearance of the general internist on academic medicine faculties has prompted much discussion by students, residents, medical subspecialists, and, not least, by general internists themselves as to what they actually do. Therefore, much attention has been directed to their wide-ranging patient care and resident teaching activities, primarily in the outpatient clinics. The general internal medicine consultation service is a major additional activity that is often overlooked or misunderstood (1, 2, 3, 4, 5). The major role of consultation medicine in the practice of general internists is emphasized by several studies of what the practicing internist does (6–9). From 20–50% of an internist's new patients are referred by other physicians for either problem-oriented consultation or for ongoing total care. Thus, relevancy of the general medicine consultation service should be made clear to residents interested in practicing general internal medicine.

A wide spectrum of unfamiliar medical problems faces the medicine resident during the general medical consultation experience. In addition, the resident must deal with the intricacies and nuances of the relationship between referring physician and consultant. Most of the medical problems dealt with on a general medicine consultation service differ categorically or in severity from those seen on the medicine wards. These differences are becoming more pronounced with the increasing activity of utilization review committees at teaching hospitals. The practice of admitting "interesting" cases for teaching purposes has become increasingly difficult due to high costs and scarce resources. Admissions to university teaching hospital medical wards now involve predominately tertiary care problems, demanding the multiple resources and technical apparatus associated with these hospitals. For example, rarely now is a patient with uncomplicated hyperthyroidism, rheumatoid arthritis, anemia, hypertension, diabetes mellitus, or even systemic lupus erythematosus admitted to the medicine service. However, these problems are often seen on the various surgical services, often unrelated to the surgical diagnosis. In addition, appropriate diagnostic techniques and care must be integrated with those of the underlying surgical illness. Understanding and managing the stress of surgery or delivery on these illnesses demands important skills, information, and insight from the medical resident different from those learned on medical wards and in clinic (2, 3).

The goals of the educationally oriented general medical consult service, then, should be:

1. Educate residents in the process of risk identification, assessment, and correction.
2. Expose residents to the problems of "interface medicine."
3. Develop the professional and social skills necessary for effective interdis-

ciplinary communication and patient care.

4. Develop an attitude that fosters continuing learning and professional development.
5. Emphasize and encourage attention to details.
6. Develop an approach that stresses efficiency, specificity, and patient advocacy.
7. Provide the understanding that the internist must have regarding the indications for surgery and the likelihood of benefit.

ATTRIBUTES OF A GENERAL MEDICINE CONSULTATION SERVICE

In the organization of an academic general internal medicine consultation service, one should carefully consider how it functions, not just what services are provided, in order to accomplish its goals. It is far too easy to discuss only the patient's medical problems with a resident and not to specifically discuss risk assessment or the interprofessional relationships involved in communicating about the case, thus losing much of the educational value of the case. Paradoxically, **the goals of teaching interprofessional relationships, risk assessment, and style of consultation are the unique aspects of the general medical consultation service** and those that require the most attention in organizing the service. The aspects that need to be considered in organizing a general medical consultation service are the patient base, resident role, faculty role, and means of teaching.

Most general medical consultation services function alongside subspecialty services. In a few hospitals, the general medical consultation service sees all consults initially and refers appropriate cases to subspecialty services. Either arrangement is satisfactory, as long as there are adequate numbers of consultations for teaching purposes (30–50 new consultations per month per resident on the ser-

vice). The service cannot gain much credibility with residents if all of the cases that involve preoperative assessment go to subspecialty services and only routine care of non-operative cases are referred to the general consult service. An important role of the faculty is to attract and maintain an adequate number and variety of cases from surgical colleagues. In general, most requests come from the orthopedic, otorhinolaryngology, neurosurgery, urology, plastic surgery, psychiatry, and obstetrics/gynecology services. Lesser numbers come from the general and thoracic surgery services (2, 3, 4).

The resident's primary responsibility on the rotation must be to the consult service in order for it to function effectively. Institutions where the residents have primary responsibilities elsewhere and are only secondarily responsible for consultations have not been able to maintain the service's teaching function. A number of services have had great success when the resident has other secondary responsibilities within the Division of General Internal Medicine during the rotation, such as clinic responsibilities for seeing new patients, evaluating preoperative outpatients, doing consultations to the emergency room, and seeing referred patients alongside faculty preceptors on a one-to-one basis. The service must maintain 24-hour availability both for service and resident teaching. Since it is impossible for a single resident to do this (most services will only have one resident), adequate cross coverage for night call and weekends must be arranged. The service should be busy enough so that it is not viewed as an "easy" rotation spent mainly in the library, but less demanding than the wards to allow adequate time for reading and assimilation of overall responsibilities. These factors must be taken into account when determining the number of residents on the service and other resident responsibilities.

The role of the faculty is crucial to the proper functioning of the service. The faculty member must see all patients in order to provide bedside teaching, adequate role modeling, and to supervise even senior residents who have little experience with or knowledge of preoperative evaluation. The faculty should emphasize review of the literature and its application to the individual patient. Aspects to be emphasized are preoperative risk assessment and the differential diagnosis and management of postoperative problems, since most residents will have an adequate background in the routine medical aspects by the time they reach the consult service. It is absolutely crucial for the faculty to discuss the interprofessional relationships involved in most cases. This involves discussing with the resident how he will communicate with the consulting service and advising on management of difficulties in professional relationships, such as when the consulting service ignores your advice. Having the faculty review and sign all consultation reports will also ensure feedback to the resident on the adequacy of the written communication. Adequate didactic material must be available to the resident, since most residents are not familiar with researching this area of the literature.

Teaching should be provided by three means. Adequate literature resources and references should be available. Routine sources, such as *Index Medicus,* do not reference consultation problems separately. We have found it useful to give the residents an outline of approaches to the most common consultation problems seen by our service, accompanied by a list of specific references and texts (9).

Conference-based teaching should be provided to the resident to efficiently teach the approach to common consultation problems. This can be done either through medicine grand rounds or through conferences of the Division of General Internal Medicine.

Most hospitals provide several other opportunities for resident teaching. Examples of such activities are: consultation

to the psychiatry service in evaluating possible medical illnesses in psychiatric patients; joint medical-obstetric clinics for pregnant patients with high-risk medical disease; consultation to surgical specialty units such as burn units; and evaluation of potential kidney donors. Such functions can be easily integrated into the more traditional inpatient consultation roles of the consultation service.

DESCRIPTION OF A GENERAL MEDICINE CONSULT SERVICE

At the Milton S. Hershey Medical Center of The Pennsylvania State University, senior medical residents rotate for 2 months on the general internal medicine consultation service. Each of the four general internists in the division spends a week at a time on the service. Rounds with the attending internist are made daily and every consultation is seen on the same day as requested. Forty to fifty new consultations are completed each month. Two-thirds of the consultation requests originate on the orthopedic, otorhinolaryngology, and neurosurgical services and the other one-third come from obstetrics/gynecology, psychiatry, urology, and general surgery. Urgent requests from the outpatient surgical clinics are also seen, and the consult resident helps to coordinate care in the emergency room for patients with medical problems needing admission or medical follow-up. In addition, a weekly high-risk obstetrics conference and clinic is attended and a weekly general internal medicine consultation conference is presented.

Continued and direct faculty participation in the consultation process provides support and direction to the medical resident, improves efficiency of patient care, and demonstrates the important interdisciplinary communication and professional skills necessary for a successful outcome. For example, in a review of 36 university teaching hospital general medicine consultation services, one-half were found to offer no ongoing faculty supervision. These were deemed by residents to be primarily service-oriented functions with little or no educational value. The other half with regular, formal faculty input were reported to be educationally rewarding and satisfying rotations (2).

We have found that the use of a structured format (Figs. 2.1, 2.2) for reporting the consultation both improves communication and provides the medical resident with an efficient means for clearly stating his impressions and recommendations. This format forces the consultant to clearly and specifically focus on the major issues, and prevents obfuscation in a lengthy novelette, which recounts the obvious and avoids answering the questions asked. By utilizing this format, we have found that relations between medical and surgical residents improve, as both are forced to deal with facts and observations rather than with loosely formed opinions. In addition, the faculty will, in almost all instances, add comments or suggestions either in writing or verbally to the consulting physician in such a manner as to indicate that they, also, have

TO	FROM	DATE OF REQUEST	TIME OF REQUEST	
				A.M.
Internal Medicine	Surgery	May, 1986		P.M.

REASON FOR REQUEST

86-year-old white male with cholelithiasis. Please evaluate for surgery and make any recommendations you feel should be followed.

PROVISIONAL DIAGNOSIS

Cholelithiasis.

REQUESTING PHYSICIAN'S SIGNATURE	PLACE OF CONSULTATION ☐ BEDSIDE ☐ OTHER	☐ ROUTINE ☐ EMERGENCY

CONSULTATION REPORT

Impressions:

1. Cholelithiasis.
2. Systolic ejection murmur—hemodynamically insignificant aortic stenosis.
3. Upper respiratory tract infection—possible sinusitis.
4. Systolic hypertension, probably secondary to PVD.
5. Probable left ventricular hypertrophy.
6. Bradycardia.
7. Question of small amount of aortic insufficiency.
8. Vertigo—questionable etiology.

Recommendations:

1. Echocardiogram to define aortic valve.
2. Bedside PFT, if patient can cooperate (doubt OBS—he was reading *Time* magazine when I examined him).
3. Room air ABGs.
4. PO antibiotic for bronchitis through weekend. Would choose Ampicillin or Tetracycline 500 PO Q-6 hours. Re-evaluate before OR Monday.

Figure 2.1. The Milton S. Hershey Medical Center Hospital Consultation Report.

Figure 2.1. (*continued*)

5. If patient has calcific aortic valve, would use antibiotic prophylaxis for abdominal surgery. Doses at the end of consult.
6. No more than 4–6 grams Na/day in perioperative period to prevent CHF.
7. S.Q. Heparin, 5000 u-Q 8 hours starting now.

Discussion:

Patient is a relatively healthy 86-year-old who denies prior cardiac or pulmonary problems and underwent general anesthesia without difficulty for bowel resection in 1984. He has a history of cardiac murmur $\times$ 60 years, but denies rheumatic fever.

He denies syncope, angina, CHF. He can walk up one flight with no problems—no orthopnea, PND, nocturia, or edema.

No history of HTN or DM or family history of cardiac disease. He does have systolic HTN now, secondary to ASPVD.
He denies productive cough and is a nonsmoker, but has felt like "he's had a cold" with stuffed up nose in hospital.

Pertinent Exam:
BP 170/70 without orthostatic changes.
Pulse 54 with occasional irregularity.
Resp. 14–22 unlabored. Afebrile.
Neck: ō JVD, carotids with decrease upstroke, but full and dicrotic.
Lungs: clear.
Cor: S_1 S_2 nl. (+) S_4 Gr. II/VI SEM aortic areas $\rightarrow$ (L) carotid.
  ? soft early diastolic blow. No S_3. No change in murmur with hand grip, valsalva, squat.
Abd: soft ō organomegaly.
Ext: ō edema.
Neuro: reflexes 2 +, =, toes ↓↓, position sense intact, mental function intact oriented $\times$ 3.

Summary:

Patient at increased risk (age 86 and possible aortic stenosis). Did tolerate general anesthesia successfully in 1984.

Would definitely get ABG's and clear up URI prior to OR.

Antibiotic: (Regarding SBE prophylaxis)

Ampicillin 1.5 g IV q 4 hours $\times$ 1 before OR and $\times$ 48 hours.
Tobramycin 1.7 mg/Kg IV q 8 hours $\times$ 1 before OR and $\times$ 48 hours.

Comments by Attending Physician: (Dr. Kammerer)

Patient seen and examined. ENT w/u "vertigo," neg; ENG —? vertebrobasilar origin. Consider ASA and dipyridamole post-op. regarding probable atherosclerotic origin of vertigo.

Carol V. Freer, M.D.	William S. Kammerer, M.D.
Medicine Resident/III	Associate Professor of Medicine

SIGNATURE OF CONSULTANT   DATE OF CONSULTATION   TIME OF CONSULTATION

A.M.

P.M.

Anna E. Smith
February 10, 1987

REF: Dr. John Jones

SUBJECTIVE: CC: Preoperative medical evaluation for cerebral arteriogram and craniotomy, because of multiple medical problems.

58-year-old white female with left falx meningioma discovered 6 weeks ago. Patient developed severe occipital headache, profound vomiting, and hypertension. An emergency CT scan showed the meningioma. Only physical finding was partial rt. homo. hemianopsia.

3 weeks ago: Early papilledema noted on opthal. evaluation and Decadron increased to 4 mg. q6h with improvement.

Medical problems include: 1. AODM on insulin; 2. Unstable angina 1/87 with finding of 30–50% LAD before 1st septal perforator, small rt. coronary & nl. LV fxn. on catheterization; 3. COPD No angina since prior hospitalization; some atypical pain (prob. noncardiac), but activity limited. No DOE, orthopnea, edema, sputum production. Insulin requirements have risen on steroids. 4. H/O pulmonary emboli.

No personal or family HX. of anesthesia problems, bleeding disorders, or transfusion reaction.

PAST MEDICAL HISTORY
ALLERGIES: None
ILLNESSES: 1. Angina (1987)
    2. AODM
    3. COPD
    4. Pulmonary Emboli
    5. Lt. falx meningioma
SURGERY: 1. T&A
    2. Cholecystectomy, 1976
    3. L5/S1 disectomy, 1986
INJURIES: 1. Back
MEDICATIONS: 1. Humulin-N insulin 45U AM 12U PM (Humulin-R coverage per schedule)
    2. Nitrodur 5 mg. Patch QAM
    3. Cardiazem 60 mg. Q6H
    4. Theodur 400 mg. Q12H
    5. TNG 0.4 mg, s1 PRN

SOC. HX. 58-year-old married secretary
 Smokes: 1PPD x26 yrs. ETOH: Rare
 Drugs: None
FAMILY HISTORY: +COPD, heart disease, cancer, diabetes
ROS: (Positives): Otherwise non-contributory.

OBJECTIVE:

VITAL SIGNS: BP RT. Arm(lie) 140/80 Pulse 76 (reg.)RR 14 Temp: 98.6 WT: 180 lbs. HT: 5'6"

GEN: Obese
NODES: Non-felt
NECK: N1. thyroid without nodules.
HEENT: Ears: N1 EAC and drums Eyes: Flat discs w/o H,E. Perrla = 3mm.
   Oropharynx: Clear w/o lesions or inflammation/discharge
HEAD: Normocephalic
CHEST: Clear to P&A; Minimal wheezes.
COR: PMI = MC1. S1&S2 normal; no murmurs, gallops, clicks, NVD or edema. Pulses all 2+/ 2+ without bruits, including carotid and pedal pulses.
ABDOMEN: N1 bowel sounds, no organomegaly, masses or tenderness.
EXTREMITIES: No cords, calf tenderness, edema. Calf (9") = 32 cm./32 cm. R/L
NEURO: M.S. Normal   GAIT: Normal
   CN: 2/12 normal, except rt field hem- CEREBELLAR: Normal
   ianopsia   DTR's: 1−2/1−2

Figure 2.2. Alternative Format for Consultation Report (Baltimore)

Figure 2.2.   *(continued)*
        MOTOR: 5+/5+ all forur ext.
        SENSORY: Normal

LABORATORY: EKG: Normal. CXR: Normal. Hct: = 46;Na$^+$ = 140.K$^+$ = 4.4 CO2 = 25.U/A Normal

ASSESSMENT:
1. Angina
2. COPD; smoker
3. AODM
4. H/O Pulmonary emboli
5. Lt. falx meningioma

No medical contraindications to planned procedures, although increased, but acceptable risk.

DISCUSSION: Multiple problems seem stable; coronary disease not critical by catheterization. Would emphasize monitoring diabetes, prevention P.E., and monitor for CV symptoms.
RECOMMENDATIONS:
1. Humulin-N 24U & ½ usual coverage day of arteriogram; D5/¼NSS @ 50 cc/hr while NPO
2. Same dose day of surgery
3. Stat Astra, acetone AM of surgery & in recovery room—call physician
3. Leg compression cuffs during surgery
4. While NPO postop, Aminophyllin 25 mg/hr continuous IV drip
5. No smoking
6. Chemstix bG ac + HS (I will write coverage); monitor chemstix q2hrs intraoperatively

Richard J. Gross M.D., F.A.C.P.

personally examined the patient and discussed specific impressions and recommendations with the resident.

Even the most senior of medical residents at the beginning of the general medicine consultation service often find themselves with little basic factual information with which to support their opinions. This is a source of much frustration, especially when their recommendations are ignored or overridden in a contest of opinions. Therefore, we try to build into our teaching program as much specific published material as is available and urge residents to research problems and complications new to them. While utilizing didactic and conference style teaching to a certain extent, we prefer to stress careful bedside observations, factual documentation of recommendations, and the importance of close patient follow-up as more effective learning techniques. Careful follow-up directly confronts the consultants with the consequences of their recommendations, reinforcing positive results, as well as spotlighting mistakes or

errors in judgment. We hope with this approach to reinforce DaCosta's dictum that, "diagnosis by intuition is a rapid method of reaching a wrong conclusion."[*] Systematic follow-up also provides us with an opportunity to identify common problems on which to concentrate our teaching, literature searches, and topics for research.

RISK ASSESSMENT

The most difficult aspect of the consultation process for many internists arises in attempting to specifically assess the risk to the patient of the proposed procedure. In large part, this develops from unfamiliarity with the physiologic stresses of anesthesia or of specific surgical procedures, and from the unpredictability of intraoperative complications. Often, this leads the internist to conclude his rec-

*From DaCosta JC: *Selections from the Papers and Speeches of John Chalmers DaCosta, MD, LLD.* Philadelphia, W.B. Saunders, 1931, p 50.

ommendations with the gratuitous and superficial reminder to "maintain blood pressure and oxygenation and avoid volume overload." Obviously, this kind of advice is rarely helpful to the physician requesting the consultation. Rather, most consultation requests are really asking the consultant to identify and define significant medical problems, to help to optimally manage them preoperatively, and to be available for close follow-up postoperatively.

The ability to function in the absence of complete data, to anticipate likely problems, and to monitor accurately and efficiently the patient's postoperative course characterizes the mature consultant. Anesthesiologists and surgeons have developed their own techniques, skills, and judgment for assessing and classifying preoperative risk factors and basically desire from their medical consultant a physician capable of identifying and correcting both obvious and subtle medical problems relevant to the patient's optimum care. Nonetheless, results of continuing study of the most frequent types of medical risks and complications in surgical patients now enables the internist to often make important recommendations regarding risk assessment and corrective measures based on clinical and physiologic observations. Listed below are some of the most frequently encountered problems and current evaluative and corrective approaches. Much of the remainder of this book will be devoted to a thorough analysis of these observations and principles.

PREDICTING AND MANAGING COMMON MEDICAL COMPLICATIONS IN SURGICAL PATIENTS

1. Postoperative pulmonary infections and insufficiency.
   a. Pulmonary preoperative evaluation: clinical evaluation *vs.* pulmonary function testing; objective predictors of risk.
   b. Concept of "prohibitive risk." More accurate preoperative prediction of postoperative pulmonary physiology; improved techniques for postoperative respiratory support.
   c. Intensive preoperative regimens to improve pulmonary function.
   d. Improved techniques for management of secretions and atelectasis.
2. Cardiac infarction, failure, arrhythmias.
   a. Timing of surgery relative to previous myocardial infarction.
   b. Assessment of cardiac risk via multifactorial clinical assessment.
   c. Preoperative physiologic profile and risk assessment via right heart Swan-Ganz catheterization.
   d. Stand-by prophylactic cardiac pacers.
3. Pulmonary emboli.
   a. Identifying the high risk patient: type of surgery, clinical status (congestive heart failure, hypotension, shock, age, weight, prior history of thrombophlebitis or pulmonary emboli, varicosities, presence of malignancy).
   b. Development of effective prophylactic anticoagulation regimens.
   c. Early ambulation, graduated pressure hose, pneumatic stockings, rocking bed.
4. Nonpulmonary infections.
   a. Prophylactic antibiotic regimens.
   b. Nutritional assessment and support.
   c. Closed-sterile drainage systems.
   d. Intravenous line care.
5. Renal failure.
   a. Early dialysis.
   b. Improved pharmacokinetic understanding of nephrotoxic drugs; nomograms.
6. Diabetes mellitus.
   a. Low-dose, constant infusion regimens for insulin.
7. Hypertension.
   a. Appropriate drug maintenance until surgery.

b. Improved management of hypertensive crisis.

SUMMARY

The well-structured and supervised general medicine consult service can provide medicine residents with a variety of skills and experiences pertinent to and important for the practice of general internal medicine. Exposure to assorted surgical disorders and to surgical judgment and decision making, as well as to various common medical problems not often seen now on medicine wards, complicated, as well, by the stress of surgery or delivery, are features of the consult service that make it educationally rewarding for the internal medicine resident.

A preoperative assessment clinic for high-risk patients, coordinating the skills of the surgeon, anesthesiologist, and internist would appear to be a natural extension of this service. When feasible, the resulting improvements in patient and physician convenience, more economical and orderly evaluations, more harmonious relations between internists, surgeons and anesthesiologists, and optimally prepared patients, would be a few of the benefits from such an approach.

READINGS

1. Byyny RL, Siegler M, Tarlov AR: Development of an academic section of general internal medicine. *Am J Med* 63:493–498, 1977.
2. Moore RA, Kammerer WS, McGlynn TJ, et al.: Consultations in internal medicine: A training program resource. *J Med Educ* 52:323–327, 1977.
3. Robie PW: The Service and Educational Contributions of a General Medicine Consultation Service. *J Gen Int Med* 1:225–227, 1986.
4. Deyo RA: The Internist as Consultant. *Arch Intern Med* 140:137–138, 1980.
5. Bomalaski JS, Martin GH, Webster JR. General Internal Medicine Consultation. *Arch Int Med* 143:875–876, 1983.
6. Johnson AC, Kroeger HH, Altman I, et al.: The office practice of internists: III. Characteristics of patients. *JAMA* 193:144–150, 1965.
7. Burnside JW: What the general internist does. *Arch Int Med* 137:1286–1288, 1977.
8. Burnum JF: What one internist does in his practice: Implications for the internist's disputed role and education. *Ann Int Med* 78:437–444, 1973.
9. Barondess JA: The Training of the Internist: With Some Messages from Practice: *Ann Int Med* 90:412–417, 1979.
10. Gross R, Kammerer WS: Medical consultation on surgical services: An annotated bibliography. *Ann Int Med* 95:523–529, 1981.

3

Evaluation of Medical Risks in the Surgical Patient

Richard J. Gross

RISK-BENEFIT: GENERAL PRINCIPLES

Evaluation of preoperative risk involves an area of the literature and a process of decision-making not covered in traditional ward rotations during internal medicine training, which also differs from routine ambulatory medicine practice. This section will cover the decision-making process in preoperative evaluation, which involves a balancing of estimated risk against the anticipated benefits of surgery.

An estimation of preoperative risk is based on a thorough history, physical examination, review of the data base available, and selectively ordered laboratory tests. Based on the data gathered from these sources, an estimation of the risk posed by medical problems for surgery can be made from the literature on preoperative evaluation (1–3) and clinical judgment. Benefits of surgery are available in standard medical and surgical texts and, very importantly, from referring surgical colleagues.

We base our decision balancing risks and benefits on five points (Table 3.1).

1. **Why was the consult really requested?** The reason for consultation is often written as a 3–4 word statement on the consultation request form, such as "angina," or "anemia, CHF, hip fracture." In each of these instances, the consultation could have been requested for numerous different purposes. The requesting physician might want approval of the patient for anesthesia or surgery; confir-

mation that a poor risk patient undergo lifesaving surgery; advice on medical management; approval of management the patient is already receiving; a document for medicolegal reasons or to satisfy the anesthesiologist; or a request for routine medical care and follow-up with no relation to the surgical procedure. In each of these cases, the surgeon may be asking for confirmation that what he is already doing is correct; for advice on one or more specific points; or for the internist to assume total care of the patient's medical problems. It is not possible to ascertain these sometimes subtle differences from the routine 3- or 4-word request. Therefore, in most cases, the reason for consultation should be briefly discussed with the referring physician to clarify the reason for the consultation. The time involved in obtaining this information will be richly rewarded in time saved and in the quality of consultation rendered to the referring physician.

Table 3.1. Decision Making in Preoperative Evaluation: Balancing Risks and Benefits

1. Why was the consult really requested?
2. What is the benefit to the patient of the proposed procedure versus no operation or an alternative procedure in terms of morbidity, disability, mortality?
3. What are the real, well-documented risks (risk estimation in order of magnitude)?
4. What is the balance of risk-benefit including both mortality and disability?
5. What are the patient's desires?

18

2. **What is the benefit to the patient of the proposed procedure or therapy?** The estimation of risk cannot be used in a vacuum. An operation presenting a 25% mortality is viewed very differently if it is a necessary life-saving procedure without which the patient would die, than if it is an elective procedure that offers the patient minimal cosmetic benefit. The recommendation for surgery may be different if an alternative procedure offering lower risk is available. The precise question usually is not "can" but "should" a patient undergo surgery.

The benefit of a planned operative procedure must be clearly understood by the consultant in order to accurately state whether the patient should undergo surgery and to interpret preoperative risk. The consultant should know the benefits of the planned procedure, any possible alternative procedure, and the natural history of the patient's problem if no operation is performed. Also vital is an understanding of how various medical risk factors relate to alternative procedures as contrasted with the proposed procedure. Benefits of surgery are often stated in terms of mortality, for which the most data are available. However, the benefit to the patient in terms of morbidity and disability is frequently more important. The consultant, therefore, should know and consider benefits in terms of quality of life as well as mortality. The final decision to undergo surgery based on benefit to the patient is usually reserved to the patient's personal physician and the surgeon. Therefore, the consultant should be tactful in communicating the effect the benefit of the procedure will have on his evaluation of the acceptability of surgical risk. However, the subject of relative benefit to the patient cannot be ignored in an accurate evaluation of preoperative risk nor in the statement of the consultant's recommendations.

3. **What are the real, well-documented risks?** The risks posed by medical problems need to be clearly stated and evaluated. Risks can be overstated, as is commonly done with older patients who are felt to be poor risks simply because of their age. Risks can be incorrectly listed, such as the patient who was felt to be a bad risk because of his age, when a treatable problem such as obstructive lung disease was the major risk factor. Risks can also be understated, as with the complicated patient in whom one or two important problems were overlooked. It is important to evaluate the problems specifically in terms of preoperative risk, since many problems have a different severity in relation to preoperative risk than in terms of clinical severity in usual practice (e.g., angina). The specific problems that affect preoperative risk should be listed, and the consultant should mentally review whether and how these affect the patient's operative status.

The risk should be estimated in terms of order of magnitude of risk. The specific percentage risk cannot be accurately used for a single patient because statistical risks based on large groups have wide variations when applied to single patients. Multiple interacting factors, biological variations, and differences in physicians' technical skills lead to major differences in "similar" patients. Thus, we find it neither accurate nor useful to state that a 25% risk is better than a 20% risk. The general order of magnitude of risk in 1990 can be classified as:

Usual or "low" risk: 0–0.01% (?0.05%) mortality
Low but increased risk: 0.01–0.9% mortality
Significant risk: 1–5% mortality
Moderate risk: 5–10% mortality
High risk: >10% mortality
Very high risk: >20% mortality

It should be realized that these figures are vastly different than they were 10–20 years ago when low risk represented 1–5% and high risk in the order of 25% mortality. This reduction in risk has been attributed to general advances in anesthesia and surgery.

4. **What is the balance of risk-benefit (including both mortality and disability)?** In deciding upon whether surgery should be undertaken, the consultant should first establish the benefits of the procedure to the patient, and secondly, the effect of increased risks due to unrelated conditions. This approach is comparable to that in medical patients where benefits are considered before side effects in deciding upon therapy. In preoperative consultations the line of reasoning is often reversed, with risk being considered of primary concern and benefit secondary.

In deference to the consulting surgeon, the internist often confines his comments to medical risk factors. Few medical disorders carry an absolutely prohibitive risk if the need for surgery is sufficient. The long-term benefits of the surgical procedure should be the basis against which short-term risks are measured, not the reverse.

5. **What are the patient's values and desires?** There are implicit value judgments in balancing risk and benefits. The value placed on life and the ability to perform certain social functions varies. An operation that offered a patient an additional year of life might be viewed much differently if it were a coronary artery bypass graft, which would render the patient asymptomatic and able to return to work, than if it were a palliative cancer operation, leaving the patient with an additional year of pain and inability to work. This balance of risk and benefit must take into account the patient's wishes. Patients' opinions should only be excluded in the rare cases where the patient is unable to communicate in any manner, or in the presence of a severe psychiatric disturbance. In these situations, the family should be interviewed for their opinion and their perception of the patient's wishes. This information

should be obtained from the patient by the referring or personal physician, rather than the consultant, in most instances. However, it is important for the consultant to be cognizant of the patient's wishes.

The preceding five-point scheme includes the total process of surgical decision making. In most cases, the consultant is mainly involved in steps 1–3, with the final decision and discussion with the patient reserved to the referring surgeon.

APPROACH TO PREOPERATIVE EVALUATION

If the decision is made to proceed with surgery, as in most cases, the risk-benefit decision must be carried over to the decision on whether to delay surgery for medical stabilization or to proceed immediately. Decisions also need to be made on which diagnostic and therapeutic recommendations are appropriate given the allotted time before the patient's surgery. Certain procedures or therapies ordinarily done in medical patients may interfere with or increase the risk of the patient's surgery. For example, an upper gastrointestinal series could not be done the afternoon before a colon resection, because of residual barium in the colon and the preoperative bowel prep.

A useful approach to preoperative decision making, balances the urgency of surgery against the evidence for significant organ system impairment (Table 3.2).

The *urgency of the surgery* is *the key controlling* factor in allowing what can be done for medical problems preoperatively: Some surgical emergencies cannot be delayed for medical problems (such as rupturing abdominal aortic aneurysm, or perforated bowel). **Conversely,** remember **elective surgery is always elective.** If the internist feels further evaluation is needed, a new problem is uncovered, or the patient is medically unstable, elective surgery should be delayed until adequate investigation, or stabilization is completed, even in the face of

Table 3.2. Approach to Preoperative Evaluation*

1. What is the status of the patient's health?**
2. If there is evidence of major organ system impairment:**
   (a) how severe is the impairment?
   (b) does the impairment affect or increase operative risk (is it relevant)?
3. *How urgent is the surgery? (Can it wait?)****
4. Will the degree of impairment be less if the surgery is delayed and the patient treated?
5. If there is no reason to delay the surgery, what specific changes in intra- and perioperative care are appropriate for the individual patient?

---

*Dr. Lourdes C. Corman, University of Florida, Gainesville, unpublished; with permission (slightly adapted).
**From Table 3.1.
***This is considered *the* most important question.

pressures to go ahead with surgery from the surgeon or family for convenience or personal reasons.

An important consideration is *whether preoperative "preparation" will reduce risk.* Often forgotten, but important, *are recommendations for intraoperative* and *perioperative care that may reduce risk.* We have found this approach (Table 3.2) to be a useful approach to deciding on whether to delay surgery and what diagnostic-therapeutic recommendations to make, once a risk-benefit decision has been made in favor of surgery.

A *special case of decision making* exists when two surgical procedures are potentially required. A common example is a patient in whom a carotid endarterectomy (first operation) may be required before major abdominal surgery, such as aortic aneurysm or colon cancer (second surgery), when the abdominal surgery was the original problem. We prefer to approach this dilemma by first establishing whether the patient would require the first procedure (carotid surgery), if the original abdominal surgery was not needed—i.e., is the carotid operation *purely prophylaxis* for the second surgery? If the patient would require carotid surgery anyway for *medical* reasons alone, then

the issue is simplified into a patient requiring two operations for *medical* reasons, and the decision is the priority of the two required operations. The priority of operations is based on: (a) the more pressing indication or which disease is more likely to worsen with delay in surgery; (b) whether one operation done first will lower or raise the risk of the second surgery; and (c) which surgery will postpone the second operation the least amount of time. This decision is fairly straightforward most of the time.

The more difficult situation occurs when the patient would *not* require the first surgery (prophylactic carotid endarterectomy in the example above), if it were not for the second surgery. This is a much more difficult decision because the first surgery usually significantly raises operative risks, and there is a paucity of data on lowering operative risk by prophylactic surgery such as is the case in the common example of carotid surgery cited above. We feel the decision should be based on a careful review of the literature regarding the established benefit of the specific prophylactic procedure for subsequent surgery, the local experience in terms of operative risks, and how urgent an indication exists for the original surgery. This is usually a much more difficult decision. In the example above, the evidence favors not doing prophylactic carotid endarterectomy for abdominal surgery in most situations (see Chapter 19).

READINGS

1. Papper EM: Some reflections on mortality due to anesthesia. *Anesthesiology* 25:454–460, 1964.
2. Rhoades JE, Allen JG, Harkins HN, et al.: The assessment of operative risk, in *Surgery Principles and Practice,* 4th Ed. Philadelphia, JP Lippincott, 1970, p 232–243.
3. Feigal DW, Blaisdell FW: The estimation of surgical risk. *Med Clin N Am* 63:1135–1143, 1979.
4. Eisman B (ed): *Prognosis of Surgical Disease.* Philadelphia, WB Saunders, 1980.
5. Bunker JP, Barnes BA, Mosteller F: *Costs, Risks and Benefits of Surgery.* New York, Oxford University Press, 1977.

4

Anesthesia: Organ Effects, Risks and General Principles

Kermit R. Tantum

The scope of anesthesiology is continually broadening and becoming more complex. The number of drugs and techniques available to the anesthesiologist is constantly increasing. These anesthetic agents and techniques routinely affect the function of many organ systems in the healthy individual and, in general, show magnified effects in patients with diseased organs, often resulting in further clinical dysfunction. The internist's management of various diseases has likewise become more complex, involving the use of an ever widening variety of potent drugs. The interaction of diseases and potent therapies with anesthetic agents and techniques is a daily problem that must be dealt with by both the anesthesiologist and the internist.

Not uncommonly, misunderstandings occur between internists and anesthesiologists with regard to their respective roles in the management of the patient who is to be anesthetized for a surgical procedure. Anesthesiologists have stated it to be a "medical insult" rather than a medical consult to be told to "avoid hypoxia and hypotension," since to do so is basic to good anesthetic care. Such advice gives little or no insight into correct anesthetic management. In general, anesthesiologists expect the internist to diagnose disease processes and optimize organ function prior to the administration of anesthesia for a surgical procedure and to give an estimate of increased risks for anesthesia and surgery posed by concomitant medical problems.

The anesthesiologist then considers it his job to select those drugs and techniques for anesthetic care that will have the least deleterious effects and result in the most favorable outcome for the patient. Optimal care of the patient with medical illness undergoing surgery requires the close cooperation of internists, surgeons, and anesthesiologists.

ANESTHETIC RISKS—MORTALITY

It is common for the internist to be asked to give "medical clearance" or more specifically, to give an estimate of anesthetic risk for an individual patient about to undergo surgery. In answering such a request, one should keep in mind that **the hazards of anesthesia cannot be considered independently of many other factors.** The overall risk is determined by a delicate balance of anesthetic agents, anesthetic technique, surgical procedure, surgical technique, and disease processes.

One extensively used system of risk assessment is the American Society of Anesthesiologists (ASA) classification of physical status. In this system, the anesthesiologist classifies the patient according to physical status before administering an anesthetic. This classification (Table 4.1) is based on the presence of systemic disturbances which may be: absent (class 1), mild (class 2), moderate (class 3), severe (class 4), or almost certain to cause death (class 5). The ASA physical status measure is a rather crude classification of physical condition and not of total sur-

Table 4.1. American Society of Anesthesiologists Physical Status Measure (ASA)

Class 1	There is no physiologic, biochemical, or psychiatric disturbance. The pathological process for which operation is to be performed is localized and not conducive to systemic disturbance. Examples: a fit patient with inguinal hernia; fibroid uterus in an otherwise healthy woman.
Class 2	Mild to moderate systemic disturbance caused either by the condition to be treated surgically or by other pathophysiological processes. Examples: presence of mild diabetes, essential hypertension, or anemia.
Class 3	Rather severe systemic disturbance or pathology from whatever cause, even though it may not be possible to define the degree of disability with finality. Examples: severe diabetes with vascular complications; moderate to severe degrees of pulmonary insufficiency; angina pectoris or healed myocardial infarction.
Class 4	Indicative of the patient with a severe systemic disorder already life-threatening and not always correctable by the operative procedure. Examples: advanced degrees of cardiac, pulmonary, hepatic, renal, or endocrine insufficiency.
Class 5	This category embraces the moribund patient who has little chance of survival but is submitted to operation in desperation. Examples: the burst aneurysm with the patient in profound shock; major cerebral trauma with rapidly increasing intracranial pressure; massive pulmonary embolus.
Emergency operation (E)	Any patient in one of the classes listed above who is operated upon as an emergency is considered to be in somewhat poorer physical condition. The letter E is placed beside the numerical classification.

reported in 1961, following review of 33,224 patients receiving anesthesia, that there were no deaths among class 1 patients. More recent data relating mortality rates to age and physical status of patients from the Massachusetts General Hospital indicated a progressively increasing incidence of mortality with higher physical status, and a smaller but progressive increase associated with age (3) (Table 4.2). It is likely that the increased mortality associated with increasing age is not related to age per se, but simply reflects the greater number of patients with significant diseases in the older age group (4).

A more specific evaluation of physical status relative to the cardiac patients has been presented by Goldman (5) in the form of a multifactorial index of cardiac risks in noncardiac surgical patients. In this study, nine factors associated with severe or fatal cardiac complications were identified (see Chapter 10). Here again, intraoperative factors were not included in the index.

A quantitative approach used in evaluating the preoperative patient that considers hemodynamic, respiratory, and oxygen transport variables has been presented by Del Geuricio (6) and by Lewin et al. (7). It is their premise that the "stress" of anesthesia and surgery requires an increase in respiratory, circulatory, and metabolic work, and that by

gical risks, since all of the factors associated with the operation itself are ignored.

Many studies, however, have been performed correlating outcome with ASA physical status. Beecher and Todd (1) reported in 1954 that there were 5 times more deaths among physical status three and four patients than among physical status one and two patients. Dripps (2)

Table 4.2. Mortality Rates by Age and Physical Status Category for All Patients at Massachusetts General Hospital, 1973–76[a]

Physical Status	Age			
	0–34	35–64	65+	All Ages
1, 2	0.1%	0.3%	1.0%	0.3%
3	5.0%	3.9%	5.2%	4.6%
4	27.5%	21.4%	31.0%	25.9%
5	70.2%	71.3%	75.8%	72.4%
All	1.0%	2.6%	5.8%	2.6%

[a] From Hirsh R, et al. (eds): *Health Care Delivery in Anesthesia*. Philadelphia, GF Stickley, 1979, p 100.

quantitating these factors preoperatively, a reasonable prediction of outcome (mortality) can be made. The evaluation involves invasive testing, utilizing the pulmonary artery catheter and determination of a physiologic profile, including cardiac output, left ventricular stroke work, peripheral vascular resistance, oxygen transport, etc. (see also Chapter 10).

Other factors important in the assessment of anesthetic risk have to do with the inherent toxicity of the anesthetic agents themselves, independent of known disease processes and the technical skill of those administering the anesthetic (8–10). Considerable controversy exists among anesthesiologists as to the relative contribution of these factors. Representing both ends of the spectrum, Keats (11, 12) and Hamilton (13) disagree as to what the relative role of drugs versus management error is in causing anesthetic mortality. It is Dr. Keats' opinion that there has been a strong bias toward attributing all unexpected deaths during anesthesia to preventable causes, i.e., accidents or misuse of anesthetic agents, such as obstructed endotracheal tubes, intubating the esophagus, failure of the oxygen supply, or obvious overdose of anesthetic drugs. He proposes that a myth has been perpetuated that anesthetic drugs are different from other drugs, i.e., absolutely safe unless someone errs. He feels that this is not in accord with what has been learned over the last decade in clinical pharmacology, and that to an undetermined extent, idiosyncratic or other adverse reactions to anesthetic drugs may account for sudden death under anesthesia. Dr. Hamilton's position is that the role of "pilot error" in sudden anesthetic deaths is much greater than that of adverse anesthetic drug reactions. At one extreme, then, is the view that all anesthetic agents are dangerous, and that it is the anesthetist's job to select the least dangerous for an individual patient. The opposite view is that any anesthetic is safe if it is administered correctly. Undoubtedly, the answer lies somewhere in between.

Considerable attention has been devoted in recent years to the preventable morbidity and mortality related to "critical incidents" in anesthesiology (14). A "critical incident" has been defined as a human error or equipment failure that could have led or did lead to an undesirable outcome, ranging from an increased length of hospital stay to death. In an attempt to minimize these preventable problems, much attention has been focused on improved monitoring in the operating room. The American Society of Anesthesiologists recently set standards for basic intraoperative monitoring (15). These standards include monitors of oxygenation, ventilation, circulation, and body temperature. Recently developed monitors now in daily use include pulse oximeters, capnographs and mass spectrometers. Coming into use at the present time are noninvasive cardiac output monitors and improved electroencephalography. It is anticipated that the improved "vigilence" brought about by these monitors will significantly reduce the preventable mishaps.

It has been documented (3) that patients who undergo surgery on an emergency basis have a higher morbidity and mortality than elective patients. There are many possible explanations for this, including: inadequate evaluation or preparation of patients, the presence of tired or less experienced personnel during off hours, and more severe surgical pathology.

In most cases, the internist will not be able to provide a precise overall evaluation of anesthetic risks, but will be able to give a reasonable assessment of the change in risk due to the disease processes that are present.

Spinal Versus General Anesthesia

There is a prevalent feeling among physicians that spinal anesthesia is inherently safer than general anesthesia and, therefore, the preferable technique for sicker patients. This idea was enhanced by Beecher and Todd (1) when they reported a lower mortality rate in a group of patients who received spinal anesthesia when compared to general anesthesia. This lower mortality reported with spinal anesthesia has been questioned, and is probably due to the inability to perform higher risk types of surgery under spinal anesthesia, such as cardiovascular and neurologic surgery.

The choice between spinal and general anesthesia depends on many factors, including: site, type, and duration of surgery; specific medical problems of the patient; and personal preference by the patient, surgeon, and anesthesiologist. Spinal anesthesia lends itself well to surgery of the lower abdomen, inguinal and rectal areas, and lower extremities. Spinal anesthesia has been used extensively in the past for upper abdominal surgery, but with better techniques of general anesthesia, this has become much less common.

Spinal anesthesia has been advocated for patients with a full stomach requiring emergency surgery; however, this technique does not guarantee that the patient will not aspirate, especially if sedatives or hypnotics are used in conjunction with the spinal anesthetic.

Spinal anesthesia has been advocated as a less invasive way of managing the patient with severe chronic pulmonary disease. While this is probably true for spinal anesthesia maintained at low levels, (i.e., adequate for a transurethral resection of the prostate), **the higher levels of spinal anesthesia required for intra-abdominal surgery may have a more deleterious effect on respiration than a carefully performed general anesthetic.** In addition, aggressive intraoperative monitoring may be more difficult under spinal anesthesia.

A major problem associated with spinal anesthesia is the hypotension induced by blocking sympathetic nerves, which becomes more pronounced the higher the level of spinal anesthesia. The correct use of fluids, pressor agents, and patient positioning can minimize this hypotension, but the potential threat must be considered, particularly in patients who are at high risk for hypotension.

Neurologic sequelae can result from spinal anesthesia and range from postspinal headache to adhesive arachnoiditis. Spinal headache is a result of cerebral spinal leakage and can be reduced to a frequency of less than 1–2% by using a 25 or 26 gauge needle. More serious complications, such as cauda equina syndrome and adhesive arachnoiditis are rare, and their incidence has been greatly lessened by the routine use of uncontaminated anesthetic solutions. With some exceptions, spinal anesthesia is contraindicated in the presence of neurologic disease. Other contraindications include: localized infections of the back, sepsis, and bleeding diatheses.

Epidural anesthesia differs little from spinal anesthesia in regards to the advantages and precautions discussed above. However, the very much larger doses of local anesthetic required for epidural anesthesia do increase the risk of adverse reactions to these agents. One popular local anesthetic, bupivicaine, is no longer utilized for obstetrical epidural analgesia in the 0.75% concentration. This is because of the cardiotoxicity, which has resulted in cardiac arrest with difficult resuscitation or deaths. Lesser concentration of this drug are still commonly used.

Same Day Admissions

In the last three years, there has been a striking increase in the percentage of total surgical patients admitted to the hospital on the day of surgery. This has been strongly encouraged (mandated) by third-party payers. Many of our earlier concerns of increased risks to these patients have been proven unfounded, providing these patients are carefully selected and prepared. Careful attention must be paid to many factors, including preadmission patient instruction, securing lab work, continuing appropriate medications, etc. While initially patients were limited to ASA class 1 and 2 status, most centers will now accept ASA class 3 patients if they are stable, and the proposed surgery and anesthetic will not destabilize them.

ANESTHESIA AND THE RESPIRATORY SYSTEM

Effects of Anesthesia

Most anesthetic agents have the potential to adversely affect respiration. These effects include alterations of: respiratory control lung volumes, distribution of ventilation and perfusion (V/Q), and respiratory muscle function (16).

RESPIRATORY CONTROL

Increasing the concentration of inhalation agents alters the normal central nervous system response to carbon dioxide. The effect is a blunting of the usual increase in minute ventilation as the arterial carbon dioxide tension rises. Narcotics also diminish this response, primarily by slowing the respiratory rate. Though originally thought to be unaffected, it is now recognized that the peripheral hypoxic reflex is even more sensitive to anesthetics (i.e., diminishes with increasing concentrations) than is the central CO_2 response. The normal cough reflex is depressed or abolished during general anesthesia.

LUNG VOLUMES

There is a uniform reduction in the functional residual capacity (FRC) of approximately 400 cc with all types of general anesthesia. This reduction in volume is frequently such that the end expiratory level falls below the closing capacity. This results in dependent areas of the lung having continued circulation but dimin-

ished ventilation, which in turn, results in venous admixture as evidenced by an increased alveolar-arterial oxygen gradient ($Pi_A - aO_2$). **This reduction in FRC occurs very rapidly after the induction of anesthesia and remains until the recovery period.** One explanation for this decrease in FRC is the relaxation of the diaphragm, which in the supine position rises into the chest.

VENTILATION, PERFUSION DISTRIBUTION

Abnormalities in the distribution of ventilation and perfusion occur regularly during anesthesia, with resultant abnormalities of oxygen and carbon dioxide exchange. When physiologic shunting and dead space are measured utilizing ordinary blood gas techniques, both of these values are found to increase during general anesthesia in the normal patient. In the normally functioning lung, regional changes in ventilation tend to be counteracted by the hypoxic-vasoconstrictor reflex (HPV), which has the effect of diverting blood away from hypoxic areas of the lung. Halothane and nitrous oxide have been shown to interfere with the HPV reflex. The distribution of ventilation within the lung varies according to the mode of ventilation utilized, i.e., spontaneous or controlled. With spontaneous ventilation, the dependent portions of the lungs are preferentially ventilated, whereas with controlled ventilation, the upper portions of the lungs are preferentially ventilated.

RESPIRATORY MUSCLE

Paralysis of the muscles of respiration is routinely produced by neuromuscular blocking agents during balanced general anesthesia. While drugs are routinely used to reverse muscle paralysis, recovery is not always complete. Various bedside tests have been devised to assess recovery from muscle relaxation. These include the head lift test, i.e., can the patient support his head off the bed for five seconds unaided, and the measurement of vital capacity, which should be greater than 10 cc/kg. The use of an electrical nerve stimulator can also be utilized in assessing patients for residual neuromuscular blockade.

The above described alterations of respiratory function can extend for a variable period of time into the postoperative period. This phenomenon, **the so-called "anesthetic tail" can be of special importance with those patients who have preexisting cardiac and pulmonary disorders.** For example, with the additional compromises in FRC and V/Q associated with major upper abdominal surgery, further clinical deterioration can be anticipated in patients with underlying cardiopulmonary disease.

Anesthetic Management

There is no one anesthetic technique of choice for patients with pulmonary disability (17). It is useful to think of the choices as ranging between "minimal interference" and maximal support." The minimal interference technique usually involves regional anesthesia or general anesthesia without an endotracheal tube. These techniques are usually used for lower abdominal and extremity procedures. With this technique, it is anticipated that the patient will maintain adequate spontaneous ventilation and that the mucociliary escalator mechanism will remain intact. It should be understood, however, that even these techniques can interfere with respiration and that many patients with respiratory diseases simply cannot lie flat, or cease coughing, for the time required for surgery. The "maximal support" technique involves a general anesthetic with tracheal intubation, artificial ventilation, suctioning, and positive pressure ventilation for an extended period of time into the postoperative period. Regional anesthesia, such as an epidural block, used intraoperatively or postoperatively for pain control may be combined with this technique.

The management of patients with bronchospasm presents special problems (18). It is important that the patient receive adequate doses of bronchodilators including beta-2 catecholamines, corticosteroids, and theophylline derivatives up to the time of induction of anesthesia. Of greatest importance is the avoidance of instrumentation of the airway, i.e., oropharyngeal and endotracheal tubes at too light a level of anesthesia. **Stimulating the upper airway without adequate regional and/or general anesthesia can precipitate severe bronchospasm.** Anesthetic agents which decrease broncho-motor tone such as halothane, enflurane, or isoflurane, are usually chosen. Atropine, while controversial, is felt by many to be a useful drug in the asthmatic undergoing surgery. Drugs stimulating histamine release are generally avoided (i.e., curare). The use of theophylline compounds during general anesthesia was at one time considered dangerous. Now with better methods of monitoring drug levels and controlling dosage, they are considered safe and, in fact, essential therapy in the operating room for treating bronchospasm. The aspiration of gastric contents into the lung is of great concern to anesthesiologists. Patients especially predisposed to aspiration include those who have recently ingested food, patients with bowel obstruction, and pregnant women. These patients are managed by utilizing such techniques as preoperative antacid and histamine blocking therapy, awake intubation, or a rapid induction with intubation in the head-up position, while holding pressure on the cricoid cartilage to prevent regurgitation.

A technique being utilized with more frequency in the operating room is that of high frequency jet ventilation (HFJV). This author has found this technique especially useful during lung resections, where excellent gas exchange can be maintained while providing the surgeon with a relatively quiet operative field.

ANESTHESIA AND THE CARDIOVASCULAR SYSTEM

Effects of Anesthesia

VENTRICULAR FUNCTION

All inhalation anesthetics in current use depress myocardial function as measured by the rate of change of ventricular pressure (DP/DT) or cardiac and stroke volume indices (19, 20). Halothane, enflurane, and isoflurane each decrease these indices progressively with increasing concentrations, with halothane showing the most cardiac depression and isoflurane showing the least. Even the less potent nitrous oxide can be demonstrated to depress myocardial function in a 40% concentration. Intravenous morphine in large doses has little direct effect on myocardial function, but may decrease cardiac output through venodilation and increased vascular capacity. Fentanyl in large doses has similar effects to those of morphine.

Diazepam has become popular as a premedicant and anesthetic induction agent and supplement. Low doses of this drug have little effect on cardiac function, while larger doses can reduce stroke volume by 30%. Ketamine has been demonstrated to enhance ventricular function in the healthy patient and patients with angina, while consistently increasing heart rate. Neuroleptic agents (droperidol combined with fentanyl) have little or no direct effect on ventricular function. Likewise, effects on ventricular function have not been demonstrated for the neuromuscular blockers.

Regional anesthetics are well known myocardial depressants in large doses. It is therefore possible with major blocks to produce ventricular depression, although this is not likely to occur with the usual and cautious use of these techniques.

MYOCARDIAL PERFUSION

Studies have been conducted in man on the effects of thiopentol, halothane, ketamine, droperidol, and fentanyl on myocardial blood flow and metabolism. In general, these have shown that coronary blood flow and oxygen consumption continue as in the unanesthetized patient to parallel changes in heart rate, systemic blood pressure, and contractile force of the heart (19). Recent data have suggested that isoflurane (compared to halothane and enflurane) may unfavorably unbalance the myocardial oxygen supply/demand ratio as evidenced by a higher incidence of myocardial ischemia. It is felt isoflurane may create an "intracoronary steal," diverting blood to normal areas of coronary circulation from ischemic beds (21).

Anesthetic agents can affect the nervous system both centrally and peripherally to produce a vasomotor depression. In addition, alterations of the baroreceptors and chemoreceptors in vascular smooth muscle can occur with general anesthesia.

While these impairments of cardiovascular function are generally minimal and tolerable in the healthy individual, they may result in hypotension and poor perfusion to critical levels in the patient with significant cardiovascular disease and a limited ability to compensate.

Anesthetic Management

ISCHEMIC HEART DISEASE

Increasing numbers of patients with myocardial ischemia are brought to anesthesia and surgery. It is essential that anesthesia interfere minimally with myocardial metabolism and function in order to reduce the incidence of postoperative myocardial infarction. In these patients, there is a delicate balance between the myocardial oxygen supply and oxygen demand. We now recognize many factors relating to anesthetic agents and techniques that tend to alter this balance. Much progress has been made in recent years in our ability to monitor patients, and to alter the oxygen supply/demand balance in a favorable direction during anesthesia (22). Traditionally, anesthesiologists have concerned themselves with oxygen supply to the myocardium, which includes such factors as coronary blood flow, oxygen saturation, and hematocrit. Recently, major attention has been directed to the factors related to oxygen demand, i.e., blood pressure (afterload), ventricular volume (preload), heart rate, and contractility. Manipulations such as laryngoscopy, tracheal intubation, and surgical stimulation elicit autonomic responses, which are more pronounced during light anesthesia. These autonomic responses increase catecholamine concentrations, which in turn cause tachycardia, hypertension, and increased systemic vascular resistance. There is, consequent to these factors, an increase in myocardial oxygen demand which can be life-threatening in critical patients.

Measurements used to evaluate myocardial oxygen demand that are commonly used in the operating room include: the rate pressure product (RPP = systolic blood pressure × heart rate) and the triple index (TI = systolic pressure × heart rate × pulmonary capillary wedge pressure). Attempts are made to keep the RPP less than 12,000 and the TI less than 150,000. The simultaneous monitoring of EKG leads II and a precordial lead have become common, as has the observation for acute changes in pulmonary-capillary wedge pressure, as methods to look for intraoperative ischemia. While none of these measurements alone have been shown to correlate closely with myocardial ischemia, it is felt that used together, a reasonable picture of myocardial oxygen balance and ischemia can be obtained.

The current philosophy and practice is to keep the cardiac pumping function and blood pressure controllably depressed. Common techniques involve relatively large doses of narcotics and muscle relaxants combined with modest levels of inhalation agents and amnesics. Nitroprusside and nitroglycerin are commonly used as supplements to reduce afterload and improve coronary circulation. Poor cardiac pumping function in the operating room is commonly managed with calcium chloride, dobutamine, dopamine or amrinone.

In the past, much concern has been expressed that beta-blockers may potentiate the myocardial depressant action of anesthetics. Some have called for discontinuation of these drugs 24–48 hours or more before anesthesia and surgery. Such discontinuation, however, may result in severe arrythmias, unstable hypertension, angina, and even myocardial infarction. More recent studies indicate that a potentiation of myocardial depressant effects with anesthesia does not occur. It is now primarily agreed that beta-blockers should be continued up until the time of anesthesia. While similar studies have not been conducted with the calcium channel blockers, the same reasoning prevails, and common clinical practice is to continue these drugs until the time of operation.

It has been common teaching for many years that elective noncardiac surgery within 3–6 months of a myocardial infarction carries a prohibitively high risk (greater than 26%) of perioperative myocardial infarction and should therefore be postponed. Recent data (23) suggest that "contemporary" management can reduce this risk to under 3% during this period. The management of these patients in this study involved use of the pulmonary artery catheter and the aggressive use of beta-blockers and vasodilator therapies. While one must have reservations about sending purely elective patients with recent myocardial infarctions to the operating room, it would seem that with proper pre- and intraoperative care, the risk to this group of patients can be significantly reduced.

HEART FAILURE

Optimum control of heart failure is mandatory before the induction of anesthesia and surgery. This control will commonly include the use of digitalis preparations. Anesthetic agents and techniques can affect individual patient tolerance to digitalis in several ways. Digitalis toxicity has been noted in the presence of low potassium, elevated PCO_2, depressed PO_2, and with the use of succinylcholine. Because of the increased liklihood of digitalis toxicity in patients undergoing general anesthesia, it has been advocated by some that this drug be withheld for 12–24 hours preoperatively. This should not be done when daily doses of digitalis are required to prevent congestive heart failure and worsening of arrhythmias, but the use of "prophylactic" digitalis should probably be condemned. Additionally, because of its toxicity, many experienced anesthesiologists will not use digitalis for its ionotropic effects in the operating room, but will choose other agents, i.e., calcium chloride, dopamine or amrinone, for this purpose.

Patients with heart failure have an increased sensitivity to both the central nervous system effects and the cardiovascular depressive effects of intravenous induction agents, i.e., thiopental. As a result, smaller doses of this drug or the use of alternate intravenous agents, such as morphine or valium, are often preferred.

Several factors that occur in the immediate post-anesthetic period can precipitate heart failure and pulmonary edema. These include: the withdrawal of positive pressure ventilation, peripheral vasoconstriction, and the increased oxygen demand created by shivering.

HYPERTENSION

Much attention has been given in the past to the relationship between antihypertensive drugs and anesthetic agents (24, 25). At one time, such agents were discontinued up to 2 weeks preoperatively in order to avoid serious hypotension in the operating room. Today, it is felt that the **reappearance of hypertension upon discontinuation of drug ther-** **apy is more of a stress and danger than continuation of the drug.** Generally, with extra care and attention, the anesthesiologist can avoid serious hypotension in patients on antihypertensive medications. One must recognize that these patients may be hypovolemic and, therefore, utilize techniques of slow induction and volume loading. The increased vascular reactivity exhibited by these patients can be managed by utilizing local anesthetic techniques, narcotics, and vasodilators.

Special problems in hypertensive patients involve the hypokalemia and hypovolemia resulting from the use of diuretics. Many anesthesiologists will refuse to administer general anesthesia to a patient with subnormal serum potassium levels because of the associated dangers of hypotension, arrhythmias, and cardiac arrest. This position has been supported by recent data demonstrating greater ventricular irritability in patients with ischemic heart disease with even minor reductions in serum potassium concentrations (26). Other recent data, which have been provided by what may be the only study on hypokalemic humans undergoing general anesthesia, found no correlation of operative arrhythmias with chronic hypokalemia (27). **My own practice is to regard modest hypokalemia (serum potassium between 3 and 3.5) as important only in patients who are digitalized or who have serious ischemic heart disease.**

A particular problem in the hypertensive patient in the immediate postoperative period is **severe hypertension upon emergence from general anesthesia.** This problem is especially likely to occur after carotid endarterectomy (20%) and abdominal aortic aneurysm resection (57%) (25). This problem may require management in the post-anesthesia recovery area utilizing such drugs as sedatives, analgesics, hydralazine, labatolol, or nitroprusside to avoid hypertensive complications (see also Chapter 10).

ANESTHESIA AND THE LIVER

Effects of Anesthesia on the Liver

Anesthetic techniques, including both general anesthesia and major block techniques reduce hepatic blood flow (HBF), as well as hepatic oxygen uptake (28). Mechanical ventilation producing an extreme of either hyper- or hypocarbia can reduce HBF. Positive pressure ventilation may also affect HBF by mechanically obstructing blood flow through the liver. Other general factors which may reduce HBF include: variations in cardiac output, splanchnic reflexes, and surgical manipulation. Each of these is a common occurrence during anesthesia and surgery. There is, however, no evidence to suggest that anaerobic metabolism occurs in the healthy individual during anesthesia. Such may not be the case, however, for patients with significant liver disease.

Numerous studies have reported abnormalities of various liver function tests following exposure to general anesthesia (29, 30). These have included abnormalities of BSP excretion, as well as elevations of serum transaminases (SGOT and SGPT) and lactic dehydrogenase (LDH). The cause of these abnormalities is, however, much more commonly related to the site of operation (near the liver) and preexisting liver dysfunction than to specific anesthetic drugs.

Two chemically related substances, chloroform and carbon tetrachloride, are known to be toxic to the liver and may cause acute yellow atrophy. For this reason, other halogenated hydrocarbons used as general anesthetics have been suspected as hepatotoxins. Halothane has received the most publicity in this regard (31), with a great concern about its ability to produce acute liver necrosis. Halothane-induced hepatic necrosis probably occurs in the range of 1 in 10,000 administrations. The weight of evidence is that intermediary metabolites of halothane are responsible for hepatic damage. Especially important is the metabolism of halothane along reductive pathways occurring under conditions of hypoxia. There are also genetic and possibly hypersensitivity contributions to this halothane liver toxicity (32). Two other commonly used halogenated hydrocarbon anesthetic agents are enflurane and isoflurane. Each of these agents are metabolized to a lesser degree than halothane and, therefore, felt to have less potential for liver toxicity. Recent data suggest that if enflurane liver toxicity exists, it is an extremely rare event (33). Isoflurance has not been demonstrated to cause specific liver injury.

Anesthetic Management

In selecting an anesthetic for a patient with liver disease, the effects of altered metabolism by the liver on the various agents administered for anesthesia must be considered. Since many of the agents used for both general and regional anesthesia are inactivated by hepatic metabolism, a more intense and prolonged action of these drugs is to be expected in patients with severely disturbed liver function. Protein binding of anesthetics is also diminished in patients with significant liver disease. Since most drugs are protein-bound at some stage, an alteration in binding sites will affect the action of these drugs. Drugs of particular importance with respect to duration and intensity of action in liver disease include: sedatives, narcotics, neuromuscular blockers, and the local anesthetics. In a practical sense, the anesthesiologists has the option of avoiding drugs, which are dependent upon normal liver function or alternatively when using such drugs, titrating them to their desired effect. Regional anesthesia may be the technique of choice in these patients when practical.

Whether halothane should be administered to patients with known liver disease is unclear. Some feel that biotransformation is lessened in the diseased liver and therefore halothane is acceptable.

However, the possibility of reductive metabolism in the diseased liver makes the choice of halothane questionable in these patients. This is particularly true when alternate agents such as enflurane and isoflurane are available. Clinical guides in the use of halothane would include: avoid its repeated exposure at short intervals in adults in the absence of a strong indication for its use, avoid its use with unexplained jaundice following a first exposure, use it with caution in obese females and in patients with a family history of problems with this agent.

Other clinical problems to be dealt with in anesthetizing patients with hepatic disease include: altered CNS function, clotting defects, risks of aspiration (especially with GI bleeding), and the often associated renal failure.

ANESTHESIA AND THE KIDNEY

Anesthetic Effects on Renal Function

Renal blood flow is uniformly diminished in the range of 30–50% by the commonly used inhalation agents halothane (38%), thiopental-nitrous oxide-narcotic (31%), isoflurane (49%) (34). This diminution is transitory and depends upon the depth of anesthesia. Additionally, there is a reduction in the glomerular filtration rate, an increase in renal vascular resistance, and a decrease in the filtration fraction. Normal autoregulation of the kidney may be interfered with by inhalation agents. These effects on renal function are probably best explained by anesthetic-induced hemodynamic alterations. Other possible explanations include: vasopressor liberation or an activation of the renin-angiotensin system with resultant aldosterone effects. Recent data, however, indicate that the vasopressor and renin abnormalities are more related to surgical stimuli under light anesthesia than to anesthetic agents themselves.

Spinal and epidural anesthesia appear to have minimal effects on renal function, even in the presence of modest hypotension.

A syndrome of high output renal failure (nephrogenic diabetes insipidus) is associated with the use of the volatile anesthetic agent methoxyflourane. This syndrome, which usually occurs after high dosages of long duration, has been determined to be due to high concentrations of fluoride ion resulting from metabolism of the agent. Most anesthesiologists no longer use this agent. Two other anesthetic agents, enflurane and isoflurane are partially metabolized with resulting free fluoride ions. While concern has been expressed for the potential renal toxicity of these agents, the degree of metabolism of enflurane is low, and for isoflurane extremely low, so that the risk of renal damage with either agent is minimal, although a few cases of high-output renal failure have been reported with enflurane.

Anesthetic Management

The importance of preoperative dialysis in improving the risk and safety of anesthesia in uremic patients cannot be overemphasized (35). A maxim in the anesthetic management of patients with diminished renal function is to use agents and techniques that will avoid further renal damage. The most important factor to be considered intraoperatively in the patient with chronic renal disease is proper fluid balance, especially the avoidance of hypovolemia resulting in intraoperative hypotension and permanent organ damage. In the patient and chronic dialysis who has no significant renal function and therefore no risk of further loss, the main intraoperative concern is avoiding hypervolemia, which may contribute to hypertension and cardiac failure. Since these patients tolerate poorly either over- or underhydration, it is essential that they be monitored for these events. In the operating room, this monitoring may take the form of minute-by-minute observations of urine output, systemic blood pressure, central venous and pulmonary capillary wedge pressures.

Equally important in this group of patients is their electrolyte balance, especially the maintenance of a normal serum potassium. Both high and low potassiums have special importance during anesthesia. A low serum potassium combined with general anesthesia may provoke arrythmias. On the other hand, a high serum potassium may be made worse by such things as the use of succinylcholine, administering cold bank blood, hypoventilation, and tissue destruction. In addition to the measurement of serum potassium levels intraoperatively, the electrocardiogram should be monitored carefully to look for changes reflecting abnormalities of serum potassium.

Most drugs used in anesthetic practice are not eliminated in their active form by the kidneys because they are weak electrolytes, which are lipid-soluble in the non-ionized state. Often these drugs are converted in the liver to water-soluble, ionized derivatives that have no pharmacological activity and are then excreted via the kidney. Included in this group are: the narcotics, most barbiturates, benzodiazepenes, phenothiazines, butyrophenone derivates, and ketamine. These drugs may be used with impunity in the face of renal failure. A few drugs used during anesthesia, however, rely upon renal excretion for termination of their action. These are highly ionized in the physiologic pH range and are eliminated unchanged via the kidney. Included in this group are nondepolarizing muscle relaxants (especially gallamine), neostigmine, atropine, and ganglionic blockers. These drugs are either not used or used with great care in this group of patients.

The anemia (as opposed to hypovolemia) commonly associated with chronic renal failure is well tolerated, and in general blood transfusions should only be given to replace blood loss, unless a hematocrit of less than 20% is present for major surgery.

Acceptable techniques for anesthesia for the patient with renal disease include: the titrated use of intravenous induction agents (which have an exaggerated effect because of decreased protein binding) combined with a potent inhalation agent i.e., isoflurane. Alternatively, nitrous oxide and a narcotic with a major tranquilizer and a depolarizing muscle relaxant will have little effect on the cardiovascular system or renal function. The reduction of inspired oxygen must be considered when using nitrous oxide in the presence of anemia, however. Narcotics also have a more intense and prolonged action in these patients, perhaps because of the often associated liver dysfunction. Muscle relaxants, which depend largely on renal excretion, should be avoided or used with great caution (gallamine, metacurine, and pancuronium).

NEW DRUGS IN ANESTHESIA

Several new drugs have been approved for use in anesthesia. These include the sedative/amnestic, midazolam, the short-acting narcotics, sufentanyl and alfentanyl, intermediate-duration muscle relaxants, atacurium and vecuronium, and a familiar drug, morphine, used in the epidural space for pain management.

Midazolam (Versed™) is a water-soluable (in vitro) injectable benzodiazepine with sedative and amnestic properties that causes little or no pain with intravenous injection. Its clinical effect usually does not last longer than two hours and it is widely used in anesthesia as a premedicant, to provide conscious sedation, and as an induction agent to general anesthesia or as a component of balanced anesthesia (36).

Sufentanyl (Sufenta) is a potent synthetic opioid with cardiovascular actions similar to fentanyl (Sublimaze) (widely used in cardiac surgery) but which may be more effective in blocking sympathetic activity during surgical stimulation. Alfentanyl (Alfenta) released in early 1987 is another synthetic opioid that has a rapid onset and brief duration of action. This agent will have use as an induction agent or as an analgesic supplement for short surgical procedures (37).

Vecuronium (Norcuron) and atacurium (Tracrium) are two new nondepolarizing muscle relaxants that have come into widespread use in the operating room. These drugs have a shorter duration (in the range of 20 minutes) than previously used muscle relaxants of this class. Vecuronium has been acclaimed because of its relative freedom from cardiovascular effects. Atacurium has a minor side effect of histamine release but is remarkable in that it is the first nondepolarizer to undergo extensive degradation to inactive breakdown products via a nonbiologic pathway i.e., it does not depend on renal or liver function for termination of activity.

Since FDA approval in late 1984, widespread use is being made of morphine (Duramorph) injected into the lumbar epidural space. Remarkable pain relief is obtained via the highly selective depressing action on nociceptive pathways without affecting motor, sympathetic, or proprioceptive pathways. Excellent pain relief can be achieved acutely in the postoperative patient (various thoraco-abdominal procedures) and chronically in patients with long-term pain syndromes (cancer pain). Side effects including nausea, vomiting, urinary retention, pruritis, and respiratory depression must be dealt with. Other narcotics are under investigation for use in the epidural space.

DRUG INTERACTIONS IMPORTANT IN ANESTHESIA

Many of the drugs used in the medical management of patients may profoundly modify a patient's response to anesthetic agents or adjuvant anesthetic drugs. Drug interactions which can be anticipated are an important part of modern anesthetic practice and are dealt with on a daily basis. Unexpected interactions, however, may be troublesome and not infrequently dangerous. **It is essential, therefore, that the anesthesiologist be informed of all medications currently or recently used** by the patient. It is rarely mandatory for drugs to be discontinued prior to anesthesia and surgery if they are a necessary part of medical management, with the exception of MAO inhibitors (though even this long held belief has been questioned) (38). Rather the on-board drugs must be known so that interactive side effects can be anticipated and managed (39, 40).

Table 4.3 lists commonly used drugs that have importance in anesthetic management. The interacting anesthetic drug, the resulting problem, and suggested management are briefly outlined.

Table 4.3. Anesthetic/Drug Interactions

Drug Class and Prototype	Anesthetic/Drug Interaction	Problem	Anesthetic Management
Diuretics (Chlorothiazide)	Volatile anesthetics and digitalis	Hypokalemia, arrhythmias	Use of balanced anesthesia; avoid alkalosis
Anti-arrhythmics Quinidine	Muscle relaxants	Prolonged	Reduced relaxant dose; monitor with nerve stimulator

Drug Class and Prototype	Anesthetic/Drug Interaction	Problem	Anesthetic Management
Amiodarone	Volatile anesthetics	Complete heart block, poor cardiac output, low systemic vascular resistance	Aggressive monitoring (pulmonary artery catheter) and consider an AV pacemaker
Digitalis		Arrhythmia	Avoid alkalosis and hypokalemia
Vasodilators (glyceryl trinitrate ointment)		Hypotension, methemoglobinemia	
Anticoagulants (Coumadin)		Bleeding	Avoid regional technique
Analgesic (non-narcotic) Aspirin		Bleeding	Caution with regional techniques
Analgesic (narcotic) Morphine		Pain tolerance in chronic users; withdrawal in undiagnosed addict	Maintain usual dose for chronic users; Use inhalation or regional; avoid pentazocine (causes withdrawal)
Myasthenia gravis drugs (Neostigmine)	Muscle relaxants	Prolonged action	Avoid or reduce use
Organophosphates (Echothiophate)	Succinylcholine, ester-type local anesthetic	Prolonged action	Avoid succinylcholine or use reduced doses with caution
Antibiotics Tetracyclines	Methoxyflurane	Renal toxicity	Avoid concomitant use; monitor with nerve stimulator; Ca^{++} gluconate; artificial ventilation
Aminoglycoside antibiotics	Muscle relaxants (Curare, pancuronium)	Prolonged action	
MAO inhibitors (Phenelzine)	Opiates, sympathomimetic	Hypertension, hypotension, convulsion, coma	Discontinue 2 weeks, avoid opiates and pressor; nitroprusside for hypertension; direct acting pressors for hypotension
Tricyclic antidepressants (Imipramine)	Volatile anesthetic	Hypotension, tachycardia, & increased intraocular pressure	Titrate anesthetic, EKG monitor, fluids, direct alpha-stimulation in small dose
	Pressors	Exaggerated response	
Lithium	Muscle relaxant, IV fluids	Prolonged action, electrolyte abnormalities, lithium toxicity	Nerve stimulator to adjust dose, less relaxant, inhalation agent for relaxation, discontinue 24–48 hr pre-op
Phenothiazines (chlorpromazine)	Apiates and other CNS depressants	Augment CNS depressant	Use less CNS depressant drugs for anesthesia; fluid and Ca^{++} for hypotension
	Droperidol	Hypotension	

Table 4.3.   Anesthetic/Drug Interactions (*continued*)

Drug Class and Prototype	Anesthetic/Drug Interaction	Problem	Anesthetic Management
Antiparkinsonism (levodopa)	Thorazine, droperidol; indirect sympathomimetics (have reduced response)	Extrapyramidal symptoms, chest wall rigidity Hypotension	Avoid droperidol and phenothiazine; muscle relaxant; Fluid for hypotension
Anticonvulsants (dilantin, phenobarbital)	Methoxyflurane, ethrane (minimal)	Enzyme inductions leading to toxic metabolites i.e., Fl$^-$	Avoid agents with toxic metabolites
Antihypertensives (Methyldopa)	Volatile anesthetics	Hypotension	Fluid, small dose of pressor
B-Blockers (Propranolol)	Volatile anesthetics	Cardiac depression, bradycardia, hypotensions, CHF, bronchoconstriction	Isoproternol, Ca^{++}, Atropine, do not reverse relaxants if bradycardic
Calcium channel blockers	Volatile anesthetics	Profound cardiovascular depression via negative ionotropism	Use low concentrations of volatile agents

READINGS

1. Beecher HK, Todd DP: A study of the deaths associated with anesthesia and surgery based on a study of 599,548 anesthetics in ten institutions, 1948–1952 inclusive. *Ann Surg* 140:2–34, 1954.
2. Dripps DR, Lamont A, Eckenhoff JE: The role of anesthesia in surgical mortality. *JAMA* 178:261–266, 1961.
3. Soper K, McPeek B: Predicting mortality for high risk surgery, in Hirsh R, Forrest WH, Orkin FK, Wollman H (eds): *Health Care Delivery in Anesthesia.* Philadelphia, George F. Stickley, 1980, pp 99–103.
4. Djokovic J, Hedley-Whyte J: Prediction of outcome of surgery and anesthesia in patients over 80. *JAMA* 242:2301–2306, 1979.
5. Goldman L, Caldera DL, Nussbaum SR, et al. Multifactorial index of cardiac risk in noncardiac surgical procedures. *N Engl J Med* 297:845–850, 1977.
6. Del Guercio LR, Cohen JD: Monitoring operative risk in the elderly. *JAMA* 243:1350–1355, 1980.
7. Lewin I, Lerner A, Green H, et al. Physical class and physiologic status in the prediction of operative mortality in the aged sick. *Ann Surg* 174:217–232, 1971.
8. Cohen EN: Toxicity in inhalation anaesthetic agents. *Br J Anaesth* 50:665–675, 1978.
9. Cullen BF: Cellular effects and toxicity of anesthetics. *ASA Refresher Courses in Anesthes* 6:43–56, 1978.
10. Steen PA, Michenfelder JD: Neurotoxicity of anesthetics. *Anesthesiology* 50:437–453, 1979.
11. Keats AS: The estimate of anesthetic risk in medical evaluation. *Am J Cardiol* 12:330–333, 1963.
12. Keats AS: What do we know about anesthetic mortality? *Anesthesiology* 50:387–392, 1979.
13. Hamilton WK: Unexpected deaths during anesthesia: Wherein lies the cause: *Anesthesiology* 50:381–383, 1979.
14. Cooper JB, Newbower RS, Kitz RJ: An analysis of major errors and equipment failures in anesthesia management: Considerations for prevention and detection. *Anesthesiology* 60:34–42, 1984.
15. American Society of Anesthesiologists House of Delegates: Standards for basic intraoperative monitoring. *ASA Newsletter* 50:12–13, 1986.
16. Rehder K, Sessler AD, Marsh M: State of the Art: General anesthesia and the lung. *Am Rev Respir Dis* 112:541–563, 1975.
17. Hirshman CA: Anesthesia and bronchospastic disease. *ASA Refresher Courses in Anesthès* 13:81–95, 1985.
18. Marsh MH: Anesthesia for patients with chronic pulmonary disease. *ASA Refresher Courses in Anesthes* 12:133–149, 1984.
19. Nagi SH: Current Concepts in Anesthesiology: Effects of anesthetics on various organs. *N Engl J Med* 302:564–566, 1980.
20. Merin RG: Effects of anesthetic drugs on myocardial performances in man. *Ann Rev Med* 28:75–83, 1977.
21. Moffitt EA, Sethna D: The coronary circulation and myocardial oxygenation in coronary artery disease: Effects of anesthesia. *Anesth Analg* 65:395–410, 1986.
22. Barash PG: Monitoring myocardial oxygen bal-

ance: Physiologic basis and clinical application. *ASA Refresher Courses in Anesthes* 13:21–32, 1985.

23. Rao TLK, Jacobs K, El-Etr AA: Reinfarction following anesthesia in patients with myocardial infarction. *Anesthesiology* 54:499–505, 1983.

24. Goldman L, Caldera DL: Risks of general anesthesia and elective operation in the hypertensive patients. *Anesthesiology* 50:285–292, 1979.

25. Martin DE, Kammerer WS: The hypertensive surgical patient. *Surg Clinics of N A* 63:1017–1033, 1983.

26. Stewart DE, Ikram H, Espiner EA, et al.: Arrhythmogenic potential of diuretic induced hypokalemia in patients with mild hypertension and ischaemic heart disease. *Br Heart J* 50:290–297, 1985.

27. Vitez TS, Soper LE, Wong KC, et al.: Chronic hypokalemia and intraoperative dysrhythmias. *Anesthesiology* 63:130–133, 1985.

28. Stoelting RK: Anesthetic considerations in the patient with liver disease. *Curr Rev Clin Anesth* 1:51–55, 1980.

29. Brohult J: Liver reaction after halothane and diethyl ether anesthesia. *Acta Anesthiol Scand* 11:201–220, 1967.

30. Klar H, Lundstrom J, Mollerberg H, et al.: The isoenzymes pattern of lactic dehydrogenase following halothane anesthesia for cholecystectomy. *Anaesthetist* 23:417–420, 1974.

31. Subcommittee on the National Halothane Study of the Committee on Anesthesia, National Academy of Science: Report: National Halothane Study (1966) possible association between halothane anesthesia and postoperative hepatic necrosis. *JAMA* 197:775–788, 1966.

32. Cousins MJ, Hall PM: Mechanisms and evaluation of hepatotoxicity. *ASA Refresher Courses in Anesthes* 13:43–57, 1985.

33. Eger EI, Smuckler EA, Ferrell LD, et al.: Is enflurane hepatotoxic? *Anesth Analg* 65:21–30, 1986.

34. Priano LL: The effects of anesthesia on renal blood flow and function. *ASA Refresher Courses in Anesthes* 13:143–156, 1985.

35. Bastron RD: Anesthetic considerations for patients with end-stage renal disease. *ASA Refresher Courses in anesthes* 13:33–41, 1985.

36. Reves JG, Fragen RN, Vinik HR, et al.: Midazolam, pharmacology and uses. *Anesthesiology* 62:310–324, 1985.

37. Bailey PL, Stanley TH: Pharmacology of intravenous narcotic anesthetics. In Miller, RD (ed): *Anesthesia,* 2nd ed. New York, Churchill Livingston, 1986, pp 781–782.

38. Michaels I, Serrins M, Shier NQ, et al.: Anesthesia for cardiac surgery in patients receiving monamine oxidase inhibitors. *Anesth Analg* 63:1041–1044, 1984.

39. Dundee JW, McCaughey W: Influence of preexisting drug therapy. In Gray CT, Nunn JF, Vetting JE (eds): *General Anesthesia,* 4th ed. Woburn, Massachusetts, Butterworths, 1979, vol. 2, pp 923–941.

40. Cascorbi HF: Perianesthetic Problems with nonanesthetic drugs. *ASA Refresher Courses in Anesthes* 6:15–30, 1978.

5

Nutritional Assessment and Support

William S. Kammerer and Barbara G. Ford

EPIDEMIOLOGY

The development of effective nutritional support techniques, simplified nutritional assessment tools, and awareness of the impact of protein-calorie malnutrition on morbidity and mortality has increased the attention being paid to the nutritional status of hospitalized patients. Bistrian and colleagues (1, 2) found that approximately 50% of hospitalized medical and surgical patients were moderately to severely malnourished. Butterworth referred to these findings as "the skeleton in the hospital closet" (3).

PATHOPHYSIOLOGY

Simple starvation due to an inability or unwillingness to eat, to malabsorption, or to iatrogenic factors (NPO, clear liquid diets, withholding meals for diagnostic tests) accounts for only a portion of the protein-calorie malnutrition seen in hospitalized patients. The balance results from physiologic responses to infection, trauma, surgery, and catabolic illnesses (COPD, cardiac cachexia, chronic renal disease, cancer, etc.). In most of these conditions, a complex interplay between insulin, glucagon, epinephrine, and glucocorticoids leads to a relative decrease in lipolysis and to an increased mobilization and utilization of somatic and visceral proteins for energy and tissue repair (4). In addition, body requirements for protein to maintain nitrogen balance increase during illness from the normal levels of 0.6–0.8 grams/kg of ideal body weight to 1.5 grams per kilogram. **The metabolic response to injury and acute infection** is characterized by an initial catabolic phase associated with an increase in nitrogen loss and oxygen consumption. It may be impossible to reverse the nitrogen loss during this phase, even with the use of parenteral nutritional support. During the second, or anabolic phase, adequate nutritional support is mandatory and may be "curative" (5–7). If the hypermetabolic process continues for too long without adequate nutritional support, protein-calorie malnutrition will result. This has been happening all too often in the sickest patients. The growing awareness by most physicians of the importance of adequate nutritional support is evidenced by the increased use of this therapy in most hospitals.

The documentation of the **increased morbidity and mortality caused by protein-calorie malnutrition** in hospitalized perioperative patients has motivated physicians to initiate preventive and corrective action. Delayed wound healing, impaired response to therapy, chronic debility and weakness also complicate and extend the patient's recovery, adding to patient suffering, an increase in morbidity and mortality, and prolonged, expensive hospital stays (8).

Impaired immunity and neutrophil function associated with moderate to severe degrees of protein malnutrition often leads to sepsis and infection (8). McClean and colleagues have convincingly correlated skin anergy with postoperative sepsis and increased mortality. They have also demonstrated that neutrophils from anergic patients or normal neutrophils incubated with serum from anergic patients show a marked inhibition of chemotaxis, explaining in part the increased susceptibility of malnourished patients to infection (9). Deficiencies (iron, zinc, vitamins A, B_{12}, pyridoxine, and folate) and excesses (essential fatty acids, vitamin E) of single nutrients, are also associated with abnormalities in immunologic function (10).

NUTRITIONAL ASSESSMENT

It is not unusual for all but the most obviously malnourished patients to be characterized as "well-nourished." Admission weights and heights are often omitted. Until recently, most physicians had little idea of how to assess nutritional status other than the height/weight ratio, one of the least sensitive measures of adequate protein nutrition in hospitalized adults.

A complete nutritional assessment includes four areas 1) anthropometric, 2) biochemical (laboratory), 3) clinical, and 4) dietary history. The assessment in each of these areas may vary in specificity and sensitivity depending on the patient. An effective assessment tool is provided in Table 5.1.

Table 5.1. Nutritional Assessment

A. Anthropometric:
  1. Height (cm) _____
  2. Current body weight (kg) _____
  3. Ideal body weight (kg) _____
    Use Metropolitan Height and Weight Tables
  4. % Ideal body weight _____

$$\% \text{ Ideal body weight} = \frac{\text{Current weight}}{\text{Ideal Weight}} \times 100$$

  5. % Weight loss _____
    % Weight loss =

$$\frac{\text{Usual weight} - \text{Current weight}}{\text{Current weight}} \times 100$$

  6. Triceps Skinfold (TSF) _____ mm
  7. Mid-arm circumference (MAC) _____ cm
  8. Arm muscle circumference (AMC) _____
    AMC = MAC (cm) − (TSF (mm) × 0.314)

Normal Values:	Males	Females
MAMC	25–27	21–23
TSF	12.5	16.5

B. Biochemical
  1. Serum albumin _____ gm/100 ml
    (normal =   3.5–5.0 gm/100 ml)

mild	2.8–3.4 gm/100 ml
moderate	2.1–2.7 gm/100 ml
severe	<2.1 gm/100 ml

  2. Serum transferrin _____ mg/100 ml

normal	250–300 mg/100 ml
mild	150–250 mg/100 ml
moderate	100–150 mg/100 ml
severe	<100 mg/100 ml

  3. Total lymphocyte count _____ mm3

normal	2500 mm3
mild	1200–2000 mm3
moderate	800–1199 mm3
severe	<800 mm3

  4. Creatinine Height Index (CHI)

$$\text{CHI} = \frac{\text{actual urine creatinine}}{\text{ideal urine creatinine}} \times 100$$
    (for patient's height)

  5. Nitrogen Balance

$$\text{Nitrogen balance} = \frac{\text{protein intake}}{6.25} - (\text{UUN} + 4)$$

  6. Delayed reactivity skin tests.

C. Clinical
  1. Physical examination of patient
  2. Medical history
  3. Social history

D. Dietary
  1. Diet history/24-hour recall
  2. Daily calorie count
  3. Assessment of Energy Needs
    Basal Energy Expenditure (Harris-Benedict)
      males: 66.5 + 13.8 (wt) + 5.0 (ht) − 6.8 (age)
      females: 655.1 + 9.6 (wt) + 1.8 (ht) − 4.7 (age)
  Activity Factor

factor	% basal calories to be added
bedrest	5–10%
ambulatory	5–20%
elevated temp	13% for each degree above normal (C)
infection, stress trauma	20%
sepsis	40%
respirator	50%
major burns	50–125%
weight gain	500–1000 additional calories per day

OR

status	Kcal/kg/IBW (33)
basal energy needs	25–30
ambulatory with wt maintenance	30–35
malnutrition with mild stress	40
severe injuries and sepsis	50–60
extensive burns	80

Anthropometric

The triceps skinfold is an indirect estimate of body fat (caloric stores). Mid-arm muscle circumference, creatinine/height index, nitrogen balance studies, cellular immunity (as measured by delayed skin hypersensitivity testing), total lymphocyte count, serum albumin, and serum transferrin levels all reflect protein nutrition. Values less than 70% of normal, along with skin test anergy, reflect severe protein malnutrition and are predictive of increased morbidity and mortality. Caloric deficiency alone is less directly associated with poor outcome.

When performing anthropometric measurements it is important to utilize a standardized procedure in order for the measurements to be reliable indicators (Fig 5.1A and B). The triceps skinfold measurement appears to be a relatively simple procedure, but best results are obtained when a trained person performs the measurement using calibrated calipers. It is also helpful if the same individual performs serial/sequential measurements using the same technique to ensure accuracy.

Other sites, such as the subscapular or supra-iliac, may be measured to assess nutritional status, but the standards for these areas are not well established.

Arm muscle circumference (AMC) is an accepted index of body protein stores. The arm muscle area (AMA) can also be estimated. Both measures may be depressed in protein malnutrition. Arm muscle area is a better indicator of change than arm muscle circumference.

The AMC and MAMC can be estimated from measures of arm circumference and triceps skinfold (TSF) (Tables 5.2 and 5.3).

Interpretation of these measurements may be accomplished by comparing them to published standards (Table 5.4). Anthropometric measurements should always be tempered with clinical judgement. They should serve to augment the total clinical picture. Serial measurements are useful as indicators of the effectiveness of nutritional intervention.

Figure 5.1A.   Measurement of Triceps Skinfold with Calipers

	Standard	90% Standard	80% Standard	70% Standard	60% Standard
Male	12.5 mm	11.3 mm	10.0 mm	8.8 mm	7.5 mm
Female	16.5 mm	14.9 mm	13.2 mm	11.6 mm	9.9 mm

Figure 5.1B.   Measurement of Mid-upper Arm Circumference

	Standard	90% Standard	80% Standard	70% Standard	60% Standard
Male	29.3 cm	26.3 cm	23.4 cm	20.5 cm	17.6 cm
Female	28.5 cm	25.7 cm	22.8 cm	20.0 cm	17.1 cm

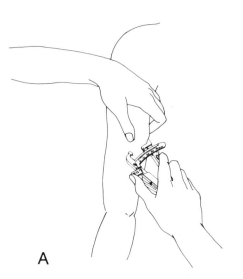

A

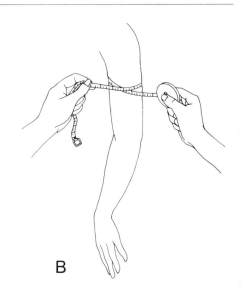

B

Table 5.2. Triceps Skinfold Norms

Age	Triceps Skinfold Percentiles (mm) for Males						
	5th	10th	25th	50th	75th	90th	95th
1–2	6	7	8	10	12	14	16
2–3	6	7	8	10	12	14	15
3–4	6	7	8	10	11	14	15
4–5	6	7	8	10	11	14	15
5–6	6	6	8	9	11	12	14
6–7	6	6	8	9	11	14	15
7–8	5	6	7	8	10	13	16
8–9	5	6	7	9	12	15	17
9–10	5	6	7	8	10	13	16
10–11	6	6	7	10	13	17	18
11–12	6	6	8	10	14	18	21
12–13	6	6	8	11	16	20	24
13–14	6	6	8	11	14	22	28
14–15	5	5	7	10	14	22	26
15–16	4	5	7	9	14	21	24
16–17	4	5	6	8	11	18	24
17–18	4	5	6	8	12	16	22
18–19	5	5	6	8	12	16	19
19–25	4	5	6	9	13	20	24
25–35	4	5	7	10	15	20	22
35–45	5	6	8	12	16	20	24
45–55	5	6	8	12	16	20	23
55–65	6	6	8	12	15	20	25
65–75	5	6	8	11	14	19	22
75–80	4	6	8	11	15	19	22

Age	Triceps Skinfold Percentiles (mm) for Females						
	5th	10th	25th	50th	75th	90th	95th
1–2	6	7	8	10	12	14	16
2–3	6	8	9	10	12	15	16
3–4	7	8	9	11	12	14	15
4–5	7	8	8	10	12	14	16
5–6	6	7	8	10	12	15	18
6–7	6	6	8	10	12	14	16
7–8	6	7	9	11	13	16	18
8–9	6	8	9	12	15	18	24
9–10	8	8	10	13	16	20	22
10–11	7	8	10	12	17	23	27
11–12	7	8	10	13	18	24	28
12–13	8	9	11	14	18	23	27
13–14	8	8	12	15	21	26	30
14–15	9	10	13	16	21	26	28
15–16	8	10	12	17	21	25	32
16–17	10	12	15	18	22	26	31
17–18	10	12	13	19	24	30	37
18–19	10	12	15	18	22	26	30
19–25	10	11	14	18	24	30	34
25–35	10	12	16	21	27	34	37
35–45	12	14	18	23	29	35	38
45–55	12	16	20	25	30	36	40
55–65	12	16	20	25	31	36	38
65–75	12	14	18	24	29	34	36

Adapted from: Frisancho, A. R. New norms of upper limb fat and muscle areas for assessment of nutritional status. *Am J Clin Nutr* 34:2540, 1981.

Table 5.3. Determination of Arm Muscle Area

$$\text{Arm Muscle Area (mm)} = \frac{(c - T)}{4} \cdot 3.14$$

T = triceps skinfold (mm)
c = arm circumference (mm)

Biochemical

Biochemical assessment of nutritional status may be accomplished using many routine laboratory tests. Serum albumin is an index of protein status, creatinine excretion is used to evaluate muscle mass, and serum transferrin reflects changes in visceral protein production. All laboratory results are best used in association with anthropometric measures and other supportive information, such as diet history and clinical signs. Many very elaborate, and often expensive, tests for vitamin and mineral status are available. Decisions regarding the treatment course and the cost/benefit ratio of these tests should be made before ordering multiple biochemical tests.

Clinical

Clinical examination is the most subjective and nonspecific part of a complete nutritional assessment. Many of the signs observed may result from nutrient deficiency or other non-nutritional causes. Any positive findings should be investigated further and confirmed with other measures of nutritional assessment. Color and condition of the skin, eyes, nails, and hair should be observed as well as the function of the musculoskeletal, cardiovascular, and gastrointestinal systems.

Clinical symptoms are best evaluated as part of an individual nutrient deficiency. The patient who has atrophic papillae, tongue fissures, and edema of the tongue is more likely to have niacin deficiency than a patient with only one of these conditions present. Confirmation of this assumption should be made using laboratory tests and diet history.

Dietary

Dietary information may be obtained by diet history and a food frequency checklist. A twenty-four hour recall of food intake is not appropriate for chronically malnourished patients unless it is felt to reflect long-term eating habits. A registered dietitian is able to obtain this information during a short patient interview and can present it to the physician to confirm other components of the nutritional assessment.

The nutritional assessment may be used to accurately predict an increase in the morbidity and mortality due to protein malnutrition in hospitalized patients. Many attempts to combine various factors into an equation to predict postoperative morbidity and mortality have been reported (11). The **Prognostic Nutritional Index** (PNI) developed by Mullen (Table 5.5) is widely used in surgical populations. As expected, multiple abnormal results are usually more sensitive than a single abnormal test and can be useful in highlighting clinically unrecognized malnutrition. Additionally, they can be used as indicators of the effectiveness of appropriate therapy and nutritional support.

DETERMINATION OF NUTRITIONAL NEEDS

All patients should be evaluated for nutritional risk within 48 hours of admission to the hospital. The initial screening process should include height, weight, weight patterns, appropriate laboratory data, medical history, and current illness. A physical exam, current diet order, chronic medications, and past weight history are also important. An interview with the patient regarding past diet modifications and practices, supplement use, and food allergies or intolerances can yield important information as well. Those at high risk of malnutrition should be further assessed. (Table 5.6).

A determination of calorie and protein needs must be made for patients requiring nutritional support.

Table 5.4 Arm Muscle Circumference and Area Norms (continued)

ARM MUSCLE AREA PERCENTILES (mm²), MALES

Age	5th	10th	25th	50th	75th	90th	95th
1–2	95.6	101.4	113.3	127.8	144.7	164.4	172.0
2–3	97.3	104.0	119.0	134.5	155.7	169.0	178.7
3–4	109.5	120.1	135.7	148.4	161.8	175.0	185.3
4–5	120.7	126.4	140.8	157.9	174.7	192.6	200.8
5–6	129.8	141.1	155.0	172.0	188.4	208.9	228.5
6–7	136.0	144.7	160.5	181.5	205.6	229.7	249.3
7–8	149.7	154.8	180.8	202.7	224.6	249.4	288.6
8–9	155.0	166.4	189.5	208.9	229.6	262.8	278.8
9–10	181.1	188.4	206.7	228.8	265.7	305.3	325.7
10–11	193.0	202.7	218.2	257.5	290.3	348.6	388.2
11–12	201.6	215.6	238.2	267.0	302.2	335.9	422.6
12–13	221.6	233.9	264.9	302.2	349.6	396.8	464.0
13–14	236.3	254.6	304.4	355.3	408.1	450.2	479.4
14–15	283.0	314.7	358.6	396.3	457.5	536.8	553.0
15–16	313.8	331.7	378.8	448.1	513.4	563.1	590.0
16–17	362.5	404.4	435.2	495.1	575.3	657.6	698.0
17–18	399.8	425.2	477.7	528.6	595.0	688.6	772.6
18–19	407.0	448.1	506.6	555.2	637.4	706.7	835.5
19–25	450.8	477.7	527.4	591.3	666.0	760.6	820.0
25–35	469.4	496.3	554.1	621.4	706.7	784.7	843.6
35–45	484.4	518.1	574.0	649.0	726.5	803.4	848.8
45–55	454.6	494.6	558.9	629.7	714.2	791.8	845.8
55–65	442.2	478.3	538.1	614.4	691.9	767.0	814.9
65–75	397.3	441.1	503.1	571.6	643.2	707.4	745.3

ARM MUSCLE AREA PERCENTILES (mm²), FEMALES

Age	5th	10th	25th	50th	75th	90th	95th
1–2	88.5	97.3	108.4	122.1	137.8	153.5	162.1
2–3	97.3	102.9	111.9	126.9	140.5	159.5	172.7
3–4	101.4	113.3	122.7	139.6	156.3	169.0	184.6
4–5	105.8	117.1	131.3	147.5	164.4	183.2	195.8
5–6	123.8	130.1	142.3	159.8	182.5	201.2	215.9
6–7	135.4	141.4	151.3	168.3	187.7	218.2	232.3
7–8	133.0	144.1	160.2	181.5	204.5	233.2	246.9
8–9	151.3	156.6	180.8	203.4	232.7	265.7	299.6
9–10	172.3	178.8	197.6	222.7	257.1	298.7	311.2
10–11	174.0	178.4	201.9	229.6	258.3	287.3	309.3
11–12	178.4	198.7	231.6	261.2	307.1	373.9	395.3
12–13	209.2	218.2	257.9	290.4	322.5	365.5	384.7
13–14	226.9	242.6	265.7	313.0	352.9	408.1	456.8
14–15	241.8	256.2	287.4	322.0	370.4	429.4	485.0
15–16	242.6	251.8	284.7	324.8	368.9	412.3	475.6
16–17	230.8	256.7	286.5	324.8	371.8	435.3	494.6
17–18	244.2	267.4	299.6	333.6	388.3	455.2	525.1
18–19	239.8	253.8	291.7	324.3	369.4	446.1	476.7
19–25	253.8	272.8	302.6	340.6	387.7	443.9	494.0
25–35	266.1	282.6	314.8	357.3	413.8	480.6	554.1
35–45	275.0	294.8	335.9	378.3	442.8	524.0	587.7
44–55	278.4	295.6	337.8	385.8	452.0	537.5	596.4
55–65	278.4	306.3	347.7	404.5	475.0	563.2	624.7
65–75	273.7	301.8	344.4	401.9	473.9	556.6	621.4

Table 5.4. Arm Muscle Circumference and Area Norms (continued)

ARM MUSCLE CIRCUMFERENCE PERCENTILES (mm), MALES								ARM MUSCLE CIRCUMFERENCE PERCENTILES (mm), FEMALES						
Age	5th	10th	25th	50th	75th	90th	95th	Age	5th	10th	25th	50th	75th	90th	95th
1–2	11.0	11.3	11.9	12.7	13.5	14.4	14.7	1–2	10.5	11.1	11.7	12.4	13.2	13.9	14.3
2–3	11.1	11.4	12.2	13.0	14.0	14.6	15.0	2–3	11.1	11.4	11.9	12.6	13.3	14.2	14.7
3–4	11.7	12.3	13.1	13.7	14.3	14.8	15.3	3–4	11.3	11.9	12.4	13.2	14.0	14.6	15.2
4–5	12.3	12.6	13.3	14.1	14.8	15.6	15.9	4–5	11.5	12.1	12.8	13.6	14.4	15.2	15.7
5–6	12.8	13.3	14.0	14.7	15.4	16.2	16.9	5–6	12.5	12.8	13.4	14.2	15.1	15.9	16.5
6–7	13.1	13.5	14.2	15.1	16.1	17.0	17.7	6–7	13.0	13.3	13.8	14.5	15.4	16.6	17.1
7–8	13.7	13.9	15.1	16.0	16.8	17.7	19.0	7–8	12.9	13.5	14.2	15.1	16.0	17.1	17.6
8–9	14.0	14.5	15.4	16.2	17.0	18.2	18.7	8–9	13.8	14.0	15.1	16.0	17.1	18.3	19.4
9–10	15.1	15.4	16.1	17.0	18.3	19.6	20.2	9–10	14.7	15.0	15.8	16.7	18.0	19.4	19.8
10–11	15.6	16.0	16.6	18.0	19.1	20.9	22.1	10–11	14.8	15.0	15.9	17.0	18.0	19.0	19.7
11–12	15.9	16.5	17.3	18.3	19.5	20.5	23.0	11–12	15.0	15.8	17.1	18.1	19.6	21.7	22.3
12–13	16.7	17.1	18.2	19.5	21.0	22.3	24.1	12–13	16.2	16.6	18.0	19.1	20.1	21.4	22.0
13–14	17.2	17.9	19.6	21.1	22.6	23.8	24.5	13–14	16.9	17.5	18.3	19.8	21.1	22.6	24.0
14–15	18.9	19.9	21.2	22.3	24.0	26.0	26.4	14–15	17.4	17.9	19.0	20.1	21.6	23.2	24.7
15–16	19.9	20.4	21.8	23.7	25.4	26.6	27.2	15–16	17.5	17.8	18.9	20.2	21.5	22.8	24.4
16–17	21.3	22.5	23.4	24.9	26.9	28.7	29.6	16–17	17.0	18.0	19.0	20.2	21.6	23.4	24.9
17–18	22.4	23.1	24.5	25.8	27.3	29.4	31.2	17–18	17.5	18.3	19.4	20.5	22.1	23.9	25.7
18–19	22.6	23.7	25.2	26.4	28.3	29.8	32.4	18–19	17.4	17.9	19.1	20.2	21.5	23.7	24.5
19–25	23.8	24.5	25.7	27.3	28.9	30.9	32.1	19–25	17.9	18.5	19.5	20.7	22.1	23.6	24.9
25–35	24.3	25.0	26.4	27.9	29.8	31.4	32.6	25–35	18.3	18.8	19.9	21.2	22.8	24.6	26.4
35–45	24.7	25.5	26.9	28.6	30.2	31.8	32.7	35–45	18.6	19.2	20.5	21.8	23.6	25.7	27.2
45–55	23.9	24.9	26.5	28.1	30.0	31.5	32.6	45–55	18.7	19.3	20.6	22.0	23.8	26.0	27.4
55–65	23.6	24.5	26.0	27.8	29.5	31.0	32.0	55–65	18.7	19.6	20.9	22.5	24.4	26.6	28.0
65–75	22.3	23.5	25.1	26.8	28.4	29.8	30.6	65–75	18.5	19.5	20.8	22.5	24.4	26.4	27.9

Adapted from: Frisancho, A. R. New norms of upper limb fat and muscle areas for assessment of nutritional status. *Amer J Clin Nutri* 34, 2540, 1981.

Table 5.5. Prognostic Nutritional Index

PNI = 158% − 16.6 (Alb) − .78 (TSF) − .2
    (Transferrin) − 5.8(DH)

Alb = Albumin gm/dl
TSF = Triceps skinfold mm
Transferrin = gm/dl
DH = 0 nonreactive
      1 <5 mm
      2 >5 mm

>50%   High Risk
40–49%   Intermediate Risk
<40%   Low Risk

Caloric Needs

Patients may have normal, elevated, or depressed energy needs during their hospitalization. A starved patient, who has adapted to a decreased food intake, will have a depressed basal metabolic rate (BMR), while a patient who has experienced trauma will have an increased BMR.

Caloric needs are dependent on the BMR, as well as on age, prior nutritional

Table 5.6. The High-Risk Patient

Gross Underweight: Weight-for-height below 80% of standard.
Gross Overweight: Weight-for-height above 120% of standard. (Due to the tendency to overlook protein and calorie requirements in the acutely ill obese patient.
Recent loss of 10% or more of usual body weight
Alcoholism
No oral intake (NPO) for over 10 days on simple intravenous solutions.
Protracted nutrient losses.
    Malabsorption syndrome
    Short-gut syndromes/fistulas
    Renal dialysis
    Draining abscesses, wounds
Increased metabolic needs
    Extensive burns, infection, traumas
    Protracted fever
Intake of drugs with antinutrient or catabolic properties: steroids, immunosuppressants, antitumor agents.

From Goodhart R, and Shills M. *Modern Nutrition in Health and Disease.* Table 22.2, p. 669, Lea and Febriger, Philadelphia, 1973. (34)

status, presence of trauma or infection, and type of nutritional support.

Several methods for determination of caloric needs are widely used. The Harris-Benedict equation is among the most accurate for calculating basal energy requirements taking age, weight, height, and sex into consideration. This formula is included in Table 5.1 Additional calories are added to the basal energy needs based on the presence of additional factors.

Protein Needs

Protein needs are influenced by metabolic rate, caloric intake, nutritional status, age, and body protein reserves. The goal of positive nitrogen balance can be achieved in the normal patient when 7–8% of the required calories are provided as protein. The hypermetabolic patient requires 16–20% of calories as protein to achieve the same goal. If inadequate protein and calories are provided, death may occur from loss of lean body mass as body protein is catabolized to meet the increased energy demands of the stressed patient. For a normal, nonstressed patient, protein requirements of 0.8–1.0 gm/kg/day are adequate. For a moderately stressed patient, the requirements are increased to 1.0–2.0 gm/kg/day and the severely stressed patient requires 2.0–3.0 gm/kg/day to prevent loss of body protein stores. Measurements of prealbumin can aid in determining whether or not the patient is receiving adequate amounts of protein and calories.

A simple method for approximating the severity of catabolic response to injury and illness and the rate of lean tissue catabolism has been proposed by Bistrian (12). The **Catabolic Index** [CI = 24-hour urine urea nitrogen (UUN) − (0.5 × dietary nitrogen + 3)]. Values of less than zero indicate no stress; 0–5, moderate catabolic stress; and above 5, severe catabolic stress. A consistent elevation of the CI indicates inadequate replacement of protein and/or calories and the need for increased nutritional support.

Adequate calories must be provided in order for protein to be used for tissue synthesis. A ratio of 1:150 of grams of nitrogen to total calories is recommended.

Records of food intake during hospitalization will help the physician to determine the adequacy of the diet in preventing catabolism and promoting anabolism. Calorie, protein, and vitamin and mineral intake can be easily calculated and compared with standards to determine dietary adequacy.

Weight change during hospitalization may also serve as a means for monitoring dietary adequacy. Initial weight gain is usually due to water retention, followed by a period of weight maintenance as excess water is diuresed and protein and fat stores are replenished. Weight gain in the third period is usually rapid as protein synthesis occurs. Gain in muscle mass is limited to approximately 250 grams/day. Weight gains greater than this amount are probably due to fluid retention and fat deposition.

Weight loss may be due to inadequate intake, increased basal expenditure or both. Weight loss is more rapid, up to 500 grams per day, after surgery, following serious infection, or with major injury. Losses greater than 500 grams per day indicate loss of lean body mass. **The greater the weight loss, the greater the morbidity and mortality.** The rate of weight loss, as well as the percentage weight loss are important factors in nutritional assessment.

NUTRITIONAL THERAPY

Adequate calories, protein, vitamins, and minerals must be supplied to the patient who is unable or unwilling to consume enough solid food. Such patients may be supported by supplemental oral feedings, feeding tubes, peripheral alimentation, or central venous hyperalimentation (total parenteral nutrition).

SELECTING A FORMULA

There are a wide variety of enteral formulas available to meet the nutritional needs of virtually all patients. These formulas vary in many ways, some subtle, others significant.

The carbohydrate (CHO) may be present as glucose, maltodextrins, or lactose. The source of CHO affects the osmolarity. Generally 50% of the calories are provided by CHO.

The protein may be present as an intact protein from food (i.e., milk), as a protein hydrolysate, or as free amino acids. Nine to twenty-four percent of the calories are provided by protein. Formulas with intact protein taste much better than those with partially hydrolyzed or free amino acids.

Butterfat (long-chain fat) or coconut oil (medium chain) provides the fat. Forty percent of calories come from fat. Fat serves to slow gastric emptying as well as provide calories.

Vitamins and minerals are generally added to these formulas to meet the Recommended Dietary Allowance if appropriate amounts of the formula are consumed.

In choosing a formula several things must be considered, including the patient's medical and nutritional status. The status of the digestive system, absorptive capacity, renal function, electrolyte balance, and route of administration must be taken into account. Palatability and acceptability are important if the formula is to be consumed orally.

Lactose content, osmolarity, viscosity, nitrogen:calorie ratio, nutritional adequacy, ease of administration, and patient tolerance must also be considered in selecting a formula. A simplified chart including various types of formulas follows in Table 5.7.

Blenderized formulas are a mixture of foods that have added carbohydrates, oils, vitamins, and minerals. They have a moderate lactose content, high viscosity, and an osmolarity of 500–800 mOsm/L.

Table 5.7. Nutrient Content Mayo Medical Center Enteral Nutrition Formulary

Formula	Kcal/ml	Non protein Kcal:gN	Osmolality mOsm	Moisture %	Volume for 100% RDA Vits(ml)	Nutrients per 1,000 ml				Nutrient Sources		
						Protein g	Total Fat (MCT fat) g	CHO g	Na/K mEq	Protein	Fat	Carbohydrate
Malabsorption and maldigestion												
Ensure Plus (Ross Laboratories)	1.5	146:1	600	76	1,600	55	53 (0)	200	50/55	Sodium & calcium caseinates, soy protein isolates	Corn oil	Corn syrup sucrose
Ensure (Ross Laboratories)	1.06	153:1	450	83	1,887	37	37 (0)	145	37/40	Sodium & calcium caseinates, soy protein isolates	Corn oil	Corn syrup sucrose
Osmolite (Ross Laboratories)	1.06	153:1	300	83	1,887	37	39 (17)	145	28/26	Sodium & calcium caseinates, soy protein isolates	MCT oil, corn oil, soy oil	Hydrolyzed corn starch
Travasorb MCT (Travenol Laboratories)	1.0 or	102:1	312	75	2,000	49	33 (26)	123	15/45	Lactalbumin, potassium caseinate	MCT oil, sunflower oil	Cornsyrup solids
	2.0	102:1	590	42	1,000	98	66 (53)	246	30/90			
Vital High Nitrogen (Ross Laboratories)	1.0	125:1	460	85	1,500	42	11 (5)	185	20/34	Whey, soy, & meat protein hydrolysates, free essential amino acids	Safflower oil, MCT oil	Hydrolyzed corn starch, sucrose
Special Formulas												
Hepatic Aid II (Kendall McGaw)	1.1	148:1	560	78	0	44	36 (0)	169	<15/<6	Crystalline amino acids (high branch-chain, low aromatic amino acids)	Soybean oil, lecithin, mono & diglycerides	Maltodextrin, sucrose

47

Table 5.7. Nutrient Content Mayo Medical Center Enteral Nutrition Formulary (*continued*)

Formula	Kcal/ml	Non protein Kcal:gN	Osmolality mOsm	Moisture %	Volume for 100% RDA Vits(ml)	Protein g	Total Fat (MCT fat) g	CHO g	Na/K mEq	Nutrient Sources Protein	Nutrient Sources Fat	Nutrient Sources Carbohydrate
Amin-Aid (Kendall McGaw)	2.0	830:1	1,095	87	0	19	46 (0)	366	<15/<6	Crystalline essential amino acids including histidine	Soybean oil, lecithin, mono & diglycerides	Maltodextrin, sucrose
Supplement Polycose (Ross Laboratories)	2.0 (3.8/g)	NA	850	NA	0	0	0	500	25/5	NA	NA	Hydrolysis of corn starch
MCT Oil (Mead Johnson Pharmaceutical)	7.7 (8.3/g)	NA	0	NA	0	0	927 (927)	0	0	NA	Fractionated coconut oil	NA
Citrotein (Sandoz Pharmaceutical)	0.66	76:1	494–515	93	1,350	41	2 (0)	122	31/18	Egg albumin	Soy oil	Sucrose, maltodextrin

NA = not applicable

From: Pemberton, C.: *Specialized Nutritional Support*, Mayo Clinic Diet Manual, p 264, Rochester, Minnesota, Mayo Foundation Publication Dept., 1988. By permission of Mayo Foundation.

This type of formula requires that digestive and absorptive function be intact. They are inexpensive and may be prepared at home or purchased commercially.

Milk-based products contain milk solids, egg albumin, caseinates, added carbohydrates, and vegetable oils. These are often used as oral supplements because of their relatively pleasant taste. The protein and lactose content is high, and they require intact digestion and absorptive function. Osmolarity is 500–700 mOsm/L.

A **lactose-free formula** is ideal for general tube feeding. It contains a mixture of protein isolates, oligosaccharides, medium chain trigylcerides, oil, vitamins, and minerals. The osmolarity, 300–400 mOsm/liter, and viscosity is low. Intact digestion and absorption is needed. These formulas are best tolerated intragastrically.

Defined formulas, or "elemental" diets, are designed for patients with short bowel or malabsorption syndrome. Proteins are provided as amino acids and/or peptides; a small amount of fat is provided as medium chain trigylcerides, and carbohydrate is present as glucose oligosaccharides. The viscosity is low but the osmolarity is high, 500–1000 mOsm/L. These formulas should be started at half-strength, and at a slow speed with close monitoring for patient tolerance. They are best given intragastrically.

Most of the defined formula diets are not tolerated for long periods of time due to their bad taste and smell and must be given by feeding tube. They must be administered slowly as their hypertonicity and hyperosmolarity predispose to gastric distention and diarrhea. Nonketotic hyperosmolar coma has been reported because of their high carbohydrate content.

Modular feedings are single nutrients supplemented with vitamins and minerals. They may be combined to produce a nutritionally complete formula or used to enhance an existing formula. They should only be used if an appropriate complete formula is not available. They are very expensive and their benefit over other formulas is low.

Special formulas are available for specific organ dysfunction. Renal formulas provide mainly essential amino acids and little of the nonessential ones. They are low in minerals and some vitamins. They are not nutritionally complete and the osmolarity is high. Hepatic formulas contain higher amounts of branched chain amino acids and fewer aromatic amino acids. They are also nutritionally incomplete and hyperosmolar.

FEEDING TECHNIQUES

For patients who are unable to eat but with normal gastrointestinal tracts, these formulas can be given by a small bore feeding tube. Nasogastric feeding may be used in alert patients who are going to resume oral intake. The gastric function must be normal in order for the formula to be administered. Usually, iso-osmolar formulas can be given full strength and at a significant volume to provide an adequate amount of calories and protein.

Nasoduodenal feeding may be used to decrease the risk of aspiration. The osmolarity should be low (400 mOsm/kg) if the feeding is to be given full strength.

For patients who will require long-term feeding, a **gastrostomy or jejunostomy feeding tube** may be preferred. Gastrostomy feeding is dependent on the patient's gastrointestinal function and the osmolarity of the formula. A jejunostomy is used when there is a proximal obstruction or total gastrectomy.

The most commonly encountered difficulty with these formulas and feeding methods is the development of diarrhea. This generally develops from administration of hyperosmolar preparations (>450 mOsm/kg) too rapidly. Most physicians find that by diluting the formula to ¼ strength and giving only ½ the final estimated volume during the first 2–3 days, and then increasing first strength, and then volume until full strength and desired volume are achieved, the gastrointestinal tract has time to adapt without the complication of diarrhea. If a patient is unable to tolerate this "go slow" approach, several iso-osmolar formulas are available (Isocal, Osmolite). For patients with lactose intolerance, a formula without this element should obviously be chosen.

Aspiration can be reduced by elevating the head of the bed, using pump infusion therapy, avoiding bolus feeding, and positioning the feeding tube in the duodenum.

PERIPHERAL ALIMENTATION

For patients who are moderately stressed and who are reasonably well nourished but who cannot eat, there are two peripheral alimentation techniques: **protein sparing and peripheral parenteral nutrition (PPN).** For those who will be able to resume adequate oral nutrition within 7–10 days, the use of 3% crystalline amino acids (30 grams of amino acid/liter) calculated to deliver approximately 90 grams of amino acid per 70 kg of ideal body weight per day, with or without 100 grams of glucose per day (protein sparing) will significantly improve nitrogen balance compared to using dextrose alone (13). In those who are marginally compensated nutritionally or in whom complications might occur that would significantly delay the return to an adequate oral intake, the added expense of this approach would be justified to delay the onset of significant protein malnutrition with its deleterious effects on wound healing, immunity, and predisposition to infection.

Partial parenteral nutrition (PPN) will supply more calories and amino acids than "protein-sparing" solutions and is appropriate for patients who are more stressed and will need nutritional support for longer than 7–10 days. When combined with even limited oral intake, amounts of protein and calories comparable to total parenteral nutrition can often be achieved. Two thousand to 2500 kilocalories can be pro-

vided using peripheral veins when fat emulsions are used.

The goal of peripheral alimentation is to meet energy needs, maintain positive nitrogen balance, assure electrolyte, vitamin and mineral status, provide fluids, and prevent essential fatty acid deficiency.

Solutions for peripheral feeding contain dextrose, amino acids, fats, vitamins, and minerals. Intravenous fat, to provide 40–50% of the calories, is given simultaneously and the flow rate adjusted so the fat infuses for the same length of time as the amino acids and dextrose. Flow rates of up to 125 cc per hour may be achieved. One liter of 10% dextrose, 1 liter of 7% amino acids, and 1 liter of 10% fat will provide about 2000 kilocalories and 70 grams of protein. Osmolarity is 500–900 mOsm/liter. Two hundred international units (IU) of heparin and 5 mg of cortisol should be added to each liter of amino acid and dextrose solution if fat emulsion is not run simultaneously.

TOTAL PARENTERAL NUTRITION

Total parenteral nutrition (TPN) is appropriate for patients who are malnourished, who are significantly stressed (catabolic index > 5: major trauma, septic, burned, etc., requiring 3000–4000 kilocalories per day), who will be unable to eat for prolonged periods, and who need to be urgently replenished. If oral feedings and peripheral alimentation are inadequate, TPN offers the most effective way to meet increased nutritional needs.

Solutions

The formulation of parenteral solutions is highly individualized. Their composition is dependent upon the calorie, protein, fluid, vitamin, and mineral needs of the patient. Solutions may be tailored to meet specific needs of the patients. Dudrick believes "It is essential for the physician to recognize that no single intravenous nutrient solution can be ideal for all conditions and all patients at all times, or for the same patients during various phases of his pathologic process" (14).

Protein solutions must meet the requirements for essential amino acids as well as total nitrogen needs. Commercial mixtures of amino acids, containing both essential and nonessential, are available in concentrations from 3–10%.

Amino acid solutions are preferred over protein hydrolysates because the protein utilization of the hydrolysates is uncertain. Up to 50% may be excreted in the urine because the hydrolysis of the protein is incomplete. The ammonia content of the hydrolysates is higher than with amino acids and the risk of hyperammonemia is greater, especially in infants.

Amino acid solutions are mixed with dextrose to produce equal volumes of amino acids and dextrose.

Protein needs for each patient should be calculated individually. A ratio of 1.0 to 1.5 grams of protein per kilogram ideal body weight per day, with a usual nitrogen to calorie ratio of 1:120 should be achieved. A ratio of 1:200 for the patient with cardiac cachexia is preferred (15).

Carbohydrate is provided as dextrose in concentrations of 5–70%. Concentrations up to 10% may be administered peripherally, but more concentrated solutions are given through a central vein.

Glucose metabolism in hypermetabolic patients may reach 1.2 grams/kilogram/hour (normal: 0.5 grams/kg/hour). The infusion of hypertonic dextrose increases insulin demand. If the pancreas is unable to produce adequate insulin, blood glucose levels may be elevated. When the renal threshold for glucose is exceeded, osmotic diuresis occurs producing glycosuria, water depletion and potential electrolyte imbalance.

Starvation, stress, trauma, infection, and shock all decrease the pancreatic response to a glucose load. This decrease in insulin production is also accompanied by insulin resistance as a result of the high circulating levels of catecholamines and glucocorticoids that are released in response to stress. Insulin should be added to the TPN solution according to serum glucose levels.

Carbon dioxide production and oxygen consumption may be increased by high carbohydrate diets leading to hypercapnia in patients with severe COPD. Using fat to replace part of the carbohydrate calories may decrease carbon dioxide production by lowering the respiratory quotient. Providing 40–60% of the daily calories as fat in the final solution will decrease this risk.

Fat is necessary to prevent or treat essential fatty acid deficiency and to provide a concentrated source of calories. Three to 4% of the total calories should be provided as linoleic acid to prevent EFAD. Total fat should not exceed 4 gm/kg/day.

Two fat solutions are currently available. One is an emulsion of soybean oil, phospholipids and glycerol (Intralipid), and the other is an emulsion of safflower oil, egg phosphatides, and glycerol (Liposyn). They are available in 10 or 20% solutions yielding 1.1 or 2.0 kilocalories per milliliter. Because they are isotonic, they may be given through either a central or a peripheral line. Fats may also lower the osmolarity of parenteral solutions given at the same time. Infusing lipid along with carbohydrate and protein improves its utilization (16).

Utilization of lipid emulsions is also dependent upon carbohydrate metabolism. If adequate carbohydrate is not provided simultaneously, fat utilization will be diminished and hyperlipidemia will occur. No more than 60% of total calories should be provided as fat.

The particles of fat in these solutions are metabolized and utilized the same way as chylomicrons, at a rate of 3–4 grams/kg/24 hours. As the serum concentration increases with the infusion, the rate of fat metabolism slows. If the infusion rate exceeds the metabolic capacity, symptoms of hyperlipidemia, gastrointestinal disturbances, impaired hepatic function, and prolonged clotting time may occur.

Vitamin requirements for TPN are not well understood, and the altered requirements of specific disease states are not well defined. Adult vitamin preparations for parenteral use contain twice the Recommended Dietary Allowance (RDA) for the water-soluble vitamins. Excess amounts of these vitamins are excreted in the urine.

Fat-soluble vitamins, which are stored in the body, are provided in amounts equal to the RDA. Excess intravenous supplementation has led to toxic levels in some patients.

Mineral requirements vary greatly in parenteral nutrition depending on the status of the patient. Body tissues are metabolized for nitrogen and other minerals during catabolism. Deficiencies may develop very quickly during this time unless supplementation is adequate. Suggestions for supplementation are included in Table 5.8.

ADMINISTRATION

Infusion of TPN solutions should begin gradually because of the high concentration of glucose. An initial rate of 1 liter per 24 hours is recommended. If the infusion is well tolerated, the rate may be doubled on the second day. The rate is increased daily until the desired caloric level/volume is achieved. Blood glucose levels should be monitored, and levels should stabilize below 200 mg%. Insulin should be added to each liter of solution for patients with hyperglycemia > 200 mg%.

Recent studies have demonstrated the stability of fat, amino acids, and dextrose when mixed together. These three-in-one mixtures have been found to be stable at 4°C when fat is added, and at room temperature for 48 hours when 50% dextrose and 8.5% amino acids are added in equal volume (17). Two- and three-liter containers are being marketed for the purpose of administering all three components from the same container but questions of stability and compatibility persist. This practice will likely increase in popularity during the next few years as these problems are resolved.

Monitoring

Careful monitoring is required for patients receiving parenteral nutrition. Assessment should be carried out daily for the first seven days of administration. After the patient is stabilized, less frequent monitoring is necessary.

Complications of TPN are minimized if management of patients is provided by an experienced team of a physician, hyperalimentation nurse, registered dietitian, and pharmacist. Strict aseptic technique, adherence to protocol, and daily follow-up are mandatory in the care of TPN patients.

Complications of TPN are generally grouped into four categories: metabolic, mechanical, infectious, and trace element deficiencies. The metabolic complications of TPN are summarized in Table 5.9.

Mechanical complications most commonly occur as pneumothorax and subclavian vein thrombosis. The frequency of pneumothorax is related to the experience and expertise of the physician inserting the catheter. Given the precarious health of the TPN candidate, catheter placement should be attempted only under expert guidance. A routine chest film to confirm proper catheter placement must be obtained before beginning TPN.

While subclavian vein thrombosis is usually not apparent clinically, occasional cases of the superior vena cava syndrome have been reported. Venous contrast studies have demonstrated that subclavian vein thrombosis is not an uncommon complication of TPN. Six thousand units of heparin per day equally divided in the TPN bottles will safely minimize this problem.

Infectious complications should occur in less than 7% of patients when proper

Table 5.8. Parenteral Mineral Supplementation for Adults

| Mineral | Basal | Amount per Kilogram Body Weight | | Comments |
		Mild to Mod. Depletion	Severe Catabolism	
Sodium	1–4 mEq	2–3 mEq	3–4 mEq	
Potassium	0.7–0.9 mEq	2 mEq	3–4 mEq	Give 5 to 6 mEq per gram nitrogen infused
Calcium	0.22 mEq	0.3 mEq	0.4 mEq	0.25 mEq/kilogram needed for calcium equilibrium. Dependent upon simultaneous administration of phosphorus and sodium not nitrogen retention
Magnesium	0.8 mEq	0.3–0.4 mEq	0.6–0.8 mEq	Give 2 mEq per gram of nitrogen infused
Phosphorus	0.3 mEq	0.8 mEq	1.2–2 mEq	Needs related to nitrogen retention which is related to calorie intake. Give 15 to 25 mEq phosphorus per 1000 nonprotein calories

Recommendations for Daily Supplementation of Trace Minerals

Minerals	Oral	Parenteral	Comments
Zinc	10–15 mg	2.5–4.0 mg	Add 4.5 to 6.9 mg if severe catabolism Add 12.2 mg/L for significant intestinal fluid loss Add 17.1 mg/kg of excessive stool or ileostomy output
Copper	1.2–3.0 mg	0.5–1.5 mg	Add up to 3.7 mg for excessive fistula loss or diarrhea
Iron	10 mg men 18 mg women	1 mg 1 mg	

From: Grant, A, and DeHoog, S. *Nutritional Assessment and Support*. Seattle: Nutritional Therapy, 1985, p 156.

aseptic technique is followed. True catheter sepsis is unusual and should occur in less than 2–3% of patients. In addition to the catheter tip, the skin, intravenous lines, and TPN solution itself should be examined in cases of TPN related sepsis. Previously, fungal organisms had been found to be responsible for more than one half of TPN-related infections but are seen much less frequently now. When catheter sepsis is suspected, the catheter can be changed over a guide-wire with appro-

Table 5.9. Complications Associated with TPN

Complication	Symptoms	Cause	Treatment
Hyperglycemia	elevated blood glucose	carbohydrate intolerance, too rapid infusion, diabetes mellitus, infection	decrease rate, treat infection, give insulin
Dehydration (Hyperosmolar Nonketotic)	hyperglycemia, elevated serum sodium and osmolality, somnolence, seizures, coma	hyperglycemia	insulin, correct free water deficit
Hypoglycemia	hypothermia, somnolence, lethargy, peripheral vasoconstriction	interruption of infusion	proper glucose infusion rate
Hypophosphatemia	paresthesias, mental confusion, hyperventilation, lethargy, decreased red blood cell function	inadequate phosphate	increase phosphate supplementation
Hypokalemia	muscular weakness, cardiac arrhythmia	excessive potassium loss, inadequate supplementation	increase potassium supplementation
Hyponatremia	lethargy, confusion	water intoxication, excess sodium loss	increase sodium supplementation, restrict free water
Hypomagnesemia	vertigo, weakness, distention, seizures	inadequate magnesium, excess losses	increase magnesium supplementation
Prerenal Azotemia	lassitude	dehydration, calorie nitrogen imbalance	correct calorie: nitrogen imbalance, insulin if hyperglycemic, correct free water deficit
Hyperchloremic, metabolic acidosis	decrease in blood pH, decrease in serum HCO_3, decrease in base excess, increase in serum Cl, increase in serum Na	excessive renal or gastrointestinal losses of base, infusion of preformed hydrogen ion, inadequate amount of base-producing substance in TPN solution to neutralize acid products of amino acid degradation, excess administration of Cl ion	decrease chloride excess in TPN solution by exchanging chloride ion with acetate ion (a base producing substance)
Hyperammonemia	elevated blood ammonia levels, somnolence, lethargy, seizures, coma	hepatic dysfunction, deficiency in urea cycle amino acids, insufficient arginine binding (Pediatrics), low non-protein-calorie to Nitrogen ratio	slow infusion rate, discontinue infusion, use arginine HCL, increase Kcal: N ratio

Complication	Symptoms	Cause	Treatment
Hypocalcemia	muscle cramps, abdominal cramps, tetany, positive Chvostek sign, convulsions	inadequate calcium administration, repletion of phosphorus without attention to the reciprocal change in calcium, albumin fluctuations, determine if it is a clinical or laboratory finding (low albumin)	add Ca Gluconate to TPN solution, infuse Ca Gluconate 10%, 10 cc STAT and prn, monitor serum calcium, phosphorus, albumin
Anemia	varies depending upon type: e.g., iron, folic acid, B_{12}	iron deficiency, folic acid deficiency, vitamin B_{12} deficiency, copper deficiency, hypophosphatemia	replace deficit of appropriate vitamin or mineral, consider trace element supplementation after 1 month of TPN (plasma protein fraction transfusion 1–2 units week)

From: Grant, A, and DeHoog, S. *Nutritional Assessment and Support.* Seattle: Nutritional Therapy, 1985, pp. 158–159.

priate cultures obtained from the catheter tip, blood, and skin. If there is no growth from the TPN apparatus or puncture site, the new catheter can be left in place. The 0.45 micron in-line filter used in adult TPN solutions will remove fungi but not bacteria. The 0.22 micron filter used in pediatric TPN systems will remove both bacterial and fungal organisms but requires pump infusion to establish an adequate flow-rate for adult patients. Intravenous tubings and filters should be replaced every 24–48 hours. Most hospitals have established protocols for equipment changes and infection control.

Trace element deficiencies are prevented with the addition of an appropriate mineral supplement. In the infancy of nutritional support with TPN, several cases of trace element deficiencies were observed. Treatment with the missing trace element cleared up the symptoms of deficiency, usually dermatitis or hematologic abnormalities. Daily supplements of copper, zinc, manganese, chromium, and cobalt are routinely provided by TPN specialists.

The administration of drugs via the TPN catheter, in addition to being a breach in aseptic technique, can lead to precipitation of mineral components of TPN solutions and should be strictly avoided. An experienced TPN pharmacist can provide invaluable advice regarding incompatibilities of compounds one might wish to add to standard TPN solutions.

TPN in Cardiac Disease

Nutritional wasting in patients with severe cardiac disease is well documented. Patients with congestive heart failure or complicated postoperative courses are at increased risk for developing cardiac cachexia.

Clinical findings in these patients include decreased heart weight in relation to body weight, hypotension, reduction in heart muscle mass and reduced cardiac output. The changes in heart size and volume induced by protein-calorie malnutrition may be a result of a wasting of the heart muscle due to decreased protein synthesis or a response to decreased blood volume and cardiac output of malnourished patients (18).

Feeding of patients with cardiac cachexia may aggravate cardiac and metabolic complications. Refeeding these patients may lead to congestive heart failure, increased cardiac output, and increased heart rates. Glucose intolerance may also be present as a result of hypermetabolism caused by stress, fever, increased catecholamine release, increased metabolic needs of respiratory and cardiac tissue or the nutritional support itself. Hyperlipidemia, often present in this population, may require modifications in the use of lipid infusions. If lipid status contradicts the use of lipid infusions, safflower oil may be applied topically to prevent essential fatty acid deficiency (19).

Diuretic therapy may increase the loss of K, Ca, and Mg important in maintaining normal cardiac status. Deficiencies of these minerals caused by diuresis or TPN may complicate recovery.

Adequate PO_4 levels must be maintained during refeeding. Cases of severe cardiomyopathy secondary to hypophosphatemia have been reported (19).

Selenium deficiency may result in congestive cardiomyopathy. Standard TPN protocols do not include selenium supplementation. It is recommended that 80–100 ug/day be provided for patients on long-term nutritional support.

In feeding patients with cardiac cachexia, the goal of nutritional support is to improve myocardial strength without unnecessary fluid or metabolic stress. The use of TPN solutions providing 1.3–1.4 kcal/cc (35% dextrose and 5% amino acids) combined with sodium restriction has been shown to prevent fluid overload (20).

Close monitoring of fluid and electrolyte balance, glucose status, and hyperlipidemia is important in these patients.

TPN in Pulmonary Disease

Malnutrition leads to a reduction in total body muscle mass, of which the respiratory musculature is included. Loss of muscle mass due to PCM or prolonged ventilatory support will compromise respiratory function. Pneumonia, atelectasis, and infection may result. It is important to provide nutritional support to ameliorate malnutrition and improve respiratory function.

Glucose, the major source of nonprotein calories, may be detrimental to patients with pulmonary failure. These patients experience increased carbon dioxide production and an increase in the respiratory quotient from 0.7 to 1.0 (19). Increased demand is placed on the respiratory muscles to remove the excess carbon dioxide. Askanazi proposes that 50% of the dextrose calories be replaced with fat calories in these patients (21). The limitation of this recommendation is the potential for decreased pulmonary diffusion capacity in adults. Monitoring of patients is important to assess pulmonary function and lipid tolerance. Total carbohydrate intake should not exceed 6 mg/kg and the fat to carbohydrate calories should be approximately a 1:1 ratio.

Anabolic needs for amino acids may affect pulmonary function by increasing the ventilatory drive response to CO_2. Dyspnea may result in patients who are unable to increase their minute ventilation.

Increased requirements for PO_4 depends on respiratory function. Hypophosphatemia has been associated with acute respiratory failure due to the inactivation of the PO_4-dependent ATP-producing enzyme responsible for oxygen transport. Other vitamin and mineral needs are not affected by respiratory failure and should be given routinely.

Feeding the patient with respiratory failure requires careful monitoring of pCO_2, pH, and respiratory quotient (RQ). The goal of nutritional support in these patients is to restore lean body mass without causing further pulmonary distress.

Solutions providing 25% dextrose and 4.25% amino acids with fat added to provide 50% of the calories are recommended. If fluid restriction is necessary, 35% dextrose or 20% fat will increase the caloric density of the solution. PO_4 supplementation of 80–100 mEq/day is recommended for hypophosphatemia.

Special considerations for patients intolerant of the large daily volumes associated with usual TPN regimens include the substitution of 70% dextrose for a 50% solution and a 10% solution of amino acids instead of 8.5%, providing adequate amounts of amino acids and dextrose in one-half to one-third the usual volume.

Patients with renal failure may be given only essential amino acids (FreAmine III, Nephramine). Patients with hepatic encephalopathy may be given an elemental amino acid formula (Hepatic-Aid) characterized by increased branch-chain amino acids (leucine, isoleucine, and valine) and decreased aromatic amino acids (tryptophan, phenylalanine, and methionine). Recent reports suggest that using branched chain amino acids may improve the mental aberrations seen in this syndrome.

Whether TPN actually improves survival of cancer patients treated with combined chemotherapy and radiation therapy is not entirely clear from the literature (22). Nonetheless, many malnourished and debilitated cancer patients who might never be able to tolerate such therapy can participate with the concomitant use of TPN. In addition, the consistent daily supply of energy and protein leads to a generalized sense of well-being and improved quality of life for these patients.

Termination of TPN

Parenteral feedings should be tapered over 48 hours to avoid hyperinsulinism seen with abrupt termination of feedings. The glucose infusion should gradually be reduced from 0.5 gm/kg/hr to .01 gm/kg/hr.

Small, frequent feedings should be given to the patients as tolerated during this period to help revitalize digestive and absorptive function. After the patient has demonstrated that near normal intakes are possible, the catheter should be heparinized and left in place for 24 hours. If food intake remains adequate, the infusion line can be removed.

OBESITY

Obesity poses a number of difficulties for the anesthetist and is associated with an increase in surgical morbidity (23, 24). **Aspiration** is more likely in the obese due to a larger gastric reservoir and to mechanical problems causing delays in the induction of anesthesia. Postoperative atelectasis is also more commonly seen in the obese. **Hypoventilation** is the rule in the obese, predisposing to cardiac arrhythmias and congestive heart failure. Due to delayed washout of anesthetic agents from large fat stores and to an increase in mechanical resistance to ventilation, especially in the morbidly obese (greater than 100% of ideal body weight), these patients ought to be supported with continued mechanical ventilation postoperatively until fully alert and capable of forceful inspiration, with a return of arterial PO_2 toward preoperative levels. This usually requires 24–48 hours.

Recovery from surgery is further complicated by an increased incidence in the obese of **wound infections, dehiscence, and incisional hernias.** While the data available are conflicting, most physicians feel that there is an increased incidence of thrombophlebitis and pulmonary embolism in the obese. A decrease in activity and mobility is thought to be partially responsible. Another theory suggests that increased levels of plasma free fatty acids in the obese cause endothelial damage, activating the clotting cascade and leading to thrombophlebitis and pulmonary emboli. A decrease in antithrombin III and fibrinolytic activity is also postulated.

A number of investigators suggest using the **ponderal index** (PI), PI = height/ the cube root of weight, as a more accurate indicator than height:weight tables for increased risk of mortality due to obesity. In epidemiologic studies, postoperative mortality begins to increase at a PI below 12.3 and dramatically increases at a PI of 11.6 or lower (25).

The **body mass index** (BMI), BMI = weight/height squared, has been reported to be a more sensitive measure of obesity than the ponderal index (26, 27) and as such might be expected to give a more accurate prediction of increased surgical morbidity and mortality, but such data does not yet exist.

MISCELLANEOUS

Numerous **drugs** affect the intermediary metabolism of protein, carbohydrate, and fat, as well as vitamins and minerals. While too numerous to discuss in this review, these are concisely examined by Yoselson (28).

"Ostomy" patients have special nutritional needs (29). The patient with a short bowel may be intolerant of fat and require medium chain triglycerides in order to avoid steatorrhea. In addition, vitamin B$_{12}$ may need to be provided parenterally. Homogenization of proteins may improve the small bowel's ability to absorb adequate amino acids, although, occasionally, synthetic amino acid preparations will need to be employed. Fat-soluble vitamin supplementation will also be required in patients with steatorrhea. Foods high in fiber and sugar content may cause excessive water loss and require compensatory increases in fluid and electrolyte intake. lactose intolerance may also be a particular problem for the ileostomy and colostomy patient. Fermented forms of milk, such as buttermilk and yogurt, or lactase added to milk should solve this problem. Fluid intake should be adequate to provide at least 1 liter of urine per day. In patients with colostomies, fecal impactions can be avoided by adequate intake

of fluids and high fiber foods. Excessive amounts of high fiber foods, however, can cause stoma obstruction. Patients with ileostomies have an increased risk for calcium oxalate renal calculi. This risk is increased by inadequate urine sodium chloride and volume. Restriction of dietary oxalate (found in high concentration in spinach, cocoa, rhubarb, chard, and beet tops) will also help to minimize this complication. Also, the addition of calcium to the diet will complex with oxalate in the intestine and render it non-absorbable.

Many detailed books are available to help the physician gain more knowledge about nutritional assessment and support (30, 31, 32). There are also intensive courses that help the member of the nutritional support team to gain practical experience in the management of TPN patients.

READINGS

1. Bistrian B, Blackburn G, Hallowell E, et al.: Protein status of general surgical patients. *JAMA* 230:858–860, 1974.
2. Bistrian B, Blackburn G, Vitale J, et al.: Prevalence of malnutrition in general medical patients. *JAMA* 235:1567–1570, 1976.
3. Butterworth C: The skeleton in the hospital closet. *Nutr Today* March/April: 4–8, 1975.
4. Blackburn G, Maini B, Pierce E: Nutrition in the critically ill patient. *Anesthesiology* 47:181–194, 1977.
5. Blackburn G, Flatt J, Clowes G, et al.: Peripheral intravenous feeding with isotonic amino acid solutions. *Am J Surg* 125:447–454, 1973.
6. Hoover H. Grant J, Gorschboth C, et al.: Nitrogen-sparing intravenous fluids in postoperative patients. *New Engl J Med* 293:172–174, 1976.
7. Greenberg G, Marliss E, Anderson G, et al.: Protein-sparing therapy in postoperative patients. *New Engl J Med* 294:1411–1416, 1976.
8. Weisner R, Hunker E, Krumdieck C, et al.: Hospital malnutrition: a prospective evaluation of general medical patients during the course of hospitalization. *AJCN* 32:418, 1979.
9. MacLean L: Host resistance in surgical patients. *J Trauma* 19:297–304, 1979.
10. Beisel W, Edelman R, Nauss K, et al.: Single-nutrient effects on immunologic functions. *JAMA* 245:53–58, 1981.
11. Baker J, Detsky A, Whiteweil J, et al.: A comparison of the predictive value of nutritional assessment techniques. *Hum Nutr and Clin Nutr* 36C:233, 1982.
12. Bistrian B: A simple technique to estimate se-

verity of stress. *Surg Gynecol Obstet* 148:675–678, 1979.

13. Silberman H, Eisenberg D: *Parenteral and Enteral Nutrition for the Hospitalized Patient.* Norwalk, Conn, Appleton-Century-Crofts, 1982.

14. Sabiston D: *Textbook of Surgery: The Biological Basis of Modern Surgical Practice.* Philadelphia, W.B. Saunders, 1972, p 162.

15. Gibbons G, et al.: Pre- and Postoperative Hyperalimentation in the treatment of cardiac cachexia. *J Surg Res* 205:439–444, 1976.

16. MacFayden B, et al.: Triglyceride and free fatty acid clearances in patients receiving complete parenteral nutrition using ten percent soybean oil emulsions. *Surg, Gynecol Obstet* 137:813, 1973.

17. Technical Information Bulletin. American McGaw No. 2, Dec 1982.

18. Heymsfield S, et al: Cardiac abnormalities in cachectic patients before and during nutritional repletion. *Am Heart Jo* 95:584, 1978.

19. Darsee J, Nutter D.: Reversible severe congestive cardiomyopathy in three cases of hypophosphatemia. *Ann Int Med* 89:867, 1978.

20. Barr L, et al.: Essential fatty acid deficiency during total parenteral nutrition. Abstract. *Ann Surg* 193:304, 1981.

21. Askanazi J, Nordstrom J, Rosenbaum S, et al.: Nutrition for the patient with respiratory failure: glucose versus fat. *Anesthesiology* 54:373, 1981.

22. Buzby G, Mullen J, Stein P, et al.: Host-tumor interaction and nutrient supply. *Cancer* 45:2940, 1980.

23. Putnam L, Jenicek J, Allen C, et al.: Anesthesia in the morbidly obese patient. *South Med J* 67:1411, 1974.

24. Strauss R, Wise L: Operative risks of obesity. *Surg Gynecol Obstet* 146:286, 1978.

25. Flewellen E, Bee D: (To the Editor) Ponderal index: Quantifying obesity. *JAMA* 241:884, 1979.

26. Cork R, Vaughn R: (To the editor) Indices of obesity. *JAMA* 242:1140, 1979.

27. Bray G: Complications of obesity. *Ann Int Med* 103(6, pt 2):1052, 1985.

28. Yosselson S: Drugs and nutrition. *Drug Intell Clin* Pharm 10:8, 1976.

29. Lewis C: Special patients: diel planning for ostomates. *Patient Care* July 15, 1977, pp 152–163.

30. Grant A, DeHoog S: *Nutritional Assessment and Support.* Seattle, Washington. Third edition, 1985.

31. Krey S, Murray R: *Dynamics of Nutrition Support.* Norwalk, Conn, Appleton-Century Crofts, 1986.

32. Rombeau J, Caldwell M: *Parenteral Nutrition.* Philadelphia, W.B. Saunders, 1986.

33. Jeejebhoy K: Total Parenteral Nutrition. *Ann R Coll Phys Surg Can.* 9:287, 1987.

34. Goodhart R, Shills M: *Modern Nutrition in Health and Disease.* Table 22.2, Philadelphia, Lea and Febiger, 1973, pp. 669.

6

Preoperative Pulmonary Evaluation

Joseph J. Trautlein

Modern anesthetic techniques allow virtually any patient to be intubated, anesthetized, and well-oxygenated intra-operatively. The challenge lies in extubating and returning the patient to totally self-generated respiration.

Anesthesia and surgery impose additional stresses on the pulmonary compromised patient including: (1) Abnormalities of gas exchange causing hypoxia, (2) respiratory depression, (3) decreased cough reflex and clearance of secretions, and (4) decreased sighing and tidal volume leading to atelectasis.

The intent of this chapter is not to review every available opinion regarding preoperative pulmonary assessment. Improvements in the quality and quantity of pulmonary function data that can be easily gathered preoperatively, as well as improvements in intra- and postoperative support and weaning techniques, antibiotics, nutritional support, and surgical practice have liberalized many of the previously determined "prohibitive" risk criteria for general surgery patients (1,2,3).

In general, then, the risk estimates for pulmonary disease in the literature should be taken as tentative because of the widely varying patient populations and more recent improvements in management and are not to be considered precise enough to be used alone to deny surgery purely on a statistical basis. There is, however, a certain irreducible minimum necessary to assure an adequate outcome. **An FEV_1 of less than 500 cc and an FVC of less than 1 liter,** regardless of operative site, are the absolute values that are most often quoted as being the dividing line between viability and imprudence.

We have tried to extract the most credible, best documented studies, and to couple these with the internist's perspective on the relationship between preoperative pulmonary testing and surgical morbidity and mortality. In broad outline, we will be dealing with general considerations in all patients, followed by discussion of certain specific high-risk situations that merit special attention.

GENERAL APPROACH TO PREOPERATIVE PULMONARY ASSESSMENT

In preoperative pulmonary assessment several general notions are useful to keep in mind. Dyspnea is a subjective phenomenon. It is a perceived imbalance between the work of breathing and tissue oxygenation. The usual bell-shaped curve of patient awareness is operative, ranging from the chronic breathlessness of the hyperventilator to the bland organicity of the chronic CO_2 retainer. Physical findings of retraction, cyanosis, clubbing, plethora, and breathlessness can be integrated with the data from the formal respiratory history. When considering general anesthesia, smoking history, history of pulmonary infections, presence or absence of sputum production and, especially, a history of asthma are crucial clues to the wary clinician (4–9).

A plausible case can be made for screening spirometry, preferably done before and after bronchodilators, for any patient over 60 who is about to undergo

Table 6.1.   Critical Historical Parameters of Operative Risks

1. Site of proposed surgery (transthoracic, trans-abdominal)
2. Duration of proposed anesthesia (greater than 2 hours)
3. Smoking history expressed in pack years
4. Previous thoracic surgery experience
5. General anesthesia within the previous year
6. History of pulmonary symptoms (dyspnea, cough, sputum production, breathlessness)
7. History of asthma
8. History of chronic bronchitis (more than 3 months per year of sputum production for more than 2 years)
9. Familial or personal history of emphysema
10. Age greater than 60 years
11. Significant obesity
12. Prior history of pneumonia, pulmonary embolus, chest trauma
13. History of personal or familial disorders of muscular function, respiratory drive or allergies
14. Dyspnea on exertion, night cough, or sedentary lifestyle that may have been forced upon the patient by cardiorespiratory compromise
15. Signs and symptoms of current upper respiratory infection

general anesthesia. The consensus of the literature is that the risks of relying primarily on the history and physical exam are false negative. That is, the patient may be significantly compromised and yet, because of lifestyle modification, denial, or unsophistication give a "negative" pulmonary history. Given the seriousness of pulmonary complications, a good pragmatic rule would be: when in doubt, get formal pulmonary function testing. When feasible, this should be coupled with arterial blood gas analysis in any patient with a history of recent pulmonary infection, asthma, smoking or prior chest surgery or in any patient who is undergoing a procedure in which postoperative deep vein thrombophlebitis is likely (Table 6.1).

Although regional anesthesia has significant cardiovascular effects, the compromise to the pulmonary system has been found to be negligible when both the patient and operator are suitable for this type of anesthesia (8,23,24).

THE IMPACT OF AGE

Aging may be viewed as a process of decreasing pulmonary compliance. The elastic recoil of the lung and accessory structures diminish as a function of chronologic age. The most significant individual variations are a function of conditioning, smoking history, weight, and cardiac status. As a general rule, the older the lung, the stiffer it is, the more difficult secretion and mobilization are, and the smaller the ventilatory reserve. Normal populations, height and weight adjusted, show a progressive diminution of forced vital capacity, FEV_1, and FEF_{25-75} as a function of the calendar (Figs. 6.1, 6.2).

A successful postoperative course, then, depends upon:

(*a*) The ability to generate a sufficient air flow to expel mucus accumulating in the postoperative period ($FEV_1 > 500$ ml, $FEF_{25-75} > 50\%$ predicted).

(*b*) Motivation sufficient to perform that maneuver (MVV > 50% predicted).

(*c*) Sufficient respiratory reserve to accommodate the predictable postoperative fall in breathing capacity.

To generate an adequate cough, the

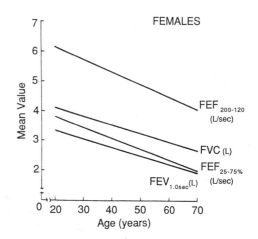

Figure 6.1. Relationship of forced expiratory measurements to age in normal women (From Morris JF, Koski A, and Johnson LC: Spirometric standards for healthy nonsmoking adults. *Am Rev Resp Dis* 103:63, 1971. Used with permission.)

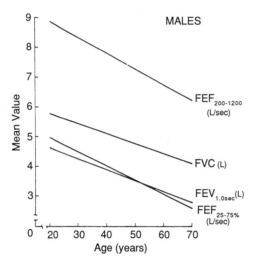

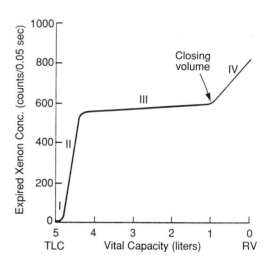

Figure 6.2. Relationship of forced expiratory measurements to age in normal men. (From Morris JF, Koski A, and Johnson LC: Spirometric standards for healthy nonsmoking adults. *Am Rev Resp Dis* 103:63, 1971. Used with permission.)

Figure 6.3. Idealized tracing of expired xenon concentration during a slow exhalation from total lung capacity (TLC) to residual volume (RV) after the previous breath has been labeled with a bolus of xenon. Closing volume (*arrow*) is the vital capacity remaining at the junction between phase III and phase IV. (From Murray JF: The Normal Lung—The Basis for Diagnosis and Treatment of Pulmonary Disease, Philadelphia, WB Saunders, 1986. Used with permission.)

maximum voluntary ventilation, which is an holistic assessment of motivation and functional reserve should be considered extremely marginal if it is below 40 liters/minute. Forced vital capacities of < 1600 cc or < 50% of predicted normals imply a degree of pulmonary impairment that virtually guarantees postoperative macro- or micro-atelectasis.

CLOSING VOLUMES AS A DETERMINATE OF OPERABILITY

In the erect, ambulatory and conscious state, basilar lung segments are maximally ventilated and receive the lion's share of perfusion. In the usual horizontal position during which surgery is performed, blood flow shifts to the dependent portion of the lung and the respirator, or the anesthetist's hand replaces spontaneous muscular action in inflating the lungs. When the patient is to be awakened, the appearance of macro-atelectasis is determined by the closing volume, that is, the lung volume at which small airway closure spontaneously occurs (Fig. 6.3).

There is substantial evidence to support the contention that even with meticulous intraoperative attention to sighing, some degree of micro-atelectasis occurs in all general anesthesia patients (11,21). In the older population this can account for a decrease of up to 30% of forced vital capacity as compared to baseline. This phenomenon clears in three to five days if there is sufficient ventilatory reserve, motivation, and postoperative respiratory care.

SURGERY IN THE OBESE PATIENT

Obesity is a risk factor from many points of view: e.g., a cardiac risk factor, an increased risk for thromboembolic disease, an increased risk for dehiscence in abdominal surgery. From a pulmonary point of view obesity is an independent risk (13–17). This is due to the fact that the obese patient starts out with a decreased expiratory reserve volume from compression of the thorax by layers of fat and compromise of diaphragmatic excursion by an oversized panniculus. Whenever possible in elective operative procedures, the patient should be strongly encouraged to initiate some attempts at weight loss, as well as physical conditioning (16,17).

PHYSICAL STATUS

The seriousness of the patient's overall condition is a further independent variable, which is evaluated by the Dripps Criteria. Dripps Criteria are a global assessment of physical status, not just pulmonary function. It provides a convenient nosology for identifying high-risk patients on the basis of history, analogous to the New York Heart Association's functional criteria. In the Dripps Criteria there are five classes (Table 6.2).

As might be expected, there are virtually no operative deaths in Class I, but the system comes up short in looking for correlations between the clinical staging of Classes II, III, IV and V as compared to objective parameter staging. For example, a patient may have significant restrictive disease on the basis of rheumatoid lung disease, even with quiescent joint symptomatology; or chest wall compliance problems such as are found in ankylosing spondylitis, previous thoracic compression fractures, or phrenic nerve injuries. The patient might be Class I or II historically, yet be an appreciable anesthetic risk.

SPECIAL CONSIDERATIONS IN NONTHORACIC SURGERY

The preoperative pulmonary status of the patient must be assessed in terms of the physiologic changes that will occur as part of the natural history of the induction of assisted ventilation. Experimental models and clinical experience have demonstrated that there are predictable alterations in regional blood flow and mucus clearing that are inherent to general

Table 6.2. Dripps Criteria for Identifying High-Risk Patients on Basis of History

Class I	There is no physiologic, biochemical, or psychiatric disturbance. The pathological process for which operation is to be performed is localized and not conducive to systemic disturbance. Examples: a fit patient with inguinal hernia or fibroid uterus in an otherwise healthy woman.
Class II	Mild to moderate systemic disturbance caused either by the condition to be treated surgically or by other pathophysiological processes. Examples: presence of mild diabetes, essential hypertension, or anemia.
Class III	Rather severe systemic disturbance or pathology from whatever cause, even though it may not be possible to define the degree of disability with finality. Examples: severe diabetes with vascular complications, moderate to severe degrees of pulmonary insufficiency, stable angina pectoris, or healed myocardial infarction.
Class IV	Indicative of the patient with a severe systemic disorder already life-threatening and not always correctable by the operative procedure. Examples: advanced degrees of cardiac, pulmonary, hepatic, renal, or endocrine insufficiency.
Class V	This category embraces the moribund patient who has little chance of survival but is submitted to operation in desperation. Examples: the burst aneurysm with the patient in profound shock, major cerebral trauma with rapidly increasing intracranial pressure, or massive pulmonary embolus.
Emergency operation (E)	Any patient in one of the classes listed above who is operated upon as an emergency is considered to be in somewhat poorer physical condition. The letter E is placed beside the numerical classification.

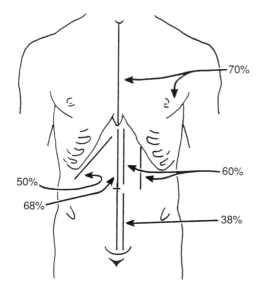

Figure 6.4. Postoperative reductions in vital capacity associated with various sites of incision. (From Fishman AP: Pulmonary Diseases and Disorders, New York, McGraw-Hill, Inc., 1988, p. 2415. Used with permission.)

anesthesia. Successful resuscitation from general anesthesia is inhibited by mechanical factors that relate to lung expansion, mucus production, and the generation of an adequate cough.

General anesthesia carries an inherent risk, which is extremely variable, ranging from 0.1% to 70% depending on the site of operation and the patient's physical status. For nonthoracic surgery, three subgroups are easily identifiable: (Fig. 6.4)

Subgroup A: Cutaneous and extremity surgery
Subgroup B: Lower abdominal surgery
Subgroup C: Upper abdominal surgery

One must distinguish between the inherent risk of general anesthesia, even if no surgery is performed, and the added physiologic stress put upon the respiratory system as a function of postoperative pain, limitation of motion and splinting, which are concomitants of the surgical procedure itself.

Regarding anesthetic risks alone, in Subgroup A, the risk is primarily that of the general anesthesia, which is generally quite low. Still, cilia are immobilized to some degree during the anesthetic phase, and mucus secretion and pooling are virtually guaranteed. The clinician is not relieved from attention to the potential for infection or pulmonary insufficiency to supervene, even though the operative site in no way interferes with the work or adequacy of respiration in the postoperative phase.

In Subgroup B, lower abdominal surgery, deep breathing is not likely to become compromised, but coughing can become excruciatingly painful. Adequate patient education prior to the procedure, the use of hand-restraining techniques, and good nursing can make the difference between an uneventful postoperative course and one fraught with complications. This is so even though, as in the case of large uterine fibroids, the "debulking" accomplished with surgery may actually result in an improvement of ventilatory function.

In Subgroup C, upper abdominal surgery, both deep breathing and coughing are voluntarily significantly inhibited postoperatively. Diaphragmatic excursions irritate the operative site and are inhibited, thereby increasing postoperative micro- and macro-atelectasis and inviting the complications of postoperative atelectasis, pneumonia, and pulmonary insufficiency secondary to mucus plugging. Instruction, motivation, and reinforcement are absolutely critical in this category of patients.

CHRONIC OBSTRUCTIVE LUNG DISEASE (COPD)

Epidemiology

Chronic obstructive pulmonary disease has been found in 10–50% of general surgical patients by pulmonary function tests. Among historical studies (Tables 6.3 and 6.4), pulmonary mortality ranged from

Table 6.3. Perioperative Mortality in Patients with Chronic Obstructive Lung Disease

Study	Population	Number	Mortality (%) Total	Mortality (%) Pulmonary
Thulbourne (1962)	Clinical COPD[a]	65	?	0
Stein (1962)	Abnormal PFT[a]	30		0
Stein (1970)	Abnormal PFT	48		8[b]
Tarhan (1973)	Clinical COPD, General anesthesia (men)	464	8	7
Gracey (1979)	Clinical COPD	157	6	3
Mean			7	4

[a]COPD = chronic obstructive lung disease; PFT = pulmonary function tests.
[b]All deaths occurred in patients undergoing thoracic surgery.

0–8%, with men being more severely affected than women.

Published studies of pulmonary complications with surgery in patients with COPD are limited by the small number of patients, varying definitions of complications, and lack of control groups. Available series (Table 6.5) show an average complication rate of 32% among patients with COPD, compared to 9% of controls. The most frequent pulmonary complica-

Table 6.4. Summary of Pulmonary Risks

	COPD	All Patients
Pulmonary mortality	4%	0–2%
Pulmonary complications	36%	9%

tion is atelectasis, with the production of purulent sputum ("bronchitis") being second. Patients with COPD have a 2–7 time increased risk of atelectasis (25–70% develop atelectasis). Severe respiratory insufficiency and the need for prolonged mechanical ventilation were rare in these series.

Risk factors for pulmonary complications include certain abnormalities of pulmonary function tests, age greater than 70, male sex, obesity, upper abdominal or thoracic surgery, duration of anesthesia of greater than 2–3 hours and repeat surgery within one year (Table 6.6).

Pulmonary function tests are the most sensitive indicators of pulmonary risk. However, while there is a loose correlation between the degree of abnormality and the pulmonary risk, there is not a precise correlation. Almost any abnormality of pulmonary testing increases the risk of atelectasis and bronchitis; whether

Table 6.5. Incidence of Pulmonary Complications

Study	Number	Population	Complications Studied[a]	Incidence (patients without prophylactic treatment)	Normal (control group) Incidence
Stein (1962)	30	Abnormal PFT[b]	A, B, D, P, R	70%	3%
Stein (1970)	48	Abnormal PFT	A, B, D, P, R	42% (60%)	10%
Thulbourne (1962)	65	Clinical COPD	B, P	33% (25%)	14%
Wrightman (1968)	53	Clinical COPD	A, B, P	26%	8%
Tarhan (1973)	464	Clinical COPD	A, B, P, R	32% (43%)	
Gracey (1979)	157	Clinical COPD	A, B, P, D, R	19%	
Mean				36%	9%
Median				32%	9%

[a]A, atelectasis, B, bronchitis (purulent sputum), D, dyspnea or bronchospasm, P, pneumonia, R, respiratory failure.
[b]PFT, pulmonary function tests.

Table 6.6. Risk Factors for Pulmonary Complications

	Studies Supportive	Studies Against
Pulmonary function test abnormalities	13, 16, 31	
Age (>70)	8, 12, 36	
Sex (male)	12	
Obesity	13, 14, 15, 16, 17	12, 28
Site of operation (abdominal-thoracic)	8, 12, 13, 14	
Upper versus lower abdominal	5, 8, 12	
Duration of anesthesia (>2–3 hr)	5, 8, 12, 16	36
Type of anesthesia General versus spinal	46, 47	
Various general agents		46, 47
Repeat anesthesia within 1 year	8	
Smoking	4, 12, 16, 44	45

the risk increases linearly with decreasing pulmonary function has not been established. Earlier reports that certain levels of pulmonary function (Table 6.7) are "prohibitive" risks for surgery are no longer universally true (10,11,16,18,19,21). **However, pulmonary function tests alone**

Table 6.7. Assessment of Risk for Postoperative Respiratory Complications by Preoperative Pulmonary Function Studies: Critical Values

For Any Surgery	Reference
More reliable	
$MEFR_{200-1200}$ <180 L/min (3 L/sec)	9, 25, 13, 31
pCO_2 >50 mm Hg	9, 13
Less reliable	
$FEV_{0.5}$ <60% FVC	53, 56
Class III or IV by history*	43, 46

*Class 0	No history of dyspnea.
Class I	DOE when walking up slight incline.
Class II	Dyspnea when walking at own normal pace on level surface.
Class III	Needs to rest after walking three blocks at normal pace.
Class IV	Needs to rest after walking two blocks at normal pace.

can neither always identify the patient who will develop serious respiratory complications, nor do they precisely correlate with the risk of minor complications.

A single pulmonary function test best predicating postoperative respiratory complications has not been established. Various studies have found complications best correlated with the maximal mid-expiratory flow rate (MEFR) (22), the maximal voluntary ventilation (MVV) and maximal breathing capacity (MBC) (4), or the forced expiratory volume in 1 second (FEV_1) (16). Adequate comparison studies have not been done except for the finding by Stein (13) that the MEFR was a better predictor of complications than the FEV_1. (Since both the FEV_1 and MEFR are closely correlated measurements derived from spirometric tracings, they should reflect similar abnormalities and Stein's finding of different predictability requires confirmation). Most studies with MVV and MBC have been done with pulmonary resection patients; less information is available for nonpulmonary thoracic and abdominal procedures. Supporters of the MVV or MBC cite its measure of patient effort and cooperation, while the detractors cite its lower reproducibility. The use of closing volumes as predictors of pulmonary risk, while theoretically inviting, has not been supported by empirical data (4,25).

In contrast, the general history and physical examination is less consistently predictive of postoperative complications, mainly due to missed cases of obstructive lung disease. A history of productive cough is the best clinical predictor of postoperative complications but is also less sensitive than spirometry.

In summary, pulmonary function tests and certain nonpulmonary factors (Table 6.8) identify a large group of patients with COPD at increased risk for atelectasis and bronchitis. While patients with abnormal pulmonary function are at a relatively increased risk of major complications or respiratory failure, a small high-

Table 6.8. Most Important Pulmonary Risk Factors for Surgery

	Minor Complications[a]	Major Complications[b]
FEV_1	Any abnormality	<1.5 L (especially <0.5 L or <20% of normal)
MVV	Any abnormality	<50%
pCO_2		>45 mm Hg
Non-pulmonary		
Age >60	Yes	Yes
Upper abdominal thoracic operation	Yes	Yes
Repeat surgery <1 year	?	Yes
Obesity	Yes	?
Duration of anesthesia >2–3 hr	Yes	Probable
Recent upper or lower respiratory infection	Yes	Probable
Concomitant cardiovascular disease, abnormal EKG	No	Probable
Poor patient effort/cooperation	Yes	?

[a]Minor complications include: atelectasis and bronchitis.
[b]Major complications include: respiratory distress, mechanical ventilation, and pulmonary insufficiency.

risk subgroup cannot consistently be identified, even in conjunction with non-pulmonary risk factors.

Diagnostic Activities and Approaches

Any history of smoking, chronic or intermittent productive cough, dyspnea, or wheezing identifies a patient at risk for chronic lung disease who requires further evaluation. This history of productive cough is the most sensitive clinical factor. A recent respiratory infection and the presence of concomitant cardiovascular disease should also be ascertained. Factors increasing oxygen consumption or delivery should be determined, including infection, metabolic abnormalities (e.g., acidosis), or anemia.

Patients meeting all three of the following criteria do not require spirometry routinely: (1) age less than 60; (2) no history of smoking or symptoms of pulmonary disease; and (3) low-risk surgery (e.g., lower abdominal, extremity, back and breast). Complete pulmonary function testing and arterial blood gases should be obtained in high-risk patients as defined in Table 6.1 Even experienced clinicians

can misjudge the severity of lung disease. In questionable cases, simple bedside spirometry for FEV_1 will often help to clarify the situation.

Remember, however, that **the estimation of pulmonary risk based on even the "best" predictors is not precise. A patient should not be denied surgery solely on the basis of statistical pulmonary risks.**

Preoperative Management

The preoperative management of the pulmonary patient can be classified into five modalities of therapy (Table 6.9). The patient should be instructed to stop smoking at least two weeks before surgery. It is important for this to be done in the ambulatory setting, as abstinence for only the 1–2 preoperative days in the hospital is probably less effective. The patient should be educated preoperatively in coughing and deep breathing, and in the use of a pillow-type splint for abdominal wounds. Instructions should also be given in the use of devices, such as the incentive spirometer that will be used postoperatively.

Table 6.9.   Preoperative Preparation of the Pulmonary Patient

1. **Patient education**
   Discontinue smoking for 2 weeks
   Cough and deep breathe with use of pillow
   Use of mechanical devices
   Tour of intensive care unit
2. **Bronchodilation**
   Nebulizer (?IPPB) (isoethrine, metaproterenol, albuterol)
   Systemic beta-2 agents (terbutaline, albuterol, metaproterenol)
   Steroids
3. **Forced lung expansion: mobilization of secretions**
   Incentive spirometry
   Back clapping and postural drainage
   IPPB (probably not effective)
4. **Humidification**
   Wide-bore O_2 system with warm moisture
   ? IPPB
5. **Infection control**
   Antibiotics

Bronchodilation

Patients should be continued on their usual bronchodilators at least through midnight the night before surgery. Patients with even mild COPD should be considered for bronchodilator therapy in order to prevent bronchospasm, especially in the immediate pre- and postoperative periods. Bronchodilators (isoethrine, metaproterenol, terbutaline, albuterol, aminophylline) can be administered systemically or by hand-held nebulizers and IPPB. Patients who have received steriods within 1 year should be appropriately covered for stress with preoperative steriods. Some patients on inhaled steriods (such as asthmatics undergoing sinus surgery) will require perioperative oral or parenteral steriods to maintain pulmonary function.

Forced Lung Expansion and Mobilizing Secretions

At the current time, incentive spirometry seems to be the best method for preventing atelectasis. Postural drainage and back clapping have also been shown, in controlled trials, to be effective techniques to increase lung expansion and mobilization of secretions. These two modalities should be combined with proper instructions to the patient in deep breathing and coughing. Blow bottles and similar devices with small moveable balls are not effective. IPPB was not effective in most controlled trials, and is more expensive (31–38).

Humidification and Delivery of Drugs

Hand-held nebulizers are as effective in delivering drugs as IPPB and substantially less expensive. Warm moisture delivered through a wide-bore tubing oxygen system is as or more effective than IPPB in delivering moisture.

Control of Infection and Antibiotics

Patients with chronic sputum production should be considered for a brief preoperative course of a broad-spectrum antibiotic in an attempt to decrease the quantity and purulence of secretions (37). The exact antibiotic selection should be guided by the gram stain and culture. **Antibiotics alone do not decrease postoperative pulmonary infections** (30,38).

Pulmonary complications were reduced by combinations of several treatment modalities in two randomized and several large retrospective studies (Tables 6.10 and 6.11). Bronchodilators alone, IPPB alone, and IPPB with bronchodilators were ineffective. Chest physiotherapy and incentive spirometry have been shown to be of benefit in most studies.

Thus, **pulmonary complications are decreased by incentive spirometry, chest physiotherapy and, especially, when multiple modalities are used.** Intraoperative factors important in decreasing complications include duration of anesthesia and anesthetic technique (intermittent sighing, control of secretions).

Table 6.10. Evaluation of Prophylactic Preoperative Pulmonary Therapy

| Study | Mortality (prep vs. non-prep) | Pulmonary Complications | | Comment |
		Prep (%)	Non-prep (%)	
Multiple modalities				
Tarhan (8)	9.5 vs. 9.0%	24	43	Men only
Stein (20)	0 vs. 27%	22	60	Randomized
Palmer (34)		9	43	Randomized
Bronchodilator only				
Palmer (34)		38	42	Randomized
Chest therapy				
Thoren (33)		12	41	Randomized
Palmer (34)		32	43	Randomized
Incentive spirometer				
Bartlett (38)		10	30	Men only, randomized
Van De Water (57)		20	40	
Dohi (32)		29	57	Randomized
Jung (36)		49	36	Randomized
IBBP (and bronchodilator)				
Baxter (35)		25	23	Randomized
Cottrell (37)		Not significant		
Blow bottles (69)				

ASTHMA

Epidemiology

Approximately 3% of Americans are affected by asthma, making it one of the most common pulmonary diseases. Specific estimates of the operative risk posed by asthma alone are not available be-

Table 6.11. Therapeutic Maneuvers Which Diminish Pulmonary Risk[a]

Preoperative cessation of cigarette smoking
Antibiotic treatment of pulmonary infection
Antibiotic treatment of chronic bronchitis
Preoperative psychological preparation
Preoperative teaching of respiratory maneuvers
Preoperative bronchodilators for asthmatics
Maintenance of good nutrition
Minimization of anesthesia time
Minimization of postoperative narcotic analgesia
Maximization of inspiration
Early postoperative mobilization
Heparin prophylaxis in selected cases

[a] From E. Harman and G. Lillington: *Med Clin North Am* 63:1289–1298, 1979. Used with permission.

cause of pooling of asthmatics with other types of lung disease in most series, with the exception of a small series of steroid-dependent asthmatics (40). The major postoperative complications are bronchospasm and inspissation of secretions. **The first few hours postoperatively are the highest risk period for an exacerbation of asthma.**

Diagnostic Activities and Approaches

Asthmatics, (especially if they are steroid-dependent) pose special problems to the anesthetist because of their peculiar hyper-responsiveness to external stimuli. The problems are increased further when parenteral atropine is used preoperatively due to drying of oral secretions, even though general surgery in itself is a good bronchodilator and inhaled atropine analogues may be additive to other bronchodilation (70).

False-negative histories are probably no better illustrated than in the case of the asthmatic patients. The extent of airway hyper-reactivity is considerably greater than the subjectively perceived existence of the asthmatic state. Methacholine provocation testing has demonstrated that there is hyper-responsiveness several orders of magnitude in excess of normal airways even with a mere history of asthma. The potential for drug-induced asthma must always be kept in mind when the word "asthma" appears in the clinical history. A small but significant subgroup of asthmatics, for example, can be put into profound bronchospasm by the ubiquitous and generally benign drug, aspirin, as well as by nonsteroidal anti-inflammatory drugs (NSAID's).

Spirometry (FEV_1 or comparable measure) should be performed in all asthmatic patients the day before operation. Arterial blood gases should be obtained for patients who are not in their stable baseline state, or with significant abnormalities in FEV_1. Blood levels of aminophylline should be obtained in all patients preoperatively and subtherapeutic or toxic levels corrected.

Additional tests useful in selected patients include sputum gram stain and culture, sputum stain for eosinophils, blood eosinophil count, and complete pulmonary function testing.

Preoperative Management

Preoperative management of the asthmatic should emphasize maintenance of adequate hydration, bronchodilators, and avoidance of allergens precipitating bronchospasm. Known allergens for the individual patient should be eliminated from the hospital environment, the most frequent offenders being soaps, fragrances, flowers, and dust. Aspirin and NSAIDs should be avoided in those sensitive to them. Smoking should be prohibited in the patient's room.

In those intermittent asthmatics maintained on oral bronchodilators, attempts should be made to optimize air flow parameters prior to surgery. One should attempt to obtain post-bronchodilator pulmonary function results essentially the same as optimal pre-bronchodilator results when using formal pulmonary function testing. Serum theophylline levels between 10 and 20 ug/ml should be maintained. The patient's usual bronchodilator should be continued until midnight the night prior to surgery. The morning dose may be given with a sip of water on the day of surgery. All asthmatics should be on a bronchodilator unless contraindicated. If the patient is to be operated on late in the day, an intravenous line should be used for administration of fluids to maintain hydration and to maintain therapeutic levels of bronchodilators. **Due to the potentiation of aminophylline toxicity by general anesthesia, aminophylline administration is usually stopped or reduced intraoperatively** and readjusted just before anesthesia is completed, with enough aminophylline over the first 30–60 minutes sufficient to restore therapeutic levels. Less severe asthmatics are usually adequately managed by giving them their last dose at midnight of a long-acting form of aminophylline and restarting intravenous aminophylline in the recovery room. Preferably, asthmatic patients should be operated on early in the morning so that adequate bronchodilator is still present and dehydration is minimized.

Sympathomimetic agents may be given orally, parenterally, or by inhalation. Selective beta-2 agonists (albuterol, terbutaline, metaproterenol, isoetharine) are preferable because of their relative lack of cardiovascular side effects and prolonged duration. Even if the patient was not using one previously, some authorities routinely administer an inhaled bronchodilator preoperatively, at least "on call" to the operating room.

Asthmatics on oral corticosteroids or those who have been on systemic steroids within the past year should receive sufficient parenteral steroids to: (*a*) cover

Table 6.12. Suggested Preoperative Regimen for Patients with Reversible Obstructive Airways Disease

1. Intravenous or oral theophylline at an approximate dose of 5.6 mg/kg load, then 0.9 mg/kg/hr, to maintain a serum level between 10–20 μg/ml.
2. Two puffs of albuterol or metaproterenol q 4–6 hr or at least "on call" to the O.R.
3. If on maintenance cromolyn or beclomethasone, prednisone 0.5–1.0 mg/kg/24 hr, or equivalent.

adrenal suppression and (b) maintain pulmonary function. Some patients on inhaled steroids will require parenteral steroids to maintain pulmonary function perioperatively as outlined previously. Adrenal suppression due to inhaled steroids is rare in the absence of recent (less than one year) systemic steroid use or nebulizer abuse. Some patients with severe asthma or a history of severe attacks may do better with prophylactic steroids perioperatively.

When in doubt, 1 mg/kg of prednisone/24 hours, begun at least six hours preoperatively is generally sufficient to block generation of leukotriene C (slow-reacting substance of anaphylaxis), the humoral mediator of bronchospasm (Table 6.12).

Postoperative Management

The most crucial period for the asthmatic is the first few hours postoperatively due to an increased risk of bronchospasm and to increased secretions. Aminophylline should be administered by continuous intravenous infusion till oral intake is resumed, except in minor procedures or in patients with stable mild disease. Other preoperatively used bronchodilators should be reinstituted. Hydration should be maintained with intravenous fluids and adequately humidified oxygen maintained until the patient resumes his normal status.

If bronchospasm occurs postoperatively, correction of systemic acidosis and the addition of inhaled ipratropium bro-mide can be lifesaving (70). Up to 8% of asthmatics are sensitive to sulfites found in parenteral medications, as well as in some bronchodilator solutions (e.g., metaproterenol). Steroid resistance has eosinophilia as a reliable marker.

LUNG RESECTION AND CHRONIC OBSTRUCTIVE LUNG DISEASE

When the operative site is the thoracic cavity, there is greater need for the application of more sophisticated pulmonary function testing. When the proposed surgery is pneumonectomy, it is imperative that the patient be left with enough functioning lung to sustain life.

On the other hand, certain thoracic operations may actually improve pulmonary function, net, in the postoperative period; for example, bullectomy in a non-emphysematous patient due to decompression of normal lung. Likewise, the resection of lobes that are perfused but not well ventilated may actually improve the ventilation-perfusion ratio with the net result, an improvement of tissue oxygenation.

Epidemiology

Generally cited mortality rates for lung resection are 3–5% for lobectomy and 10–15% for pneumonectomy. The mortality and morbidity rates for lung surgery vary widely, depending upon: (1) patient selection (age, pulmonary function); (2) type of operation (pneumonectomy, lobectomy, segmental resection); (3) experience and skill of the surgical team and (4) the availability of postoperative intensive respiratory care facilities and personnel.

The use of the following criteria to select surgical candidates for lung resection has reduced mortality from 20–50% to 10–15% for high-risk patients. Unlike previous criteria, these criteria have made it possible to reduce operative mortality without eliminating large numbers of patients.

For pneumonectomy, the major general criteria for operability are a Forced Ex-

Table 6.13.   Major Criteria for Pneumonectomy

1. $FEV_1 > 2$ L
2. MBC $> 50–55\%$ predicted
3. FVC $> 50\%$ predicted

If any of three criteria not met → split function tests.

piratory Volume in one-second $(FEV_1) > 2$ liters, a Maximal Breathing Capacity (MBC) $> 50\%$ predicted, and a Forced Vital Capacity (FVC) $> 50\%$ of the predicted value (Table 6.13). Patients that meet all three criteria will tolerate pneumonectomy.

Patients that do not meet one or more of those criteria should undergo split pulmonary function studies and/or physiologic assessment with pulmonary artery balloon occlusion (Table 6.14).

Split studies will show the proportion of ventilation and perfusion going to the areas of lung to be resected, and, thus, predict residual pulmonary function. Patients requiring split function studies have a higher mortality than those meeting all major criteria, but the mortality is still within acceptable limits for surgery. **While a large number of "minor" criteria have correlated with operative mortality (Table 6.15), these are not as useful as the major criteria plus split function and physiologic studies, and**

Table 6.14.   Split Pulmonary Function and Pulmonary Artery Occlusion Studies for Pneumonectomy

	Reference
1. Predicted post-pneumonectomy or lobectomy $FEV_1 > 800$ ml	47
2. After ipsilateral pulmonary artery occlusion by balloon catheter and exercise with bicycle	
a. Mean contralateral pulmonary artery pressure < 35 mm Hg	
b. Systemic $PaO2 > 45$ mm Hg	47, 48

Table 6.15.   Minor Criteria for Pneumonectomy (Negative)

1. Age > 60 (especially if FEV_1, < 2 L)
2. $FEV_1 < 50\%$ FVC
3. $DL_{co} < 50\%$
4. MVV $> 50–70\%$
5. VC $< 70\%$
6. FVC < 0.5 (predicted postoperatively)
7. Abnormal EKG and MBC
8. Abnormal heart on chest x-ray
9. N_2 washout abnormal ($<3\%$)
10. RV/TLC $> 50\%$ predicted
11. EKG (PVCs, infarction, coronary insufficiency, non-specific ST-T changes)
12. FVC $< 50\%$
13. PaCO2 > 45 mm Hg

should not be used to deny a patient surgery.

Patients not meeting major criteria and split function tests for pneumonectomy may tolerate lobectomy or segmental resection. In these cases, split function studies should define the proportion of ventilation/perfusion going to both the lobe or segment to be resected and the whole lung.

Preoperative Evaluation

Patients not meeting all major criteria (Table 6.13) should be referred to a center performing split function and/or physiologic pulmonary artery occlusion studies. The quantitative perfusion lung scan is the split function test most commonly performed, and correlates at least as well as more invasive studies (59) with postoperative morbidity and mortality. A predicted FEV_1 of $> 0.8–1.0$ liters in the remaining lung is the criterion of operability for both pneumonectomy and lesser resection.

SUMMARY

For any patient about to undergo major surgery, functional assessment, both historically and objectively can identify most of those at high risk, and, in some instances, indicate pre- and postoperative maneuvers to minimize the risks of a bad outcome.

READINGS

1. Pett SB, Wernly JA: Respiratory function in surgical patients. Perioperative evaluation and management. *Surg Ann* 20:311–329, 1988.
2. Mohr DN, Jett JR: Preoperative evaluation of pulmonary risk factors. *J Gen Intern Med* 3:277–287, 1988.
3. Jackson CV: Preoperative pulmonary evaluation. *Arch Intern Med* 148:2120–2127, 1988.
4. Tisi GM: Preoperative evaluation of pulmonary function. *Am Rev Resp Dis* 119:293–310, 1979.
5. Harman E, Lillington G: Pulmonary risk factors in surgery. *Med Clin N Am* 63:1289–1298, 1979.
6. Rehder K, Sessler AD, Marsh HM: General anesthesia and the lung. *Am Rev Resp Dis* 112:541–563, 1975.
7. Block AJ, Olsen GN: Preoperative pulmonary function testing. *JAMA* 235:257–258, 1976.
8. Tarhan S, Moffitt EA, Sessler AD, Douglas WW, Taylor WF: Risk of anesthesia and surgery in patients with chronic bronchitis and chronic obstructive pulmonary disease. *Surgery* 74:720–726, 1973.
9. Pearce AC, Jones RM: Smoking and anesthesia: Preoperative abstinence and perioperative morbidity. *Anesthesiology* 61:576–584, 1984.
10. Williams DC, Brenowitz JB: Prohibitive lung function and major surgical procedures. *Am J Surg* 132:763–766, 1976.
11. Okinaka AJ, Glenn F: The surgical patient with emphysema and CO_2 retention. *Arch Surg* 90:436–443, 1965.
12. Wightman JAK: A prospective survey of the incidence of postoperative pulmonary complications. *Br J Surg* 55:85–91, 1968.
13. Stein M, Koota GM, Simon M, Fran HA: Pulmonary evaluation of surgical patients. *JAMA* 181:765–770, 1962.
14. Gracey DR, Divertie MB, Didier EP: Preoperative pulmonary preparation of patients with chronic obstructive pulmonary disease. *Chest* 76:123–129, 1979.
15. Diament ML, Palmer KNV: Spirometry for preoperative assessment of airways resistance. *Lancet* 1:1251–1253, 1967.
16. Latimer RG, Dickman M, Day WC, et al.: Ventilatory patterns and pulmonary complications after upper abdominal surgery determined by preoperative and postoperative computerized spirometry and blood gas analysis. *Am J Surg* 122:622–632, 1971.
17. Miller WF, Wu N, Johnson RL Jr: Convenient method of evaluating pulmonary ventilatory function with a single breath test. *Anesthesiology* 17:480–493, 1956.
18. Diament ML, Palmer KNV: Postoperative changes in gas tensions of arterial blood in ventilatory function. *Lancet* 2:180–182, 1966.
19. Cain HD, Stevens PM, Adaniya R: Preoperative pulmonary function and complications after cardiovascular surgery. *Chest* 76:130–135, 1979.
20. Stein M: Pulmonary evaluation and therapy prior to surgery. *Int Anesth Clin* 9:3–19, 1971.
21. Gaensler EA: Preoperative evaluation of lung function. *Int Anesth Clin* 3:249–275, 1965.
22. Hodgkin JE, Dines De, Didier EP: Preoperative evaluation of the patient with pulmonary disease. *Mayo Clin Proc* 48:114–118, 1973.
23. Ravin MB: Comparison of spinal and general anesthesia for lower abdominal surgery in patients with chronic obstructive pulmonary disease. *Anesthesiology* 35:319–322, 1971.
24. Hendolin H, Lahtinen J, Lansimies E, et al.: The effect of thoracic epidural analgesia on respiratory function after cholecystectomy. *Act Anaesthesiol Scand* 31:645–651, 1987.
25. Askrog VF, Smith TC, Eckenhoff JE: Changes in pulmonary ventilation during spinal anesthesia. *Surg Gynecol Obstet* 119:563–567, 1964.
26. Paskin S, Rodman R, Smith TC: The effect of spinal anesthesia on the pulmonary function of patients with chronic obstructive pulmonary disease. *Ann Surg* 161:35–40, 1969.
27. Boutros AR, Weisel M: Comparison of effects of three anaesthetic techniques on patients with severe pulmonary obstructive disease. *Can Anaesth Soc J* 18:286–292, 1971.
28. Crape, RD, et al.: Spirometry as a preoperative screening test in morbidly obese patients. *Surgery* 99:763–767, 1986.
29. Bartlett RH, Gazzaniga AB, Geraghty TR: Respiratory maneuvers to prevent postoperative pulmonary complications. *JAMA* 224:1017–1021, 1973.
30. Thulbourne T, Young MH: Prophylactic penicillin and postoperative chest infections. *Lancet* 2:907–909, 1962.
31. Stein M, Cassara EL: Preoperative pulmonary evaluation and therapy for surgery patients. *JAMA* 211:787–790, 1970.
32. Dohi S, Gold MI: Comparison of two methods of postoperative respiratory care. *Chest* 73:592–595, 1978.
33. Thoren L: Postoperative pulmonary complications: Observations on their prevention by means of physiotherapy. *Acta Chir Scand* 107:193–205, 1954.
34. Palmer KNV, Sellick BA: The prevention of postoperative pulmonary atelectasis. *Lancet* 1:164–168, 1953.
35. Baxter WD, Levine RS, Rapids G: An evaluation of intermittent positive pressure breathing in the prevention of postoperative pulmonary complications. *Arch Surg* 98:795–798, 1969.
36. Jung R, Wight J, Nusser R, Rosoff L: Comparison of three methods of respiratory care following upper abdominal surgery. *Chest* 78:31–35, 1980.
37. Cottrell JE, Siker ES: Preoperative intermittent positive pressure breathing therapy in patients with chronic obstructive lung disease: Effect on postoperative pulmonary complications. *Anesth Analg* 52:258–262, 1973.
38. Bartlett RH, Gazzaniga AB, Geraghty T: The yawn maneuver: Prevention and treatment of

postoperative pulmonary complications. *Surg Forum* 22:196–198, 1971.

39. Valentine MD: The asthmatic patient as a surgical risk. *Surg Clin N Am* 50:631–635, 1970.
40. Oh SH, Patterson R: Surgery in corticosteroid-dependent asthmatics. *J Allergy Clin Immunol* 53:345–351, 1974.
41. Schlenker JD, Hubay CA: Colonization of the respiratory tract and postoperative pulmonary infections. *Arch Surg* 107:313–317, 1973.
42. Hobbs BB, Hinchcliff WA, Greenspan RH: Effects of acute lobar atelectasis on pulmonary hemodynamics. *Invest Radiol* 7:1–9, 1972.
43. Schlenker JD, Hubay CA: The pathogenesis of postoperative atelectasis. *Arch Surg* 107:846–850, 1973.
44. Mittman C: Assessment of operative risk in thoracic surgery. *Am Rev Resp Dis* 84:197–207, 1961.
45. Boushy SF, Helgason AH, Billig DM, Gyorsky FG: Clinical, physiologic, and morphologic examination of the lung in patients with bronchogenic carcinoma and the relation of the findings to postoperative deaths. *Am Rev Resp Dis* 101:685–695, 1970.
46. Boushy SF, Billig DM, North LB, Helgason AH: Clinical course related to preoperative and postoperative pulmonary function in patients with bronchogenic carcinoma. *Chest* 59:383–391, 1971.
47. Olsen GN, Block AJ, Swenson EW, Castle JR, Eynne JW: Pulmonary function evaluation of the lung resection candidate: A prospective study. *Am Rev Resp Dis* 111:379–387, 1975.
48. Boysen PG, Block AJ, Olsen GN, Moulder PV, Harris JO, Rawitscher RE: Prospective evaluation of pneumonectomy using the ^{99m}technetium quantitative perfusion lung scan. *Chest* 72:422–425, 1977.
49. Lockwood P: The principles of predicting the risk of post-thoracotomy function-related complications in bronchial carcinoma. *Respiration* 30:329–344, 1973.
50. Lockwood P: The relationship between pre-operative lung function test results and post-operative complications in carcinoma of the bronchus. *Respiration* 30:105–116, 1973.
51. Lockwood P: Respiratory function and cardiopulmonary complications following thoractomy for carcinoma of the lung. *Respiration* 29:468–479, 1972.
52. Lockwood P: Lung function test results and the risk of post-thoracotomy complications. *Respiration* 30:529–542, 1973.
53. Simonsson BG, Malmberg R: Differentiation between localized and generalized airway obstruction. *Thorax* 19:416–419, 1964.
54. Ali MK, Mountain CF, Ewer MS, Johnston D, Haynie TP: Predicting loss of pulmonary function after resection for bronchogenic carcinoma. *Chest* 77:337–342, 1980.
55. Reichel J: Assessment of operative risk of pneumonectomy. *Chest* 62:570–576, 1972.
56. Wang KC, Howland WS: Cardiac and pulmonary evaluation in elderly patients before elective surgical operations. *JAMA* 166:993–997, 1958.
57. Van De Water JM, Watring WG, Linton LA, Murphey M, Byron RL: Prevention of postoperative pulmonary complications. *Surg Gynecol Obstet* 135:229–233, 1972.
58. Uggia LG: Indications for and results of thoracic surgery with regard to respiratory and circulatory function test. *Acta Chir Scand* 111:197–212, 1956.
59. Olsen GN, Block AJ, Tobias JA: Prediction of postpneumonectomy pulmonary function using quantitative magroaggregate lung scanning. *Chest* 66:13–16, 1974.
60. Schwartz HJ, Lowell FL, Melby JC: Steroid resistance in bronchial asthma. *Ann Int Med* 69:493–499, 1968.
61. Chester EH, Belman MJ, Bahler RC, et al: The effect of physical training on cardiopulmonary performance in patients with chronic obstructive pulmonary disease. *Chest* 72:695–702, 1977.
62. Ellul-Mecalleff R, Fenech FF: Effect of intravenous prednisolone in asthmatics with diminished adrenergic responsiveness. *Lancet* 2:1269–1270, 1975.
63. Plafsky KM, Ofilvie RI: Dosage of theophylline in bronchial asthma. *N Engl J Med* 292:1218–1221, 1975.
64. Ribon A, Parikh S: Drug-induced asthma: A review. *Ann Allergy* 44:220–224, 1980.
65. Rosenthal RR (ed): Bronchoprovocation: State of the art. *J Allergy Clin Immunol* 64:569–674, 1979.
66. Pierce AK, Robertson J: Pulmonary complications of general surgery. *Ann Rev Med* 28:211–221, 1977.
67. Shnider SM, Papper EM: Anesthesia for the asthmatic patient. *Anesthesiology* 22:886–892, 1961.
68. Boutros AR, Weisel M: Comparison of effects of three anaesthetic techniques on patients with severe pulmonary obstructive disease. *Can Anaesth Soc J* 18:286–292, 1971.
69. Iverson LIG, Ecker RR, Fox HE, May IA: A comparative study of IPPB, the incentive spirometer, and blow bottles: The prevention of atelectasis following cardiac surgery. *Ann Thorac Surg* 25:197–200, 1978.
70. Gross NJ: Drug therapy. Ipratropium bromide. *New Engl J Med* 319:486–494, 1988.

7

Basic Mechanical Respiratory Support

Larry B. Grossman

Mechanical respiratory support is generally considered when the clinician is aware of either one or more of four basic situations compromising the patient: the patient is unable to secure the quantity of oxygen required; unable to adequately remove carbon dioxide; unable to protect the airway; or unable to clear secretions. The technical aspects of mechanical ventilation will be dealt with in some detail, emphasizing the "how to" aspects. Complications will be discussed with concern for prevention and prompt recognition. Due to the breadth of this chapter, the specifics and mechanics rather than theory will be emphasized. Abbreviations used are presented in Table 7.1.

EPIDEMIOLOGY

There are several specific situations in which respiratory failure requiring mechanical ventilation is more likely to occur. An appreciation of the most common risk factors that lead to hypoxemia and/or hypercarbia will aid in anticipation and prompt corrective action.

The patient with a history of an obstructive airway abnormality will have impaired gas exchange as a result of increased airway resistance and the trapping of air with small airway abnormalities (e.g., asthma, emphysema, and bronchitis), or from increased large airway resistance due to tumor or tracheal stenosis. The **flow-volume loop** is useful in determining whether the obstruction is due to large or small airway obstruction by the graphic presentation of the data. Pulmonary function tests provide quan-

Table 7.1. Abbreviations

A-aDO$_2$	Alveolar-arterial oxygen tension difference
ABG	Arterial blood gas
CPAP	Continuous positive airway pressure
CVP	Central venous pressure
FiO$_2$	Inspired oxygen fraction
HFJV	High frequency jet ventilation
HFO	High frequency oscillation
HFPPV	High frequency positive pressure ventilation
IMV	Intermittent mandatory ventilation
NIF	Negative inspiratory force
PaCO$_2$	Arterial carbon dioxide tension
PaO$_2$	Arterial oxygen tension
PEEP	Positive end expiratory pressure
SIMV	Synchronized IMV
VC	Vital capacity
V$_D$/V$_T$	Ratio of dead space to tidal volume

titative information that can determine the degree of impairment, the response to bronchodilators, and progressive changes in the patient's chronic ailment. Clinically, the compromised patient exhibits an increased effort to ventilate, an increased heart rate, a decreasing PaO$_2$ with an increasing PaCO$_2$ and a decreasing pH. **The pH** is an indicator of the progressive severity of the clinical situation. Bronchodilators are usually the first line of therapy in the effort to avoid intubation in the patient with small airway obstruction, but if the situation deteriorates, then mechanical support is often required.

Inadequate gas exchange due to an acute parenchymal disease may require respiratory support. A high oxygen gradient and low compliance are characteristic of processes such as pneumonia, atelectasis, and pulmonary edema. Generally, the problem is more of oxygenation than ventilation, but both are seen. In any case, the patient must dramatically increase his work of breathing.

Ventilatory failure (hypercarbia) can be due to several different or combined situations. Hypoventilation can be the result of a neurological problem, as in the case of muscle weakness or central depression (1). Preoperative evaluations and the past clinical history can alert one to possible postoperative respiratory compromise for patients with neuromuscular weakness. Guillain-Barré syndrome is but one example of a diagnosis that can be followed by serial clinical signs to indicate whether ventilatory support is necessary. An iatrogenic cause of muscle weakness is the use of muscle relaxants in the operative period. One must check the anesthesia report for documentation, as well as clinical signs, that the muscle relaxants have been adequately reversed. A basic evaluation would be to check the patient's grip and ability to lift his head for five seconds. In addition, a nerve stimulator is often used by the anesthesiologist to evaluate the effect of the neuromuscular blocking agents. In cases in which succinylcholine has been used, postoperative muscle weakness could possibly be the result of a pseudocholinesterase deficiency. Whatever the cause, mechanical respiratory support should be used as long as the respiratory status is compromised.

Cranial surgery or trauma may alter the respiratory pattern and level of consciousness. Artificial hyperventilation to a $PaCO_2$ of approximately 30 torr can decrease cerebral blood flow and aid in decreasing cerebral edema. The neurologist or neurosurgeon may request the patient to be ventilated to a lowered $PaCO_2$ as a treatment modality. This is often fine tuned by monitoring intracranial pressures. Also, since medications may be used to sedate the neurological patient, respiratory support may be required. If the patient is obtunded, one must protect the airway from the risk of aspiration or obstructed breathing.

Narcotics are the medications that classically cause a patient to hypoventilate or even to obstruct the airway. Narcotics will alter the carbon dioxide response curve so that a higher carbon dioxide tension is required to promote a ventilatory response. Other sedatives may act with the narcotics to further alter the response curve and cause hypoventilation. When one reverses a narcotic with an antagonist, one must be vigilant to the fact that the duration of the reversal agent and the narcotic may differ. If the effect of the antagonist dissipates before the narcotic, the patient may become renarcotized.

The specific type of surgery or trauma is a major factor regarding the need for respiratory support, as previously noted with cranial surgery. The chest can be effected by pneumothorax, hemothorax, or hydrothorax. Similarly, chest wall instability can cause hypoxia, a decreased vital capacity, hypoventilation, and an increased work of breathing. Upper abdominal surgery may affect ventilation by impairing diaphragmatic excursions. Also, incisional pain and the requirement for narcotics can be major factors resulting in shallow breathing and atelectasis.

The respiratory problems of the obese patient will be magnified after surgery. Since the work of breathing is increased for these individuals, the addition of drugs, position in bed, and incisional pain will compound the problem. The obese patient generally ventilates more easily in a sitting position, due to the large abdomen and its contents not pressing against the diaphragm.

Poor nutrition is often the factor that upsets a marginal situation. With further postoperative deterioration in nutrition, the marginal patient may not be able to maintain the work of breathing.

There is also the problem of **restric-**

tive diseases that limit the ventilatory capacity. Patients with significant scoliosis, ankylosing spondylitis, etc., must be protected from all the factors that might compromise their already decreased vital capacity. A restrictive abnormality can be temporarily improved by removing ascites or effusion.

The addition of surgery can add factors that cause the marginal patient to require mechanical respiratory support. Kofke (2) describes why pulmonary dysfunction is seen after major abdominal and thoracic surgery. The significant reduction in the functional residual capacity is accompanied by the loss of expiratory reserve volume and inspiratory reserve. There is also a decrease in the forced vital capacity and maximal expiratory flows. This low lung volume situation results in small airway closure and atelectasis.

One study that specifically sought to identify the risk factors associated with postoperative respiratory morbidity concluded that the factors were a productive cough, purulent sputum, a low one second forced expiratory volume, upper abdominal surgery, a previous history of postoperative respiratory problems, and the presence of a nasogastric tube (3).

When a high probability of respiratory failure is evident, the patient should remain intubated and be given respiratory support postoperatively. The patient can be extubated when it will not be deleterious; for example, the patient after heart surgery who should have a stable cardiovascular system prior to extubation.

INDICATIONS FOR INTUBATION AND MECHANICAL SUPPORT

The indications for intubation and/or mechanical support will be discussed together since intubation requires mechanical support of varying degrees. We will consider four areas: **oxygenation, ventilation, pulmonary toilet, and airway protection.** It should be noted that the criteria for intubation (or mechanical ventilatory support) may be considered as the opposite of those for weaning from ventilatory support and extubation (see Table 7.4, p 86).

Whereas the apneic patient obviously requires intubation and mechanical support, those patients with lesser degrees of respiratory failure must be individually evaluated. To determine the **adequacy of oxygenation,** one uses arterial blood gas (ABG) values, alveolar-arterial oxygen tension differences (A-aDO$_2$), or a comparison of the inspired oxygen (FiO$_2$) to the PaO$_2$. An increase in the A-aDO$_2$ is detrimental and can be due to right to left shunting of blood past alveoli that are perfused but not ventilated (true shunt) or as a result of incomplete oxygenation of blood passing by alveoli that are poorly ventilated (a ventilation-perfusion inequality). When a patient is being followed with pulse oximetry, a sudden and pronounced decrease in the oxyhemoglobin saturation may indicate an event necessitating additional respiratory support. The section on technical aspects presents values and data concerned with oxygenation.

Ventilation can be evaluated in several ways. One technique is to determine the PaCO$_2$ and pH. Another method is to consider whether the patient must or can increase his work of breathing as determined by serial minute ventilation data. Fatigue and abrupt decompensation may ensue if this is not evaluated or anticipated. The excess work of breathing may also cause detrimental effects in other areas, primarily the cardiovascular system.

The pH and PaCO$_2$ may appear normal, but the work involved to keep the values normal may be too much for the patient to maintain. Generally, a PaCO$_2$ greater than 55 torr is hypoventilation requiring intubation, unless there is chronic hypercapnia with a normal pH. A respiratory rate of greater than 35/minute indicates a current ventilatory problem and surely puts the patient at risk once he tires. A vital capacity (VC) less than 15 ml/kg of body weight indicates an inadequate ventilatory reserve and a limited ability to cough productively. Inefficient ventilation can be determined by an increased dead space to tidal volume ratio (V_D/V_T) where 0.3 is normal. Clinically, one looks for ineffective or mechanically uncoordinated ventilation.

A depressed level of consciousness identifies a patient who is not able to **protect his airway** from obstruction or aspiration. Since aspiration can precipitate a rapid respiratory arrest, the obtunded patient must be carefully evaluated for laryngeal reflexes. One must be aware that if a nasogastric tube in an obtunded patient becomes obstructed or if the patient develops active emesis, the nasogastric tube can cause the cardio-esophageal sphincter to be less competent, making aspiration a significant risk. In these situations, the endotracheal tube is an effective way to protect the airway.

The endotracheal tube also provides a means for satisfactory **pulmonary toilet** in the patient who cannot cough adequately. The patient with thick or copious secretions may not be able to clear the secretions if he cannot generate a negative inspiratory force (NIF) of at least 25 cm of H_2O or has a VC of less than 15 ml/kg of body weight. If the patient is not able to take a deep breath, he will be at risk for not keeping the alveoli expanded and clearing secretions. The chest x-ray should be examined for areas of atelectasis and pneumonia. Fiberoptic bronchoscopy is sometimes required in addition to routine suctioning.

In summary, an increasing $PaCO_2$, a decreasing PaO_2 and pH, respiratory fatigue, risk of aspiration or airway obstruction, and an ineffective cough would each suggest the need for careful evaluation for intubation and mechanical respiratory support (4, 5).

SOURCES OF INFORMATION FOR VENTILATORY PLANS

The individual undertaking postoperative ventilatory care can gather considerable information by consulting the anesthesiologist's preoperative evaluation note and the anesthesia record from the operation. This will provide data as to whether the patient is a likely candidate for respiratory failure and the immediate indications for mechanical ventilation. The pertinent preoperative information will often mention preexisting respiratory problems, responses to therapies, chest x-ray reports, results from pulmonary function tests and arterial blood gases, and prior surgical experiences. The prior records may reveal past surgical and postoperative respiratory complications, and successful or unsuccessful treatment of problems. They may also alert the physician to anticipate or prevent adverse situations during the present admission. Based on the preoperative evaluation, recommendations might include bronchodilators, chest physiotherapy, alerting the patient to the possibility of postoperative intubation, and instructing the patient in postoperative respiratory plans.

The anesthesia record should note the surgical procedure and complications, fluid replacement, the ventilation technique with volumes and rate, the type of anesthetic, intubation approach and difficulties, intraoperative laboratory tests ordered, the reversal of muscle relaxants and/or narcotics, and the stability of various systems. The agents used for the anesthetic are important due to their different actions and durations. An asthmatic patient may have had clear breath sounds during the surgery due to the bronchodilator effects of a halogenated gas, but postoperatively his intrinsic disease and the irritation of the endotracheal tube may require the immediate use of bronchodilators. When reviewing an anesthetic using a narcotic approach, the

Table 7.2.   Preoperative and Operative Information That Might Be Useful Postoperatively

ANESTHESIA PREOPERATIVE EVALUATION DATA BASE

History and Physical   Orders
    Laboratory results
Chest X-ray reports   ABG results
Pulmonary function tests: with and without
    bronchodilators
Respiratory Problems: treatment and re-
    sponse to treatment
Previous anesthetics: operative and postop-
    erative problems

ANESTHESIA RECORD

Operative procedure   Complications
Ventilator settings: FiO_2, volumes, rates
Intubation: difficulties, size of endotracheal
    tube
Anesthetic technique and agents: halogen-
    ated agents, narcotics, muscle relaxants
Fluids   Invasive monitors   Nasogastric tube
Temperature   Operative laboratory tests

length of action of the agent and amount used are key concerns. The patient's temperature during and after the procedure may effect the oxygen consumption, metabolism, and reversability of the relaxants. Table 7.2 lists some pertinent information that may be available by reviewing the preanesthesia evaluation sheet, past records, the chart, and the anesthesia record. Verbal communication with the anesthesiologist is an excellent approach, but the records should always be reviewed. Communication with the respiratory therapists and nurses is also essential.

TECHNICAL ASPECTS OF MECHANICAL VENTILATION

The technical aspects of mechanical ventilation can be approached by considering the specific indications requiring the mechanical support. Although various needs will overlap and must be integrated into the overall plan, this approach provides a starting point.

Oxygenation is a priority in the postoperative period. The color of the patient's skin, mucous membranes, and nailbeds provides the basic clinical sign. However, cyanosis is an unreliable indicator of hypoxemia since a sufficient amount of reduced hemoglobin must be available, the finding is subjective, and peripheral cyanosis may be due to the patient being cold postoperatively. Therefore, a high index of suspicion and clinical signs will alert the physician to gather more information. A PaO_2 will further delineate the situation when required. Since the patient is usually receiving supplemental oxygen, the FiO_2 and PaO_2 can be compared to determine if the FiO_2 is adequate. When the patient arrives from the operating room with an endotracheal tube in place, one usually starts with the FiO_2 used in the operating room, and then changes are made according to the PaO_2. The pulse oximeter is often useful as a noninvasive means by which the oxyhemoglobin saturation of functional hemoglobin can be monitored. The accuracy of the pulse oximeter may be compromised by significant levels of dysfunctional hemoglobins (e.g., carboxyhemoglobin and methemoglobin). Continued intubation is usually required if the A-aDO_2 is greater than 350 torr or if the PaO_2 is less than 60–70 torr with supplemental oxygen. Of course, the clinical impressions and signs must be correlated with the laboratory values. The FiO_2 should be analyzed to be certain that the system is actually delivering the oxygen concentration desired.

One must check the intubated patient for proper positioning of the endotracheal tube. Bilateral breath sounds and possibly a chest x-ray will determine that one is not ventilating only one lung (generally the right lung) and causing a massive shunt due to the perfusion of both lungs with the ventilation of only one lung. When listening for bilateral breath sounds, one must listen along the mid-axillary lines in order to determine that the breath sounds are equal for both lungs. If the endotracheal tube impinges on the carina, the patient may continue to cough and be uncomfortable. Also, one will not be able to satisfactorily suction both lungs. The endotracheal tube should be 3–5 cm above the carina. If for any reason fiberoptic bronchoscopy is necessary, the tube position can also be verified during the procedure.

Since one would like to achieve a PaO_2 that permits nearly full hemoglobin saturation, a minimum PaO_2 of 60 torr is required in the acutely ill. Of course, the patient with severe chronic obstructive pulmonary disease is often an exception to this rule of thumb. Due to the concern of oxygen toxicity, one attempts to decrease the FiO_2 as long as the PaO_2 is not a problem. **Oxygen toxicity** due to prolonged high inspired oxygen tensions causes a deterioration of pulmonary function (6). There is an increased right to left shunt, decreased pulmonary compliance, and a decreased functional residual capacity. Structurally, there is a loss of the capillary endothelial integrity, interstitial edema, hemorrhage, and fibrosis. The tolerance to an increased FiO_2 is variable, and there are no definite limits for safety. Generally, it is felt that clinically significant changes occur if the patient with normal lungs receives 48 hours of exposure to an FiO_2 equal to or greater than 0.6 at one atmosphere. However, an FiO_2 above 0.5 in a critically ill patient has the potential of causing significant damage. Since the safest elevated FiO_2 for continuous administration has not been clearly defined, we usually seek an FiO_2 less than 0.5 and preferably 0.4. Register (7) studied the results of mechanically ventilating patients with an FiO_2 of 0.5 for 16–24 hours and found that there may be an impairment of pulmonary gas exchange after extubation. He recommended that supplemental oxygen be administered at the lowest possible level that will provide an oxyhemoglobin saturation greater than 90%.

By using positive end expiratory pressure (PEEP) or continuous positive airway pressure (CPAP), one can generally decrease the FiO_2 to safer levels. Most patients can be started on PEEP at 5 cm H_2O since PEEP is useful in intubated patients who are at risk for developing decreased lung volume. **The contraindications to PEEP** are: an unstable cardiovascular system in which impeding venous return could be deleterious, emphysematous bullae, or an increased intracranial pressure. PEEP is titrated against the cardiovascular effects and the desired oxygenation. In the difficult case, one may need to consider cardiac output, PaO_2 and mixed venous PO_2. Since the PEEP can have a negative effect on cardiac output, one titrates to seek the "best" PEEP. This means that 10 cm H_2O of PEEP may not be better than 5 cm. The "more is better" concept does not work in this situation. One seeks the lowest PEEP that enables one to use a "safe" FiO_2 to provide a satisfactory PaO_2. If the mixed venous oxygen tension decreases with PEEP, the problem of tissue hypoxia may not be improved until cardiac output is improved. One must then work to improve the cardiovascular hemodynamics with the appropriate therapies (i.e., vasopressors, fluids, etc.). The basic goal is to lower the FiO_2 to 0.4 or less while achieving an acceptable PaO_2 (8).

Often, preoperative pulmonary function tests with and without bronchodilators will suggest that one consider intravenous or nebulized agents in the postoperative period to optimize bronchodilation. With an endotracheal tube in place, the normally minimally reactive preoperative airway may now require a bronchodilator.

VENTILATORY EQUIPMENT AND ITS MANAGEMENT

Basically there are two types of ventilators. The **pressure cycled ventilator** delivers an inflation until the direct preset pressure is achieved and then a passive expiration ensues. Since the tidal volume is determined by the inspired gas flow, preset pressure, and the patient's compliance, the tidal volume can vary with this approach.

The **volume-limited ventilator** delivers a preset volume regardless of the pressure, although there is a peak pressure pop-off valve as a safety measure. The volume-limited ventilator is generally preferred because of the constant tidal volume. One can set the ventilator with a tidal volume of 12 ml/kg of body weight (range of 10–15 ml/kg) and observe the movement of the chest wall to be certain the initial volume appears adequate. The exact tidal volume and rate can be fine tuned with arterial blood gases (ABGs).

The four approaches to the respiratory rate are: **controlled, assist/control, intermittent mandatory ventilation (IMV),** and **synchronized IMV (SIMV).** Table 7.3 compares the basics of the various modes of ventilation. Controlled ventilation is basically a set rate with no spontaneous ventilation permitted by the patient. Although the assist/control mode allows a full tidal volume whenever the patient initiates an inspiration, it guarantees a preset rate even if not initiated by the patient. IMV allows spontaneous ventilation of variable volume between the mandatory ventilations. The SIMV mode synchronizes the positive-pressure inspiration with the patient's spontaneous breaths. It should be noted that there has not been shown any physiologic advantages to the SIMV concept. Some advocates of IMV point out the greater ease of weaning the patient from ventilatory support. Those individuals advocating the assisted mode see this method as a safeguard, since full volumes are guaranteed or generated with less effort.

Cane and Shapiro (9) have presented an excellent review article that logically presents and compares the four modes of ventilation by their ability to minimize disruption of cardiopulmonary physiology. They point out that full ventilatory support (i.e., the ventilator provides all the energy for effective alveolar ventilation) can be provided by all four modes, but partial ventilatory support (i.e., the patient and the ventilator provide the ef-

Table 7.3. Basic Comparison of Mechanical Ventilation Methods as Reviewed in the Text

I. Pressure-Cycled
- inflation to preset pressure
- passive expiration
- tidal volume can vary

II. Volume-Limited
- preset volume
- constant tidal volume
- peak-pressure pop-off valve

1. Controlled
   - preset rate
   - no spontaneous ventilation
   - can provide full ventilatory support

2. Assist/control
   - preset rate
   - full tidal volume with patient initiated inspiration
   - can provide full ventilatory support
   - advocates point out safety of guaranteed volumes

3. Intermittent mandatory ventilation (IMV)
   - spontaneous ventilation of variable volume between mandatory ventilations
   - advocates point out use in weaning
   - can provide full and partial ventilatory support
   - less disruption of cardiopulmonary physiology

4. Synchronized IMV
   - synchronizes the positive-pressure inspiration with the spontaneous breaths
   - can provide full and partial ventilatory support
   - less disruption of cardiopulmonary physiology
   - concern that the demand valve increases the work of breathing at rates <4

III. High Frequency Ventilation
- lower mean airway pressure

1. High Frequency Positive Pressure Ventilation (HFPPV)
   - 60–120 breaths/minute
   - no entrainment of additional gas

2. High Frequency Jet Ventilation (HFJV)
   - 80–300 breaths/minute
   - entrainment of additional gas

3. High Frequency Oscillation (HFO)
   - 600–3000 breaths/minute
   - higher flow of oxygen must be provided

fective alveolar ventilation) can only be managed by IMV or SIMV. They present information that shows that partial ventilatory support has advantages of less disruption of cardiac output and ventilation-perfusion relationships, that it is very effective in conjunction with PEEP, and that less sedation may be needed. There is some concern that the demand valve used with SIMV may increase the work of breathing at ventilator rates of four per minute or less.

One technique is to start with an IMV rate of 10/min and wean as tolerated. This provides full support until the patient's status allows increased spontaneous ventilations. The inspiration to expiration ratio is usually initially set as 1:2. The patient with chronic obstructive pulmonary disease or asthma may require a longer expiratory phase. By checking an ABG approximately 20 minutes after a setting change, one can aggressively titrate as required and accomplish weaning as permitted. One seeks a normal pH with a $PaCO_2$ at 35–40 torr. Obviously, the vital signs should be monitored during the changes. A pulse oximeter is a useful continuous monitor of oxyhemoglobin saturation. If the patient is not in phase with the ventilator or in any way is struggling with the ventilator, one must immediately check that the circuit is not the cause of hypoxia or hypoventilation, and decide whether sedation is necessary.

A method of displaying CO_2 concentration changes during respiratory cycles is referred to as **capnography.** The instruments usually used are infrared capnographers and mass spectrometers. In his review article, Carlon (10) and his fellow authors point out that capnography is a qualitative rather than quantitative technique and discuss some examples of the clinical use of capnography. The ability to monitor mechanical failures and changes during weaning are being studied. Capnography may have a monitoring role in intensive care units.

In very special circumstances when muscle relaxants are deemed necessary, there must be total vigilance with ventilator alarms, appropriate monitors, and notification of participating staff. One example of the use of neuromuscular blocking agents is in head trauma to reduce intrathoracic pressure and venous pressure in order to decrease intracranial pressure. One must be constantly concerned about inadequate analgesia or sedation in patients that are on neuromuscular blocking agents. Paralysis puts the patient at risk for disconnection from the ventilator, pulmonary emboli from immobility, lack of a cough reflex, and peripheral nerve injury from careless positioning (11).

Since the obtunded patient cannot communicate, he is dependent on alarms and monitors to indicate faulty ventilation. Conversely, one can help the alert patient communicate his concerns for comfort by providing writing implements or word charts, and appropriate sedation or pain medication. The patient with a tracheostomy might benefit from a "talking tracheostomy tube," using an external airflow directed to the larynx for speech, or an electric artificial larynx device, or other artificial voicing systems.

Proper pulmonary toilet is essential in the intubated patient since the patient will be unable to clear his secretions. Where appropriate, the patient must be turned to different positions as tolerated and percussed in order to mobilize secretions. Hourly hyperinflation with an anesthesia bag and suctioning with sterile techniques is essential for satisfactory pulmonary toilet. Hyperinflation was also thought to be necessary since the endotracheal tube prevents the patient from sighing effectively. In patients with otherwise normal lungs, hyperventilation will reverse the deterioration of lung function caused by prolonged mechanical ventilation. However, this routine clinical practice was shown to be of no value in patients with respiratory failure on prolonged ventilation (12). Suctioning must be done carefully to avoid complications. **Endotracheal suctioning** can cause bradycardia and hypotension in some individuals. Winston's study (13) compared the prophylactic use of either nebulized (0.05 mg/kg) or parenteral (1 mg) atropine to prevent cardiovascular problems. Both preparations prevented the hypotensive response, but there was more tachycardia with parenteral use. At no time should the catheter be down the endotracheal tube for a prolonged period of time. A safe method by which to accomplish this task is to manually ventilate with oxygen, place the suction catheter into position, apply suction on withdrawal, and resume ventilation. Also available is a double-lumen suction catheter that simultaneously insufflates oxygen at 10 L/min while suctioning (14). One may instill 1–2 ml of sterile saline between ventilations if the secretions are particularly thick. If a routine for pulmonary toilet is not adhered to, the patient is at risk for atelectasis, pneumonia, and inspissated secretions. The chest x-ray will assist the physician in ordering chest physiotherapy in the best position to drain affected areas of the lungs (15). Fiberoptic bronchoscopy is useful for diagnosis, suctioning, and lavaging in difficult or persistent situations.

Since the endotracheal or tracheostomy tube bypasses the patient's humidification system and dry gases affect ciliary action, one must humidify the gas in order to prevent the drying of secretions and mucosal irritation. Devices for bubble diffusion, jet nebulization, or passover humidification can be used to provide heated humidification.

The choice of an oral endotracheal tube versus a nasal endotracheal tube depends on the consideration of a number of factors. Generally, the nasal tube is better tolerated by the patient for longer periods. The nasal tube has less movement on the trachea and less accidental extubations. However, one must take care to prevent nasal necrosis. The oral tube must be securely taped to the upper lip to decrease mobility. The nasal tube would be contraindicated where there is risk of nasal hemorrhage (as in the anticoagulated patient), risk of sinus infection, or if there is a leakage of cerebral spinal fluid from the nose. One usually seeks an endotracheal tube that will be large enough to prevent airway resistance and small enough to not apply excessive pressure to the laryngeal area, and that has a cuff of the high compliance/low pressure type. Every day the cuff pressures need to be checked (<25 cm H_2O). The cuffs on the endotracheal tube must have just enough volume for a seal. This can be accomplished by letting volume out of the cuff until a small leak is heard with positive pressure ventilation, and then adding a small volume to just seal the system. If a tracheostomy tube is in place, it can be changed weekly once the stoma is developed. However the elective change of any tube should not be scheduled after a feeding, as one is risking a possible emesis and aspiration.

When to **convert from an endotracheal tube to a tracheostomy tube** has often been primarily a question of time. The appropriate length of time for the endotracheal tube to be in place is changing due to the low pressure cuffs now being used. Bishop (16) notes that a tracheostomy is best utilized in the patient who will require prolonged intubation and will benefit from the increased comfort, since it is no longer routine to perform a tracheostomy after 1 week of intubation. Direct fiberoptic visualization of the cuff site is now also possible. Generally, one might wait approximately 10–12 days before considering a tracheostomy. However, if there is a possibility that the patient might be extubated in a few days, one would probably delay the tracheostomy and weigh the relative risks.

Prior to removing a tracheostomy tube, one must determine that there is no requirement for positive pressure to augment oxygenation and ventilation, that pulmonary toilet can be accomplished without the tracheostomy, and that the patient can protect his airway. Certainly the patient who lacks a gag reflex is going to have difficulty protecting his airway. A simple test for determining protection of the airway can be accomplished by deflating the cuff, having the patient sip some very dilute methylene blue (a drop in a glass of water), and then checking to see if there is any blue suctioned from the trachea. If blue is noted, the patient did not pass the test. However, if no blue is noted, this is no guarantee that an aspiration could not occur. If the patient fails the test, one can encourage him to exercise his laryngeal apparatus by talking while the cuff is deflated and then retest. When the patient qualifies for removal of the tracheostomy tube, one can then insert a fenestrated tracheostomy tube. Since this tube does not have a cuff but does have an opening to allow free exchange from the oropharynx to the lungs, one can determine if the patient can handle his added dead space by plugging the exterior part of the tube. This allows the stoma to remain patent while testing the added dead space. Once the patient shows that he can handle the dead space and secretions, the fenestrated tube can be removed and a dressing applied.

PROBLEMS DUE TO MECHANICAL VENTILATION

The endotracheal tube can create problems if one is not attentive to details. Proper placement of the tube must be checked by auscultation and, if necessary, by chest x-ray to prevent intubation of the right mainstem bronchus or obstruction of the right upper lobe orifice. If the tube encroaches on the carina, the patient may cough and struggle due to discomfort. Since the tube must be patent to function properly, one must order humidification and suctioning to prevent inspissated secretions. Also, observe the tube for compression or kinking. The cuff on the endotracheal tube must be checked

for leaks or overinflation, as previously discussed.

Generally, an endotracheal tube with an internal diameter of 7.5–8.5 mm will be adequate for an adult. Laryngeal damage is usually related to large tube size, mobility of the tube, duration of intubation, local sepsis, and decreased vascularity in the area due to decreased cardiac output. Irritation and pressure causes edema, erosion, ulceration, and occasionally fibrosis when healing. Hoarseness or stridor can be caused by edema of the vocal cords. Obstruction can develop from subglottic edema. A flow volume loop pulmonary function test may aid in this diagnosis. The severity of the obstruction will determine whether conservative treatment, reintubation, or tracheostomy is required. Conservative treatment may entail humidification, oxygen, and possibly nebulized racemic epinephrine (0.5 ml in 1.5 ml of normal saline) every 2 hours. Some authors have recommended steroids for edematous obstruction. If the vocal cords or subglottic areas develop granulation or fibrosis, then surgical treatment may be required.

Tracheal complications are due to irritation and pressure causing edema, erosion, ulceration, and fibrosis. The irritation is a result of high cuff pressures and mobility of the tube. Erosion can cause a fistula or erode a major vessel with resulting catastrophic hemorrhage. Severe problems with ventilation develop when tracheomalacia causes collapse of the airway and obstruction. Tracheal stenosis is usually noted within 2 months of decannulation. **Generally, stridor indicates an airway narrowed to 5 mm or less.** In summary, the complications of intubation can be decreased by using low pressure cuffs and by securing the tube so that there is limited movement.

The patient who does not receive satisfactory nutrition may not be able to maintain the work of breathing. When tolerated, nasogastric or gastrostomy feedings are preferable to total parenteral nutrition. There is now data showing that total parenteral nutrition may increase CO_2 production and therefore may cause respiratory distress in the patient with already compromised ventilation. Increased ventilatory demands due to total parenteral nutrition may be alleviated by using more fat emulsion and less glucose than are contained in the standard hyperalimentation formulas. By measuring CO_2 production in expired gases or indirect calorimetry, appropriate changes in glucose could be made and followed.

The patient in the intensive care unit is at risk for stress gastritis and gastrointestinal hemorrhage. The use of steroids adds to this concern. Although the exact mechanism by which stress ulceration occurs has not been defined, the basic approach to prevention has been to decrease the gastric acidity. High potency antacids and histamine-2 receptor antagonists are used to achieve a gastric pH of >4 in order to decrease the incidence of bleeding from stress gastritis. When Noseworthy (17) and his colleagues evaluated medications for controlling the gastric pH, they concluded that intravenous ranitidine hydrochloride in a dosage of 200 mg/ day was as effective as antacids (Maalox and Amphogel) in reducing acidity. Increasing the dose of ranitidine did not provide additional control. Certainly any clinician using H-2 receptor antagonists should be aware of the side effects and contraindications.

Many authors have detailed the psychological problems of being in an intensive or critical care environment. Some patients with lengthy periods of mechanical ventilation are described as becoming **"ventilatory dependent."** The patient may hyperventilate or become agitated when he does not have the familiar sense of a functioning ventilator assisting him. This problem often requires consultation with a psychiatrist, emotional support by the staff, and subtle variations in using the ventilator. One advantage of the IMV technique is to allow the gradual decrease in the mechanical rate. In order to provide the patient with a psychologic sense of security, one may even be required to artificially cycle the machine while the patient is actually breathing spontaneously and unassisted.

Although oxygen toxicity was discussed previously, it is worthwhile repeating that using the least amount of FiO_2 required is best. In addition, one must be prepared to evaluate and treat the patient for a pneumothorax due to barotrauma or the misplacement of central intravenous lines.

Since infection of the respiratory tree can be caused by instrumentation of the airway, sterile techniques must be strictly adhered to when suctioning or during bronchoscopy. All respiratory equipment must be changed every 24 hours. Infection is also a consideration when using invasive monitors such as arterial lines, central intravenous lines, and Foley catheters.

One cannot orchestrate ventilatory support without a concern for fluid management. By following serial body weights, central venous pressures, pulmonary capillary wedge pressures, and fluid input and output, one can make an educated estimate about changing the variables. Although the kidneys and the lungs often seem to have the opposite requirements, the data will usually enable one to respond appropriately.

CRITERIA FOR EXTUBATION

The criteria for extubation involve various clinical and laboratory evaluations. Clinical judgment will ultimately be based on experience with the criteria. The physician must ascertain that the clinical situation is stable or improving before considering extubation. The patient's level of consciousness must be considered since the comatose or obtunded patient will not be able to protect his airway from obstruction or aspiration. The confused patient may not be able to cooperate with voluntary coughing and deep breathing in order to prevent atelectasis. The patient who cannot clear thick and copious secretions could be at risk for post-extubation decompensation. The stability of the cardiovascular system should be evaluated by noting the need for medications, arrythmias, abnormalities of blood pressure or pulse rate, elevated central venous pressures, and the related renal status. Certainly a chest x-ray should be examined for areas of atelectasis so that the problem can be treated prior to extubation. It is embarrassing to extubate a patient and then realize on reviewing a post-extubation x-ray that a condition exists that could have been improved prior to the removal of the tube. If bronchospasm is a problem, one should consider the timing of the bronchodilator treatment so as to optimize the extubation process. **Nutrition** should be carefully considered in patients that are difficult to extubate since both decreased nutrition and increased caloric intake can be problems. The use of enteral or parenteral alimentation can prevent the consequences of starvation. However, excessive calories on the day of weaning may lead to an increased respiratory effort to handle the carbon dioxide produced and may not be well tolerated by some patients. Therefore, prior to weaning, calories might need to be decreased and the carbohydrates limited in order to decrease the production of carbon dioxide (18).

Table 7.4 lists the **guidelines that can be used for weaning and extubation.** The list is divided into three categories. **Category I** has the basic criteria that should be met before the patient undertakes the weaning process leading to extubation. **Category II** lists the evaluations at the end of weaning that will be met by the majority of the patients that can be extubated. **Category III** lists the more sophisticated criteria that may be useful in more difficult cases or in those of academic interest.

Prior to weaning, the patient should be able to accomplish the levels of pul-

Table 7.4. Guidelines for Extubation

Category I: Criteria to qualify for weaning

Vital capacity (ml/kg body weight)	>15
Inspiratory force (cm H_2O)	>25
PaO_2 (mm Hg or torr) with $FiO_2 \leq 0.4$	65–75
$PaCO_2$ (mm Hg or torr)	<55 with normal pH
pH	7.35–7.45
Resting minute ventilation	<10 L
Ability to double the minute ventilation	

Category II: Criteria to qualify for extubation after weaning

PaO_2 (mm Hg or torr) with FiO_2 at 0.6	>80
$PaCO_2$ and pH as listed in category I	
Respiratory rate	<35; preferably <25

Category III: Additional criteria

V_D/V_T (normal 0.3)	<0.6
A-a$DO_2^{1.0}$ (mm Hg or torr)	<350

monary performance that are listed under Category I. The vital capacity will give one a method to determine whether the patient can keep his alveoli expanded and secretions cleared. The VC should be at least 10 ml/kg of body weight, but preferably 15 ml/kg (or greater) of ideal body weight. A negative inspiratory force greater than 25 cm of water is another important consideration since it relates to the strength of the respiratory muscles (19). The inspired oxygen fraction (FiO_2) should be 0.4 or less with a PaO_2 of at least 65–75 torr. This generally guarantees sufficient arterial hemoglobin saturation. PEEP should not be essential for satisfactory oxygenation. Prior to weaning, an ABG should show no respiratory acidosis or carbon dioxide retention. Scroggin describes checking for a resting minute ventilation of less than 10 liters and then testing the patient's ability to double the resting minute ventilation during a 15 second test. This is felt to indicate adequate ventilatory reserve (20).

Weaning should be started early in the day after the patient has had the night to rest. Table 7.5 provides a flow sheet that further explains the process of weaning and extubation. Where possible, the patient should have his trunk elevated 30–40 degrees to improve ventilation. If the patient meets the previously mentioned weaning criteria, the patient can be placed on spontaneous T-tube ventilation with an FiO_2 of 0.6. Some authors suggest increasing the FiO_2 provided by the ventilator by 10–20% for the weaning period. Past experience has shown us that using an FiO_2 at 0.6 is a simple and effective approach. The patient is continuously observed for cardiovascular stability (i.e., pulse rate, blood pressure, cardiac rhythm), respiratory rate and effort, and level of consciousness. A pulse oximeter can be used to follow oxyhemoglobin saturation during the weaning process. After approximately one half hour or more, the ABG is evaluated. If the PaO_2 is greater than 80 torr with an FiO_2 of 0.6, then after extubation the patient will generally have a satisfactory PaO_2 with a high humidity oxygen mask with

Table 7.5. Flow Chart for Weaning and Extubation

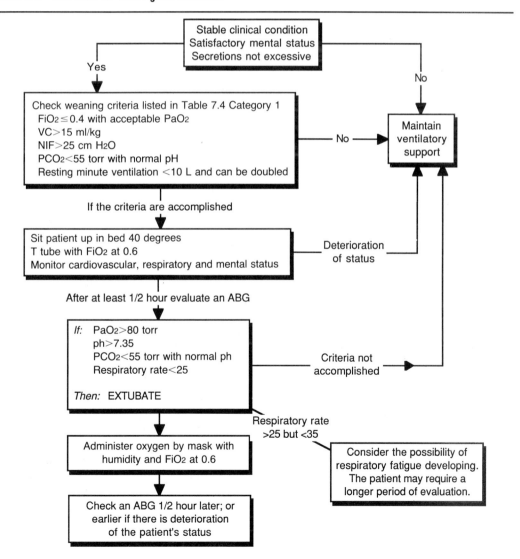

an FiO_2 of 0.6. The concept of a PaO_2 greater than 80 torr with an FiO_2 of 0.6 is a simple way of considering the $A\text{-}aDO_2$. If the $A\text{-}aDO_2$ is calculated, then the $A\text{-}aDO_2$ should be less than 350 torr. The pH should be normal, or at least not acidotic. The $PaCO_2$ should be 35–40 torr, although higher values may be tolerated if the pH is normal (as seen in chronic hypercapnia). Since a respiratory rate greater than 35 per minute will generally be associated with post-extubation ventilatory failure, one seeks a rate of approximately ≤ 25. A V_D/V_T may be helpful in a borderline case if the ratio is significantly less than 0.6 and, preferably, closer to 0.3. If the patient does not meet the above criteria or if one's clinical judgment is negative, then the IMV is set to support the patient and the trial is repeated when the situation improves (21, 22, 23). If the patient has been receiving 5 cm or less of PEEP during the weaning, the PEEP or CPAP does not have to be removed for the trial. In fact, maintaining 5 cm or less of CPAP during the trial has been felt to be advantageous. Prior to extubation, the patient is hyperinflated and suctioned. By giving a positive pressure ventilation while removing the tube, one can often successfully cause secretions lying above the cuff to be blown upward into the pharynx where they can be removed by oral suctioning. **Someone skilled in intubation should be present at all extubations.**

Nichoff (24) and her associates evaluated the efficacy of pulse oximetry and capnometry in postoperative weaning. The two modalities were felt to be useful in monitoring respiratory status during postoperative weaning and could result in less frequent ABGs; but capnometry appeared to be relatively insensitive to hypercarbia. A review of this article noted that although the results of noninvasive monitoring could be useful, the physician should continue to use conventional parameters at his discretion (25).

When patients fail to be successfully weaned, mechanical ventilation should be resumed while the physician considers what might be the cause of the failure and possible therapies to improve the situation. One has to evaluate the initial indications for the mechanical support and any new problems that developed during the intubation (e.g., infections, psychological concerns, nutrition, cardiovascular hemodynamics, etc.).

The inability to sustain spontaneous ventilation because of excessive respiratory work may be a reason for a failed weaning trial. With increased respiratory work, there is usually respiratory muscle fatigue and deterioration of gas exchange. Researchers have found that indirect calorimetry is a relatively simple and reliable bedside method to evaluate the oxygen cost of breathing, which appears to be a predictor of weaning in patients recovering from respiratory failure. Further studies are needed to evaluate the use of the oxygen cost of breathing to identify, monitor, and assess patients with weaning problems. Lewis (26) suggests that this means of measurement might be useful in evaluating the ventilatory effects of nutritional programs, respiratory muscle conditioning, and weaning strategies.

Jannace (27) has reported on cyclic hypercarbia that occurred in a patient on cyclic total parenteral nutrition. After evaluating the patient with indirect calorimetry and then changing to a continuous infusion, the patient tolerated periods of unassisted ventilation.

The period after extubation requires several specific activities and orders. The patient should not be fed for a period of time (8–24 hours) in order to prevent aspiration due to laryngeal incompetence that develops from having a tube in place for an extended period. In addition, if the patient requires reintubation, then delaying oral intake will prevent the problem of intubating a patient with a full stomach who is at increased risk of vomiting and aspiration. The patient can be started on an incentive spirometer if his vital capacity is adequate (at least 15 ml/kg of body weight). If the vital capacity is borderline, then IPPB (intermittent positive-pressure breathing) is often used. Various studies have questioned the efficacy of IPPB since the incentive spirometer is generally more beneficial to the patient. In order to prevent atelectasis, orders are written for deep breathing, percussion, coughing, and position changes. Supplemental oxygen with humidification is provided as necessary.

HIGH FREQUENCY VENTILATION

High frequency positive pressure ventilation is a form of mechanical ventilatory support that is still being investigated (28). The original investigations of high frequency ventilation were conducted while searching for an improved method of ventilation for laryngoscopy and bronchoscopy. The technique was then adapted for general mechanical ventilation. There are basically three types of ventilation that are included in the concept of high frequency ventilation. **High frequency positive pressure ventilation** (HFPPV) uses a frequency greater than 60 breaths per minute and may increase up to 120 breaths per minute. With HFPPV, the tidal volumes are considerably less than the tidal volumes used in conventional ventilation. There is no entrainment of additional gas in this technique. **High frequency jet ventilation** (HFJV) uses a frequency that may range from 80–300 breaths per minute; with rates of 100–200 per minute more common. An injector is used to accelerate the gas flow provided by the ventilator. Gas from a high pressure source is cycled by a mechanism such as a solenoid. By developing the Bernoulli effect, the accelerated flow entrains a parallel flow of gases to increase the tidal volume provided. This enhanced tidal volume may provide the advantage of not increasing the peak inflation or airway pressure. One manipulates the driving pressure, inspiratory times, and frequency. An attempt

to develop a universal formula using the patient's weight to determine the jet ventilator's driving pressure or tidal volume to achieve normocarbia was unsuccessful. The authors (29) recommended caution in determining the settings based on patient weight. **High frequency oscillation** (HFO) provides less bulk gas flow than the other two methods. This technique uses a piston, bellows, or loudspeaker to create a to-and-fro movement that pushes gas into the airway. Higher flows of oxygen must be provided to guarantee the proper oxygenation. HFO usually uses frequencies between 600–3000 breaths per minute. When using HFO in adults, there is a problem with leakage. Most of the studies of HFO in human subjects are in neonates. Froese points out that the nature of the expiratory phase in high frequency ventilation may be altered to occur by passive recoil of the lung and chest wall or by active manipulation. Since the various approaches using passive expiration may risk pulmonary hyperinflation, he feels that it should be noted in the terminology whether the high frequency ventilation modality uses a passive or active expiratory cycle (30).

Some mechanical ventilators are able to provide frequencies up to 100 breaths per minute. However, since these are basically conventional ventilators, the clinician must ascertain that the valve systems in this equipment can operate safely at substantially higher frequencies. These ventilators are providing a form of ventilation similar to HFPPV.

HFJV is the method of high frequency ventilation most used clinically. Only HFJV has been approved by the Food and Drug Administration with the limit of a frequency less than 150 breaths per minute. The Food and Drug Administration has stated that the specific uses for HFJV are presently bronchopleural fistula, bronchoscopy, and tracheal or laryngeal surgery. HFJV has been tried in other clinical problems, but the other uses remain limited and investigative (31). Kahn

(32) and his colleagues have reported on their successful use of HFPPV on two patients who would have required independent lung ventilation. They recommended a trial of HFPPV for patients with unilateral lung disease who fail conventional management.

The specifics of "how to" use high frequency ventilation will not be discussed due to the different methods being used and developed, the specifics of the equipment, the ongoing investigations, and presently the limited clinically approved uses for high frequency ventilation. However, this topic is presented since high frequency ventilation is a different concept in mechanical ventilation and does have some specific indications. High frequency ventilation should not be used where there is obstruction of the expiratory outflow of gas from the lung. Adequate training is needed in order to understand the characteristics of each high frequency approach, to evaluate the appropriate situations in which it should be used, and to anticipate the possible complications.

The conventional views of alveolar ventilation do not explain how high frequency ventilation provides satisfactory oxygenation and elimination of carbon dioxide. Various theories of convention and diffusion gas flow concepts are used to explain its effect. However, there is no definite agreement on how gas transport occurs with this method. This is complicated by the different means of providing high frequency ventilation and the various equipment.

NEW MODES OF MECHANICAL VENTILATION

Some new methods of ventilatory support are being developed to solve various problems with more specific approaches. These techniques are beyond the scope of this chapter, but they will be briefly noted for completeness. The definitive studies and evaluations of these newer modes are pending.

Differential lung ventilation enables one to ventilate each lung individually. With this technique PEEP could be administered selectively to one lung. The inverse ratio method involves a longer inspiratory than expiratory time in order to improve the distribution of the mechanical ventilation. By using pressure support ventilation with a predetermined level of positive pressure, the overall work of breathing may be decreased and weaning improved. (33, 34).

READINGS

1. O'Donohue WJ, Baker JP, Bell GM, et al.: Respiratory failure in neuromuscular disease. *JAMA* 235:733–735, 1976.
2. Kofke A: Postoperative respiratory care techniques, in Kofke A, Levy JH (eds): *Postoperative Critical Care Procedures of the Massachusetts General Hospital.* Boston, Little, Brown and Co., 1986, p. 32.
3. Michell C, Garrahy P, Peake: Postoperative respiratory morbidity: identification and risk factors. *Aust N Z J Surg* 52:203–209, April, 1982.
4. Lecky JH, Ominsky AJ: Postoperative respiratory management. *Chest* 2:50S–57S, 1972.
5. Pontoppidon H, Geffin B, Lowenstein E: Acute respiratory failure in the adult (three parts). *N Engl J Med* 287:690–698; 743–752; 799–806, 1972.
6. Otto CW: Respiratory intensive care, in Lebowitz PW (ed): *Clinical Anesthesia: Procedures of the Massachusetts General Hospital.* Boston, Little, Brown and Co., 1978, pp. 384–414.
7. Register SD, Downs JB, Stock MC, et al.: Is 50% oxygen harmful? *Crit Care Med* 6:598–601, 1987.
8. *Annual Refresher Course Lectures by the American Society of Anesthesiologists.* Philadelphia, JB Lippincott. Some specific lectures are: (*a*) John B. Downs, Physiologic Alterations of Mechanical Ventilation, #230, 1979; Physiological Effects of Mechanical Ventilatory Support, #133B, 1977; Weaning the Ventilator Dependent Patient, #142, 1984. (*b*) H. Barrie Fairley, Adult ARDS: Clinical Aspects, #117, 1976; Respiratory "Fine Tuning": PEEP, CPAP, IMV, etc., #103A, 1978. (*c*) Robert Kirby, Respiratory "Fine Tuning": PEEP, CPAP, IMV, etc., #103B, 1978; Indications for and appropriate uses of PEEP/CPAP, #141, 1984. (*d*) Jerome Modell, Patterns of Respiratory Support Aimed at Pathophysiology, #223A, 1976; Update on Means of Mechanical Ventilatory Support, #401, 1984. (*e*) Barry A. Shapiro, PEEP Therapy in Acute Lung Injury, #173, 1985; Clinical Management of the Patient with ARDS, #412, 1987. (*f*) Ronald A. Harrison, Ventilation of the Critically Ill Patient, #243, 1987.

9. Cane RD, Shapiro BA: Mechanical Ventilatory Support. *JAMA* 254:87–92, 1985.

10. Carlon GC, Ray C, et al.: Capnography in mechanically ventilated patients. *Crit Care Med* 16:550–556, 1988.

11. Willatta SM: Paralysis for ventilated patients? Yes or No? *Int Crit Care Dig* 4:9–10, 1985.

12. Novak RA, Shumaker L, Snyder JV, et al.: Do periodic hyperinflations improve gas exchange in patients with hypoxemic respiratory failure? *Crit Care Med* 12:1081–1085, 1987.

13. Winston ST, Gravelyn TR, Sitrin RG: Prevention of bradycardic responses to endotracheal suctioning by prior administration of nebulized atropine. *Crit Care Med* 11:1009–1011, 1987.

14. Kelly RE, Yao FSF, Artusio JF: Prevention of suction-induced hypoxemia by simultaneous oxygen insufflation. *Crit Care Med* 9:874–875, 1987.

15. Burton EG (ed): *Respiratory Care: A Guide to Clinical Practice.* Philadelphia, JB Lippincott, 1977.

16. Bishop MJ: Endotracheal tubes and tracheotomies: risks and benefits in the OR and ICU, #262 in *Annual Refresher Course Lectures by the American Society of Anesthesiologists.* Philadelphia, JB Lippincott, 1987.

17. Noseworthy TW, Shustack A, Johnston RG, et al.: A randomized clinical trial comparing ranitidine and antacids in critically ill patients. *Crit Care Med* 9:817–819, 1987.

18. Beaton N, Bone CB: Criteria for weaning your patients from respirators. *J Resp Dis* April 1985, pp 80–83.

19. Marini JJ, Smith TC, Lamb V: Estimation of inspiratory muscle strength in mechanically ventilated patients: The measurement of maximal inspiratory pressure. *J Crit Care* 1:32–38, 1986.

20. Scroggin CH: The technique of weaning from mechanical ventilation. *J Crit Illness* June 1986, pp 59–69.

21. Feely TW, Headley-White J: Weaning from controlled ventilation and supplemental oxygen. *N Engl J Med* 17:903–906, 1975.

22. Sahn SA, Lakshminarayan S, Petty TL: Weaning from mechanical ventilation (Special Communication). *JAMA* 235:2208–2212, 1976.

23. Hall JB, Wood LDH: Liberation of the patient from mechanical ventilation. *JAMA* 257:1621–1628, 1987.

24. Nichoff J, et al.: Efficacy of pulse oximetry and capnometry on postoperative ventilatory weaning. *Crit Care Med* 16:701–705, 1988.

25. Tasch MD: Commenting on "Efficacy of pulse oximetry and capnometry on postoperative ventilatory weaning." Literature Scan: *Anesthesiology* vol 11, n 6, p 7, Dec. 1988.

26. Lewis WD, et al.: Bedside assessment of the work of breathing. *Crit Care Med* 2:117–122, 1988.

27. Jannace PW, et al.: Total parenteral nutrition—induced cyclic hypercapnia. *Crit Care Med* 16:727–728, 1988.

28. Sjostrand U: High frequency positive-pressure ventilation (HFPPV): A review. *Crit Care Med* 6:346–364, 1980.

29. Bayly R, et al.: Driving Pressure and arterial carbon dioxide tension during high-frequency jet ventilation on postoperative patients. *Crit Care Med* 1:58–61, 1988.

30. Froese AB: High-frequency ventilation: Uses and abuses, in Barash PG (ed): *Refresher Courses in Anesthesiology.* Philadelphia, JB Lippincott, 1986.

31. Gallagher TJ: Current status of high frequency ventilation, #171 in *Annual Refresher Course Lectures by the American Society of Anesthesiologists.* Philadelphia, JB Lippincott, 1986.

32. Kahn RC, Koslow M, Weinhouse G: High-frequency positive pressure ventilation for unilateral lung disease. *Crit Care Med* 16:814–816, 1988.

33. Wissing DR, Romero MD, George RB: Comparing the newer modes of mechanical ventilation. *J Crit Illness* 2(3):41–49, 1987.

34. Cohen AT, Parsloe MRJ: Modes of ventilation: SIMV for all? *Inten Care World* 4(2):58–62, June 1987.

8

Invasive Physiologic Monitoring

John M. Field

RIGHT HEART CATHETERIZATION

INTRODUCTION

Right heart catheterization and pulmonary artery pressure monitoring with balloon-tipped catheters have significantly advanced the care of certain critically ill patients. Therapeutic plans and response to treatment can now be objectively guided, obviating a clinical trial and error technique which is not always optimal in a hemodynamically or clinically unstable patient.

Initially, the use of the **Swan-Ganz catheter** was directed at the complicated cardiac patient. The current widespread use of this monitoring method and its application to other medical and surgical conditions make familiarity with it a necessity for the consulting internist.

INDICATIONS FOR PULMONARY ARTERY MONITORING

In general, insertion of a pulmonary artery catheter is indicated when the data to be obtained will be needed to clarify a clinical situation and guide or direct a therapeutic plan. In most cases, invasive monitoring occurs in the complicated cardiac patient who is a candidate for interventional therapy for optimizing preload and afterload. It is rare that invasive monitoring is indicated in uncomplicated myocardial infarction and may be stressful to the patient (1). Patients with severe congestive heart failure, refractory to standard therapy may also be candidates for invasive monitoring. It may also be necessary to obtain hemodynamic data to separate **cardiogenic from noncardiogenic pulmonary edema** (2).

Patients suspected of major **structural complications of myocardial infarction** are often catheterized both for monitoring and diagnostic purposes. The two most common complications recognized clinically are **rupture of the ventricular septum** (O_2 step-up at right ventricular level) and **papillary muscle dysfunction or chordal tear** (absence of O_2 step-up; prominent V waves in the pulmonary artery or wedge tracing; greater than 10 mm Hg mean PCW pressure). Rupture of the left ventricular free wall with cardiac tamponade and papillary muscle rupture are usually suddenly fatal.

While echocardiography can effectively diagnose pericardial effusion, pulmonary artery catheterization is often needed to confirm clinically life-threatening **tamponade physiology** prior to emergent intervention or surgical therapy. Pulmonary artery catheterization is occasionally necessary to quantitate **pulmonary hypertension,** although qualitative estimates from Doppler-Echo are improving and may substitute for most clinical purposes.

Most patients who undergo **cardiac surgical procedures** are candidates for invasive monitoring during the immediate recovery period. Some clinicians advocate the perioperative monitoring of cardiac patients undergoing major noncardiac surgery (e.g., thoracic, abdominal, vascular). Such monitoring should be discontinued promptly when filling pressures are judged adequate or stable. The

Table 8.1. Indications for Invasive Monitoring

- **complicated cardiac patient**
  clarification of hemodynamic status
  cardiogenic shock
  refractory congestive heart failure
  mechanical complications of infarction
- **cardiac tamponade**
- **diagnosis of cardiogenic vs. non-cardiogenic
  shock**
  adult respiratory distress syndrome
  septic shock
- **cardiac surgery**
- **major surgical procedures in the cardiac
  patient**
  thoracic-abdominal
  vascular
- **major surgical procedures in the elderly**
  risk stratification
- **chronic heart failure**
  acute exacerbations failing initial therapy

use of pulmonary artery pressure monitoring is also felt to be indicated in patients with noncardiogenic pulmonary edema and the adult respiratory distress syndrome. One study, which performed preoperative invasive monitoring, found a high percentage of elderly patients with abnormal hemodynamics. In 85% of patients, abnormalities were present which were not detected on clinical preoperative assessment. A subgroup of 23% of patients were felt not to be elective surgical candidates due to unacceptable risks (3). This study recommends routine preoperative invasive evaluation for risk stratification and intervention in elderly patients.

The most common clinical indications for invasive monitoring of pulmonary artery pressures are listed in Table 8.1. A consideration of those indications which are diagnostic, guide therapy, or alter prognostic indications are mandatory for physicians who perform right heart catheterization (4).

PRINCIPLES OF RIGHT HEART CATHETERIZATION

Bedside catheterization of the heart was first described by Swan et al. in 1970 (5).

This technique consisted of the introduction of a balloon-tipped catheter, which was flow-directed through the right heart. Subsequently, the addition of a special Teflon catheter with thermistors allowed for measurement of cardiac output as well as right-sided heart and pulmonary artery pressures (6).

Although originally introduced via antecubital veins, many catheters are now introduced through subclavian, supraclavicular, or internal jugular routes. While more comfortable for the patient, these routes of introduction carry with them the complications commonly associated with central venous access method.

Rapid placement of the catheter affords measurement of the pulmonary artery pressure (PA), pulmonary artery occlusion pressure (pulmonary capillary wedge pressure or PCW), and thermodilution cardiac output. However, when feasible, all right heart pressures (right atrial, right ventricular, pulmonary artery [phasic & mean], pulmonary capillary wedge [phasic & mean] should be measured and recorded as well as right atrial, ventricular, and pulmonary artery oxygen saturations. These may be helpful in the evaluation of certain differential diagnoses, e.g., VSD versus mitral insufficiency. A simultaneously obtained arterial oxygen saturation allows for calculation of the arterial-venous oxygen difference, an indirect measure of cardiac output.

The above information constitutes a complete right heart catheterization and should be obtained when clinical circumstances permit. For most practical monitoring situations, serial PA pressures, serial PCW pressures and cardiac output determinations are most often employed. A list of normal pressures, cardiac output and A-V O_2 difference is given in Table 8.2.

INTERPRETATION OF DATA

A detailed discussion of data interpretation is beyond the scope of this chapter

Table 8.2.   Normal Right Heart Data

Pressures		O₂ Sat
site	normal range (mmHg)	
right atrium	1–5	75%
right ventricle		75%
peak systolic	32	
end-diastolic	5	
pulmonary artery		
		75%
peak systolic	32	
end-diastolic	13	
average mean	15	
pulmonary artery wedge	4–12	97%
v wave	<10 mmHg mean	

Thermodilution Cardiac Output

cardiac index	3.5 Liters/min/M²

A-V O₂ Difference

4.1 volumes %

and the reader is referred to several works evaluating findings in both cardiac and noncardiac patients (7,8,9). An example of low and high filling pressure patterns complicating myocardial infarction is given in Figure 8.1.

However, it should be noted that one of the major pitfalls in the management of critically ill patients is the misinterpretation of right heart pressure and hemodynamic data base. Limitations of the technical system, the reproducibility of results, technical calibration, and catheter systems are common problems. Further, while initial data may be semiquantitative, serial management of the patient should view the changing data base as qualitative and require clinical collaboration to avoid the above listed pitfalls. Use of the Swan-Ganz catheter should be tempered by the limited conditions in which monitoring is useful, and recognition of complications, and discomfort for the patient.

The physician managing a patient with a pulmonary artery catheter should also have a thorough understanding of the tracing and wave forms in the usual recording and with other modifications such as artifact, dampening, and frequency response variations (10).

COMPLICATIONS

Atrial and ventricular arrythmias have been reported. Short episodes of ventricular tachycardia are not uncommon and ventricular fibrillation may occur (11). Passage of the catheter across the ventricular septum has caused right bundle branch block and transient complete heart block. Left fascicular blocks have also been reported (12). These rhythms have been transient and often terminate with repositioning or catheter withdrawal. Patients with left bundle branch block should be managed cautiously.

As noted above, certain complications

Example 1

patient with anterior wall infarct, high filling pressure, and low output state (cardiogenic shock)

RA	8 mmHg
RV	40/8 mmHg
PA	40/28 mmHg
PCW	28 mmHg
CI	1.9 L/Min/M²

Example 2

patient with inferior wall infarct, low filling pressure, and low output state (volume dependent)

RA	2 mmHg
RV	15/2 mmHg
PA	15/4 mmHg
PCW	4 mmHg
CI	2.2 L/Min/M²

Figure 8.1. Two examples of acute infarction, which by clinical exam exhibited a low output state. The pulmonary exam in both patients was complicated by chronic pulmonary disease.

are a result of the choice of insertion site and include local infection, pneumothorax (usually with subclavian approach), air embolism, and inadvertent arterial puncture and sheath placement. Use of the internal jugular vein has minimized pneumothorax.

Pulmonary complications include ischemic and embolic events. One study found an incidence of 7.2% pulmonary focal ischemic lesions felt to be associated with wedging the Swan-Ganz catheter. More serious and potentially fatal complications include **hemoptysis and pulmonary artery rupture** (13,14). These complications have been significantly reduced with careful monitoring of the wedge and pressure tracing.

The incidence of primary **catheter related sepsis** is low, about 1–2%. A prospective study identified three factors related to positive blood cultures: bacteremia, three or more repositionings of the catheter, and catheterization for longer than 72 hours (15).

Rupture of the catheter balloon can also occur, usually when overinflated. When recognized, this is not associated with serious complications, except in patients with a right to left shunt. If unrecognized, air embolism of the pulmonary artery segment is possible with repeated attempts at balloon inflation. Intracardiac knotting of the catheter is rare (16).

Perhaps the most significant factor in the prevention of complications is the presence of an experienced physician during insertion and positioning of the catheter. Also, proper attention should be given to the accuracy of the hemodynamic measurement attained and their limitations. A knowledge of cardiopulmonary hemodynamics and fluid-filled catheter mechanisms is important for correct interpretation.

ARTERIAL LINES

Arterial indwelling catheters are indicated for continuous monitoring of blood pressure and for frequent sampling of arterial blood to avoid multiple traumatic punctures of arterial sites.

When properly performed arterial line placement is safe and has few immediate complications. Major complications include hand and digital ischemia. This can often be prevented by performing an Allen's test prior to insertion and monitoring skin color and temperature after placement. Use of a 20-gauge catheter instead of an 18-gauge catheter has also been demonstrated to reduce thrombotic complications (17).

The rate of catheter sepsis is approximately 4% (18). Most arterial lines are now placed percutaneously with lower rates of sepsis. Higher rates are observed with surgical cutdown technique. Local infection and poor technique during arterial sampling will increase the risk of infection. Placement of the catheter for longer than four days has also been reported to increase infection and sepsis (19).

SUMMARY

Right Heart Catheterization with pulmonary artery pressure monitoring is a valuable adjunct to the management of critically ill patients. The consulting internist should have a firm understanding of the indications and complications associated with the use of these catheters. Patient management requires an in depth understanding of cardiac hemodynamics and alterations in specific pathologic states. Knowledge of the technical systems utilized is helpful in avoiding pitfalls in interpretation.

READINGS

1. Spodick DH: Physiologic and prognostic implications of invasive monitoring: undetermined risk/benefit ratios in patients with heart disease. *Am J Cardiol* 46:173–175, 1980.
2. Goldenheim PD, Kazemi H: Cardiopulmonary monitoring of critically ill patients. Part 2. *New Engl J Med* 311:776–780, 1984.

3. Del Guercio LRM, Cohn JD: Monitoring operative risk in the elderly. *JAMA* 243:1350–1355, 1980.

4. Matthay M, Chatterjee K: Bedside catheterization of the pulmonary artery: Risks compared with benefits. *Ann Intern Med* 109(10):826, 1988.

5. Swan HJC, Ganz W, Forrester J, et al.: Catheterization of the heart in man with the use of a flow-directed balloon-tipped catheter. *New Engl J Med* 283:447–451.

6. Ganz W, Donoso R, Marcus H, et al.: A new technique for measurement of cardiac output by thermodilution in man. *AJC* 27:392–396, 1971.

7. Grossman W: Cardiac catheterization and angiography: Part VI Profiles of hemodynamic and angiographic abnormalities in Specific Disorders. Philadelphia, Lea & Febiger, 1986.

8. Forrester JS, Diamond G, Chatterjee K, et al.: Medical therapy of myocardial infarction by application of hemodynamic subsets. *New Engl J Med* 295:1356–1362, 295:1404–1413, 1975.

9. Connors AF Jr, McCaffree DR, Gray BA: Evaluation of right heart catheterization in the critically ill patient without myocardial infarction. *New Engl J Med* 308:263–267, 1983.

10. Grossman W: Cardiac catheterization and angiography. Pressure measurement. Philadelphia, Lea & Febiger, 1986.

11. Cairns JA, Holder D: Ventricular fibrillation due to passage of a Swan-Ganz catheter. (letter to the editor) *Am J Card* 35:589, 1975.

12. Castellanos A, Ramirez A, Cortes A, et al.: Left fascicular blocks during right heart catheterization using the Swan-Ganz catheter, the flow directed balloon-tipped catheter. *New Engl J Med* 290:927–931, 1974.

13. Golden M, Pinder T Jr, Anderson W, et al.: Fatal pulmonary hemorrhage complicating use of a flow-directed balloon-tipped catheter in a patient receiving anticoagulant therapy. *Am J Cardiol* 32:865–867, 1973.

14. Pape LA, Haffajee CI, Markis JE, et al.: Fatal pulmonary hemorrhage after use of the flow-directed balloon-tipped catheter. *Ann Intern Med* 90:344–347, 1979.

15. Applefeld J, Caruthers T, Reno D, et al.: Assessment of the sterility of long-term cardiac catheterization using the thermodilution Swan-Ganz catheter. *Chest* 74:4377–379, 1978.

16. Lipp H, O'Donoghue K, Resnekov L: Intracardiac knotting of a flow directed balloon catheter. (letter to the editor) *New Engl J Med* 284:220, 1971.

17. Davis FM, Stewart JM: Radial artery cannulation: a prospective study in patients undergoing cardiothoracic surgery. *Br J Anesthesiology* 52:41–46, 1980.

18. Band JD, Maki DG: Infections caused by arterial catheters used for hemodynamic monitoring. *Am J Med* 67:735–741, 1979.

19. Maki DG, Hassemer CA: Endemic rate of fluid contamination and related septicemia in arterial pressure monitoring. *Am J Med* 70:733–738, 1981.

9
Pulmonary Embolism and Venous Thrombosis

Thomas J. McGlynn, Jr.

PULMONARY EMBOLISM, EPIDEMIOLOGY AND OVERVIEW

Approximately 600,000 symptomatic episodes of pulmonary emboli contribute to the deaths of 50,000 or 9% of United States patients each year. Proper treatment reduces mortality from 30% to 5–9% (1, 2). Two-thirds of patients die before acute intervention (embolectomy, streptokinase) can be effective. Prophylactic measures and changing practice habits (early ambulation and discharge) may reduce the incidence of fatal emboli.

Pathophysiology

Venous endothelial tears due to excessive reflex vasodilation, and a transient decrease in venous flow volume and pulsatility occur with general anesthesia and surgery. At both the venous endothelial and systemic levels, anesthesia and the release of tissue thromboplastin and other factors result in a hypercoagulable state. Platelet aggregates develop behind venous valves of the deep pelvic, thigh and calf veins, and progress into thrombi (3–5).

Approximately 20% of deep venous thrombi of the thigh or pelvis embolize (6). Calf thromboses rarely, if ever, embolize, but about 20% can propogate into the deep veins of the thigh. Embolus size, antecedent cardiopulmonary reserve, and the patient's ability to regain hemodynamic stability within 1 hour of the onset of symptoms correlate best with outcome.

Prolonged, severe cardiopulmonary compromise is uncommon in the absence of massive emboli, which occlude 50% or greater of the pulmonary vascular bed.

Acute decreased pulmonary blood flow due to reflex pulmonary vasoconstriction, humoral effects, or mechanical obstruction of pulmonary vasculature can precipitate: pulmonary hypertension, right heart strain, decreased cardiac output, peripheral hypoxia, and hypotension. Over a few hours, emboli fragment and redistribute downstream; a small number resorb completely within days. Ninety percent resolve completely over several weeks to months and leave no residual lung scan, standard pulmonary function, chest x-ray or clinically significant residual deficits. Small perfusion scan defects persist 1 year after an episode among 10% of the patients. Rare patients develop thrombotic casts in major pulmonary arteries and progressive symptomatic pulmonary hypertension.

All diagnostic studies should be completed within 48 hours of an acute event. Blood gas abnormalities and specific EKG patterns often resolve over minutes to a few hours. Perfusion scan abnormalities, most diagnostic of emboli, become less distinct and less interpretable within a few days.

Symptoms and Signs

Evaluate all patients, especially those with associated increased risk, for **unexplained dyspnea, chest pain, shock,**

Table 9.1. The Risk of Phlebitis/Thromboembolism Related to Type of Surgery and Clinical Risk Factors (Adapted from Rose SD, 1979 and Coon WW, 1976)

A. Type of Surgery	Prevalence of Venous Thromboembolic Disease by Phlebography and ^{131}I-Fibrinogen
General surgery, age less than 40	16–42%
General surgery, age over 60 or patient has a malignancy	40–61%
Gynecologic surgery	10–26%
Thoracic surgery	12–25%
Neurosurgery	4–40%
Urologic surgery	10–58%
Orthopaedic surgery	40–78%

B. Clinical Risk Factors	Relative Increased Risk of Thromboembolic Disease
Age greater than 60	2-fold increase compared to patients under 60
Estrogen contraceptive agents	4–7-fold ⎫ increase compared to non-pregnant peer
Pregnancy	5-fold ⎭ group
Obesity	½- to 2-fold increase compared to non-obese patients
Heart disease	3½-fold increased risk compared to patients without heart disease (except hypertensive and congenital heart disease patients under age 30)
Malignancy	2–3-fold increased risk among all patients with cancer
Prior venous thromboembolic disease	2-fold increased risk
Trauma	All patients at increased risk; pelvic and leg fractures highest risk
Paralysis, prolonged bed rest, and immobilization	Degree of increased risk varies with clinical circumstances and patient characteristics
Myeloproliferative disorders, thrombocytosis, paroxysmal nocturnal hemoglobinuria, and ulcerative colitis	Best available evidence indicates significant increased risk

cardiopulmonary deterioration, major arrhythmias and syncope. The clinical manifestations of emboli are frequently transient, inconstant, nonspecific, and at times deceivingly benign. Dangerously large emboli can produce few symptoms and only one sign. Dyspnea and tachypnea are the only symptoms and signs found in more than 80% of the patients. Chest pain and apprehension occur among slightly more than half of the patients; cough, hemoptysis, fever among less than half. Among physical findings, rales, fever, increased second sound, and tachycardia occur in about half of the patients. An S3 or S4, diaphoresis, clinically evident phlebitis, edema,

Table 9.2. Symptoms and Signs of Pulmonary Embolism (Adapted from Urokinase Trial (4) by permission)

Symptoms	%	Signs	%
Dyspnea	81	Tachypnea (>16)	87
Pleuritic pain	72	Rales	53
Apprehension	59	Increased pulmonic second sound	53
Cough	54	Tachycardia (>100)	44
Hemoptysis	34	Fever (>37.8)	42
Sweats	26	S3, S4 gallop	34
Syncope	14	Diaphoresis	34
		Phlebitis	33
		Peripheral edema	23
		Murmur	23
		Cyanosis	18

new heart murmurs and cyanosis occur in a third or fewer patients. Syncope, cyanosis, hypotension and an increased P2 occur more commonly among those with large emboli, but each of these findings may be absent even with massive emboli (7–10).

Diagnostic Evaluation

A reliable diagnosis can be made on the basis of lung scans alone in about 50% of the patients. The remainder require angiography. **Diagnostic perfusion defects** should be: visible on at least two views; multiple, segmental, or lobar in size, and sharply marginated with convex inner margins in areas of the scan that are not associated with chest x-ray defects. Scans with one or more large segmental or greater defects and a ventilation mismatch, predict the presence of emboli with greater than 90% accuracy and do not require further study. Subsegmental defects with matching ventilation defects usually indicate an absence of emboli (87%) and may not require further study if the clinical situation is only mildly suggestive of emboli. Normal scans eliminate emboli. Subsegmental defects (half of a lung segment or less) and matching ventilation defects, or defects in the same location as chest x-ray defects (except perfusion defects much larger than x-ray defects) are difficult to interpret and require angiographic clarification (11).

Ventilation scans increase the specificity of lung perfusion scan interpretation. The absence of an associated ventilation defect (the common finding in other lung diseases) on ventilation scan suggests that perfusion scan deficits are due to emboli. This finding is not 100% specific. Multiple segmental and larger defects without associated ventilation defects are 90% predictive of emboli. Some patients with emboli develop both perfusion and ventilation defects. These findings may need angiographic clarification. Table 9.3 summarizes the results of the best major prospective study of scan criteria.

The chest x-ray must be available to interpret scans. X-rays demonstrate common disorders (pneumonia, emphysema and blebs, congestive heart failure, tumor, effusion, etc.) that provide alternative explanations for perfusion scan defects. They are abnormal in a widely varying number of patients with emboli (less than half to 90%). Four signs are most common and support the diagnosis: effusions, elevated hemidiaphragm, infiltrate, and atelectasis. a few uncommon signs are highly suggestive (a convex density over the diaphragm—Hamptom's hump) and at times easily overread (regional oligemia—Westermark's sign). The small sympathetic effusions that occur after any abdominal surgery or childbirth are not associated with perfusion defects.

Multiple view **pulmonary angiography** with selective magnification and injection clarifies the findings of abnormal but equivocal lung perfusion scans. Well marginated, intraluminal defects with streaming of the dye around them or sharp cut off of vessels 2.5 mm or greater are most reliably diagnostic. Other criteria can be used but are less specific for emboli and require careful interpretation. In experienced hands morbidity and mortality of the procedure are far lower than the risks associated with untreated emboli or unnecessary anticoagulation.

Several studies provide ancillary data. Nine of ten patients develop nonspecific **EKG abnormalities.** Specific diagnostic patterns suggesting right heart strain or cor pulmonale occur in less than 10% of the cases. The most common abnormalities are nonspecific ST and T wave changes. Low voltage, bundle branch blocks, arrhythmias, and a Q wave infarct pattern can result from emboli.

Almost nine of ten patients demonstrate arterial hypoxemia associated with hypocarbia and alkalosis due to tachypnea. **Blood gas determinations** lack specificity and sensitivity. Hypoxemia due

Table 9.3. Radionucleotide Scans and Pulmonary Embolism

Finding	Interpretation and Recommendation
Perfusion Scans Alone	
Normal	Emboli eliminated
One or more large defects	71% Probability emboli present (if risks of therapy high or suspicion of emboli low, go to angiography)
One or more small defects	27% Probability emboli present (angiography necessary)
Indeterminant	17% Probability emboli present (angiography necessary)
Perfusion and ventilation scan	
One or more large Perfusion defects + Ventilation mismatch	86–91% Probability of emboli or DVT (angiography unnecessary)
One or more large Perfusion defects + Ventilation match	23–40% Probability of emboli or DVT (angiography necessary)
One or more small Perfusion defects + Ventilation mismatch	27% Probability of emboli or DVT (angiography necessary)
One or more small Perfusion defects + Ventilation match	LOW probability of emboli (13%) (angiography may be unnecessary if risks are low and suspicion of emboli is low)
Indeterminant	Variable probability of emboli or DVT (17 to 58%). (angiography necessary)

From Hull et al., Annals of Internal Medicine, Vol 98, 891–899, 1983. This is the best prospective evaluation of diagnostic criteria and a well done study. Retrospective studies suggest that the specificity and predictive values of this study might have been greater if two other diagnostic criteria were used (defects on scans seen on two views, two or more defects present).

to asymptomatic chronic lung disease, age or other lung disorders limit the screening value of this test. Age alone reduces the PO_2 of many normal patients ($PO_2 < 80$ torr by age 60 is normal). Even large emboli may not produce hypoxemia.

Occasionally, the presence of acute thrombophlebitis can be demonstrated with **contrast venography, impedance plethysmography or other studies** and anticoagulation therapy is justified. Negative studies do not exclude the presence of emboli. Pulmonary angiography must be used to clarify the nature of perfusion scan defects in these patients. A **diagnostic thoracentesis** can also be useful if it demonstrates the presence of a sanguinous effusion (2 of 3 effusions due to emboli) and lung tumor, tuberculosis, or chest trauma are absent.

DEEP VENOUS THROMBOSIS, OVERVIEW AND PATHOPHYSIOLOGY

Patients often complain of a "charley horse" like constant discomfort or of a "heaviness" in the leg. **Calf pain, tenderness, edema, cording, a positive Homan's sign, etc. are unreliable indicators of phlebitis (19).** Fifty percent of hospitalized patients with deep vein thrombosis (DVT) have no physical findings; at least one-third of the patients suspected on clinical grounds do not have DVT. The diagnosis is always confirmed, in all but the most florid cases, by noninvasive studies or venography.

Deep venous thromboses begin as multicentric or single locus platelet and thrombin deposits proximal to valve cusps in the veins of the calf, thigh, or pelvis.

Initially localized disease can propagate rapidly over 24 hours. Venous flow volume, pulsatility and the degree to which the venous system will accommodate an increased volume and empty after occlusive pressure is applied to the system, are altered by the presence of DVT. Diagnostic studies identify these abnormalities, and their sensitivity varies according to the location of the thrombosis, the stage of disease development, the degree of venous occlusion, the presence or absence of extensive venous collaterals and technical aspects of each test, including observer experience.

Diagnostic Studies for DVT

Electrical impedance plethysmography and phleborheography are sensitive and specific for deep venous thrombi of the thigh and pelvis and first-line diagnostic studies. When clinical signs and symptoms suggest DVT, test sensitivity is 96–100%, specificity 94% (20). Studies can be repeated every other day until leg symptoms resolve or a positive test indicates a need for therapy (21). The sensitivity of both studies is substantially reduced when disease is mild and limited to the calf. Contrast venography is indicated in the presence of equivocal noninvasive studies, when the patient cannot be re-evaluated over several days and when an immediate definitive answer is required. Doppler ultrasound and I-125, fibrinogen scans provide complimentary diagnostic information. Radionuclide venography is not widely used.

Impedance plethysmography measures the flow and change in flow of small electrical currents across the venous system. These parameters vary according to the volume of blood in the venous system and the change in venous flow after pressure is applied through a leg cuff and released during the study. Sensitivity and specificity are decreased by technical errors, early disease with partial venous occlusion, the presence of large collaterals

and disease limited to the distal calf veins. Two trials have confirmed the validity of serially studying patients and withholding therapy in the absence of positive results.

Phleborheography compares current and previous, right and left leg tracings of venous pulsations and flow volumes after venous flow is occluded with pressure cuffs applied at several levels of the leg (22). Overall sensitivity is 83–93%, with a sensitivity of 92–96% for disease above the knee. Specificity is 87–97%. Loss of respiratory waves, elevation of the baseline after distal compression, poor foot emptying, and prominent arterial pulse waves suggest acute disease. A return of respiratory waves, less prominent baseline elevation, improved foot emptying, and loss of arterial pulsations suggest chronic disease. The sensitivity of the test for early disease limited to the calf may be 50% or lower.

The **venous Doppler test** depends on the interpretation of sound waves reflected from moving cells at rest and after flow augmentation following the application of external cuff pressure. Sensitivity (87–98%) and specificity (76–100%) are best for well-developed proximal (thigh) disease but vary widely depending on observer technique and experience. Sensitivity decreases in the presence of partial obstruction to flow, in disease in the lower calf and in the presence of large collaterals. The test is therefore considered complimentary to other studies and cannot be relied upon as a single definitive study.

The **I-125 fibrinogen** study is very sensitive to calf disease but inadequately sensitive to evaluate clinically more important thigh disease. False negative and positive rates average 8–12%. After thyroid block is achieved through potassium iodide administration, the nucleotide is injected, and baseline counts over the legs are obtained 4 hours later. Subsequent increases in counts of over 20%, which persist for 24 hours, identify hot spots that require additional diagnostic studies. False positive studies occur with any active fibrin deposition: cellulitis, trauma, fracture, edema, etc.

Contrast venography provides the definitive test (23). Sensitivity approaches 100% if all veins are filled through the judicious use of tourniquets and the iliofemoral vein is adequately visualized. The most specific criteria is a lucent intraluminal defect with dye streaming around it. Venous cutoff and wall irregularity provide less specific positive criteria.

Radionuclide venography involves the injection of technetium labeled albumin and visualization of the venous system using standard nuclear medicine techniques. Although the sensitivity and specificity of the technique have been reported as high as 93 and 100% respectively in one small study, technical aspects and the definition of the best diagnostic criteria inhibit the widespread use of this approach. It provides a reasonable diagnostic alternative in the hands of experienced and skilled individuals.

Treatment of Emboli and Deep Venous Thrombosis (DVT)

The **acute treatment** of life-threatening, massive emboli consists of supportive measures: fluids for hypotension, oxygen for hypoxia, bronchodilators for significant bronchospasm, anti-arrhythmic agents for arrhythmias, etc. Embolectomy or streptokinase infusions should be considered if the patient cannot be stabilized within 1 hour and diagnostic studies clearly establish the diagnosis. An inferior venacaval umbrella is indicated in three situations: (*a*) when there is an absolute contraindication to anticoagulation therapy, (*b*) when angiographically documented recurrences occur during adequate full-dose anticoagulant therapy, or (*c*) when a patient with marginal reserve is deemed incapable of survival in the event of a small recurrence. Mild to moderate edema or stasis sequela occur among 40% of patients (usually those with antecedent clinical evidence of stasis), insert migration occurs in less than 1%, and recurrent emboli are reduced to about 6% (26). Resolving and fragmenting emboli produce dramatic lung scan changes, even on the opposite side of the lung. For this reason, recurrent emboli should be angiographically documented.

Streptokinase is a proteolytic agent that dissolves thrombi. It is contraindicated in the presence of systolic pressures over 200 mm Hg, diastolic pressures over 110 mm Hg, major trauma, recent delivery, and surgery within 10 days, possible internal bleeding, cerebrovascular accident (CVA) within 2 months, pregnancy, age over 75 years, cavitary lung disease, inflammatory bowel disease, bacterial endocarditis, and intracardiac thrombi. All anticoagulants should be discontinued and coagulation studies should be near normal. A complete coagulation profile should be obtained and, invasive procedures should be avoided. The patient should be placed on a unit that permits close observation. Blood drawing should be minimized 22-gauge needles should be used.

The standard loading dose is 250,000 international units (IU) in normal saline over 30 minutes followed by a maintenance dose of 100,000 IU per hour for 12 to 24 hours for emboli. Longer courses (24 to 72 hours) for large venous thromboses can be given. The thrombin time should be 2–5 times normal and checked after 4 hours, (along with a hematocrit), to assure thrombolytic effect. If excess resistance to streptokinase is present (thrombin time < 1.5 times normal control), the infusion should be stopped. If bleeding occurs, one can give oral or intravenous **e-amino-caproic acid** (5-gram loading dose, then 1 gram per hour). Post-infusion, full-dose anticoagulation should begin after coagulation studies have returned to normal. The drug insert should be reviewed for additional recommendations before use.

The treatment of the vast majority of patients with emboli and deep venous thrombosis (calf and thigh) is the same—preventing propagation of venous thrombi and the recurrence of emboli through **full-dose intravenous anticoagulation.** Active bleeding, diastolic blood pressure of 115 or greater, cerebral vascular hemorrhage, recent vascular or neurosurgery, surgery or invasive procedures within 24 hours, pericarditis, vasculitis, and bacterial endocarditis contraindicate acute heparin therapy. If diagnostic studies must be delayed more than a few hours, begin continuous intravenous heparin therapy using an IVAC or Harvard pump. Continuous infusion reduces major bleeding complications to less than 1%, minor bleeding to less than 10% and is more effective than subcutaneous treatment in the prevention of recurrences. The drug insert should be reviewed for additional recommendations.

Administer a 5,000 unit loading bolus and then infuse heparin at a rate of 20 units/kilogram/hour or 1,000 to 2,000 units per hour. Measure the activated partial thromboplastin time (APTT) every 4–6 hours, adjusting the infusion rate by 500 units per hour until the APTT is at an optimum level of 1.5 to 2.0 times normal (optimum whole blood clotting time 25–30 seconds). Once regulated, measure the APTT daily. Decreased doses are frequently necessary after 72–96 hours. Maintain the heparin infusion for 7–10 days, and maintain bed rest for about 5 days to assure cessation of clot propagation and fixation of the clot to the vessel wall.

Warfarin therapy is continued for 3 months and occasionally longer to reduce recurrences of emboli to 2% or less. It is associated with a 4% bleeding complication rate. Begin oral coumadin therapy on the 5th day of heparin therapy. Since the prothrombin time may increase to a therapeutic range 72 hours before adequate coumadin-induced anticoagulation, continue both the heparin and coumadin

therapy at least 4 days (31). Begin therapy on the 5th to 7th day with 10–15 mg on day one, and adjust subsequent doses according to the prothrombin time response. Coumadin requirements vary from 2.5–25 mg daily. Optimum therapy (adequate anticoagulation with minimum bleeding) is achieved with a prothrombin time of 1.5 times normal (18–21 seconds). The incidence of anticoagulant associated bleeding can be reduced by maintaining the prothrombin time (PTT) at 1.5 times normal during warfarin therapy or prescribing subcutaneous heparin. Twice daily subcutaneous heparin which is adequate to increase the PTT to 1.5 times normal 4 hours after injection provides another alternative. No monitoring is necessary for this therapy, but many patients refuse to use daily injections.

Ambulatory patients with suspected DVT but negative noninvasive studies can be followed with alternate day phleborheography or impedance plethysmography for 7–10 days. Anticoagulant therapy is not required unless a positive test (indicating DVT above the knee) is obtained, in which case the patient is treated acutely for 10 days and with anticoagulation for 3 months thereafter. Unadjusted dose subcutaneous heparin (5000 IU every 12 hours) for 6 weeks provides adequate prophylaxis for patients with disease limited to the calves. Steptokinase is not indicated for calf vein thromboses, and the indications for streptokinase in DVT remain uncertain. It can be used early in the course of severe extensive DVT, such as phlegmasia dolens where extensive thrombosis and inflammation produce a pale, painful, grossly swollen and tender leg due to venous and arterial compromise.

Selection of Patients for Prophylaxis

Postoperative and hospitalization-associated DVT (and assumably emboli) can be reduced through mechanical intervention (Turbigrip stockings, pneumatic compressive devices, electrical calf stimulators, inferior vena cava umbrellas) and pharmacologic intervention (fixed-dose low-dose subcutaneous heparin, adjusted low-dose heparin, full-dose heparin, two-step warfarin therapy and intravenous dextran). Other regimens have been less well studied. Estrogens increase the risk of DVT several fold and, whenever possible, should be discontinued 3 weeks prior to surgery.

The efficacy of various regimens has been established for patients undergoing different types of surgery. The risk of postoperative DVT varies from low to high. The relative patient risk is determined primarily by the type of surgery, the type and duration of anesthesia, and the number of associated risk factors. A precise definition of exactly how much increased risk is incurred with the presence of some conditions is not possible.

Compressive stockings and early ambulation provide useful adjuncts in the prophylaxis of all patients, but alone are not effective among moderate- to high-risk patients. One early, controlled but nonrandomized autopsy study demonstrated a 50% decrease in autopsy proven deaths associated with emboli among a general surgical population using compressive stockings. Careful fitting is essential, and graded compressive stockings appear to be most effective.

External pneumatic compressive devices (EPC) employ pump stockings with variable cycles of inflation to optimize venous flow and pulsatility. Generally, they are started at surgery and maintained until the patient is ambulatory. Mild skin damage, sweating, and loss of ambulation present practical problems with use. They are advantageous in situations where anticoagulation is contraindicated (neuro- and ophthalmologic surgery) and in high-risk situations (prostate surgery, elective knee and hip surgery). **Electrical calf stimulators** use low-voltage currents to initiate muscle

contractions and optimize venous flow. Practical aspects have inhibited widespread use.

Fixed dose low-dose heparin (LDH) provides effective prophylaxis for most moderate-risk surgical and medical patients. Beginning 2 hours before surgery, 5,000 units of heparin should be administered every 8–12 hours. Therapy should be maintained until the patient is ambulatory.

Adjusted dose low-dose heparin (ALDH) provides protection for high-risk (elective hip surgery) patients (35). Prior to surgery, an initial dose of 3500 units is given subcutaneously and the APTT is measured after six hours, and at least once daily throughout therapy. Heparin is administered every 8 hours and additional units are added until the APTT is maintained at 31.5–36 seconds. Continue therapy for 8 days. Contraindications include bleeding disorders, trauma or surgical procedures where the risks of bleeding are unacceptable, and drug hypersensitivity. The incidence of hematomas or significant bleeding is very low.

Dextran (D) 40 (Gentran) or 70 (Gentran 70) decreases platelet aggregation through platelet coating and is generally about as effective as low-dose heparin but more expensive and cumbersome to use. They rarely causes anaphylaxis but occasionally aggravate congestive heart and renal failure. Dextran 70 is administered as 10ml/kg or 1000 ml loading dose on the day of surgery, followed by 500 ml daily for the next 2 or 3 days and then every other or third day until the patient is ambulatory or up to 2 weeks.

Two-step warfarin therapy (W) inhibits vitamin K dependent coagulation factors. Ten days before surgery, a dose adequate to increase the protime 1.5 to 3 seconds above baseline is given. Postoperatively, the dose is adjusted so that the prothrombin time is 1.5 times the control (38).

Table 9.4 categorizes patients into low-

Table 9.4. Perioperative Prophylaxis for Thromboembolism

Surgery, Risk of Thromboembolism and Patient Characteristics	Prophylaxis

ABBREVIATIONS: ALDH—Adjusted low-dose heparin, S&A—Stockings and early ambulation, D—Dextran, EPC—External compressive devices, LDH—Low-dose heparin, W—Two step warfarin. RISK ASSESSMENTS: L—Low, M—Moderate, H—High.

GENERAL

L—age <40, anesthesia <0.5 hrs., no other risk factors	none or S&A
M—age >40 or obesity, malignancy, past DVT/PE, complicated procedure	LDH, D
H—advanced age and malignancy, 3 or 4 risk factors	S&A + LDH or D

ORTHOPEDIC

H—elective hip surgery and knee reconstruction	ADLH, W, D
—hip fracture	EPC, D, S&A
M—all other types of orthopedic surgery	LDH, D

UROLOGIC

M—age >40, urologic surgery, transurethral prostatectomy	LDH, EPC
H—advanced age, transvesicle prostatectomy	LDH and or EPC

GYNECOLOGIC AND OBSTETRIC

L—<40 yrs., anesthesia <0.5 hrs.	S&A
M—age 40–70 yrs. no other risk factors	LDH, EPC, D
H—gynecologic malignancy or age >40 and other risk factors (D/C estrogens 3 weeks prior to surgery whenever possible)	LDH + EPC, W, D + EPC
M—pregnancy and prior DVT/PE	LDH
—pregnancy plus other risk factors	LDH + EPC, or individualized regimen

NEUROSURGERY AND NEUROLOGY

H—craniotomy patients	EPC
H—extracranial surgery	EPC or LDH, or both
H—nonhemorrhagic stroke	LDH
H—other strokes	EPC

TRAUMA

H—hip fractures (see orthopedics)	

Surgery, Risk of Thromboembolism and Patient Characteristics	Prophylaxis
H—head and spinal cord injuries	EPC, S&A
?—severe musculoskeletal trauma	LDH, S&A, EPC

MEDICAL CONDITIONS

M—myocardial infarct, congestive failure, pulmonary infections	LDH

RISK FACTORS

INHERITED: antithrombin III, protein C or S deficiencies, dysfibrinogenemia, plasminogen and plasminogen activator disorders

ACQUIRED: Lupus anticoagulant, nephrotic syndrome, paroxysmal nocturnal hemoglobinuria, cancer, stasis (congestive heart failure, myocardial infarction, constrictive pericarditis, anasarca), advanced age, estrogen therapy, sepsis, immobilization, stroke, polycythemia rubra vera, inflammatory bowel disease, obesity (> 40% above ideal body weight), prior DVT/PE, thrombocytosis

Adopted from National Institutes of Health Consensus Development Conference Statement, Volume 6, No. 2 March 1986. For estimates of actual risk levels see above reference.

moderate- and high-risk groups and identifies regimens that have reduced the incidence of DVT and/or emboli in proper trials.

READINGS

1. Dalen JE, Alpert JS: Natural history of pulmonary embolism. *Prog Cardiovasc Dis* 17:259–270, 1975.
2. Alpert JS, Smith R, Carloon J, et al.: Mortality of patients treated for pulmonary embolism. *JAMA* 236:1477–1480, 1976.
3. Camerato DJ, Stewart GJ, White JV: Combined dihydroergotamine and heparin prophylaxis of postoperative deep vein thrombosis: proposed mechanisms of action: *Am J of Surg* 150:39–44, 1985.
4. Cotton CT, Roberts VC. The prevention of deep vein thrombosis with particular reference to mechanical methods of prevention. *Surgery* 81:228–235, 1977.
5. Kakkar VV: Pathophysiologic characteristics of venous thrombosis. *Am J Surg* 150 (4A):1–6, 1985.
6. Moser KM, Le Moine JR: Is embolic risk con-

ditioned by location of deep venous thrombosis: *Ann Intern Med* 94:439–444, 1981.

7. Bell WR, Simon TL, De Mets DL: The clinical features of submassive and massive pulmonary emboli. *Am J Med* 62:355–359, 1977.
8. Tow DE, Wagner HN: Recovery of pulmonary arterial blood flow in patients with pulmonary embolism. *N Engl J Med* 276:1053–1059, 1967.
9. Spies WG, Spies SM, Mintzer RA: Radionuclide imaging in diseases of the chest (Part 1). *Chest* 83:122–127, 1983.
10. Sasahara AA, Hyers TM: The urokinase pulmonary embolism trial. *Circulation* 47:1–198, 1973.
11. Hull RD, Hirsch J, Carter CJ, et al.: Pulmonary angiography, ventilation lung scanning, and venography for clinically suspected pulmonary embolism with abnormal perfusion lung scan. *Ann Intern Med* 98:891–899, 1983.
12. Neumann RD, Sostman HD, Gottschalk A: Current status of ventilation-perfusion imaging. *Seminars in Nucl Med* X:198–217, 1980.
13. Light RW, George RB: Incidence and significance of pleural effusions associated after abdominal surgery. *Chest* 69:621–625, 1976.
14. Dantzker DR, Bower JS: Alterations in gas exchange following emboli. *Chest:* 81:495–498, 1981.
15. Sorbini CA, Grassi V, Solinas E, et al.: Arterial oxygen tension in relation to age in healthy subjects. *Respiration* 25:3–13, 1968.
16. Dalen JE, Brooks HL, Johnson LW, et al.: Pulmonary angiography in acute pulmonary embolism: Indications, techniques, and results in 367 patients. *Am Heart J* 81:175–185, 1971.
17. Bynum LJ, Wilson JE III: Characteristics of pleural effusions associated with pulmonary embolism. *Arch Intern Med* 136:159–162, 1976.
18. Stein PD, Dalen JE, McIntyre KM, et al.: The electrocardiogram in acute pulmonary embolism. *Progr in Cardiovascular Dis* XVII:247–257, 1975.
19. Barnes RW, Wu KK, Hoak JC: Fallibility of the clinical diagnosis of venous thrombosis *JAMA* 234:605–607, 1975.
20. Wheeler HB: Diagnosis of Deep Vein Thrombosis. *Am J Surg* 150:4A,7–13, 1985.
21. Huisman MV, Buller HR, Ten Gate JW, et al.: Serial impedance plethysmography for suspected deep venous thrombosis in outpatients. *New Engl J Med* 314:823–827, 1985.
22. Camerota AJ, White JV, Katz ML: Diagnostic methods for deep vein thrombosis: Venous doppler examination, phleborrheography, iodine-125 fibrinogen uptake, and phlebography. *Am J Surg* 150:4A, 14–24, 1985.
23. Hull R, et al.: Clinical validity of a negative venogram in patients with clinically suspected venous thrombosis. *Circulation* 64: No. 3,622–625, 1981.
24. Uphold RE, Knopp R, dos Santos PAL: Radionuclide venography As an outpatient screening test for deep venous thrombosis. *Ann Emerg Med* 9:613–616, 1980.

25. Gomes AS, Webber MM, Buffkin D: Contrast venography vs. radionuclide venography: A study of discrepancies and their possible significance. *Radiology* 142:219–228, 1982.
26. Greenfield LL, Alexander EL: Current status of surgical therapy for deep vein thrombosis. *Am J Surg* 150:4A,64–70, 1985.
27. Moser KM, Longo AM, Ashburn WL, et al.: Spurious scintiphotographic recurrence of pulmonary emboli. Am J Med 55:434–443, 1973.
28. National Institutes of Health Consensus Development Conference, Thrombolytic Therapy in Thrombosis. *Ann Int Med* 93:141–144, 1980.
29. Salzman EW, Deykin D, Shapiro RM, et al.: Management of heparin therapy: Controlled prospective trial. New Engl J Med 292:1046–1050, 1975.
30. Hull RD, Raskob GE, Hirsh J, et al. Continuous intravenous heparin compared with intermittent subcutaneous heparin in the initial treatment of proximal-vein thrombosis. *New Engl J Med* 315:1109–1114, 1986.
31. Hull R, Hirsh RJ, Carter C, et al.: Different intensities of oral anticoagulant therapy in the treatment of proximal vein thrombosis. *New Engl J Med* 307:1676–1681, 1982.
32. Hull R, Delmore T, Carter C, et al.: Adjusted subcutaneous heparin versus warfarin sodium in long-term treatment of venous thromboembolism. *New Engl J Med* 306:189–194, 1982.
33. Simon TL, Hyers TM, Gaston JP, et al.: Heparin pharmacokinetics: Increased requirements in pulmonary embolism. *Br J Haematol* 39:111–120, 1978.
34. Basu D, Gallus A, Hirsch J, et al.: A prospective study of the value of monitoring heparin treatment with the activated partial thromboplastin time. *N Engl J Med* 287:325–327, 1972.
35. Leyvraz PF, Jacques R, Fedor B, et al.: Adjusted versus fixed-dose subcutaneous heparin in the prevention of deep-vein thrombosis after total hip replacement. *New Engl J Med* 309:954–958, 1983.
36. Hull R, Delmore T, Genton E, et al.: Warfin sodium vs. low-dose heparin in long-term treatment of venous thrombosis. *New Engl J Med* 301:855–888, 1979.
37. National Institutes of Health Consensus Development Conference, Thrombolytic Therapy in Thrombosis. *Ann Int Med* 93:141–144, 1980 or write to NIH for: NIH Consensus Development Conference Statement, *Prevention of Venous Thrombosis and Pulmonary Embolism,* Vol 6, No 2, 1986.
38. Francis CW, Marder VJ, Evarts CM, et al.: Two step warfarin therapy. *JAMA* 294:374–378, 1983.
39. Bergqvist, D: *Post-operative Thromboembolism.* New York, Springer Verlag, 1983.
40. Goldhaber, SZ: *Pulmonary Embolism and Deep Venous Thrombosis.* Philadelphia, WB Saunders, 1985.
41. Shamma GVRK, Schoolman Michael, Cells C, et al.: Pulmonary embolism: Part II, *Circulation* 67:474–477, 1983.

10

Cardiovascular Disease and Hypertension

Richard J. Gross and David E. Kern

Cardiovascular disorders are the medical problems that most commonly require perioperative assessment and management. Most frequent are hypertension and ischemic heart disease. Intermediate in frequency are congestive heart failure, dysrhythmias, conduction abnormalities, valvular heart disease, and previous cardiac surgery. Patients with pericardial disease are occasionally encountered. The reported prevalence of cardiac disease in surgical patients is summarized in Tables 10.1 and 10.2.

The clinical data available on the cardiac risk of surgery is extensive. In reviewing conclusions from clinical series, the marked differences in patient population, in definition of heart disease, in measurement of complications, and in methods of analysis should be remembered.

The first section of this chapter (General Evaluation of the Cardiovascular Patient) describes the approach to the cardiac patient. It will be useful to read this first before reference to more detailed sections on specific problems.

GENERAL EVALUATION OF THE CARDIOVASCULAR PATIENT (SEE ALSO CHAP. 23)

Epidemiology

Most studies designed to identify cardiac risk factors have utilized postoperative myocardial infarction and cardiac death as endpoints. The risk factors for congestive heart failure are different and less clearly defined. Predictors of postoperative angina have not been studied.

Patients with *"cardiac disease,"* usually defined as ischemic heart disease (IHD),

Table 10.1. Prevalence of Cardiac Disease in Surgical Patients[a]

Study	Number	All Cardiac Disease	Coronary Artery Disease	Prior MI	Prior Angina
Nachlas, 1961	6,059	3.3%	3.3%		
Knapp, 1962	8,984[b]			5%	
Topkins, 1964	12,712			5%	
Hunter, 1968	141	18%	17%	4%	8%
Tarhan, 1972	32,877			1.3%	
Steen, 1978	73,321			.8%	
Rosen, 1966	506			1.6%	
Goldman, 1977	1,001[b]		27%	10%	

[a] Data from Refs. 1, 9–11, 14–15, 18, 20)
[b] All patients over age 40.

Table 10.2.   Prevalence of Coronary Artery Disease in Vascular Surgery Patients by Cardiac Catheterization and Clinical Criteria[a]

			All Patients		Subcategories of Patients by Clinical Findings	
Study	Total # of Pts.	Type of Surgery	% CAD by Cardiac Cath	% Severe Operable[b] CAD by Cardiac Cath	High Risk[c] % Severe Operable CAD by Cardiac Cath	Low Risk[c] % Severe Operable CAD by Cardiac Cath
Hertzer (1984)	1,000	All	91%	25%	34%	14%
Hertzer (1985)	506	Carotid	93%	28%	37%	16%

[a] Abbreviations: CAD = coronary artery disease; Cath = cardiac catheterization, ETT = ECG stress test.
[b] "Severe operable" CAD = greater than 70% coronary stenosis, but anatomy suitable for coronary artery bypass surgery.
[c] High risk = + clinical history/exam or ETT for CAD[d]
Low risk = − clinical history/exam or ETT for CAD[d]
[d] + (or −) Clinical or ETT = all patients either with (or without) clinical findings, laboratory abnormalities, or abnormal ECG exercise stress test, suggesting the presence of coronary artery disease.

have a 3–4-fold increased perioperative mortality and 5–6-fold increased risk of postoperative myocardial infarction compared to patients without cardiac disease (Tables 10.3–10.5). Cardiac mortality comprises one third to three-quarters of total mortality in cardiac patients (1–4). Post-operative cardiac deaths are about equally distributed between sudden death and cardiogenic shock (2).

The factors which independently correlate with life-threatening or fatal perioperative cardiac complications have been elucidated by Goldman (1, 2) and others. They include recent myocardial infarction, decompensated congestive heart failure or history of pulmonary edema, significant aortic stenosis, dysrhythmia, age greater than 70, emergency surgery, surgery involving the aorta, peritoneal or

Table 10.3.   Summary of Perioperative Cardiovascular Risk in Patients with Ischemic Heart Disease[c]

Patient Status (Preoperative)	Mortality (Range)		Postoperative Myocardial Infarction
	Total	Cardiac	
No "cardiac disease"[a]	3% (0.2–10%)	?[b]	0.8% (0.1–2%)
"Cardiac disease" present[a]	11% (5–20%)	?	5% (2–8%)
Angina (stable)	4% (4–12%)	?	4% (?)
Past myocardial infarction (MI)			
All	5–15%	5%	7%
Within 3 months	25–40% ⎫ 15–25%[d]	?	35% ⎫ 25%[e]
Between 3–6 months	5–20% ⎭	?	17% ⎭
More than 6 months	2.5%	?	5%
Unknown	?	?	10%

[a] Cardiac disease data based mostly on patients with ischemic heart disease.
[b] ? = data not available or uncertain.
[c] See also Table 10.4
[d] Recent figures show postoperative mortality may be less (see footnote e and Table 10.4) (4).
[e] Recent studies indicate current risk of reinfarction may be about 2–6%, using modern hemodynamic monitoring and anesthesia (Table 10.4) (60–61).

Table 10.4. Surgery After Myocardial Infarction (MI): Risk in Recent Studies[a]

| Time From Prior MI | % Postop Reinfarction | | % Total Mortality |
	Wells, 1976 (61)	Rao, 1977–82 (60)	Foster, 1978–81 (4)
0–3 mos.	0%	6%	}5–17%[b]
3–6 mos.	—	2%	

[a]Year in parenthesis denotes year study performed (not published).
[b]Includes 0–6 months. 0%[0/13] patients having CABG between MI and noncardiac surgery died postoperative the second surgery. 17%(1/6) patients without CABG died.

thoracic cavities, significant intraoperative hypotension, and poor general medical condition (Table 10.6).

Risk factors in other studies but not found by Goldman (1, 2), include severe or unstable angina, possible angina, and multiple other measures of congestive heart failure (Table 10.7) (4–6).

Factors which do not independently correlate with these life-threatening or fatal cardiac complications include sex, type and length of anesthesia, valvular

Table 10.5. Risk of Perioperative Death and Myocardial Infarction in Patients with "Cardiac" Disease

| Study | Total Number (Number with Cardiac Disease) | Postoperative Myocardial Infarction | | | Postoperative Deaths (All Causes) | | | Postoperative Cardiac Death[e] | Notes[a] |
		Cardiac Disease	Without Cardiac Disease	Total	Cardiac Disease	Without Cardiac Disease	Total		
Nachlas, 1961	6,059 (200)				10.5%	3.5%	3.5%		
Driscoll, 1961	496 (NS)			2.4%					B
Knapp, 1962[b]	8,984 (427)	6%	0.7%	0.9%					A
Arkins, 1964[c]	1,005 (1,005)	5%			22%			10%	C
Chamberlain, 1964	217 (NS)	2%							
Topkins, 1964[b]	12,712 (658)	6.5%	0.7%	1%					A
Skinner, 1964	766 (766)				13%				A
Hunter, 1968	141 (26)	7.6%	0.9%	2%			1.4%	0%	
Mauny, 1970	365 (NS)	8%							
Tarhan, 1972[b]	32,877 (422)	6.6%	0.13%	0.2%					
Sapala, 1975	416 (416)	2.4%			5.3%			3.8%	
Goldman, 1977[b]	1,001 (NS)	3.0%	2%	1.8%			5.9%	1.9%	
Goldman, 1977[e]	1,001 (NS)	8.9%	3%	3.2%					
Steen, 1978[b]	587 (587)	6.1%			5.1%				
Cooperman, 1978[d]	566 (NS)						8.5%	4.1%	
Plumlee, 1972	18,013 (NS)			0.1%					
Rosen, 1966	506 (74)	7%	0.4%	1.2%					
Mean		5.8%	1.1%	1.4%	11.2%	3.5%	4.8%	4.0%	

[a]A = patients over age 50, only males, or both. B = myocardial infarction diagnosed by electrocardiogram only (other studies used clinical criteria). C = patients with cardiac disease only.
[b]Cardiac disease limited to previous myocardial infarction.
[c]Cardiac disease limited to coronary artery disease.
[d]Series limited to one surgical disease.
[e]Cardiac death redefined as myocardial infarction plus cardiac death.
[f]Data from Refs. 1-3, 7-21.

Table 10.6. Independent Preoperative Risk Factors for Major Cardiac Complications[a]

	Relative Points
1. History	
a. Age > 70	5
b. MI within 6 months	10
2. Physical	
a. S3 gallop or JVD	11
b. Significant aortic stenosis	3
3. EKG	
1. Arrhythmia or PACs	7
b. >5 PVCs/min	7
4. General medical condition	
a. $pO_2 < 60$, $pCO_2 > 50$	
b. K < 3.0, $HCO_3 < 20$ meq/dl	
c. BUN > 50, CR > 3.0 mg/dl	3
d. Chronic liver disease or abnormal SGOT, or	
e. Bedridden from non-cardiac causes	
5. Operation	
a. Intraperitoneal, intrathoracic, or aortic	3
b. Emergency	4
Total possible	53

[a] Life-threatening and fatal cardiac complications defined as postoperative pulmonary edema, myocardial infarction, ventricular tachycardia, or cardiac death. (From Goldman L, et al: Multifactorial index of cardiac risk in noncardiac surgical procedures. *N Engl J Med* 297:845, 1977. Used with permission.)

Table 10.7. Other Independent Preoperative Risk Factors for Major Cardiac Complications (Found in Subsequent Studies, But Not By Goldman)

Risk Factor	Refs.
1. *Angina*	5
Class III, IV (CCS)[a]	6
Unstable (<6 months)	6
2. *Congestive heart failure* (CHF)	
Pulmonary edema (<1 week)	5, 6
Pulmonary edema (ever)	5, 6
Any CHF (ever)	5
Other measures[b]	4

[a] CCS = Canadian Cardiovascular Society
[b] See reference for list of measures.

rhythmias, cardiac conduction abnormalities, valvular and pericardial disease are factors that are discussed at length in later sections of this chapter.

Goldman (1, 2) found that age over 70 years was an independent risk factor for myocardial infarction and cardiac death. Previous studies (7) had shown nonsignificant trends (8–9) or no change in risk (10–11) with increasing age.

Noncardiac disease may increase the cardiac risk of surgery. *Poor general medical condition* (defined as $pO_2 < 60$, $pCO_2 > 50$, serum potassium < 3.0, serum bicarbonate < 20 meq/dl, BUN > 50, creatinine > 3.0 mg/dl, chronic liver disease or an abnormal SGOT, or being bedridden from noncardiac causes) was independently associated with serious cardiac complications, including death, in Goldman's series (1). An increased risk has been suggested when ischemic heart disease and chronic obstructive lung disease coexist. Presumably, some of the hypoxic or hypercarbic patients in the Goldman study represented patients with chronic lung disease. The increased mortality with electrolyte abnormalities, renal disease, liver disease, and debility has not been investigated in other studies.

The *type and location of surgery* is important. Emergency surgery increases the risk of both postoperative infarction and

lesions other than aortic stenosis, presence of rales, peripheral vascular disease, first degree, mono- and bifascicular heart block, mild to moderate hypertension, stable mild to moderate angina pectoris, nonspecific electrocardiographic changes, left ventricular hypertrophy, smoking, hyperlipidemia, and diabetes. The increase in surgical risk due to severe, unstable, or postinfarction angina pectoris or severe hypertension (especially when associated with end organ or ischemic heart disease) remains inadequately studied, and not determined with certainty, despite additional recent studies (Table 10.7).

Hypertension, intraoperative hypotension, previous myocardial infarction, congestive heart failure, angina, dys-

cardiac death (2). Cardiac risk is increased in operations involving the peritoneal or thoracic cavity or aorta (1, 3, 7–18). There is an increased mortality when a second and third operation is performed during a single hospitalization for the same problem. Certain types of minor surgery have low risk even in patients with severe ischemic heart disease (excluding recent myocardial infarction). Low-risk procedures include dental work under local anesthesia, transurethral prostate resection, eye surgery, and uncomplicated hernia repair.

The effect of the *type of anesthesia* on cardiac risk is more complex. Spinal and general anesthesia carry the same risk of postoperative myocardial infarction and cardiac death (1, 8–11, 17–19). Congestive heart failure, however, is more frequently seen after general than after spinal anesthesia (2). Local or regional anesthesia carries a very low risk of any cardiac complications. The high complication rates for local anesthesia in many studies reflect use of this technique in very poor risk patients, rather than the effect of the anesthesia itself. Most minor surgery under local anesthesia can be accomplished at very low risk.

Whether there is a relationship between *duration of anesthesia* and cardiac complications is unclear. The duration of anesthesia and operation has been related to cardiac complications in some studies (1, 7, 9–10, 20), but not in others (1, 8, 11, 18, 20). The length of anesthesia was not an independent risk factor in Goldman's study (2). The relationship between type of procedure and duration of anesthesia may explain some of the conflicting results (2, 10). Some recent studies have found that cardiac complications only increased for very long anesthesia times of more than 3–5 hours or in certain types of surgery (2, 10). Prolonged anesthesia time may be associated with increased risk of congestive failure and noncardiac death or infarction (2). Confounding variables (e.g., type of operation,

location of operation) and methodologic differences (e.g., complications measured, method of measuring anesthesia duration) in and among studies prevent more definitive conclusions regarding the risk of prolonged anesthesia.

Risk factors for developing coronary artery disease, such as diabetes mellitus, hyperlipidemia, smoking, left ventricular hypertrophy, and hypertension, do not affect operative risk (1–3, 11, 18, 21). These findings would suggest that there is not a major increased risk in patients with "subclinical" coronary artery disease.

An increased risk of cardiac complications has not been convincingly demonstrated for patients with *peripheral vascular disease* or *cerebrovascular disease* (2, 3).

Nonspecific electrocardiographic changes did not correlate with postoperative myocardial infarction in Goldman's study (2). While an association was demonstrated between nonspecific electrocardiographic changes and cardiac death, it was not an independent one. By multivariate analysis, the risk attributable to other related factors was removed and the relationship did not persist.)

In order to provide an overall measure of perioperative cardiac risk, Goldman developed a relative point scale for nine independent risk factors which he called the *Cardiac Risk Index* (Tables 10.6 and 10.8) (1). Other authors (5–6, 22–23) (Table 10.7) have suggested additional risk factors, but inadequate information is available to evaluate these against the original Goldman scale. If confirmed, the findings of independent risk for categories of angina would be "new"; the congestive heart failure variables represent different ways of measuring failure rather than a new risk factor. Four classes of risks were constructed based on the total number of points (Tables 10.8 and 10.9). The number of life-threatening complications and cardiac deaths rose progressively from Class I to Class IV.

Several recent studies (24–27) (Tables

Table 10.8.   Goldman's Cardiac Risk Index: Relationship to Perioperative Cardiac Complications [a]

Class	Point Total	No or Only Minor Complication (N = 943)	Life-threatening Complication (N = 39) [b]	Cardiac Deaths (N = 19)
I(N = 537)	0–5	532 (99%)	4 (0.7%)	1 (0.2%)
II(N = 316)	6–12	295 (93%)	16 (5%)	5 (2%)
III(N = 130)	13–25	112 (86%)	15 (11%)	3 (2%)
IV(N = 18)	≥26	4 (22%)	4 (22%)	10 (56%)

[a] Figures in parentheses denote percentage of patients in class with complications or death. (From Goldman L, Caldera DL, et al.: Multifactorial Index of Cardiac Risk in Non-cardiac Surgical Procedures. *N Engl J Med* 297:845, 1977. Used with permission.)
[b] Documented intraoperative or postoperative myocardial infarction, pulmonary edema, or ventricular tachycardia without progression to cardiac death.

10.10 and 10.11) have confirmed the validity of Goldman's Cardiac Risk Index. The sensitivity (Fig. 10.1) of the CRI has been questioned (28). Other authors have modified the index (5–6) (Table 10.7) with claimed increased accuracy; additional studies will need to clarify which index is superior.

Two other classifications have been used in determining the cardiac risks for surgery. The *New York Heart Association (NYHA) Functional Classification* is useful in assessing the surgical risk for postoperative congestive failure and mortality. The *Dripps American Society of Anesthesiologists (ASA) Classification* (see

Table 10.9.   Comparison of Goldman's Cardiac Risk Index (CRI) and ASA Classification [a]

Classi-fication	Number of Each Group		Cardiac Deaths		Life-threatening Complications	
	CRI	ASA	CRI	ASA	CRI	ASA
I	537	129	1 (0.2%)	0 (0%)	4 (0.7%)	0 (0%)
II	316	408	5 (2%)	3 (1%)	16 (5%)	7 (2%)
III	130	323	3 (2%)	8 (2%)	15 (11%)	13 (4%)
IV	18	112	10 (56%)	6 (5%)	4 (22%)	19 (17%)

[a] Percentages are percentage of patients in class with complications or death. Note: Since Goldman's CRI was derived from the above data and the ASA classification was applied prospectively to it, the comparison is biased in favor of the CRI. (Adapted From Goldman L, et al.: Multifactorial Index of Cardiac Risk in Non-cardiac Surgical Procedures. *N Engl J Med* 297:845, 1977. Used with permission.)

Table 10.10.   Goldman Cardiac Risk Index: Relationship to Perioperative Cardiac Death in Subsequent Studies

CRI Class	Study (% Cardiac Deaths)				
	Goldman (1)	Nichols (24)	Zeldin (26)	Waters (27)	Average (Mean)
I	.2%	.0%	2%	.1%	.1%
II	2%	1.6%	1%	.6%	1.3%
III	2%	2.9%	4%	5.6%	3.6%
IV	56%	0%	26%	0%	[20%]*

*Average may not be meaningful because 0% mortality in some studies may be due to very small numbers of patients in the class IV group.

Table 10.11.   Goldman Cardiac Risk Index: Relationship to Postoperative "Major" Complications in Subsequent Studies[a]

CRI Class	Study (% Major Complications)					
	Goldman (1)	Jeffrey (25)[b]	Zeldin (26)	Nichols (24)	Waters (27)	Average (Mean)
I	.7%	7%	.5%	.7%	.6%	1.9%
II	5%	11%	2%	7.4%	3.8%	5.8%
III	11%	38%	11%	31%	9.3%	20%
IV	22%	—	4%	50%	20%	[24%][c]

[a] Major complications ("life-threatening" complications as defined by Goldman [2]) are myocardial infarction, pulmonary edema, or ventricular tachycardia, without cardiac death.
[b] Includes cardiac death unlike other studies; only patients have abdominal aortic aneurysm repair. These differences may account for much higher complication rates in this study.
[c] Average may not be meaningful because of very small numbers of patients in Class IV group in most studies.

p. 22) is predictive of cardiac complications but may not be as precise as Goldman's Cardiac Risk Index (Tables 10.9, 10.10, and 10.11).

EKG stress tests provide some degree of separation of risk (28, 31–32, 34, 46–49).

Dipyridamole-thallium scan "stress" tests had a high degree of accuracy in predicting postoperative cardiac complications in several studies (using *intravenous* dipyridamole) (Table 10.12) (29–40) of vascular surgery. Patients undergoing vascular surgery with positive dipyridamole-thallium tests had an average 52% risk of postoperative myocardial infarction; patients with negative tests had a 0% risk (Table 10.12). However, patients with negative dipyridamole-thallium scans have had postoperative myocardial infarctions (35–36). The dipyridamole-thallium test provides a useful separation of cardiac risk, at least in a high-risk population; further studies need to be done in lower risk groups, such as general surgical patients. Larger numbers of patients and different types of surgery need to be studied to confirm these findings. Only studies using *intravenous* dipyridamole have been adequately done; the intravenous preparation is not yet FDA approved or commercially available at this time. The use of *oral* dipyridamole for thallium testing (41) has not been adequately standardized or studied; concerns remain about variable oral absorption rate affecting test accuracy. The use of oral dipyridamole for thallium stress testing is not currently recommended until more information is available.

The combination of clinical information and dipyridamole-thallium stress test results better predicts cardiac complications in vascular surgery patients than either does alone (35).

Ejection fraction by radionuclide scan also provides some separation of risk (Table 10.13) (42–45) for vascular surgery, but less data are available. Low ejection fraction ($\leq 35\%$) itself is not a prohibitive contraindication to surgery, but risk is significantly increased (43).

Holter monitoring for ischemia (by ST-depression criteria) also has been shown to be predictive of postoperative cardiac complications in preliminary studies (38, 50–52) (Table 10.13A). Holter monitor ischemia may be nearly as predictive as dipyridamole-thallium stress tests, but no direct comparison has been done (38). Most of the holter monitor recorded ischemic episodes were silent ischemia (52).

The role of cardiac catheterization in establishing risks in surgical patients with cardiac disease has not been well studied. Cardiac catheterization has identified patients with coronary disease missed clin-

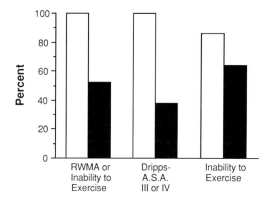

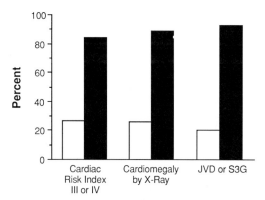

Figure 10.1. Sensitivity (*open bars*) and specificity (*solid bars*) of selected preoperative predictors in patients with and without perioperative cardiac complications. Dripps-A.S.A. = Dripps-American Society of Anesthesiologists; RWMA = regional wall motion abnormality. (From Gerson MC, et al.: Cardiac prognosis in noncardiac geriatric surgery. *Ann Intern Med* 103:834, 1985. Copyright 1985 American College of Physicians, used with permission.

Table 10.12. Dipyridamole-Thallium Scan as Predictor of Postoperative Cardiovascular Complications (Vascular Surgery)

Study	No. of Patients	% Postop. MI	
		Thallium +[a]	Thallium −[a]
Cutler (31)	116	26%	0%
Boucher (33)	48	50%	0%
Leppo (29)	69	94%	?
Eagle (30)	111	45%	0%
Lette (37)	66	43%	0%
Average of all studies		52%	0%

[a] + = abnormal; − = normal.

Table 10.13. Ejection Fraction (Radionuclide) as Predictor of Postoperative Cardiovascular Complications (in Vascular Surgery)

Ejection Fraction	Study	MI	Deaths
≥55%	Pasternak (1984, 1985)	0%	0%
≥35%	Pasternak (1984, 1985)	9%	0%
	Kazmers (1988)	3%	4%
≤35%	Pasternak (1984, 1985)	80%	20%
	Kazmers (1988)	29%	14%
	Kazmers (1988)	18%	4%

ically in high-risk vascular surgery (4, 53–54, 57). The accuracy of clinical (see also p. 628) parameters is better for estimating risk of cardiac death rather than major cardiovascular complications. The current best estimate is that clinical determination has about a 75% sensitivity. Studies of non-invasive testing do not provide enough information to estimate the *increment* of improvement *after* taking the clinical examination into account, but preliminary studies (28, 30, 35) indicate

Table 10.13a. Holter Monitoring for Ischemia as Predictor of Postoperative Cardiac Complications (Vascular Surgery)

Study	Patients	% Postop Cardiac Events[a,b]	
		Ischemia Positive	Ischemia Negative
Raby (52)	176	38%	1%

[a]Postop = postoperative
[b]Post cardiac events = cardiac death, myocardial infarction, unstable angina, pulmonary edema.

Table 10.14.   Risks of Routine Coronary Angiography (N = 1,000)[a,b] Prior to Vascular Surgery

1) "Severe CAD" = 598 (60%)
2) Cardiac Operation (N = 226)
—CVS Mortality = 12 (5.3%)
—PVS Mortality = 1 (0.8%)

3) All Patients PVS Mortality = 21 (2.6%)

[a] Data from ref. 53.
[b] Abbreviations: CAD = coronary artery disease; CVS = cardiovascular surgery; PVS = peripheral vascular surgery.

surgical risk. The risk of the catheterization itself is small (about 1:1500).

The sensitivity of *overall clinical assessment* (excluding non-invasive studies and cardiac catheterization) for identification of cardiac risk for noncardiac surgery has been estimated in several small studies (Tables 10.2, 10.15) (1, 28, 30, 35, 53–54, 57). The accuracy of clinical (see also p. 628) parameters is better for estimating risk of cardiac death rather than major cardiovascular complications. The current best estimate is that clinical determination has about a 75% sensitivity. Studies of non-invasive testing do not provide enough information to estimate the

increment of improvement *after* taking the clinical examination into account, but preliminary studies (28, 30, 35) indicate that it is less impressive than when the non-invasive tests are evaluated in isolation.

Preoperative Evaluation (Tables 10.16 and 10.17)

Regardless of the specific types of heart disease, preoperative evaluation should include a complete *history and physical exam* (see p. 614). When the patient has had a recent complete history and physical exam, a shortened preoperative evaluation should include, at a minimum, a complete cardiovascular and pulmonary history, smoking history, medication history, allergic and bleeding history, vital signs, including any postural changes, weight, and examination of the nose, mouth, throat, respiratory and cardiovascular systems. Factors that increase cardiac work or decrease cardiac performances should be sought such as fever, anemia, hypertension, hypervolemia, hypovolemia, hypoxia, hypercarbia, acid-base or electrolyte disorders, uncontrolled diabetes, smoking, and medications.

Table 10.15.   Sensitivity of Preoperative Clinical Assessment at Identifying Postoperative Cardiac Complications

Study	Clinical Measure[a]	Endpoint or Criterion[a]	Sensitivity of Clinical Assessment
Yeager (57)	Clinical	CV death	100%
Eagle (30)	Clinical	Postoperative "ischemic event"	100%
Eagle (257)	Clinical	Postoperative "ischemic event"	83%
Gerson (28)	CRI "indicator"	Postop CV complication	77%
Hertzer (54)	Clinical	Coronary Angiography	77%
Hertzer (53)	Clinical	Coronary Angiography	79%
Goldman (1)	CRI Class III/IV	CV death	69%
		Major CV complication	36%

[a] Abbreviations: CRI = Goldman Cardiac Risk Index; clinical = variable combinations of history, physical, non-invasive testing; CV = cardiovascular.

Table 10.16.   Preoperative Evaluation in the Patient with Cardiac Disease

ALL PATIENTS
  History: Emphasizes cardiovascular and respiratory systems, smoking history, medication history.
  Physical exam: Emphasizes vital signs including postural changes in blood pressure and pulse, weight, volume and hydration status, ENT, respiratory and cardiovascular systems
  Laboratory: Chest x-ray, EKG, CBC, electrolytes, glucose, BUN, or creatinine
  Classification of risk: NYHA, Dripps-ASA, Goldman's CRI (see text)
PATIENTS ON DIGOXIN OR ANTIARRHYTHMICS
  Serum drug levels
PATIENTS WITH HISTORY OF SMOKING OR CHRONIC LUNG DISEASE
  Spirometry, arterial blood gases
SPECIAL CIRCUMSTANCES
  Arterial blood gases, stress testing, holter monitor, echocardiography, gated blood pool scan, thallium scanning, dipyridamole thallium stress testing, cardiac catheterization

Basic laboratory tests include an electrocaradiogram, chest x-ray, hematocrit, electrolytes, glucose, and urea nitrogen or creatinine. Serum levels should be obtained for digoxin and antiarrhythmic drugs. Although toxic levels in asymptomatic patients are not diagnostic of clinical drug toxicity, serum levels provide an estimate of the risk of subsequent toxicity. Spirometry and arterial blood gases are indicated for people who smoke regularly or who have lung disease.

Table 10.17.   Factors Which Increase Cardiac Work or Adversely Affect Cardiac Performance

Fever
Anemia (hematocrit < 30)
Electrolyte disorders; ↓ CA, ↓ Mg
Acid-base imbalance
Hypoxia, hypercarbia, pulmonary dysfunction
Hypervolemia, hypovolemia, or dehydration
Hypertension
Smoking
Medications
Pain, anxiety

Non-invasive tests of cardiac function are most useful when the existence, type, or severity of cardiovascular disease is uncertain. There is insufficient evidence to support the routine screening with non-invasive tests of clinically low-risk patients for cardiac disease. Some authorities would not routinely screen asymptomatic patients even for high-risk surgery (28, 30, 32, 38, 58–59); although some authors and data reach the opposite conclusion specifically for high cardiac risk vascular surgery (33, 40, 46, 53). The specific role of most non-invasive tests in predicting surgical risk for the cardiac patient remains inadequately studied.

Stress testing is useful in quantitating exercise tolerance, confirming the diagnosis, and estimating the severity of ischemic heart disease. Echocardiography is most useful in evaluating valvular heart disease; an estimate of ventricular function is also obtained. Gated blood pool scanning gives the best non-invasive estimate of ventricular function. Thallium scanning may confirm a prior myocardial infarction, quantitate damage, and estimate severity of ischemic disease (especially when done as part of an electrocardiogram (EKG) stress test).

The use of cardiac catheterization to confirm and quantitate coronary and valvular heart disease is discussed on pages 133 and 156.

The *Goldman Cardiac Risk Index, NYHA Functional Classification,* and the *ASA classification* are useful adjunctive data, especially in patients with multiple risk factors. None of these indices should be the sole criteria for surgical decisions.

The *final diagnostic impression* should clearly state (*a*) the diagnoses that represent cardiac risk factors for surgery, (*b*) the certainty with which these diagnoses are established, and (*c*) an overall estimate of surgical risk. Accurate assessment of cardiac risks for surgery cannot be based upon a vague, imprecise diagnosis of ischemic heart disease nor on conditions, such as mild hypertension, which do not increase surgical risk.

Patients should generally be classified as *high*, *medium*, or *low risk* in making decisions about surgery. Patients with recent myocardinal infarction, unstable angina, decompensated congestive heart failure, significant aortic stenosis, or poor Goldman, NYHA, or ASA classification should be considered high risk. Only urgent, life-saving surgery should be undertaken in these patients until their heart disease is improved. Patients with moderately severe, stable angina, significant arrhythmia or conduction disturbance, controlled but moderately symptomatic congestive heart failure, myocardinal infarction over 6 months old (without risk factors) or intermediate Goldman, NYHA, or ASA classifications should be considered medium risk. Patients with a stable mild to moderate angina, with controlled symtomatic congestive heart failure, or with favorable Goldman, NHYA, or ASA classification should be considered low risk.

Surgical decisions must consider not only the risk of cardiac disease, but the magnitude of the surgery. Operations involving the thoracic and peritoneal cavities or aorta clearly represent increased risk. Conversely, low-risk surgery includes most operations on the extremities, head and neck (excluding radical neck dissection), breasts, and skin. Miscellaneous low-risk procedures include uncomplicated hernia repair, hemorrhoidectomy, and transurethral prostate resection. Minor procedures done under local or regional anesthesia probably entail less risk than the same procedures done under general or spinal anesthesia.

The final judgment regarding the advisability of surgery rests upon the simultaneous consideration of several factors: the medical status of the patient, the type of operation, the need for surgery, and the type of anesthesia required. This decision is best made after thorough discussion among internist, surgeon, and anesthesiologist.

Management

Once the decision to operate has been made, efforts should be directed toward minimizing controllable risks. Smoking should be discontinued 2 weeks prior to surgery. Factors that increase cardiac work or decrease cardiac performance (Table 10.17), such as fever, anemia (hematocrit less than 30), hypoxia, hypercarbia, acid-base or electrolyte disturbances, and severe hypertension should be corrected whenever possible. Hypervolemia, hypovolemia, hypotension, and dehydration should be tested. Medication use should be reviewed, potential adverse effects and interactions anticipated, and adjustments made when necessary.

In general, the higher the risk, the more intensive should be the perioperative cardiac monitoring. High-risk, patients will usually require an intensive care unit bed during the immediate postoperative period.

Selected high-risk patients may benefit from hemodynamic monitoring with pulmonary artery (Swan-Ganz) catheters (see pp. 133, 140, and Chapter 8, p. 92).

Management of specific cardiovascular risk factors are discussed in subsequent sections of this chapter.

PREOPERATIVE HYPERTENSION

Epidemiology

With a prevalence of approximately 10% in the adult population, sustained hypertension is one of the most common medical problems encountered in the preoperative patient. Although associated with other potential and proven preoperative risk factors (such as congestive heart failure, coronary artery disease, cerebrovascular disease, renal failure, and hypokalemia secondary to diuretic therapy), mild to moderate hypertension per se has not

Table 10.18. Hypertension and Surgery[a]

Study Group	Number	Mean Systolic	Complications			
			Cardiac Death	Non-fatal Major Complication	Intra-operative Hypotension Requiring Treatment	Perioperative Hypertension[b]
Goldman and Caldera (prospective) (2)						
Normotensives, no history of hypertension	431	126	1 (0.2%)	10 (2%)	82 (19%)	33 (8%)
Treated hypertensives, BP normalized	79	136	1 (1%)	6 (8%)	16 (20%)	21 (27%)
Treated hypertensives, BP ≥ 160 systolic or ≥ 90 diastolic	40	154	0 (0%)	0 (0%)	13 (33%)	10 (25%)
Untreated hypertensives	77	161	1 (1%)	1 (1%)	21 (27%)	15 (20%)

Study Group	Number	Systolic	Total Mortality
Skinner and Pearce (retrospective: patients with cardiac disease (8)	368	101–140	11%
	331	141–200	14%
	55	>200	14%

[a] Modified from Goldman L, Caldens DL: Risks of general anesthesia and elective operations in the hypertensive patient. *Anesthesiology* 50:285, 1979; and Skinner JF, Pearse ML: Surgical risk in the cardiac patient. *J Chronic Dis* 17:57, 1964, (Pergamon Press), with permission.
[b] Significant difference between normotensive and hypertensive patients (regardless of treatment or degree of control).

been shown to be an independent predictor of perioperative morbidity or mortality.

The unimportance of mild to moderate hypertension as an independent preoperative risk factor is supported by existing clinical epidemiologic data (1–3, 8, 18, 20, 65) (Table 10.18), although conflicting data exists (3, 51, 125). In Goldman and Caldera's prospective study (65) of nonemergency procedures in 196 hypertensive and 480 normotensive patients, neither preoperative systolic nor diastolic hypertension independently increased the chances of perioperative cardiovascular complications (death, infarction, ischemia, failure, arrhythmias), intraoperative hypotension requiring therapy, or postoperative renal failure. Thus, preoperative hypertension was independently correlated with neither cardiac complications nor cardiac death (1, 2). In a retrospective study of 627 vascular surgery patients, Cooperman et al. (3) also failed to identify preoperative hypertension as a risk factor for postoperative cardiovascular complications. Skinner and Pearce (8) reported similar findings in an earlier retrospective study of 857 operations in cardiac patients. Hypertension by itself was not associated with increased perioperative mortality, although hypertensive heart disease was. Two early, large prospective studies by Chamberlain and Edmonds-Seal (21) and Rosen et al. (18) failed to demonstrate increased risk of myocardial ischemia or electrocardiographic deterioration in hypertensives compared to normotensive patients undergoing surgery. Other studies (4, 10, 66) which have reported increased perioperative mortality or morbidity in hypertensives compared to normotensive patients, were retrospective and failed to control for associated risk factors.

Uncontrolled hypertensives do experience a *greater relative intraoperative blood pressure decrease* than controlled hypertensives or normotensives, but *the absolute level of blood pressure nadir is not lower* (65, 67). Furthermore, there is no evidence that the greater decrease in blood pressure is associated with a poorer clinical outcome. In Prys-Robert's careful pre-, intra-, and postoperative hemodynamic studies of 43 patients (67–68), however, electrocardiographic evidence of transient ischemia not infrequently accompanied the intraoperative blood pressure falls, especially in untreated or poorly controlled hypertensives. Goldman et al. did not confirm this finding in their larger study (1, 2, 65), but intraoperative monitoring and recording was less intensive and their patients had more mild hypertension than those of Prys-Roberts. Goldman et al. were unable to demonstrate a significant relationship between the presence or severity of preoperative hypertension and the need for treatment of intraoperative hypotension with adrenergic agents or fluid challenges.

Another finding of unproven clinical importance is the *increased risk of perioperative hypertensive episodes* in patients who have a history of preoperative hypertension. In the study by Goldman et al., (1, 2, 65), perioperative hypertensive events (defined as a systolic blood pressure of over 200, a rise in systolic blood pressure of over 50, or the use of intravenous antihypertensive therapy) were more likely in hypertensive than normotensive patients (23% vs. 8%), regardless of whether preoperative blood pressure was adequately controlled (Table 10.18). A history of markedly increased blood pressures (diastolics > 110) further increased the chance of perioperative hypertension. Prys-Roberts (69), in reviewing his experience with over 200 hypertensive patients, has also concluded

that postoperative hypertension (defined as systolic blood pressure over 250 or diastolic over 140) is more common among patients who have previous histories of severe hypertension, regardless of whether or not the blood pressure was under control prior to anesthesia.

It should be emphasized that while there is substantial data on mild and moderate hypertension, very few severely hypertensive patients (diastolic $\geq$ 110 mm Hg) have been included in major studies. The demonstration of transient myocardial ischemia associated with relatively large intraoperative blood pressure falls in severely hypertensive patients suggests a possibly increased perioperative risk (69) in these patients.

Data has accumulated over the past three decades on the use of antihypertensive agents in the immediate perioperative period. Early fears of drug interactions, blockade of vasomotor reflexes with consequent intraoperative hypotension, unresponsiveness to pressor agents, and depression of cardiac output by betablockers, were based upon incomplete physiologic and pharmacologic knowledge and uncontrolled clinical reports (70–72). Early recommendations were that antihypertensive agents be withdrawn prior to elective surgery (70–72). Subsequent larger and better designed studies have demonstrated that reserpine (73–75) and other antihypertensive agents (65, 76) can be safely continued up to the time of surgery (77).

Beta-blockers were of special concern because of negative inotropic and chronotropic effects up to 36 hours and hypersensitivity to subsequent adrenergic stimulation 24–48 hours after cessation of therapy (78–80). However, experience in coronary bypass surgery (81–84) and more limited experience on noncardiac surgery (2, 85–88) has demonstrated that propranolol can be given safely within 24 hours of surgery. Discontinuation of propranolol in patients with coronary artery disease 24–72 hours preoperatively may result in increased risk of perioperative ischemia (82). In one study of anesthetized hypertensive patients given the beta-blocker practolol plus atropine intravenously, no significant difference could be demonstrated between pre- and post-drug heart rate, cardiac output, or mean arterial pressure (89). The patients receiving practolol showed significantly attenuated tachycardia and hypertensive responses to laryngoscopy and intubation and fewer dysrhythmias and ischemic changes than controls.

Abrupt discontinuation of clonidine may occasionally precipitate a withdrawal syndrome manifested by hypertension and tachycardia (91–92).

In summary, uncomplicated mild and moderate hypertension does not seem to be a risk factor for perioperative morbidity or mortality. However, preoperative hypertension, whether controlled or uncontrolled, does predispose to postoperative hypertension. Preoperative uncontrolled hypertension is associated with relatively large intraoperative blood pressure reductions that are of questionable clinical significance. Whether severe preoperative hypertension independently increases perioperative morbidity and mortality is unknown. It is safe to continue most antihypertensive drugs until the time of surgery.

Evaluation

Of particular concern during the preoperative assessment of the hypertensive patient is the detection of associated surgical risk factors. Hypertension has been etiologically linked to coronary artery disease, congestive heart failure, cerebrovascular disease, and renal disease. Diuretic-associated hypovolemia, hypokalemia, and alkalosis should also be detected preoperatively. Primary aldosteronism and hyperadrenalism are rare causes of hypertension associated with hypokalemia, Pheochromocytoma, another rare cause of hypertension, is of major concern periop-

Table 10.19. Preoperative Assessment Pertinent to the Hypertensive Patient

History
  1. Assess associated risk factors and end organ damage: coronary artery disease, congestive heart failure, cerebrovascular disease, renal disease, pheochromocytoma
  2. Medication history
  3. Blood pressure on and off medication
Physical exam
  1. Blood pressure and pulse (supine, sitting, and standing; both arms)
  2. Evaluation of hydration and intravascular volume, especially if on diuretics
  3. Fundoscopy
  4. Cardiovascular exam
  5. Respiratory exam
Laboratory
  1. EKG
  2. Chest x-ray
  3. Electrolytes (especially if on diuretics)
  4. BUN/creatinine
  5. Urinalysis

eratively (see page 296). In the hypertensive patient, the preoperative history, physical examination, and laboratory evaluation should be oriented toward the detection of these risk factors (Table 10.19).

Since many antihypertensive agents have the potential for intraoperative drug interactions with anesthetics, pressors, or neuromuscular blocking agents, the consulting internist should familiarize him/herself with the relevant pharmacology of the patient's drugs (76, 93–95) (see p. 34). For example, preoperative use of diuretics may cause hypokalemia, which can be accentuated by intraoperative hyperventilation or hypovolemia, which will make the patient more sensitive to intraoperative blood loss. Agents that block adrenergic transmission may render the patient more sensitive to direct-acting and less sensitive to indirect-acting pressor agents. The names, dosages, and schedules of the patient's medications should be clearly listed and available to the anesthesiologist. The range of preoperative blood pressures on and off antihypertensive therapy should be recorded for future reference.

Management (Table 10.20)

Patients with controlled or partially treated hypertension who have diastolic pressures < 110 should in general be continued on their antihypertensive medication until the time of surgery. Patients with untreated mild to moderate hypertension (diastolics < 110) may undergo most elective surgery, with institution of antihypertensive therapy electively postoperatively.

Certain special surgical procedures may require control of even mild hypertension. For example, mild hypertension has been said to increase the risk of bleeding in certain retinal surgery, brain surgery, and wound hematomas in plastic surgery. Most of the increased risk is based on clinical experience without firm data, except for preliminary data for wound hematomas in plastic surgery.

Patients with severe hypertension (diastolic ≥ 110 mm Hg) or with hypertension causing significant cardiac, neurologic, or renal compromise should probably have their blood pressures at least partially controlled before non-urgent surgery. In patients requiring preoperative control of hypertension, blood pressure should be lowered with careful attention to the time necessary to achieve maximal

effects of the drugs used. For the oral agents used in most cases, this involves week(s) and, practically, discharge and readmission of the patient. Rushed "control" of blood pressure with rapid increases in medication over several days may result in volume depletion, hypokalemia, or hypotension at the time of surgery.

Urgent and emergency surgery should not be delayed because of severe hypertension, except in the presence of hypertensive encephalopathy, hypertensive-induced acute cardiac decompensation, or other hypertensive emergencies. When blood pressure control is needed urgently preoperatively, nitroprusside can be used. Intermediate acting agents such as apresoline can be used when a few days are available.

While most antihypertensive agents can be continued up to and including the morning of surgery (given with small sips of water), a few deserve special consideration. Because of the potential for serious drug interactions (including hypertensive crises) MAO inhibitors should be discontinued at least 2 weeks prior to surgery. Guanethidine is also usually withdrawn 2 weeks prior to surgery because of its profound interference with circulatory reflexes, although not all authorities agree with this strategy (76). Clonidine should generally be given the morning of surgery and resumed immediately postoperatively to minimize the risk of a withdrawal syndrome. When a prolonged period of postoperative nasogastric suction is required, parenteral methyldopal may be substituted for oral clonidine in the reasonable but unsubstantiated expectation of preventing a withdrawal syndrome; clondine patches can also be used. When a prolonged period of postoperative nasogastric suction is anticipated preoperatively, consideration should be given to gradually tapering clonidine prior to surgery. Generally, an alternative medication should be substituted for any antihypertensive drug discontinued preop-

Table 10.20.   Suggested Preoperative Management of the Hypertensive Patient

Antihypertensive therapy
  May be continued until time of surgery, provided anesthesiologist is aware of medications. MAO inhibitors and perhaps guanethidine should be discontinued 2 weeks before surgery.
Uncontrolled hypertension
  Mild to moderate hypertension need not be controlled preoperatively. Need for preoperative control of severe hypertension (diastolic > 110), and hypertension complicated by significant CNS, cardiac, or renal disease is uncertain, but recommended prior to elective surgery. Hypertensive emergencies should be treated preoperatively.
Associated risk factors
  Should be recognized and managed (see text).

eratively. Beta blockers are usually continued until the morning of surgery.

There is some theoretical concern that patients treated with angiotensin converting enzyme (ACE) inhibitors such as captopril might have difficulty maintaining their blood pressure if there was significant blood loss during surgery. In practice, however, many patients receiving ACE inhibitors have undergone major surgery without difficulty. If a hypotensive episode were aggravated by an ACE inhibitor, this could be counteracted easily with volume expansion. ACE inhibitors do not interfere with the action of commonly used general anesthetics. It is currently recommended that ACE inhibitors be continued until the morning of surgery.

The extent of intraoperative monitoring, including the use of intra-arterial, central venous, and/or Swan-Ganz catheters, should depend upon the severity and lability of the patient's blood pressure, as well as the presence of associated disease factors. The routine use of precordial V_4 or V_5 lead, as well as limb leads, may enhance the detection of intraoperative ischemia (90, 96–97) associated with marked blood pressure changes.

INTRAOPERATIVE AND POST-OPERATIVE HYPERTENSION

Epidemiology

The incidence of perioperative hypertension is dependent upon how it is defined, the intensity of blood pressure monitoring, and the population being monitored. In Goldman and Caldera's series of 676 non-emergency procedures in 617 patients who were closely monitored except during intubation and laryngoscopy, 82 patients (13%) experienced intraoperative or recovery room hypertension defined as a systolic blood pressure of over 200 mm, a systolic blood pressure rise of over 50 mm, or the use of intravenous medications to lower blood pressure (65). Factors that predisposed to perioperative

hypertensive episodes were preoperative hypertension, regardless of control or treatment (23% or hypertensives vs. 8% of normotensives), and type of surgery. The frequency of hypertensive episodes during or after surgery was 57% for abdominal aortic aneurysm resections, 29% for peripheral vascular procedures, 8% for intraperitoneal or intrathoracic procedures, and 4% for all other procedures. When all 1001 patients, including those undergoing emergency procedures, were included in the analysis, the findings were similar (1). In a study of 1844 recovery room patients monitored at 10-minute intervals, 60 (3.25%) experienced hypertensive episodes defined as at least two consecutive measurements of systolic blood pressure > 190 and diastolic > 100 (98). In one report, hypertension (defined as systolic blood pressure over 150 mm Hg) was listed as a complication in only 485 or 1.6% of 29,583 routinely monitored recovery room patients (99).

Intraoperatively, laryngoscopy and intubation are usually associated with mean arterial pressure rises of 20–30 mm or more (100–102). The hypertensive response can be attenuated somewhat by the use of surface anesthesia* (100) or beta-blocking agents (101). Other common causes of intraoperative hypertension include too light anesthesia, overreplacement of intravenous fluids, ventilatory inadequacy ($\uparrow pCO_2$ or $\downarrow pO_2$), organ manipulation (especially kidney or brain), and the use of pressor agents.

Postoperatively, hypertension is frequently seen in the anesthetic emergence period (58, 103). Other common postoperative causes of hypertension are pain secondary to inadequate analgesia, ventilatory insufficiency, overreplacement of intravenous fluids, reaction to an endotracheal tube, and residual effects of va-

---

*Defined as transcricothyroid injection of topical anesthetic, bilateral superior laryngeal nerve block, and topical anesthetic spray of the pharynx, larynx, and trachea.

sopressor drugs (98). Over half the patients have a history of preoperative hypertension (65, 98). Postoperative hypertension is more common after vascular surgery (58, 104). Approximately one-third of the patients have no obvious cause for their increased pressure (98). Increased sympathetic nervous system activity may be the mechanism in postoperative hypertension in at least some patients (103).

While definitive data are not available, the existing literature and clinical experience suggest that perioperative hypertensive episodes are usually easily managed, often self-limited, and infrequently a cause of significant morbidity or mortality.

Evaluation

Evaluation of perioperative hypertension is directed toward answering two questions: (a) What is the cause of the hypertension? and (b) How severe is the hypertension? A search for the cause of perioperative hypertension (Table 10.21) should begin with an assessment of ventilatory adequacy (observation, respiratory exam, arterial blood gases), an evaluation of the depth of anesthesia, determination of the surgeon's activities in the operative field, review of perioperative drug use, evaluation of the patient's volume status (postural blood pressure, jugular, central venous; pulmonary wedge pressure; or cardiovascular exam), and knowledge of a preoperative history of

Table 10.21.   Common Causes of Intraoperative and Postoperative Hypertension

Laryngoscopy/intubation
Too light anesthesia
Inadequate analgesia
Ventilatory inadequacy
Overreplacement of intravenous fluids
Organ manipulation
Medications
Emergence from anesthesia
Preoperative hypertension (risk factor)
Type of surgery (risk factor)

hypertension or other rare risk factors (pheochromocytoma, hyperthyroidism).

The severity of the hypertension should be assessed by measurement of the blood pressure and determination of the blood pressure rise, fundoscopy and evaluation of CNS status, cardiovascular examination with review of the EKG and/or electrocardiographic monitor, and evaluation of renal function.

Management

Management of perioperative hypertension episodes should, if possible, be directed toward their etiology. Adequate ventilation and oxygenation must be assured. The depth of anesthesia may need to be increased, or adequate analgesia provided. Hypervolemia can be treated with diuretics or by not replacing fluid losses. Nonspecific measures such as positive pressure ventilation may decrease blood pressure by interfering with venous return. Tilting the patient may be helpful by inducing postural hypotension.

Parenteral hypotensive therapy is infrequently required, but in the presence of hypertensive-induced encephalopathy, congestive heart failure, angina, infarction, or arrhythmia, it will be needed. Immediate and smooth blood pressure control can be established with intravenous nitroprusside (Nipride), trimethaphan (Arfonad), or nitroglycerin. All three need intensive supervision, and the trimethaphan's effects are very sensitive to postural changes. Intravenous nitroglycerin may be preferable when acute myocardial ischemia is present, because it will improve the ischemia, which has not been shown with the other agents. Intravenous diazoxide (Hyperstat) will provide prompt although less controllable blood pressure reduction, with maximal effect at 5 minutes and a duration of 2–24 hours. It requires less intensive supervision, but may precipitate EKG ischemic changes. In semi-acute situations, parenteral hydralazine can be used with maximal effect

Table 10.22.   Parenteral Availability of Commonly Used Antihypertensive Drugs

Drugs Available in Parenteral Form	Parenteral Form Not Available	
	Drug	"Equivalent" in Same Class
Furosemide, Bumetanide, Ethacrynate	Thiazide diuretics	Furosemide, Bumetanide, Ethacrynate IV
Reserpine	Clonidine, guanabenz, guanfacine (central acting)	Methyldopa IV; clonidine patch
Methyldopa	Minoxidil (vasodilator)	Hydralazine IM or IV
Hydralazine	Prazosin (peripheral alpha adrenergic blocker)	Hydralazine IM or IV
Propranolol, Metoprolol, Labetolol	Atenolol, Nadolol, Timolol[c] (beta-blocker)	Propranolol, Metoprolol,[a] Labetolol, Esmolol[a] IV
Enalaprilat	Nifedipine, Verapamil, Diltiazem, Nicardipine (calcium channel blockers)	Nifedipine s.l.[b]
Nitroglycerin[a]	Captopril, Lisinopril (angiotension inhibitor)	Enalaprilat IV
	Guanethidine (ganglionic blocker)	None
Patches Clonidine Nitroglycerin		

[a] Not FDA approved for this use; limited published experience.
[b] Hypotension a potential problem with nifedipine sublinguinal. Although available in parenteral form, verapamil intravenously has not been used for hypertension and dosing guidelines are not available.
[c] Also acebutolol, pindolol.

in 20–40 minutes and a duration of effectiveness of 3–8 hours. Reflex tachycardia may occur and require control. Both hydralazine and diazoxide may increase dP/dt and sheering forces, and are less desirable after aneurysm or vascular surgery. Intravenous labetolol has been used with success (105–106). Sublinguinal nifedipine may also be used (107), but is less controllable and may produce profound hypotension.

When the hypertension is not directly responsible for any serious sequelae, therapy can usually be withheld while the episode is allowed to spontaneously resolve, or if the hypertension persists, until oral medication can be given. The short-term risk of severe asymptomatic postoperative hypertension is not well defined. Therefore, the decision whether to put parenteral therapy in this circumstance should be made after consideration of the potential benefits versus hazards for each individual patient, including the height and expected duration of the rise in blood pressure, and preexisting cardiac and vascular disease.

In the chronic severely hypertensive patient (diastolic 110), antihypertensive therapy should be resumed within 12–24 hours of surgery, if the patient is stable, neither hypotensive nor hypovolemic, and able to take oral medication. Parenteral therapy may be considered for severely hypertensive patients who will be unable to take oral medication for prolonged periods of time. Most classes of antihypertensives have at least one agent available in parenteral form (Table 10.22). While logical and often preferable it is not requisite that a parenteral agent in the same class be used.

Recent studies have shown that a continuous infusion of propranolol* averaging 3 mg/hr can be used for postoperative blood pressure maintenance (49, 58, 108–111). We have found a somewhat lower dose of ½–3 mg/hr to be effective, so that it may be prudent to start at a lower dose until more experience is available (112).

_____

*This is not an FDA approved method of administration.

Some experience is needed to learn to adjust the continuous infusions, but once experience is gained, there is less hypotension and bradycardia than by standard methods of administration such as intermittant intravenous doses (comparison studies have not been done).

Moderately hypertensive patients (diastolic 100–110) *may* require parenteral antihypertensive agents for blood pressure control before they are able to resume oral medication. Many moderate hypertensive patients can be managed by sodium restriction similar to mildly hypertensive patients. Mildly hypertensive patients (diastolics < 100, systolics < 180) may be initially managed by sodium restriction and observation, thus avoiding the risks or trouble of parenteral agents, especially if they will be able to resume oral medications within 1 week. Other factors may reduce the need for treatment. A mild degree of blood pressure lowering occurs in some patients after general anesthesia and may last from hours to more than a week. Bedrest also lowers blood pressure.

In summary, parenteral antihypertensive therapy should be considered after treatment of hypervolemia, hypoxia, or hypercapnia, pain, anxiety, and other stressful or contributory states. Then the decision whether to follow or treat hypertension, when the patient cannot take oral medication, should be based upon the magnitude of postoperative blood pressure elevation, the presence of end organ disease (e.g., congestive heart failure), the time before the patient will be able to take oral agents, and the ability to monitor the patient.

INTRAOPERATIVE AND POSTOPERATIVE HYPOTENSION

Epidemiology

Although little sound epidemiologic data has been published on the causes of intra- and postoperative hypotension, most textbooks seem to agree on its most common causes (98, 113–115) (Table 10.23).

Table 10.23. Causes of Intraoperative and Postoperative Hypotension

Common
Hypovolemia, secondary to blood loss, diuretic, or fluid loss/redistribution
Inadequate ventilation or oxygenation
Induction of anesthesia
Excessive anesthesia
Spinal anesthesia
Medications
Interference with venous return secondary to surgical manipulation or positive pressure ventilation
Reflex response to surgical manipulation
Postural changes
Reflex response to endotracheal manipulation or unrelieved pain
Less common
Myocardial failure or infarction
Dysrhythmia
Pulmonary embolism
Acid-base or electrolyte imbalance
Sepsis
Transfusion or allergic drug reaction
Pneumothorax
Rare
Adrenocortical insufficiency or other endocrine disorders
Pericardial tamponade
CNS disease

Some degree of blood pressure fall is a frequent intraoperative occurrence. Usually there is a hypotensive response to the induction of anesthesia (101–102), and intraoperative blood pressures often remain lower than preoperative values (113). Choice of anesthesia is one factor. For example, blood pressure reduction secondary to vasodilation and myocardial suppression often accompanies halothane anesthesia, while blood pressure tends to be maintained at higher levels during cyclopropane anesthesia. Mild reduction in blood pressure can be regarded as a physiologic response to anesthesia and does not require treatment as long as perfusion is adequately maintained.

Significant intraoperative hypotension, however, is independently associated with a 5-fold increase in cardiac mortality (2, 113). It may also increase the risk of myocardial infarction (7) and ischemia (67).

In most studies, significant intraoperative hypotension has been defined as a 33% or greater fall from baseline for at least 10 minutes, or an absolute decrease in blood pressure of 50% or greater. The duration of hypotension may be as or more important than the degree of hypotension (9, 21), unless a very profound fall in blood pressure occurs. The increased risk is limited to unexpected falls in blood pressure; patients undergoing planned hypotension by the anesthesiologist do not have increased cardiac risk (2).

Unplanned intraoperative hypotensive episodes are common. In one study (65), hypotension requiring intraoperative fluid challenges or pressor agents occurred in 23% of 617 patients over the age of 40 undergoing 676 non-emergency procedures. Variably defined, significant intraoperative hypotensive episodes have been observed in 15–32% of patients with known ischemic heart disease (7, 21). In 7%, blood pressure actually falls to shock levels (9).

The most common cause of significant intraoperative hypotension is hypovolemia, usually secondary to blood loss. Other common causes include excessive anesthesia, intraoperative medications (e.g., neuromuscular blocking agents), excessive or interacting preoperative medications, reflex response to surgical or endotracheal manipulation, interference with venous return by surgical manipulation and/or positive pressure ventilation, inadequate ventilation (hypoxia or hypercarbia), hypocapnia secondary to hyperventilation, paralysis of sympathetic vasoconstrictors by spinal anesthesia, use of excessive local anesthesia, and postural changes. Less common causes include myocardial failure or infarction, dysrhythmia, pulmonary embolism, sepsis (especially in the already infected patient), electrolyte or acid-base imbalance, and transfusion or drug reactions. Infrequent to rare causes include central nervous system disease, cardiac tamponade, adrenocortical insufficiency, and other endocrine disorders.

Postoperative hypotension, defined as a systolic blood pressure less than 100, was reported in 4.6% of 29,583 routinely monitored recovery room patients (99). The most common etiologies of significant hypotension in the immediate postoperative period are: *(a)* hypovolemia due to blood loss with inadequate volume replacement, and *(b)* inadequate ventilation or oxygenation. Other frequent causes are the residual effects of anesthesia and perioperative medications, positional changes, acid-base or electrolyte imbalance, dysrhythmia, myocardial failure or infarction, and pulmonary embolism. Interference with venous return by positive pressure ventilation or iatrogenic pneumothorax and vagal reflex responses to unrelieved pain or endotracheal manipulations may also contribute to postoperative hypotension. Septic shock usually occurs a few days into the postoperative period, but may occur early after contaminated surgery. Causes of postoperative hypotension after the first or second postoperative day are similar to the causes in other medical patients.

Evaluation

The initial evaluation of hypotensive patients is directed at determining the clinical significance of the hypotension. The actual blood pressure, as well as the magnitude of the fall, should be noted. The adequacy of perfusion should be ascertained by palpating the pulses, observing the warmth and color of the skin, viewing the operative field in the anesthetized patient for changes in rate of bleeding and color of the blood, checking urine output, and in the unanesthetized patient assessing cerebral function.

Once the presence of significant hypotension has been established, there should be an attempt to establish an etiology (Table 10.23). This will involve a determination of the adequacy of ventilation and oxygenation (observation, respiratory exam, arterial blood gases), an assessment of the patient's volume status, a review of medications and anesthetic concentration (if intraoperative), a look at the operative field to rule out obstruction to venous return or excessive manipulation, a look at the patient's EKG or electrocardiographic monitor, an examination for cardiac failure, and the ruling out of infection. Arterial blood gases and electrolytes can be drawn if needed. Central venous pressure (CVP) or pulmonary wedge pressure should be measured when significant hypotension is not quickly reversible and when the etiology is uncertain or knowledge of central pressures would be important for diagnosis or treatment (Table 10.24).

Although most forms of shock are associated with signs of peripheral vasoconstriction (cold, pale, clammy skin) and excessive sympathetic activity (diaphoresis, tachycardia), it should be remembered that shock can exist in the presence of peripheral vasodilation. So called "warm shock" is often associated with sepsis, metabolic disorders, toxins, spinal anesthesia, and neuropathic phenomena.

Management

Treatment of significant perioperative hypotension is directed toward its etiology (Table 10.23). When the cause is unknown and the patient's volume status is uncertain, a fluid challenge may be given (300–500 cc of normal saline or Ringer's lactate) rapidly over 5–15 minutes and repeated once or twice if necessary. If there is no response, a central venous or Swan-Ganz catheter should be inserted for initial diagnosis (Table 10.24) and subsequent management. The measured pressure will then guide replacement of fluid to high normal central venous or pulmonary wedge pressure.

Intraoperatively, when the cause is unknown, the concentration of anesthesia is then usually decreased and the oxygen is increased. If there is any question of adrenal insufficiency, steroids should be given.

If there is no response to the fluid challenge and alteration of anesthetic and

Table 10.24.   Central Pressure in Intraoperative and Postoperative Hypotension

Usually elevated central pressure
   ($\uparrow$ CVP, $\uparrow$ PWP)[a]
Cardiac
   Cardiogenic shock (myocardial infarction)
   Left ventricular failure
   Right ventricular failure (normal or low PWP)
   Pericardial tamponade
   Constrictive pericarditis
Pulmonary embolism (normal PWP)
Positive pressure respiration (normal to low PWP)
Usually reduced central pressure
   ($\downarrow$ CVP, $\downarrow$ PWP)
Hypovolemia
   Blood loss
   Fluid deficits: vomiting, NG suction, third-spacing, polyuria, adrenal insufficiency
   Loss of vascular tone
      Direct effects of medication/anesthesia
      Vagal response to surgical or endotracheal manipulation
      Hypercarbia and hypoxia
      CNS disease
      Anaphylaxis
      Adrenal insufficiency
   Interference with venous return secondary to surgical manipulation
Either elevated or reduced central pressure
   ($\uparrow$ or $\downarrow$ CVP, $\uparrow$ or $\downarrow$ PWP)
Hypoxia
Sepsis

[a] CVP, central venous pressure; PWP, pulmonary capillary wedge pressure.

oxygen concentrations, a pressor agent should be given while the search for etiology continues. Several pressor agents are available. Dopamine at low dosage (<10 μg/kg/min) increases cardiac output through beta-adrenergic stimulation with relatively modest effects on heart rate, while producing renal, mesenteric, coronary, and cerebral vasodilation through a specific action on dopamine receptors. At higher doses ($\geq$20 μg/kg/min) it causes vasoconstriction through alpha-adrenergic stimulation. Dobutamine, a predominantly beta-agonist ($\beta_1 > \beta_2$), increases cardiac output in low dosage with relatively little effect on blood pressure or heart rate, while decreasing left ventricular filling pressure. Isoproterenol is a β_1- and β_2-adrenergic stimulator which raises cardiac output by positive inotropic and chronotropic effects, while producing skeletal, renal, and mesenteric vasodilation. Drugs that act indirectly through release of nor-epinephrine at nerve terminals, as well as directly through receptor stimulation, include ephedrine, mephenteramine (Wyamine), and metaraminol (Aramine). Mixed alpha- and beta-receptor stimulation is achieved by ephedrine and mephenteramine (Wyamine). Metaraminol (Aramine) and levarterenol (Levophed) have predominant alpha-adrenergic effects, while methoxamine (Vasoxyl) and phenyephrine (Neo-Synephrine) are pure alpha-adrenergic stimulators. With the varying mechanisms of action of the different sympathomimetic agents, there is ample opportunity for individualization of therapy. For example, when the problem is vasodilation as in neurogenic shock or hypotension secondary to spinal anesthesia, and volume expansion alone is insufficient, an agent with predominant alpha stimulation may be preferred. When the treatment goal is to increase cardiac output and peripheral perfusion without markedly increasing myocardial oxygen demand, dopamine or dobutamine may be the drug of choice. In the presence of anesthetics such as cyclopropane and halothane, which sensitize the myocardium to catecholamines, sympathomimetics, which are less dysrhythmogenic such as dopamine are preferred to the more dysrhythmogenic agents, isoproterenol and norepinephrine. Anesthesiologists usually prefer indirect-acting pressors, which they feel are also less likely to cause dysrhythmias.

The necessity of treating perioperative shock may be avoided by its prevention. Every effort should be made to prevent significant hypotension by careful drug, anesthetic and ventilatory management, by correction by preoperative hypovolemia, by prompt replacement of volume losses, and by appropriate evaluation and treatment of infections. An hypotensive event may be especially harmful in the patient with atherosclerotic heart disease in whom coronary blood flow is more dependent on perfusion pressure and less responsive to local hypoxia.

PREOPERATIVE ISCHEMIC HEART DISEASE (ANGINA, MYOCARDIAL INFARCTION)

Epidemiology

The data available on the surgical risk of patients with angina pectoris is summarized in Table 10.25. In a prospective series (1, 2), stable mild to moderate angina pectoris did not independently increase the risk for postoperative myocardial infarction or cardiac death. The observed increased risk was due to other concomitant risk factors, rather than the stable angina itself. Two retrospective (9, 18), and one prospective (5) series showed an increased number of complications in patients with angina compared to those without heart disease. Among the small number of patients with angina who have undergone surgery and been reported in the literature, 5% have had postoperative myocardial infarctions and 4–12% have died. Cardiac complications are not markedly increased in patients with both stable angina and a myocardial infarction more than 6 months old (2, 8, 10, 19). Unstable or severe angina were independent risk factors in a recent study (6). The risks of unstable, severe, or post-infarction angina are not well established, despite a recent new study, since few patients have been reported and criteria for stability has not been stated.

A previous myocardial infarction substantially raises the risk of postoperative mortality and postoperative myocardial infarction (Tables 9.2, and 10.26–10.29). The total mortality of all patients with prior myocardial infarction who undergo surgery ranges from 5–15%, which is 2–3 times the 0.2–6% for all patients. About one-third of the total mortality is due to cardiac causes (7). Thus, the cardiac mortality of the post-infarction patient is about

Table 10.25. Risk of Non-cardiac Surgery in Patients with Angina[a]

Study	Design[b]	Number[c]	Postoperative Myocardial Infarction	Postoperative Death (All Causes)	Type of Angina[c]
Goldman, 1977	P	70	2 (3%)	3 (4%)[d]	Definite
		139	5 (3.6%)	5 (3.6%)[d]	Definite; possible
Nachlas, 1961	R	41		12.2%	Not stated
Rosen, 1966	P	18	1 (5.5%)		Not stated
Sapala, 1961	R	99		5 (5%)	Angina
		55		6 (11%)	Angina and MI
Skinner, 1964	R	192		(11%)	All angina cases
		70		(9%)	Angina and hypertensive heart disease
		61		(16%)	Angina and healed myocardial infarction
		20		(10%)	Unstable angina
Steen, 1978	R	200	14 (7%)		Angina and myocardial infarction
Larsen, 1987	P	229		8 (3.5%)[d]	Stable angina
	P	9		1 (11%)[d]	Unstable angina
Mean			(5%)	(9%)	

[a] Data from Refs. 1, 5, 8–10, 18–19.
[b] P, prospective; R, retrospective.
[c] Number with angina.
[d] Cardiac deaths only.

5% (2). The risk of postoperative myocardial infarction averages 7% in studies of patients with prior preoperative myocardial infarction, as compared to 0.1–2% for all patients.

There is a generally accepted relationship between risk and time since prior myocardial infarction (Tables 10.3, 10.4; see also Table 10.30). The perioperative risk is very high for the patient with a "recent" myocardial infarction (occurring within 6 months of surgery) (1–2, 8, 10,

Table 10.26. Risk of Postoperative Death or Myocardial Infarction in Patients with Prior Myocardial Infarction[a]

Study	Number with Prior MI	Total Mortality (%)	Cardiac Mortality (%)	% Post-operative MI
Arkins, 1964	267	24		
Topkins, 1964	658		4.7	6.5
Tarhan, 1972	422			6.6
Steen, 1978	587		4.3	6.1
Goldman, 1977	101		6.9	2.8
Knapp, 1962	427		3.5	6.1
Nachlas, 1961	54	13.5		
Sapala, 1975	227	9.2		
Skinner, 1964	180	16		
Hunter, 1966				7.6
Rosen, 1966				0.6
Mean		16	5	5

[a] Data from refs. 1, 8–12, 14–15, 18–20.

Table 10.27.   Risk of Cardiac Complications by Preoperative Cardiac Status[d]

	Postoperative Myocardial Infarction			Postoperative Death	
Study	No Prior History MI	Angina-No Prior MI	Prior MI	No Prior History MI	Prior MI
Knapp, 1962	0.7%[a] (59)[b]		—[c](26)		
Topkins, 1964	0.7% (79)		6.5% (43)		
Hunter, 1968	0.9% (1)		7.6% (2)		
Tarhan, 1972	0.08% (27)	0.05% (16)	6.6% (28)		
Goldman, 1977	2% (15)	3% (2)	2.8% (3)	1% (12)	7% (7)
Steen, 1978			6% (36)		
Rosen, 1966	0.6% (3)		0.6% (3)		
Vonknorring, 1981	.09% (12)				

[a] Percentage of patients with complications.
[b] Number of patients with complications.
[c] Data not available.
[d] Data from Refs. 1, 11, 14–15, 20, 116

Table 10.28.   Risk of Perioperative Cardiac Death in Patients with Ischemic Heart Disease[d]

Study	Design[a]	Patient Group	Number with Heart Disease[c]	Total Mortality N (%)	Cardiac Mortality N (%)
A. All patients					
Nachlas, 1961	R	All patients	(6059)	(3.5%)	
Hunter, 1968	R	All patients	(141)	2 (1.4%)	0 (0%)
Goldman, 1977	P	All patients	(1001)	59 (5.9%)	19 (1.9%)
Rosen, 1966	P	Non-random sample; all patients	(506)	1 (0.2%)	
Nichols, 1987	P	All patients	?		0.5%
B. Arteriosclerotic heart **disease (ASHD)**					
Nachlas, 1961	R	ASHD	200	(10.5%)	
Arkins, 1964	R	ASHD	1005	225 (22%)	101 (10%)
Skinner, 1964	R	ASHD; valvular heart disease, congestive heart failure	766	100 (13%)	
Sapala, 1964	R	ASHD	416	22 (5.3%)	16 (3.8%)
C. Preceeding myocardial **infarction**					
Arkins, 1964	R	MI patients only[b]	267	65 (24%)	
Nachlas, 1961	R	MI patients only	52	(13.5%)	
Skinner, 1964	R	Healed + acute MI patients only	180	(16%)	
Sapala, 1964	R	MI patients only	227	15 (6.6%)	
Goldman, 1977	P	MI patients only, age > 40	101		7 (6.9%)
Steen, 1978	R	MI patients	587	30 (5.1%)	
Topkins, 1964	P	MI males, > age 50	658		(4.7%)
Knapp, 1962	R	MI males, > age 50	427		(3.5%)

[a] R, retrospective; P, prospective.
[b] MI, myocardial infarction.
[c] Total sample size in parenthesis.
[d] Data from Refs. 1, 8–10, 12, 14–15, 18–20, 24.

Table 10.29. Risk of Postoperative Myocardial Infarction in Patients with Ischemic Heart Disease[a]

Study	Design[b]	Patient Group	Number	Total Postoperative Myocardial Infarction N (%)	Mortality of Postoperative Myocardial Infarction N (%)
A. All patients					
Driscoll, 1961	P	All patients	496	12 (2.4%)	2/12 (17%)
Knapp, 1962	R	Males > age 50	8,984	85 (0.9%)	26/85 (30%)
Topkins, 1964	P	Males > age 50	12,712	122 (1%)	52/122 (42%)
Hunter, 1968	P	All patients	141	3 (2%)	0/3 (0%)
Tarhan, 1972	R	All patients	32,877	71 (0.2%)	44/71 (62%)
Goldman, 1977	P	All patients	1,001	18 (1.8%)	5/18 (28%)
Goldman, 1977	P	All patients > age 40	1,001	18 (1.8%)	5/18 (28%)
Plumlee, 1972	R	All patients	18,013	24 (0.1%)	20/24 (83%)
Rosen, 1966	P	Non-random sample; all patients	506	3 (0.6%)	
Alexander, 1961	R	All patients undergoing cholecystectomy	100	9 (9%)	(77%)
B. Arteriosclerotic heart disease (ASHD)					
Arkins, 1964	R	ASHD	1,005	55 (5%)	38/55 (69%)
Chamberlain, 1964	R	ASHD; hypertensive heart disease	217	5 (2%)	
Mauney, 1970	P	Abnormal EKG	365	30 (8%)	16/30 (53%)
Tarhan, 1972	R	MI; coronary artery disease	422	44 (10%)	29/44 (66%)
Sapala, 1975	R	ASHD	416	10 (2.4%)	
C. Prior myocardial infarction (MI)					
Knapp, 1962	R	MI males > age 50	427	26 (6%)	15/26 (58%)
Topkins, 1964	P	MI males > age 50	658	43 (6.5%)	31/43 (70%)
Tarhan, 1972	R	MI	422	26 (6.6%)	15/28 (54%)
Goldman, 1977	P	MI	101	3 (3%)	1/3 (33%)
Steen, 1978	R	MI	587	36 (6.1%)	25/36 (69%)
Rosen, 1966	P	MI	8	0 (0%)	

[a] Data from Refs. 1, 3, 7–9, 10–21.
[b] R = retrospective; P = prospective.

12, 116–117). Available data suggest that the risk of perioperative death is 15–25% and of recurrent infarction, 25%.

Recent studies suggest the risk of recurrent myocardial infarction and death perioperatively in patients with prior infarction is currently much lower (Table 10.4) (4, 60–61). The risk of perioperative death has fallen from 15–25% to 5–17% and of recurrent infarction from 25% to 2–6%. The authors attribute the decline to better hemodynamic monitoring (i.e., the Swan-Ganz catheter), drug treatment of asymptomatic hemodynamic abnormalities, but concomitant changes in an-esthetic and surgical techniques may have also contributed. These studies were not randomized and have been criticized (64, 118). Other studies of general hospital series (Table 10.9, p. 112) (24, 26–27) have not shown a general decline in cardiac deaths in the same time period, but these studies did not give particular attention to hemodynamic monitoring. Until randomized trials are done, a reasonable conclusion is the risk of perioperative myocardial reinfarction in the post-infarct patient *may be* lower with intensive hemodynamic monitoring and current anesthetic/surgical techniques, but further

Table 10.30.   Risk of Postoperative Myocardial Infarction in Patients by Time since Prior Myocardial Infarction[b]

Study	Design[a]	Patient Group	Number	Total Postoperative Myocardial Infarction (No. with Prior MI)	Time since Prior Myocardial Infarction						
					0–3 mo	4–6 mo	7–12 mo	1–2 yr	2–3 yr	>3 yrs	Un-known
Knapp, 1962	R	Males > age 50	8,984	85 (26)	←— 100% —→		33%	41%	12%	0%	
Arkins, 1964	R	Coronary artery disease	1,005	55 (?)	40%	←— 22% —→					
Topkins, 1964	P	Males > age 50	12,712	122 (43)	←— 55% —→	25%	22%	6%	1%		
Tarhan, 1972	R	All patients	32,877	71 (28)	37%	16%	5%	4%	←— 5–10% —→		
Goldman, 1977	P	All patients	1,001	18 (3)	8%	0%	←— 0% —→		4%		
Steen, 1978	P	Prior MI	587	36 (36)	27%	11%	6%	4%	←— 4–12% —→		
Von Knorring, 1981	R	All patients	12,654	116	←25%→			18%	15%	←10%—→	

[a] P, prospective; R, retrospective.
[b] Data from Refs. 1, 11–12, 15, 20, 116.

studies will be required to confirm this and definitely establish the level of current risk.

The risk of postoperative cardiac complications was greater between 0–3 months than between 3–6 months in all four series (2, 10–12) providing data on these intervals (Tables 10.3 and 10.30). We have interpreted this data as suggesting that risk drops after 3 months. Other authors reviewing the same data have concluded that the risk does not drop until after 6 months, based upon the lack of statistical significance (117). The controversy over a difference in risk between 0–3 and 3–6 months is not likely to be resolved, because of the huge number of patients that would be required for adequate statistical analyses. (The Mayo Clinic study (10) of 73,321 patients contained only 33 patients who had a myocardial infarction within 6 months of surgery.)

After 6 months, the surgical risk of patients with prior myocardial infarction becomes much lower (total mortality of 2.5%, recurrent infarction in 5%) and plateaus without much decline thereafter (Tables 10.3 and 10.4; see also Table 10.30). Even then the risk of reinfarction, if not death, remains elevated compared to the risk in patients without heart disease (Table 10.3. see p. 108).

It should be remembered that patients with previous myocardial infarction are a small percentage of all surgical patients. While patients without previous myocardial infarctions are at much lower risk, they still account for about two-thirds of postoperative myocardial infarction (Table 10.27) and the majority of cardiac deaths because of their larger numbers. Other risk factors (e.g., Table 10.6) must be searched for in this patient group. Preliminary data (119) indicate that intraoperative ischemia and its relationship to anesthetic management is an important risk factor; this needs to be confirmed in general surgical patients.

The data relating silent ischemia by holter monitor or ECG stress test to the risk of noncardiac surgery is given on p. 113.

Preoperative Evaluation

The preoperative evaluation should be conducted as described in Table 10.16 (p.

116). Because of their proven or potential prognostic importance, the history of a recent myocardial infarction, the presence of unstable or severe angina pectoris, congestive heart failure, and aortic stenosis should be clearly documented. Factors that could adversely affect cardiac performance (Table 10.17) should be searched for.

The use of ECG stress tests to subcategorize risk of *recent* post myocardial infarction restraints has been suggested (19a) but never evaluated.

A clear role has not been established for cardiac catheterization with coronary angiography in assessing surgical risk of patients with ischemic heart disease. Noncardiac surgery can be safely performed 6 or more weeks after coronary artery bypass grafting, (see also p. 158), but whether bypass grafting lowers surgical risk has not been demonstrated by randomized prospective trials. Cardiac catheterization is not indicated in most patients with mild to moderate stable angina pectoris because of no or minimal increase in cardiac risk. Likewise, patients with healed myocardial infarction older than 6 months without angina would not be expected to benefit from preoperative bypass grafting. Studies have not separately examined subgroups of patients with ischemic heart disease that might benefit from preoperative bypass grafting, such as patients with post-infarction, severe, or unstable angina despite optimal medical management, or substantial silent ischemia. At present, the decision on cardiac catheterization must be individualized.

Management

Non-urgent surgery should be deferred until 6 months post myocardial infarction. If surgery cannot be postponed for 6 months, some benefits may be gained by deferring surgery for at least 3 months. *The guidelines for postponing surgery remain unchanged even with the more recent indication of lower surgical risk post myocardial infarction (Table 10.4), since the risk still remains elevated (although less so) for 6 months, as compared to after 6 months.*

Angina should be controlled preoperatively, except in the most urgent circumstances, using long-acting nitrates, beta-blocking agents, and/or calcium channel blockers. The degree of control of angina must be individualized depending upon the severity of the patient's disease and the type of surgery and anesthesia planned. A reasonable general goal is the absence of angina at rest and on mild exertion. Medications should be continued up until the time of surgery and are usually given the morning of surgery with a sip of water; this includes beta blockers (see pp. 34, 622). A decision should be made on whether aspirin should be discontinued depending on the severity of angina and the type of surgery. Usually aspirin should be discontinued 7 days before surgery to allow return of normal platelet function (see pp. 325, 622).

A consensus has not been achieved on indications for Swan-Ganz pulmonary artery and radial artery catheterization (see pp. 92, 133, 140). General guidelines include *consideration* of Swan-Ganz catheters in patients with recent myocardial infarction (within 6 months), with severe coronary artery disease, with major complicating risk factors (e.g., congestive heart failure), or in patients in whom large volume shifts are anticipated (e.g., abdominal aortic aneurysms).

Aggravating factors (Table 10.51) should be treated and prevented. Associated cardiac conditions should be identified and managed as described in other sections of this chapter.

The role of coronary artery bypass grafting (CABG) and coronary angioplasty specifically to reduce risk for general surgery is uncertain. Although the risk of surgery after *prior* CABG *for other reasons* is low and less than that for non-bypassed patients (see p. 158), the combined risk of coronary surgery and non-cardiac surgery may equal or exceed the risk with coronary bypass (Table 10.14). (The risk of the CABG must be taken into account if it is done only to reduce subsequent general surgical risk.) (see p. 114) Angioplasty has not been studied specifically in the preoperative setting. Although seemingly ideal, the significant risk of re-stenosis soon after angioplasty, the need for antiplatelet anticoagulation, and the implications of a failed procedure leading to emergency bypass surgery all raise major problems for a patient requiring subsequent noncardiac surgery. Until these issues are resolved by careful studies, coronary bypass and angioplasty must be decided on an individual basis. If a patient requires coronary angioplasty or bypass for the usual medical indications, then the decision becomes one of a patient requiring two surgical procedures. A decision will need to be made on which comes first, remembering that subsequent noncardiac surgery should wait 1½–3 months after cardiac surgery (see p. 21).

Postoperatively, patients should be monitored for cardiac complications, especially angina, myocardial infarction, arrhythmias, and congestive heart failure. The extent and duration of monitoring depend on the patient's risk, the type of surgery, and the intraoperative and initial postoperative course. We recommend placing high-risk patients in an intensive care unit and obtaining routine electrocardiograms and cardiac enzymes as described on page 137. All patients with a cardiac history should be monitored routinely for cardiac symptoms and signs. Even in the low-risk patient without clinical findings, an electrocardiogram should be obtained on the 5th or 6th postoperative day or immediately prior to discharge and before any further surgery.

The use of the intra-aortic balloon pump has been described in a few extremely high-risk patients, but substantial experience is lacking (121, 129, 135).

Special Considerations

CHRONIC OBSTRUCTIVE PULMONARY DISEASE

Chronic obstructive pulmonary disease commonly coexists with ischemic heart disease since smoking is a common risk factor. The presence of chronic lung disease in addition to ischemic heart disease adds significantly to operative risk (2, 8). The decision to undertake major surgery should be carefully considered in patients with concomitant moderate to severe heart and lung disease.

POSTOPERATIVE ISCHEMIC HEART DISEASE

Epidemiology

Myocardial infarction occurs in the postoperative period in about 1% of all surgical patients (Tables 10.3 and 10.5). The highest risk of postoperative myocardial infarction (25–35%) occurs when surgery is done within 6 months of a previous myocardial infarction (p. 128). Factors that increase the risk for postoperative myocardial infarction and death are discussed on pages 128–134.

The mortality from postoperative myocardial infarction is high: 50–80% in most series for reinfarctions in patients with prior preoperative myocardial infarction and about 38% in patients without prior myocardial infarction. Two recent studies have found a lower mortality rate for postoperative reinfarction in prior myocardial infarction patients of 28–36% (60, 116), but most authorities remain unconvinced that the mortality rate has dropped for this very high risk subset. (Tables 10.31 and 10.32). Insufficient patients have been studied to indicate whether there is a difference in mortality between transmural and subendocardial infarction in surgical patients (2). The 2–3 times higher mortality in surgical as compared to medical patients has been attributed to the failure to include prehospital deaths in medical statistics, the added stress of the postoperative state, and the lack of inten-

Table 10.31. Mortality of Postoperative Myocardial Infarction[a]

Study	Year	Number	No. with Postoperative Myocardial Infarction	Mortality of Postoperative Myocardial Infarction
		All Patients		
Driscoll	1961	496	12	2 (17%)
Knapp	1962	8,984	85	26 (30%)
Arkins	1964	1,005	55	38 (69%)
Topkins	1964	12,712	122	52 (42%)
Alexander	1966	100	9	(77%)
Hunter	1968		3	0 (0%)
Mauney	1970	141	30	16 (53%)
Tarhan	1972	365	7	44 (62%)
Plumlee	1972	32,877	24	20 (83%)
Goldman	1977	18,013	12	5 (28%)
		1,001		
Becker	1987	30,000	28	12 (43%)
Von Knorring	1981	12,654	50	16 (32%)
MEAN				(45%)
		Patients with Previous Myocardial Infarction Only		
Knapp	1962	427 (8,984)	36	15 (58%)
Topkins	1864	658 (12,712)	43	31 (70%)
Tarhan	1972	422 (32,877)	28	15 (54%)
Goldman	1977	101 (1,001)	3	1 (33%)
Steen	1978	587	36	25 (69%)
Rao	1983	733 (?)	14	5 (36%)
MEAN				(53%)

[a] Data from Refs. 1, 7, 10–17, 20, 60.

Table 10.32. Mortality of Postoperative Myocardial Infarction[a]

	Prior MI (%)	No Prior MI (%)
Arkins, 1964	25	
Goldman, 1978	33	27
Goldman, 1978[b]	78	52
Knapp, 1962	58	19
Steen, 1978	69	
Tarhan, 1972	54	67
Topkins, 1964	70	27
Von Knorring, 1981	28	36
Rao (Study 1) 1983	57	
(Study 2) 1983	36	
Range	25–78	19–67
Mean	51%	38%

[a] Data from Refs. 2, 10–12, 15, 20, 60, 116.
[b] Including sudden cardiac deaths as MI.

sive monitoring. The first and second explanations may be the best ones. The last explanation is not particularly satisfying, since even studies done in the era of intensive monitoring (1, 2) have not shown a marked decrease in mortality, nor have retrospective comparison studies of postoperative patients admitted to intensive care units (10). The results of these studies are not conclusive, however, since an increased number of poor-risk patients have been operated on in recent years, and poor-risk patients tend to be admitted to intensive care units. Despite high mortality, deaths after postoperative myocardial infarction represent only a proportion of postoperative total deaths or cardiac deaths (Table 10.33).

Table 10.33. Postoperative Mortality[a]

Study	Number	Total Deaths	Post-operative Cardiac Deaths	Deaths After Post-operative MI only
Driscoll, 1961	496			0.4%
Knapp, 1962	8,984			0.3%
Arkins, 1964	1,005	22%	10%	4%
Topkins, 1964	12,712			0.4%
Hunter, 1968	141	2%	0%	0%
Tarhan, 1972	32,877			0.13%
Goldman, 1977	1,001	5.9%	1.9%	0.5%
Steen, 1978	587			4.2%
Plumlee, 1972	18,013			0.1%
Becker, 1987	30,000			0.04%
Nichols, 1987	609		0.5%	
Zeldin, 1984	1,140		1.2%	

[a] Data from Refs. 1, 10–15, 17, 20, 26, 116, 124.

The clinical presentation of myocardial infarction may differ in the postoperative as compared to the medical patient. Chest pain is the presenting complaint in only about one-half of the patients with myocardial infarction (2, 11, 13, 17, 122–123) (Table 10.34). Most other patients have congestive heart failure or hypotension. A few patients will have supraventricular tachycardia as the presentation (2, 11, 65, (122–123). Probably only a small percentage of patients with postoperative infarction have no symptoms or findings (1) (Table 10.34), although several series (10, 13, 18) have found 22–50% of postoperative infarctions were asymptomatic. The differences in percentages of asymptomatic patients are due in part to differences in clinical follow-up of patients and frequency of routine postoperative electrocardiograms. Incidences of asymptomatic myocardial infarction may be overestimated by studies using routine electrocardiograms, since cardiac isoenzymes and nucleide scans were not obtained.

Postoperative myocardial infarction can occur throughout the first postoperative

Table 10.34. Presentation of Myocardial Infarction in the Postoperative Period (see also Refs. 94, 95)[c]

Study	No. of Postoperative MI	Presentation				No Symptoms (Routine EKG)	Other
		Chest Pain	Hypo-tension	CHF	SVT		
Goldman, 1978	18	50%	17%	28%	6%	6%	
Driscoll, 1961	12	17%	33%[a]			50%	8% bronchospasm
Plumlee, 1972	24	12%					"Most" other patients had hypotension, cardiac arrest, or EKG changes
Tarhan, 1972	28[b]	78%					22% "other clinical findings"
Steen, 1978	36	30%					25% cardiac arrest; 11% no symptoms; 22% occurred in operating room
Becker, 1987	28	39%	39%	25%	18% (?)		4% cardiac arrest 4% hypertension, nausea 7% change in mental status
Von Knorring, 1981	35	58%					8% cardiac arrest
Median[d]		40%	30%	26%	12%	22%	

[a] Included intraoperative hypotension.
[b] Patients with reinfarctions only.
[c] Data from Refs. 1, 10–12, 17, 116, 124.
[d] Total exceeds 100%.

Table 10.35.   Occurrence of Postoperative Myocardial Infarction by Postoperative Day[d]

Study	No. of Postoperative MIs	Postoperative Day				Uncertain Time
		0[a]	1–3	4–6	≥7	
Goldman	18	11%	33%	44%	11%	
Tarhan[b]	71	NS[c]	62%	38%		
Plumlee	24	50%	25%	4%	13%	8%
Becker	28	39%	53%	4%	4%	
Von Knorring	38	13%	74%	10%	3%	
Median		26%	53%	10%	8%	

[a] Myocardial infarction on day of operation.
[b] Included only infarctions within one week of surgery.
[c] NS, not stated.
[d] Data from Refs. 1, 11, 17, 116, 124.

week. It peaks at the 3rd to 5th postoperative day (2, 9, 11, 122–123) (Table 10.35). More recent studies (25, 52) using more frequent EKG's and cardiac enzymes suggest that most myocardial infarctions occur within the first 48 hours of surgery with a peak incidence as close as 24 hours. Raby et al. (52) have hypothesized the later peak incidence at day 3–5 in older studies was an "artefact" due to less frequent monitoring of EKGs and creatine kinase.

The frequency of and risk factors for postoperative angina have not been well studied (4). Angina, as well as myocardial infarction, may present atypically in the postoperative period. Transient cardiac ischemia may be manifested by hypotension, arrhythmia, or dyspnea.

Transient ST-T wave changes without myocardial infarction develop in about 5% of patients postoperatively.

Evaluation

For the reasons discussed above, myocardial infarction should be suspected not only in patients complaining of chest pain, but also in those developing congestive heart failure, hypotension, or new supraventricular tachycardias postoperatively (although other explanations for these symptoms will be found in most instances).

In patients identified preoperatively as high risk (p. 128), we obtain routine electrocardiograms and cardiac isoenzymes although data on yield is controversial. Since the major risk of postoperative myocardial infarction extends to the 5th or 6th postoperative day, with a peak at the 3rd to 5th day, routine monitoring should extend until the 5th to 6th postoperative day.

Neither the height of rise nor pattern of cardiac enzymes (total CPK, SGOT, LDH) will differentiate myocardial infarction from operative trauma, especially in the first 3 days after major surgery (125–127). CPK isoenzymes should be obtained, since they reliably separate heart and skeletal muscle CPK. An occasional patient with massive trauma or electrical damage to muscle may have a positive or equivocal CPK-MB band using some clinical assays. These patients usually have a strikingly high total CPK. LDH isoenzymes may also be helpful. Another useful diagnostic technique is cardiac scanning using [99]technitium or [108]thallium. These scans have a high sensitivity for transmural infarctions, but will miss many subendocardial infarctions. They are not affected by abdominal and most noncardiac thoracic surgery (128).

Patients with postoperative cardiac ischemia should be evaluated for aggravating factors (Table 10.17), as well as congestive heart failure and arrhythmias.

Management

Postoperative patients who develop chest pain, hypotension, congestive heart failure, supraventricular tachycardia, or suspicious changes on routine electrocardiograms should be admitted to an intensive or coronary care unit. Admission to an ICU or CCU is warranted by the difficulty in making the diagnosis in patients without chest pain and by the high mortality of postoperative infarction. About one-half of the deaths from postoperative myocardial infarction occur suddenly due to arrhythmias, and thus are potentially salvagable in monitored intensive care units.

Management of postoperative myocardial infarction or angina is similar in perioperative and medical patients. Aggravating factors (Table 10.17), congestive heart failure, and arrhythmias are treated in the usual manner. Some authorities advocate administering prophylactic lidocaine during the first 24–48 hours of infarction, in view of the high mortality due to arrhythmias. In the patient who is unable to take oral medication, chest pain should be treated with parenteral narcotics, sublingual short- or long-acting nitrates, topical long-acting nitrates, intravenous nitroglycerin, sublingual nifedipine, intravenous propranolol or metoprolol. Nitrates and propranolol can also be given prophylactically for anginal pain. The intravenous dose of propranolol is 1–3 mg given at no more than 1 mg per 5 minutes, repeated every 4–6 hours; a continuous infusion of ½–3 mg/hr has also been described (see p. 124). No exact correspondence between oral and intravenous doses of propranolol has been established.

Swan-Ganz and radial artery catheterization should be considered in the patient with congestive heart failure or hypotension and postoperative infarction or ischemia (see also p. 92).

Invasive monitoring should also be considered in the patient with postoperative moderate to severe angina or myocardial infarction who is not doing well or stabilizing; or whom also has marked fluid shifts. Catheterization allows precise control of fluid status which may decrease the need for pressor agents. It allows more precise titration of pressor agents when they are required for the treatment of hypotension, of afterload reducing agents when they are used for the treatment of congestive heart failure, and anti-anginal agents by monitoring their hemodynamic effects and precise control of intravascular volume.

PREOPERATIVE CONGESTIVE HEART FAILURE

Epidemiology

Preexisting congestive heart failure increases the risk of postoperative congestive heart failure, pulmonary edema, cardiac death, and perhaps dysrhythmia (2). The worse the failure, the greater the risk.

While Cooperman (3) reported that 33% of 43 patients with congestive heart failure developed undefined "cardiac complications" and Skinner (8) observed that the worse a patient's NYHA functional class the higher the perioperative mortality, a more comprehensive evaluation of risk awaited Goldman's study (1, 2) (Tables 10.36 and 10.37). Patients with a history of heart failure, who are no longer in failure preoperatively, and patients categorized as NYHA functional Class 1 or 2 experienced little, of any, increased perioperative cardiac risk when compared to controls. On the other hand, patients with a past history of pulmonary edema (regardless of preoperative status), patients with an S_3 or jugular venous distension, and patients categorized as NYHA functional Class 3 or 4 all had marked and significantly increased risk compared to controls. Of 35 patients with a 3rd heart sound or jugular venous distension, 14% developed nonfatal life-threatening

Table 10.36.   Risks of Developing Congestive Failure (CHF) in Surgical Patients[a]

Predictor	No. of Patients	All CHF[b]	Pulmonary Edema
No prior CHF	853	4%	2%
Past CHF			
Now compensated	87	16%	6%
Past pulmonary edema (regardless of current status)	22	32%	23%
Decompensated CHF preoperatively	66	21%	16%
Preoperative physical findings			
S3 gallop	17	47%	35%
JVD	23	35%	30%
NYHA Class			
I	935	5%	3%
II	15	7%	7%
III	34	18%	6%
IV	17	31%	25%

[a] Modified from Goldman L, et al.: Cardiac risk factors and complications in non-cardiac surgery. *Medicine* 57:357, 1978, with permission.
[b] New or worsened postoperative heart failure with or without pulmonary edema.

complications, 20% died cardiac deaths, and 35–47% experienced new or worsened postoperative failure (most frequently pulmonary edema). A preoperative S_3, jugular venous distension, or

Table 10.37.   Relationship of New York Heart Association (NYHA) Functional Class to Perioperative Mortality[a,b]

Functional Classification	Total No. of Cases	Mortality (%)	Intrathoracic and Intra-abdominal	
			Cases	Mortality (%)
Class I	46	4	9	11
Class II	569	11	199	21
Class III	145	25	59	42
Class IV	6	67	1	100

[a] From Skinner JF, Pearce ML: Surgical risk in the cardiac patient. *J Chronic Dis* 17:57, 1964, Pergamon Press, with permission.
[b] See also ref. 34a.

history of pulmonary edema was significantly associated with postoperative cardiac death, but not postoperative myocardial infarction. The development of intra- or postoperative supraventricular tachycardia occurred more frequently in patients with congestive heart failure (8–13%) compared to the entire surgical population (3.9%).

Evaluation

The preoperative evaluation should be conducted as described on page 115 (Table 10.16). Because of their prognostic importance, a past history of pulmonary edema, the presence of an S_3 or jugular venous distension, the NYHA functional class, and an assessment of the severity and degree of control of the patient's congestive heart failure should be clearly recorded.

Gated blood pool scanning estimates of ejection fraction may help refine risk estimation in patients whose status is uncertain. Low ejection fraction (<35%) by scan does not represent an absolute contraindication to surgery, but indicates increased risk (43).

Patients with adverse prognostic factors despite optimal therapy must be considered high risk, and judgments regarding the advisability of non-urgent surgery should be adjusted accordingly.

Factors which adversely affect cardiac performance (Table 10.1) should also be detected. Of particular concern in the patient with congestive heart failure is the possibility of complications from therapy. Diuretics may cause hypovolemia, hypokalemia, hyponatremia, and alkalosis. Thus, a careful assessment of volume and electrolyte status should be performed close to the time of operation. Secondly, the risk of digitalis toxicity is increased during surgery, in part due to the dysrhythmogenic effects of anesthetics. Serum levels of digoxin or digitoxin should therefore be obtained in patients receiving these drugs.

Management

Patients with poorly controlled congestive heart failure should have all but emergency, life-saving surgery postponed and be treated with diuretics, digoxin, and afterload reducing agents according to general medical guidelines. Care should be taken to avoid overdiuresis with resulting hypovolemia and the risk to perioperative hypotension. Surgery is preferably postponed several days to a week to diminish the risk of drug toxicity (e.g., electrolyte disturbance) and overdiuresis, and to allow resolution of all abnormalities, because resolution of some abnormalities (e.g., increased lung water) may lag behind the rapid hemodynamic changes produced by morphine and diuretics. Important parameters to follow include orthostatic blood pressure and pulse changes, respiratory rate, input and output, weight, neck vein distension, central venous or pulmonary wedge pressure when necessary, heart and lung exam, blood urea nitrogen, and electrolytes.

Regardless of the status of the patient's failure, abnormalities which could adversely affect cardiac performance (Table 10.17) should be corrected whenever possible.

Digoxin is usually withheld on the morning of surgery to diminish the risk of drug toxicity. It should be continued postoperatively, starting the day of surgery. Digoxin may be given intravenously in patients unable to take oral medication, but the dosage should be reduced by about one-third to compensate for incomplete oral absorption. The role for prophylactic digitalization in patients with a previous history but no present evidence of heart failure is discussed on pages 152.

Diuretics are likewise usually withheld on the morning of surgery and resumed postoperatively. When the immediate postoperative period is characterized by major volume shifts, diuretics should be administered as necessary and the dosage should be based upon continued clinical assessment of fluid balance. In such patients, the keystone to management is meticulous attention to the control of intravenous fluids, with diuretic therapy playing a secondary role. The parameters mentioned above (p. 138) should be carefully monitored.

When afterload reduction is necessary and the patient is unable to take oral medication, available agents include topical and parenteral nitroglycerine, parenteral hydralazine, and parenteral nitroprusside.

Preoperative pulmonary artery (Swan-Ganz) catheter insertion should be seriously considered in patients with moderate to severe congestive heart failure (NYHA Class 3 or 4, S_3, jugular venous distention, or measured ejection fraction <35% despite therapy), and in some patients with lesser risk undergoing surgery which requires major volume replacement. Monitoring of central pressures allows accurate replacement of blood and fluid losses, and early treatment of volume overload.

POSTOPERATIVE CONGESTIVE HEART FAILURE

Epidemiology

Limited information (2, 143, 151) is available on the risk of developing congestive heart failure perioperatively. In Goldman's prospective series of 1001 patients over age 40 (1, 2), 6.3% developed new or worsened congestive heart failure and 3.6% progressed to cardiogenic pulmonary edema. Eighty-six per cent of observed postoperative pulmonary edemas were cardiac in origin, 14% noncardiac. Postoperative pulmonary edema from all causes was recognized in 1 per 4500 anesthesias in a retrospective series of patients not selected for age (probably an underestimate by the investigator's own admission) (152).

There are several risk factors for the development of postoperative heart failure. *The best predictor of both postoperative new or worsened failure and pulmo-*

nary edema is preoperative heart failure (pp. 138–139).

Postoperative new or worsened heart failure developed in about 20% of patients with significant mitral or aortic valve disease in Goldman's series (2). Patients at risk included those with history or physical examination evidence of significant aortic stenosis, aortic regurgitation, or mitral stenosis. The presence of a grade 2 or louder murmur of mitral regurgitation carried a similar risk.

However, about two-thirds of the patients developing new or worsened heart failure or pulmonary edema had neither preoperative heart failure or valvular disease (2). Other factors which were less predictive of but did correlate with the development of pulmonary edema and significant new or worsened congestive heart failure included: (*a*) age greater than 60, (*b*) intra-abdominal, intrathoracic, or aortic surgery, and (*c*) nonspecific electrocardiographic changes (2, 152). These factors, however, did not predict the development of mild failure. Six of 21 patients (29%) in Goldman's series (2) who suffered postoperative myocardial infarction also developed pulmonary edema. Postoperative congestive heart failure or pulmonary edema did not develop in any patient receiving spinal or regional anesthesia in two reported series (2, 152). There was no difference in the incidence of postoperative failure among patients receiving different general anesthetic agents. Excessive fluid administration was implicated in one-half of the cases of postoperative pulmonary edema in Cooperman's series (152).

Pulmonary edema tends to develop either intraoperatively or immediately postoperatively. In one study (152), three-quarters of the cases had developed by one-half hour and 95% by one hour after the completion of surgery. No information is available on the time course for the development of mild to moderate failure.

The clinical presentation of postoperative congestive heart failure or pulmonary edema is usually characterized by tachypnea and often by rales. The presenting sign is wheezing without rales in one-quarter of cases (152). Hypertension and tachycardia are present in most patients. Neck vein distension was not present in one-half of patients in a series that included noncardiac causes of pulmonary edema (152). Acute respiratory insufficiency is a manifestation in one-half of patients.

The mortality of postoperative pulmonary edema is high and ranges from 20–57% depending on the series (2, 152). Of these deaths, 70% are due to cardiac causes and 30% to noncardiac reasons (2). Patients who develop postoperative mild to moderate congestive failure do not have an increased risk of cardiac death, but the mortality from other causes (15%) is high (2).

Evaluation

The diagnosis of congestive heart failure is based upon history, physical examination, and chest x-ray findings. The approach is similar in postoperative and medical patients. Two postoperative situations, however, many complicate the diagnostic process.

First, symptoms of postoperative heart failure and postoperative respiratory complications may be similar. Postoperative pulmonary edema may present first as wheezing, tachypnea, or respiratory insufficiency. The presence of an S_3 gallop or unequivocal jugular venous distension strongly favors the diagnosis of congestive failure. Postoperative hypertension is common in postoperative pulmonary edema, but may occur with respiratory problems. Useful clues include the presence of preoperative risk factors for congestive heart failure (see above) and the absence of antecedent lung disease. Chest x-ray examination is often very helpful. Occasionally, insertion of a pulmonary artery (Swan-Ganz) catheter is required for diagnosis.

Second, when pulmonary edema develops postoperatively, the etiology may be unclear. Yet the differentation of cardiogenic from non cardiogenic pulmonary edema is important for management. The findings of an S_3 gallop, jugular venous distension, prior history of failure, or postoperative myocardial infarction favor a cardiac etiology. The presence of sepsis favors a noncardiac cause, but cardiac failure can also occur in this setting. A trial of diuretic therapy is a reasonable diagnostic modality, as long as the patient is not hypotensive and is closely watched. Insertion of a pulmonary artery catheter is often necessary, especially when the patient does not improve or becomes hypotensive with diuretic therapy.

Once the diagnosis of cardiac failure has been established, those factors which can precipitate or worsen failure (Table 10.1) should be searched for. A careful review of all records of intake, output, and serial weights is especially helpful in establishing the role of fluid overload in precipitating failure. Myocardial infarction must be ruled out in patients with pulmonary edema, since a small but significant number will have myocardial infarction.

Management

The management of patients with postoperative congestive heart failure and pulmonary edema follows usual clinical guidelines with use of diuretics, oxygen, morphine, afterload reducers, and inotropic agents (digoxin, dopamine). Patients in severe distress in the immediate postoperative period may be stabilized by reintubation and positive pressure respirators. Mild failure can usually be managed with diuretics and sodium restriction alone.

After the acute episode of failure or pulmonary edema is over, postoperative management should be based on careful monitoring of fluid administration and volume status (see p. 111), diuretics, and

in some cases, digitalization and afterload reduction.

Factors precipitating failure or worsening cardiac performance (Table 10.17) should be corrected.

PREOPERATIVE DYSRHYTHMIAS

Epidemiology

Preoperative dysrhythmias are encountered occasionally in the general surgical population and more frequently in the subgroup of patients with heart disease (Table 10.38).

The presence of preoperative dysrhythmia is associated with increased perioperative morbidity and mortality (Table 10.39). Goldman (1, 2) demonstrated that the presence of frequent premature ventricular contractions (more than 5 PVCs per minute), non-sinus rhythm, or premature atrial contractions (PACs) predicted an increased perioperative cardiovascular morbidity and death, even after other risk factors had been controlled. Nonfatal life-threatening cardiac complications† occurred in 16% of the patients with frequent PVCs and 10% of the patients with PACs or non-sinus rhythm versus 3.3% and 3% in the respective control groups. Cardiac deaths occurred in 14% of the patients with PVCs and 9% of the PAC non-sinus group, versus 1.4% and 1% of the respective control groups. Both >5 PVCs per minute and the presence of non-sinus rhythm or PACs were independently correlated with cardiac death; only the former was independently associated with postoperative myocardial infarction.

Other authors have confirmed the increased perioperative morbidity in patients with preoperative dysrhythmias. Cooperman (154) in a retrospective study of 566 patients undergoing peripheral vascular surgery found a 33% incidence

---

†Defined as documented intra- or postoperative myocardial infarction, pulmonary edema, or ventricular tachycardia not resulting in cardiac death.

Table 10.38.   Incidence of Preoperative Dysrhythmias

Study	Goldman (1, 2)	Skinner (8)	Morrison (153)	Morrison (153)	Cooperman (139)
Population	General Surgical (Age > 40)	Cardiac Disease	Rheumatic Heart Disease	Atherosclerotic Heart Disease	Peripheral Vascular Disease
Number	1001[a]	857[b]	189[b]	485[b]	566[a]
Abnormal rhythm	6.5%			17.9%	3.7%
Atrial fibrillation	4.8%	11.6%	11.8%	12.8%	
Atrial flutter		0.5%		1.2%	
PVCs[c]	4.4%[c]				
PACs	5.2%				

[a] Patients.
[b] Operations.
[c] Over five premature ventricular contractions per minute after bedside examination and review of history, medical record, and preoperative electrocardiogram.

of cardiovascular complications in patients with preoperative dysrhythmia versus 9% in patients with normal rhythm; the association was statistically significant. Skinner and Pearce's retrospective study (8) of surgery in cardiac patients found that 13% of 99 patients with atrial fibrillation who underwent major operative procedures died, versus 7% of 76 patients with a normal EKG; the difference, however, is not statistically significant. Morrison (153) found that operative mortality increased from 4–18% when atrial fibrillation (20 operations) accompanied rheumatic heart disease (total of 189 operations). There was a less impressive and not statistically significant increase from 15–18% when non-sinus rhythm (87 operations), mostly atrial fibrillation, accompanied ischemic heart disease (total

of 485 operations). In a study (155) without a comparison group, 60 patients with chronic atrial fibrillation who underwent 76 major operations had a 5% mortality rate, a rate closer to that reported by Goldman.

The perioperative risk of arterial embolization in patients with atrial fibrillation is unknown. Using data from Morrison (153), however, one can calculate that the risk lies between 0 and 1.6% in patients with atrial fibrillation and atherosclerotic heart disease, and between 0 and 9% in patients with atrial fibrillation and rheumatic heart disease. Unfortunately, only the risk for all patients with atherosclerotic heart disease (0.3%) and rheumatic heart disease (1.3%) was given; the embolization rate for the subgroups with atrial fibrillation was not reported.

Table 10.39.   Perioperative Mortality in Patients with Preoperative Dysrhythmia[a]

Study	Goldman (1)	Skinner (8)	Morrison (153)	Finkbeiner (155)
Non-sinus rhythm	9% (65)[b]		18% (109)[c]	
Atrial fibrillation	6% (48)[b]	13% (99)[c]		5% (60)[b]
>5 PVCs/min	14% (44)[b]			
PACs	8% (52)[b]			

[a] Goldman, cardiac mortality; others, total mortality.
[b] Percentage mortality (number of patients with dysrhythmia).
[c] Percentage mortality (number of operations in patients with dysrhythmia).

Whether dysrhythmias are causally related to morbidity and mortality or simply serve as markers of severe underlying cardiopulmonary disease is uncertain. The available evidence favors the latter explanation. Goldman (1, 2) found, for example, that the patients with PACs who died from cardiac causes were all elderly, had major operations, and were frequently unstable. The presence of PVCs did not correlate with the development of ventricular tachycardia, but 43 of the 44 patients with PVCs had other signs of important heart disease. Sapala et al. (19) found mortality to be higher among heart patients with a previous myocardial infarction complicated by dysrhythmia, block, or failure (10% of 61 patients) than among heart patients with dysrhythmia, block, or failure without previous infarction (2.2% of 90 patients). Vanik and Davis (156) found the incidence of serious intra- and postoperative dysrhythmias unrelated to the presence of preoperative dysrhythmia but increased in patients with heart disease without preoperative dysrhythmia.

Evaluation

Preoperative evaluation of the patient with dysrhythmia should be directed toward determining the cause of the dysrhythmia and detecting the presence of associated risk factors. Most commonly this will involve a search for cardiac disease, pulmonary disease, electrolyte or acid-base disorders, and dysrhythmogenic drug use. The routine preoperative evaluation should be conducted as described in (Tables 10.16 and 10.17) (p. 115). A prolonged rhythm strip and/or a 24-hour Holter monitor may be helpful in diagnosing, quantitating, and estimating the prognostic importance of a dysrhythmia.

Management

Management of dysrhythmia in preoperative and nonsurgical patients is similar. If possible, etiologic factors should be corrected, such as uncompensated heart failure, hypoxia, hypocarbia or hypercarbia, hypokalemia or other electrolyte imbalance, acid-base imbalance, and the use of dysrhythmogenic drugs. Associated conditions, such as myocardial infarction, valvular heart disease, idiopathic hypertrophic subaortic stenosis (IHSS), or chronic lung disease, should be managed as discussed elsewhere in this text. There is no evidence that the suppression of preoperative dysrhythmias, which otherwise need not be treated, reduces surgical morbidity or mortality. The indication for anti-arrhythmic drugs is no different in the preoperative than in the nonsurgical patient.

Dysrhythmias that should generally be treated include: ventricular tachycardia, multiform complex or frequent PVCs, especially in the presence of heart disease, PVCs associated with recent myocardial infarction, atrial fibrillation or flutter with rapid ventricular response, other paroxysmal supraventricular tachycardia, sick sinus syndrome, and any rhythm that significantly impairs cardiovascular function.

Necessary anti-arrhythmic drugs should generally be continued to provide protection until surgery. A preoperative dose should usually be given early the morning of surgery with a small sip of water.

Because of the possibility of drug interactions, the anesthesiologist must be informed of all the patient's preoperative medications. Quinidine, procainamide, and lidocaine, for example, potentiate the action of skeletal muscle relaxants (see p. 148).

Since digitalis preparations may increase the risk of intra- and postoperative dysrhythmia (see pp. 152–155), we generally withhold maintenance digoxin during the 12 hours before surgery, unless it is needed to control ventricular rate, and resume it postoperatively. Digitalis is not given to patients with pre-excitation syndromes (e.g., Wolff-Parkinson-White syndrome), since it increases refractoriness at the AV junction and enhances conduction through the accessory pathway. Should atrial fibrillation develop, a dangerously rapid ventricular response might ensue which could degenerate into ventricular fibrillation. Digitalis is also avoided in patients with IHSS because of its positive inotropic effect which could increase outflow obstruction.

Symptomatic bradyarrhythmia requires pacemaker insertion (see p. 148). Preoperative pacemaker insertion would also be expected to benefit the asymptomatic patient with severe bradyarrhythmia whose rate does not increase with exercise or stress (see p. 148).

INTRAOPERATIVE AND POSTOPERATIVE DYSRHYTHMIAS

Epidemiology

Several studies (2, 156–179) have documented the frequency of intraoperative and postoperative dysrhythmias. Because of differences in patient populations, types of surgery, classifications of rhythm disturbances and methods of monitoring, reported incidences of dysrhythmia vary widely among studies, ranging from <1% in the unmonitored postoperative period (165) to >80% in the continuously monitored intraoperative period (159).

Intraoperative dysrhythmias are quite common, occurring in from 18–84% of patients in reported series (156, 159–160, 162–164, 166–168, 180). Bradydysrhythmias, nodal rhythm, AV dissociation, wandering pacemaker, and simple ventricular and atrial premature contractions are the most frequently observed intraoperative dysrhythmias. Tachyarrhythmias occur in only a small percentage of patients. Intraoperative cardiac arrest occurs in about 0.1% of patients (range 0.03–0.4%) (156, 162, 181–186), asystole being the cause slightly more often than ventricular fibrillation (162, 183, 187).

Supraventricular tachydysrhythmias (atrial fibrillation, atrial flutter, paroxys-mal supraventricular tachycardia) are the most commonly reported postoperative dysrhythmias. They occur in only a few percent (less than 1–4%) of the general surgical population (2, 157, 165), but in about 10–20% of patients who have undergone intrathoracic surgery (Table 10.40). Atrial fibrillation is observed 3–4 times more frequently than either atrial flutter or paroxysmal supraventricular tachycardia. The majority of postoperative dysrhythmias occur within 4–5 days of surgery. Premature ventricular and atrial contractions have been reported less frequently than supraventricular tachydysrhythmias (170–171, 173, 176, 179). Ventricular tachycardia is uncommon (≤1% of thoracic surgery cases) (161, 170–178).

Factors which are associated with an increased likelihood of intraoperative and/or postoperative dysrhythmias (Table 10.41), include type of surgery (intrathoracic, intra-abdominal, major vascular) (2, 157, 162, 165), type of anesthesia (cyclopropane > halothane, methoxyflurance, enflourane > ether, nitrous oxide > local, epidural), heart disease (especially congestive heart failure) (pro: 1, 2, 156–157, 159, 162, 167, 172, 174; con: 160, 171), chronic lung disease (2, 157), old age (pro: 2, 156, 161, 164, 170, 172, 174, 176, 178; con: 160, 162, 171), use of digitalis preparations preoperatively (see p. 152), the use of spontaneous rather than controlled ventilation (166, 168), and infection (157, 187). Rare predisposing factors are thyrotoxicosis and pheochromocytoma. Procedures during surgery that may precipitate dysrhythmia include induction, intubation, organ manipulation (especially the oculocardiac reflex), excessive concentration of anesthetic agent, over- or underventilation, hypotension and use of sympathomimetics or succinylcholine (156–160, 166, 179). Sympathomimetic drugs that are most likely to produce dysrhythmia in the presence of cyclopropane or halogenated hydrocarbon anesthesia include epinephrine and nor-

Table 10.40.   Postoperative Supraventricular Tachydysrhythmias: Frequency and Mortality

Study	Type of Population	Total Number	No. (%) with SVT[a]	Deaths (%)	Deaths Contributed to or Caused by SVT[a] (%)	% of Deaths Contributed to or Caused by SVT[a]
Goldman (157a)	General surgical	916	35 (4%)	17 (49%)	0 (0%)	0%
Rogers (165)	General surgical		50 (?%)	?	6 (12%)	
Stougard (170)	Thoracic surgery	260	51 (20%)	?	0 (0%)	
Beck-Nielsen (171)	Thoracic surgery	300	38 (13%)	1 (3%)	0 (%)	0%
Mowry (172)	Thoracic surgery	574	22 (4%)	2 (9%)	0 (0%)	0%
Ghosh (173)	Thoracic surgery	100	18 (18%)	?	?	
Cohen (174)	Thoracic surgery	92	13 (14%)	?	?	
Cerney (175)	Thoracic surgery	76	12 (16%)	1 (8%)	1 (8%)	100%
Krosnik (161)	Thoracic surgery	82	10 (12%)	2 (20%)	2 (20%)	100%
Massie (166)	Thoracic surgery	120	9 (8%)	1 (9%)	?1 (9%)	0–100%
Bailey (177)	Thoracic surgery	78	9 (12%)	0 (0%)	0 (0%)	
Currens (178)	Thoracic surgery	56	12 (21%)	3 (25%)	1 (8%)	33%
Rose (179)	Cardiac surgery	50	35 (70%)	?	?	
Cheanvechai (176)	Cardiac surgery	397	58 (15%)	?	0 (0%)	
Wisoff (188)	Cardiac surgery	200	20 (10%)	0 (0%)	0 (0%)	
Tyras (169)	Cardiac surgery	140	26 (19%)	1 (4%)	?	
Totals (thoracic and cardiac surgery only)		2525	282 (11%)	11 (7%)	5 (3%)	
Totals (general, thoracic, and cardiac surgery)						15–19% (4–5/27)

[a] SVT, supraventricular tachycardia.

epinephrine (158, 166); low-dose dopamine, methoxamine, phenylephrine, and mephenteramine are probably less dysrhythmogenic. Electrolyte-acid-base imbalance and hypoxia are additional factors that may facilitate the development of dysrhythmias. Central venous or Swan-Ganz catheters may occasionally trigger dysrhythmias.

Most studies do not explicitly relate the occurrence of intraoperative and postoperative dysrhythmia to morbidity and mortality. Intraoperative dysrhythmias, while extremely common, are generally transient, self-limited, and benign. In Vanik's study (156) which reported a 17.9% frequency of intraoperative dysrhythmia, only 0.9% were judged to be serious (defined as new onset of atrial fibrillation, nodal bradycardia <30 beats per minute, nodal tachycardia >170 beats per minute,

complete AV dissociation, bundle branch block, ventricular tachycardia or fibrillation, persistent multifocal ventricular premature contractions, "bizarre ventricular rhythms," or cardiac arrest). Intraoperative bradydysrhythmias, which occur in 10–15% of patients (2, 160, 163), are nearly always self-limited or respond easily to atropine or adrenergic agents (2). Among the intraoperative dysrhythmias, only cardiac arrest is associated with a high mortality (50–93%) (182–185). The likelihood of successful resuscitation decreases with worsening ASA class (183) (see p. 22 for description of the American Society of Anesthesiologist's classification system).

Unlike intraoperative rhythm disturbances, postoperative supraventricular tachydysrhythmias are associated with substantial mortality, at least in the non-

Table 10.41. Factors Predisposing to Intraoperative and Postoperative Dysrhythmias

Causes
  Induction and/or intubation
  Organ manipulation
  Excessive anesthesia
  Hyperventilation and hypoventilation
  Hypoxia
  Hypotension
  Drugs
  Electrolyte imbalance
  Acid-base imbalance
  Myocardial infarction
  Congestive heart failure
  Pulmonary embolism
  Irritation by central catheters
Risk factors
  Old age
  Chronic lung disease
  Congestive heart failure, heart disease
  Intrathoracic, intra-abdominal, or major vascular
    surgery
  Type of anesthesia (see text)
  Preoperative digitalization
  Thyrotoxicosis
  Pheochromocytoma

thoracic, noncardiac surgery population. However, death is usually not attributable to the dysrhythmia; it most often is caused by the patient's underlying disease or other postoperative complications (Table 10.40). For example, of the 35 patients who developed new postoperative supraventricular tachydysrhythmias in Goldman's series (157), 16 (46%) had other acute cardiac conditions, 11 (31%) had major infections (154), 10 (29%) had preexisting hypotension, 8 (23%) had metabolic derangements, 8 (23%) had dysrhythmias associated with parenteral drug therapy, and 7 (20%) were hypoxic. In 94% the rhythm returned to normal sinus; 40% required no new therapy; only two patients (6%) required cardioversion. Although mortality was 49%, no deaths were contributed to or caused by dysrhythmia.

Evaluation

The approach to the patient who develops an intraoperative or postoperative dysrhythmia involves determining the (*a*) diagnosis, (*b*) cause, and (*c*) significance of the dysrhythmia. Dysrhythmias should be documented by printed rhythm strip in addition to the oscilloscope monitor. A rapid assessment of hemodynamic significance of the dysrhythmia should include measuring of blood pressure, palpating of pulses, observing the warmth and color of the skin, viewing the operative field in anesthetized patients for changes in rate of bleeding, checking urine output, and examining cerebral function in awake patients. Cardiac failure can be detected by history, physical examination, and review of the central venous pressure, pulmonary wedge pressure, and cardiac output if relevant monitoring equipment is in place. History and a 12-lead electrocardiogram will aid in the detection of myocardial ischemia.

Examination for the cause of the dysrhythmia should include a determination of the adequacy of ventilation and oxygenation (arterial blood gases), an assessment of the depth of anesthesia, a look at the operative field to rule out excessive or unusual organ manipulation, and review of medication use. Hypertension, hypotension, electrolyte, or acid-base imbalance, myocardial failure, and ischemia should also be excluded as the cause of dysrhythmia.

Management

Most intraoperative dysrhythmias are transient, do not require anti-dysrhythmic drugs, and respond to correction of the underlying cause or adjustment of the anesthetic technique. Ventilatory abnormalities, hypoxia, too light or deep anesthesia, and excessive organ manipulation can readily be corrected. Offending medications can be discontinued. Heart failure, electrolyte and acid-base abnormalities, hypotension, and hypertension can be treated.

The indications for and methods of antidysrhythmic drug use or cardioversion are similar in surgical and nonsurgical patients. Quinidine, procainamide, and, to a much lesser extent, lidocaine should be used cautiously in the immediate postoperative period, since they could cause respiratory depression by potentiating the effects of muscle relaxants given intraoperatively.

CONDUCTION ABNORMALITIES

Epidemiology

The risk of anesthesiology and surgery in the presence of cardiac conduction abnormalities has been best defined for patients with chronic bifascicular and monofascicular block. Bifascicular block is more common in hospitalized patients than in the general population, and in one series (2) was present in 4.5% of 1001 preoperative patients over age 40 (2.3% with right bundle branch block (RBBB) and left anterior hemiblock (LAH), 2.0% with left bundle branch block (LBBB), and 0.2% with RBBB and left posterior hemiblock). In the nonsurgical population, bifascicular block progresses to more advanced atrioventricular (AV) block at a modest

rate (about 6% per year for RBBB and LAH) (189–192). Whether unexplained symptoms (dizziness, syncope) or abnormal conduction in the His-Purkinje system (HPS) increase the rate of progression is controversial (192–194). Bifascicular block alone does not seem to significantly increase the risk of developing intraoperative or postoperative complete heart block (CHB). Reported in the literature are 316 patients with bifascicular block who underwent 409 procedures (2, 195–201; 186, 191, 211); only one developed complete heart block (Table 10.42), which occurred during intubation and was transient. Monofascicular block, like bifascicular block, is more frequent in hospitalized than in healthy populations. It is several times more common than bifascicular block. Of the 1001 preoperative patients in Goldman's study (2), LAH was present in 9% and RBBB in 3%. In nonsurgical populations, monofascicular block progresses at a considerably slower rate than bifascicular block (202–203). Clinical data suggest that there is also little chance of progression to CHB during or after surgery. Among 90 pa-

Table 10.42. Risk of Operation in Bifascicular Block[g]

Study	RBBB + LAH	LBBB	RBBB + LPH	Total Number of Procedures	Progression to CHB
Goldman (2)[a]	23	20	2	45	0
Ventkataraman (195)[b]	38	0	0	73	0
Rooney (196)	27	0	0	44	0
Pastore (197)[c]	44	0	0	52	1[d]
Berg (198)[e]	26	4	0	36	0
Kunstadt (199)[f]	21	3	0	38	0
Gertler (200)	0	10	0	23	0
Bellocci (201)	48	40	10	98	0
Total	227	77	12	409	1

[a] Seven patients with prolonged P-R.
[b] Five patients with prolonged P-R, two with history of syncope.
[c] Five patients with prolonged P-R, one with history of syncope.
[d] CHB transient during intubation but temporary pacemaker inserted.
[e] Four patients with prolonged P-R and LBBB, 12 with history of syncope of dizziness.
[f] Four patients with prolonged P-R and LBBB.
[g] See text for definition of abbreviations.

tients with LAH and 63 with RBBB undergoing operation, none progressed to CHB (2, 200). Finally, in terms of perioperative cardiovascular morbidity and mortality, monofascicular or bifascicular block did not emerge as an independent risk factor in Goldman's series of 1001 surgical patients, 202 of whom had an abnormal QRS pattern (2). Cardiovascular mortality was slightly higher, however, for this subgroup when compared to the entire series (5% versus 2%).

First-degree AV block is more common than monofascicular or bifascicular block in healthy populations (204–205). It generally does not progress to higher degrees of block and usually reflects conduction abnormalities above the HPS (207). Among 24 patients with first-degree AV block in addition to bifascicular block who underwent surgery, there was no progression to CHB (2, 195, 197–199).

Unlike first-degree AV, monofascicular, and bifascicular block, the presence of untreated chronic complete heart block is thought to substantially increase operative risk. In the nonsurgical population with chronic complete heart block unrelated to myocardial infarction or digitalis toxicity, 1-year mortality may be as high as 40% without a pacemaker (208–209). Prognosis is improved substantially by pacemaker implantation (209–210). Patients with bifascicular block who previously experienced transient complete heart block during myocardial infarction may also be at substantially increased risk of subsequent sudden death if not treated with a pacemaker (211). In a report by Vandam and McLemore (212), before pacemakers were available, 22 patients with constant or intermittent CHB unrelated to infarction underwent general anesthesia and surgery. Five experienced circulatory arrests consistent with asystole, and in four asystole was documented. One respiratory arrest occurred. There were no deaths, and all patients were resuscitated with drug therapy. The risk of circulatory arrest was 36% (4 of

11) in patients with and 9% (1 of 11) in patients without a previous history of Stokes-Adams attacks.

In a review of the literature, we could not find adequate data on operative risk for patients with advanced (high-grade), Mobitz Type II, or Mobitz Type I second-degree AV block. Advanced second-degree AV block is said to be prognostically indistinguishable from CHB (213). Mobitz Type II second-degree block almost always reflects disease in the HPS, and it is therefore generally believed to have high potential for progression to Stokes-Adams attacks (207). There is some clinical evidence that this belief is valid (214, 215), with 13 of 24 patients in one poorly defined retrospective series (214) progressing to CHB and three more dying suddenly. In the absence of sufficient perioperative data, it is prudent to assume that both advanced and Mobitz Type II second-degree AV block increase operative risk. On the other hand, Mobitz Type I AV block more frequently represents disease in the AV node, which is thought to have a relatively benign course (207), and therefore would be expected to carry little operative risk. However, a minority of Mobitz Type I patients may have disease in the HPS (207).

Evaluation

Evaluation of the preoperative patient with a cardiac conduction abnormality includes (a) definition of the conduction defect and determination of its prognostic significance, (b) detection of reversible or treatable etiologic factors, and (c) assessment for associated operative risk factors.

The conduction defect is first classified as to type, chronicity, and presence/absence of associated symptoms. The routine preoperative evaluation (pp. 115–117, Table 10.16), should be performed to identify the cause of the conduction disturbance and the presence of associated preoperative risk factors. The electrocardiogram, including rhythm strip, chest x-ray, electrolytes, digoxin and anti-ar-rhythmic drug levels, and other indicated tests, should be reviewed. Common etiol-ogies of conduction abnormalities include: atherosclerotic and hypertensive heart disease, myocardial infarction, idiopathic, congenital, cardiomyopathy, valvular heart disease, drug toxicity electrolyte distur-bances, and previous cardiac surgery. As-sociated preoperative risk factors include recent myocardial infarction, congestive heart failure, and arrhythmias. Twenty-four-hour Holter monitoring can identify higher degrees of block that may be missed on a standard tracing. Atrial pacing or electrophysiologic testing of the HPS are helpful in selected instances in defining the significance and site of block or brad-yarrhythmia.

Management

Recommended indications for preoper-ative temporary or permanent pacemaker placement rest primarily on expert opin-ion (117, 216–217), reasoning from the incomplete data already discussed, and consideration of the possible adverse ef-fects of pacemaker placement such as ventricular irritability, pneumo- or hem-othorax, infection, myocardial perfora-tion, etc. (197, 218–220).

Our recommendations are listed in Ta-ble 10.34. Temporary pacemaker implan-tation is advisable in patients with unex-plained symptoms and bifascicular block, who cannot be fully evaluated preopera-tively. If a pacemaker is not placed pre-operatively in patients in the "probably indicated" or "probably not indicated" cat-egories, a temporary pacemaker should be immediately available in the operating room for emergency insertion if needed. In addition, a syringe containing atropine and an intravenous solution of isoproter-enol should be immediately available.

Conduction abnormalities appearing in the setting of an acute myocardial infarc-tion have different prognostic and thera-peutic implications and are not discussed in this book.

Associated preoperative risk factors should be managed as discussed else-where in this chapter.

PACEMAKERS

Epidemiology

It is estimated that over 100,000–200,000 individuals in the United States (0.05–0.1% of the population) have per-manent cardiac pacemakers (221–222). Because of an increased likelihood of heart disease, an older average age, and the occasional prophylactic use of temporary pacemakers, the prevalence of pace-makers among preoperative patients is undoubtedly higher than in the general population, although exact figures are not easily accessible.

Perioperative morbidity and mortality are probably not significantly increased because of the presence of a pacemaker (58, 223–224). Potential difficulties do ex-ist. Electrocautery or other electromag-netic interference may interfere with EKG monitoring, suppress pacemaker func-tion, trigger dysrhythmias, or, in the presence of inadequately insulated exter-nal pacemaker wires, result in myocar-dial cauterization and inability to pace (221, 223, 225–230). The cautery can also reprogram the pacemaker (230). Demand pacemakers are more sensitive than fixed rate models, and pacemakers with uni-polar electrodes more sensitive than ones with bipolar electrodes. Even in the ab-sence of electrical interference, the use of temporary transvenous pacing may in-crease ventricular irritability (197). Per-ioperative conditions that may lower the pacing threshold and increase suscepti-bility to dysrhythmia or electrical inter-ference include: hypoxia, the use of sym-pathomimetic amines, and myocardial ischemia. Perioperative conditions that can raise pacing threshold and cause irregularity in or cessation of pacing include: hyperkalemia, acidosis, alkalosis, and the use of succinyl choline. With ventricular pacing, cardiac output may be particularly sensitive to drops in venous-filling pressure caused by perioperative blood loss because of the loss of effective atrial contraction. Another potential problem is electrode displacement, which is most likely to occur within 24–48 hours of transvenous insertion. Finally, it should be remembered that patients requiring pacemakers often have underlying heart disease, which may independently increase surgical risk.

Evaluation

The routine preoperative evaluation should be conducted as described on pages 115–117 (Table 10.16). Attention should first be focused on a search for associated factors, which independently increase perioperative risk, such as recent myocardial infarction, congestive heart failure, and dysrhythmia. Secondly, pacemaker function should be evaluated and possible perioperative risks noted, such as the planned use of diathermy. In addition to the 12-lead electrocardiogram, a rhythm strip should be obtained. The most important information to record for the anesthesiologist is *type of pacemaker, pacing mode, pacing rate,* any unusual or potential problems in the individual patient, and where the internist or cardiologist can be reached at the time of surgery if problems occur. When demand pacemaker function is persistently suppressed by an intrinsic cardiac rhythm, the pacemaker can be converted from demand to fixed rate with the use of magnet and interspike intervals measured. A slowing in rate, failure to pace, failure to capture, failure to sense, or oversensing suggest pacemaker malfunction and the need for further evaluation and correction before surgery. The use of medications or presence of electrolyte, acid-base, or hypoxic

disorders that could affect pacemaker function should be noted.

Interference with pacemaker function by electrical equipment (especially electric cautery) during surgery is "possible and should be considered before the procedure." (230).

Management

Indications for perioperative pacemaker insertion are discussed on pages 148–150 and summarized in Table 10.43.

Intraoperative pacemaker management includes careful insulation and grounding of all electrical wires and equipment, continuous electrocardiographic monitoring, immediate availability of atropine and of isoproterenol, a magnet that can convert from demand to fixed rate modes, and an alternative tem-

Table 10.43. Indications for Preoperative Temporary or Permanent Pacemaker Placement

Definitely indicated
Present or past history of complete heart block[a]
Present or past history of high-grade AV block
Present or past history of Mobitz Type II AV block
Mobitz Type I second-degree AV block due to HPS disease (uncommon)
Symptomatic or significant sinus node dysfunction
Symptomatic or significant bradyarrhythmia
Idioventricular rhythm
Symptomatic/high suspicion and unable to evaluate preoperatively (emergency operation)
Probably indicated
Unexplained symptoms and bifascicular block
Trifascicular block with severe underlying heart disease (some cases)
Probably not indicated but uncertain
Bifascicular block with prolonged P-R interval (most cases)
Mobitz Type I second-degree AV block thought not to be due to HPS disease (common)
Not indicated
Asymptomatic bifascicular block
Symptoms and bifascicular block, symptoms explained by cause not requiring pacemaker
First-degree AV block

[a] Except for past history of transient CHB associated with inferior myocardial infarction and unaccompanied by post-infarction bifascicular block.

porary pacemaker for emergency insertion.

Electrocautery should be avoided when possible. If it must be used, the ground plate should be located as close to the operative site and as far (at least 15 cm) from the pulse generator as possible. The cautery should not be used within 12 inches of the pacemaker, because the pacemaker may be directly damaged (230). A well-shielded pacemaker should be used (see manufacturer's specifications). If demand mode suppression occurs, the frequency and duration of electrocautery can be limited to bursts of 1 sec duration more than 10 sec apart. Alternatively, the pacemaker can be converted to fixed rate in an attempt to avoid electrical interference with demand function.

The method of conversion to a fixed rate varies with the pacemaker type. Most older demand, non-programmable pacemakers can be converted by a magnet. These units are becoming less frequently encountered in practice. A magnet should *NOT* be used for more modern programmable pacemakers, because it may reprogram the pacemaker, or convert dual chamber to a single chamber ventricular pacemaker. Because of the multiple types and complexity of current pacemakers, and their different responses when exposed to electrical "noise" in the operating room, a cardiologist should be involved preoperatively in deciding on how to manage the pacemaker intraoperatively and postoperatively (usually this will be the cardiologist who inserted or monitors the pacemaker).

Since diathermy can interfere with electrocardiographic recording, palpation of the pulse, arterial pressure, or esophageal stethoscopic monitoring will be necessary during cautery use. During use of electric cautery, the monitor should be intermitantly checked specifically to assess if the pacemaker is functioning properly.

The danger of electrode dislodgement or perforation should be minimized by delaying surgery until 48 hours after permanent pacemaker insertion when possible and by avoiding sudden movements, positions, or traction that might predispose to this complication.

Good supportive care such as the avoidance of hypovolemia, hypoxia, and electrolyte and acid-base imbalance should be stressed. Although pulse generators are equipped with protective circuits to guard against externally applied high-voltage discharge, damage can occur. Therefore, the minimum necessary voltage should be used for cardioversion and defibrillator paddles should not be placed directly over the pulse generator during cardioversion or defibrillation.

In patients with pacemakers that can be programmed, the pacing rate may be increased when needed to suppress dysrhythmias or increase cardiac output.

Finally, antistaphylococcal antibiotic prophylaxis is recommended for pacemaker implantation (221, 231).

The risk of endocarditis from unrelated surgery in patients with indwelling transvenous pacemakers appears to be low (212, 221, 222, 232). Some recommendations clearly favor not giving prophylaxis in this situation (221, 231), while the American Heart Association Committee Report (232) does not take a position, by stating that "dentists and physicians may choose to employ prophylactic antibiotics to cover dental and surgical procedures in these patients."

PREOPERATIVE DIGITALIZATION

Epidemiology

General agreement exists that digitalis glycosides are indicated preoperatively in the treatment of congestive heart failure and atrial fibrillation or flutter with rapid ventricular response (58, 117, 233–234).

The value of "prophylactic" preoperative digitalization to prevent intraoperative and postoperative failure or arrhythmia is controversial (235–237). Disputed indications for preoperative digitalization include: history of previous heart failure, cardiomegaly without clinical failure, history of previous or recurrent supraventricular tachycardia, cardiac or intrathoracic surgery, presence of coronary artery, myocardial, or significant valvular disease, and age over 60. These conditions have been shown (1) or can reasonably be expected to increase the risk of intraoperative and postoperative supraventricular arrhythmia or failure.

The arguments of the proponents of prophylactic digitalization include the following. First, digitalis preparations have been shown in normal man to increase myocardial contractility (238–239), even though they may not raise cardiac output (237); in the dog, digitalis reduces the negative inotropic effects of anesthetic agents (238–242). Postoperatively, an increase in cardiac output is often required (243–245). It, therefore, seems reasonable prophylactically to administer a positive inotropic agent to patients at increased risk of developing heart failure during the stresses of surgery and the postoperative state. Secondly, digitalis has been shown to control, at least partially, the ventricular rate in patients developing intra- or postoperative supraventricular dysrrhythmias (246–249). Furthermore, it may provide partial protection against the development of supraventricular dysrhythmia, although the data is conflicting (pro: 247–248, 250–253; con: 2, 249, 254–255). Prophylactic digitalization is therefore advocated by its proponents for patients at increased risk to prevent the development of supraventricular dysrhythmias or, at least, to better control the ventricular rate if they develop.

Those who caution against prophylactic digitalization in the preoperative patient offer the following arguments. (a) Digitalis glycosides are drugs with low toxic to therapeutic ratios. Surgical patients are frequently exposed to conditions that increase the changes of digitalis toxicity, such as hypoxia, hypokalemia, and acid-base disturbances. There is suggestive clinical evidence that digitalized patients do experience an increased risk of perioperative ventricular and supraventricular dysrhythmias including bradydysrhythmias (2, 117, 156, 236, 249, 254, 256–257). Furthermore, it may be difficult to determine whether a new perioperative dysrhythmia represents digitalis toxicity or not, thus complicating treatment. (b) The clinical data supporting the value of prophylactic digitalization is weak. There is no convincing evidence (247–255) that digoxin prevents perioperative congestive heart failure or mortality. The data regarding its effectiveness in the prevention of supraventricular tachycardia are conflicting (247–255). Although digitalized patients who do develop atrial fibrillation or flutter have lower ventricular rates, the difference in rates is not very large (mean 160 in 30 undigitalized patients versus mean 129 in 41 digitalized patients versus mean 129 in 41 digitalized patients (246, 248–249). Over 50% of digitalized patients required additional digitalis (although 50–75% less than undigitalized patients) or other treatment (246–249). The benefit of this latter advantage in terms of reduced morbidity is uncertain. (c) When a dysrhythmia arises which requires cardioversion because of hemodynamic compromise, a non- or underdigitalized patient is preferred both because of the danger of cardioversion in the presence of digitalis toxicity and because of the relative refractoriness of digitalis toxic rhythms to cardioversion (258–259). (d) Selecting an optimal dose of digitalis in a patient without dysrhythmia or evidence of failure is difficult (236) since there are no clinical parameters to follow and one is forced to rely solely on serum digitalis levels or standard dosages. In summary, the opponents would argue against prophylactic digitalization because of inherent difficulties in its use, its potential for causing toxicity or complicating perioperative care, and the lack of proven significant benefits from its use.

The decision whether to use preoperative prophylactic digitalization should be guided by an assessment of the potential risks versus benefits. The risk of the development of postoperative congestive heart failure in 1001 general surgical patients was approximately 6% (1); over half of these developed pulmonary edema with an attendant high mortality. Factors that increased the risk of perioperative failure were preoperative failure (30–47% risk), significant aortic or mitral valvular disease (20% risk), age over 60, more than nonspecific EKG abnormalities, and major surgery (see pp. 138–142). Neither angina nor preoperative myocardial infarction was independently correlated with postoperative cardiac failure. The value of prophylactic digitalization in preventing postoperative failure is unproven; in fact, the majority of studies show no such benefit (2, 248–250, 252–255). The risk of prophylactic digitalization is also poorly defined. While several studies suggest an increased risk of arrhythmia (2, 156, 236, 249, 254, 256), the risk is quantitated in only two (249, 254). In several other studies, digitalis toxicity was not found to be a major problem (247–248, 250, 252). In summary, cardiac failure is a serious postoperative complication that occurs in a few percent of the general hospital population and a higher percentage of certain risk groups. Neither the risks nor benefits of prophylactic digitalization have been adequately established.

The risk of intraoperative or postoperative supraventricular tachycardia is approximately 4% for the general surgical population, about 10% for patients who are over age 70 or have congestive heart failure, chronic obstructive pulmonary disease, or an abnormal EKG, and between 10 and 30% for patients undergoing intrathoracic pulmonary or cardiac surgery (2, 249). The relationship of new perioperative supraventricular tachycardia to morbidity has not been explicitly evaluated. However, since it can adversely affect cardiac function and raise

Table 10.44. Effect of Preoperative or Postoperative Prophylactic Digitalization on Frequency of Supraventricular Tachycardia (SVT)[a]

	Number	SVT	% SVT
Digitalized	130	20	15.4%
Not digitalized	163	32	19.7%

[a] Pooled data from controlled randomized prospective studies (248–249, 252). $p > 0.25$ (NS).

myocardial oxygen demand, its presence must be considered undesirable. As noted above, there is conflicting evidence regarding the benefit of prophylactic digitalization in the prevention of arrhythmia. Most studies are retrospective and have not controlled for preoperative risk factors (247, 250–251, 253–255). There are three prospective randomized clinical trials (248–249, 252), one of which utilized postoperative digitalization and has been published in only abstract form (252). Pooling data from these studies (Table 10.44), no significant benefit is seen for preoperative prophylactic digitalization. In summary, supraventricular tachycardia represents a mild to potentially serious perioperative complication in from 10–30% of selected patients. There are neither proven clinical benefits or risks to the use of prophylactic digitalization.

Management

Based upon the available evidence and a weighing of potential risks versus benefits, *we do not routinely recommend preoperative digitalization in cardiac patients without failure or present or past supraventricular dysrhythmia; in patients undergoing intrathoracic surgery; or in the elderly. Our recommendations for digitalis use are the same in preoperative patients as in nonsurgical patients:* (a) chronic atrial fibrillation or flutter with rapid ventricular response, (b) congestive heart failure, and (c) past history of atrial fibrillation or flutter with persistence of the predisposing etiologic factor, such as mitral stenosis or ischemic heart disease. Digitalis or other antiarrhythmic drugs are used in patients with recurrent paroxysmal atrial or nodal tachycardias. Digitalis is avoided in patients with associated idiopathic hypertrophic, subaortic stenosis or Wolff-Parkinson-White syndrome.

VALVULAR HEART DISEASE AND IDIOPATHIC HYPERTROPHIC SUBAORTIC STENOSIS (IHSS)

Epidemiology

Data on perioperative risk in valvular heart disease is limited. Reported series (2, 8, 153) include small numbers of patients, and very few patients with severe lesions. *The risk of surgery seems to vary with the valve affected (aortic vs. mitral), the type of lesion (stenosis vs. insufficiency), and the severity of the lesion (Tables 10.45 and 10.46).* Aortic disease appears to pose a greater risk than mitral disease (2, 8, 260). In Goldman's series (1, 2), of all aortic and mitral lesions, only true aortic stenosis (not systolic ejection murmurs) served as an independent risk factor for perioperative cardiac death. While mitral regurgitant murmurs were associated with postoperative infarction and cardiac death, the significance of the association did not persist after other risk factors had been controlled, suggesting that mitral regurgitant murmurs may serve more as a marker of underlying cardiac disease than as causes themselves of perioperative morbidity or mortality. About 20% of patients with mitral regurgitant murmurs grade II or louder, significant aortic regurgitation, significant mitral stenosis, or significant aortic stenosis developed new or worsening congestive heart failure in the postoperative period. A reasonable general rule seems to be that surgical risk parallels the severity of the valvular lesion as measured by history, physical examination, laboratory evaluation, and New York Heart Association Functional Classification (1, 2, 8, 117, 153). In Morrison's series of 150 patients with rheumatic heart disease (153), morbidity and mortality were increased when atrial fibrillation, cardiomegaly, or poor NYHA Functional Classification accompanied the underlying valvular disease.

No specific data exist for perioperative risk of patients with prolapsed mitral valve

ble 10.45. Valvular Heart Disease: Mortality of Non-cardiac Surgery

alve	Lesion	Goldman (2) N	% Cardiac Death	Skinner (8) N	Total Mortality	N	Total Mortality (Thoracic and Abdominal Procedures Only)	Morrison (153) N	Complication Excluding Death	Mortality	O'Keefe (260) N	Total Mortality	Complications
tral	Stenosis	14	7%	35	6%	9	0%	147	4.1%	4.8%			
	Insufficiency	55	7%										
rtic	Stenosis	23	13%	59	10%	15	20%				48	0%	14%
	Insufficiency	12	8%										
mbined mitral and aortic rheumatic heart disease				17	6%	4	25%	41	2.4%	4.9%			
								189	3.7%	3.7%			

Table 10.46. Valvular Heart Disease: Risk of Postoperative Infarction and Cardiac Death[a]

Risk Factor	Number	Postoperative Infarction	Cardiac Death
Mitral regurgitation murmur (grade II/VI or louder)			
No	946	13 (1%)	15 (2%)
Yes	55	5 (9%) $p < 0.001$	4 (7%) $p < .05$
Mitral stenosis			
No	987	17 (2%)	18 (2%)
Yes	14	1 (7%) NS[b]	1 (7%) NS
Aortic systolic ejection murmur (grade II/VI or louder)			
No	730	13 (2%)	11 (1%)
Yes	248	5 (2%)	5 (2%)
Yes, with true aortic stenosis	23	0 (0%) NS	3 (13%) $p < .01$
Aortic regurgitation			
No	989	17 (2%)	18 (2%)
Yes	12	1 (8%) NS	1 (8%) NS

[a] From Goldman L, Calden DL, et al: Cardiac risk factors and complications in non-cardiac surgery. *Medicine* 57:357, 1978, with permission.
[b] NS, not significant.

(Barlow's syndrome), or tricuspid disease (58). It seems reasonable to assume that the risk for prolapsed mitral valve parallels the severity of the mitral regurgitation.

A small series (N-35) of patients with IHSS undergoing major surgery experienced no perioperative deaths and one myocardial infarction ("related to" coronary disease and spinal anesthesia) (261). Fifteen percent developed significant dysrhymias. The types of arrthymias included PVC's, sinus bradycardia, paroxysmal atrial tachycardia, and increased rate in atrial fibrillation. There was no predominant dysrhythmia, with no one arrthymia occurring in more than three patients. The authors recommended avoiding spinal anesthesia based on their one patient, one other patient in the literature, and the physiology of spinal anesthesia and IHSS (19, 135).

Evaluation

The preoperative evaluation should be conducted as described on pages 115–117 (Table 10.16). The nature and severity of the valvular lesions and the presence of associated cardiac risk factors (e.g., congestive failure, dysrhythmia) should be clearly noted.

Non-invasive tests of cardiac function may supplement history, physical examination, and routine laboratory findings.

Two dimensional and M-mode echocardiography is a useful adjunct in diagnosing and quantitating the severity of mitral stenosis and IHSS, and may provide findings suggestive of a bicuspid aortic valve, aortic insufficiency, or mitral regurgitation. Valvular calcification detected by echocardiography or fluoroscopy is an especially helpful clue to the significance of aortic systolic murmurs in elderly patients. Combining doppler flow with echocardiography gives a more precise assessment of the severity of valvular lesions of all types. Gated blood pool scanning gives a reliable estimate of ventricular function.

Cardiac catheterization should be considered in consultation with a cardiologist when (*a*) the diagnosis or hemodynamic significance of a valvular lesion remains uncertain, and (*b*) the information gained from catheterization would influence the decision whether to perform valvular before noncardiac surgery or whether to operate at all.

Management

Prophylaxis for bacterial endocarditis should be given to all patients with valvular heart disease, septal defects, or IHSS (p. 387). Concomitant congestive heart failure, arrhythmias, and coronary artery disease should be managed as described on pages 128, 138, and 145, respectively. Factors that could impair cardiac performance (p. 116, Table 10.17) should be corrected. When valvular surgery is indicated, it generally should be performed prior to elective noncardiac surgery. Patients on prophylactic anticoagulation for mitral stenosis and atrial fibrillation should be managed as described on page 160 (see Table 10.50).

Hemodynamically significant IHSS is of particular concern perioperatively and should be managed in connection with a cardiologist. Treatment with beta-blocking agents should be continued up until the time of surgery and resumed immediately postoperatively. When the patient is unable to take oral medications, intravenous propranolol may be substituted. Perioperative monitoring of left ventricular filling pressures (with a Swan-Ganz catheter) may be helpful in preventing volume depletion with consequent increased obstruction to ventricular outflow, reduction in cardiac output and hypotension. Hypotension, when it occurs, should be treated first with volume expansion. Inotropic agents such as isoproterenol and dopamine are best avoided, since they may also increase outflow obstruction, while pure alpha-adrenergic agents may occasionally be useful. When paroxysmal atrial fibrillation occurs, it should be cardioverted because of the adverse hemodynamic consequences of the loss of atrial contribution to left ventricular filling. The use of digoxin should be avoided.

PERICARDIAL DISEASE

Epidemiology

We are aware of no published clinical data quantifying the operative risk of noncardiac surgery in patients with pericardial disease. It is reasonable, however, to anticipate an increased perioperative morbidity and mortality in certain types of pericardial disease. Patients with tamponade or constrictive pericarditis (now rare) may initially maintain their cardiac output by compensatory tachycardia (262). Cardiac output may fall if the tachycardia is prevented, the degree of tamponade increases, myocardial contractility is suppressed, filling pressures fall, or peripheral resistance and blood pressure increase. Potential intraoperative dangers include bradycardia, the cardiodepressant effects of general anesthetics, hypovolemia with reduced filling pressures, and the hypertensive response to laryngoscopy and intubation. Patients with tamponade or constrictive pericarditis may also be at increased postoperative risk. Cardiac output, which normally may decrease during anesthesia, often rises postoperatively; patients whose cardiac outputs remain low may experience increasing acidosis and a higher postoperative mortality (243–245). Finally, when myocarditis accompanies pericarditis, dysrhythmia, heart block, or congestive heart failure may be present and increase perioperative risk.

Evaluation

Preoperative evaluation should be directed at determining the etiology of the pericardial disease and excluding the presence of tamponade, constrictive disease, or associated risk factors. The differential diagnosis of pericardial disease includes: idiopathic, viral, bacterial, mycobacterial, drug-related (e.g., hydralazine, procainamide), renal failure, post-myocardial infarction, post-pericardiotomy, trauma, dissecting aneurysm, malignancy, rheumatic fever, collagen vascular disease, radiation, sarcoidosis, hypothyroidism, and protein malnutrition. The possibility of tamponade or constrictive disease should be evaluated by checking the blood pressure and pulse contour, measuring pulsus parodoxus, observing the jugular veins for Kussmaul's sign and a prominent X and/or Y descent, auscultating the heart for diminished heart sounds or a pericardial knock, checking for edema, hepatomegaly, and ascites, assessing the adequacy of tissue perfusion, echocardiography, and if suspicion remains, by right heart catheterization. Tamponade without significant paradoxus can be seen in the presence of left ventricular failure (263). Pericardial effusion should be routinely searched for by echocardiogram. It may be suggested by an increase in the cardiac silhouette on current compared to previous x-rays. A complete cardiovascular history and physical exam and electrocardiogram are also essential parts of the preoperative assessment as described on pages 115–117 (Table 10.16).

Management

Elective surgery should generally be delayed until therapy for the pericardial disease is undertaken and the process resolves. Pericarditis by itself is not an absolute contraindication to urgent lifesaving surgery. Cardiology consultation should be obtained, the patient's hemodynamic status carefully assessed, and the need for surgery carefully considered.

In the event of actual or impending tamponade, preoperative pericardiocentesis or operative drainage should be performed. A falling cardiac output secondary to tamponade can be bolstered temporarily with saline infusions, inotropic agents (isoproterenol or dopamine),

and/or afterload reduction (nitroprusside or hydralazine) while definitive treatment is being arranged. When pericardial effusion is present, we recommend preoperative right heart catheterization to rule out subclinical tamponade. Anticoagulation is contraindicated because of the danger of hemopericardium. Intraoperative management of patients with preoperative pericarditis should include arterial pressure and electrocardiographic monitoring and monitoring of cardiac output, and right heart and pulmonary artery diastolic and wedge pressures with a triple-lumen Swan-Ganz catheter.

OPERATIONS IN PATIENTS WITH PRIOR CARDIAC SURGERY

Epidemiology

An increasing number of patients are undergoing cardiac surgery for coronary artery bypass grafts or valve replacement. Mean survival now exceeds 5 years for most cardiac valve and bypass surgery. Subsequent noncardiac surgery is likely, therefore, to be performed in significant numbers of cardiac surgery survivors.

The major concern for *patients with coronary artery bypass grafts* during noncardiac surgery is postoperative infarction and cardiac death. In seven reported series (16, 264–267), comprising 1,463 patients and 1,570 procedures, there was a 1% total and 0.3% cardiac mortality (Table 10.47). The total mortality after bypass grafting is close to the 0.8% mortality for the population as a whole. Most of the deaths were related to the primary noncardiac disease or to surgical problems. The most common cardiac complications were transient arrhythmias. There were only twelve postoperative myocardial infarctions, with no reported postinfarction cardiac deaths (264–265). These results are impressive, especially since many of the patients were in NYHA Class III or IV prior to bypass grafting (264).

Table 10.47. Surgery after Coronary Artery Bypass Grafts[a]

Study	Number	Time since Bypass Grafting	Mortality Total	Mortality Cardiac	Cardiac Complications
Crawford, 1978	358	10 days–89 months	1%	0%	6 postop MI
					14 arrhythmias
Mahar, 1978	99	2 days–84 months		0%	No arrhythmias "requiring
					treatment"
McCollum, 1977	60	12 days–24 months	0%	0%	0 MI
					1 pulmonary edema
					7 SVT
Scher, 1976	20	3 weeks–68 months	5%	0%	1 postop MI
					3 arrhythmias
Edwards, 1978	53	1 day–48 months	4%	4%	4 arrhythmias
Foster, 1986	743	?	0.9%	.5%	5 postop MI
					25 arrhythmias
					10 CHF[2]
Hertzer, 1984	130	?	0.8%	?	
Total					
Patients	1,463		1%	0.3%	
Procedures	1,700		0.8%	0.2%	

[a]Data from refs. 4, 16, 53, 264–265, 266–267.

It remains unclear whether noncardiac surgery is more risky when performed *early compared to late* after bypass grafting. Most of the reported perioperative deaths (6 of 9) have occurred in patients operated on within 30 days of bypass surgery (Table 10.48). However, the increased risk may be more related to the nature of the surgery rather than its timing. Four of the six reported deaths in this early period occurred after emergency surgery (16, 264, 268), and most were due to infectious or surgically related causes. None of the deaths were cardiac, although "significant numbers" of cardiac complications were reported in one series (264) of patients operated on within 30 days of bypass surgery. Elective surgery performed 6–12 weeks after bypass had a low risk (1% mortality) in one small series (264) (Table 10.48) similar to that of surgery performed later.

Table 10.48. Surgery within 3 Months of Coronary Artery Bypass Grafting[a]

Study	Type of Surgery	Number	Time since Bypass Grafting	Total Mortality	Cardiac Deaths	Complications
Crawford, 1978	Elective	70	6–12 weeks	1%	0%	"No cardiac complications"
	Not Stated	18	<30 days	11%[b]	0%	"Many cardiac complications: arrhythmias, MI"
Lucas, 1980	Urgent	8	3–16 days	25%	0%?	1 atrial arrhythmias
Edwards, 1978	Elective	4	Same hospitalization	0%	0%	
	Urgent	1	1 day	100%	?	Ventricular arrhythmias, progressive renal failure, sepsis

[a]Data from refs. 16, 264, 268.
[b]One of three deaths occurred during emergency operations.

Noncardiac surgery may also be required after cardiac valve replacement. No reported series have measured the risks of congestive heart failure, arrhythmias, bacterial endocarditis, myocardial infarction, or angina in patients with prosthetic valves who undergo noncardiac surgery. The incidence of endocarditis is presumably small, since patients are routinely given prophylactic antibiotics. The frequency of the cardiac complications probably relates to the functional status of the prosthetic valve as well as the presence of associated cardiac disease.

Most patients with prosthetic, non-tissue valves require long-term anticoagulation. During later noncardiac surgery, there is a risk of bleeding if anticoagulation is continued and thromboembolism from the artificial valve if anticoagulation is discontinued.

Three reported series describe the management of anticoagulation in 279 patients with prosthetic valves undergoing noncardiac surgery (Table 10.49) (269–271). Although management varied among and within the three series, most patients had their coumadin discontinued from 1–3 days preoperatively to 1–5 days postoperatively.

In 155 patients with aortic valve prostheses, there were no instances of embolization when anticoagulation was discontinued for a total of 1–7 days perioperatively. All investigators concurred that anticoagulation can be stopped for a total of about 5–7 days in patients with aortic valve prostheses.

The magnitude of the risk of temporary cessation of anticoagulation in patients with mitral valve prostheses is less certain, and their anticoagulant management more controversial. Two fatal emboli occurred among 95 patients with mitral valve prostheses in whim anticoagulation was discontinued periopera-

Table 10.49.   Management of Anticoagulation during Noncardiac Surgery in Patients with Prosthetic Valves[a]

Study	Total Procedures (Patients)	Valve Type	Method	Complications
Katholi, 1976	44 (36)	31 aortic	25 Discontinued; resumed post-op days 3–5	None
			6 continued anticoagulation	3 "massive hemorrhages"
		13 mitral or combined	10 discontinued 3–5 days	2 fatal emboli
			3 continued anticoagulation	1 hemorrhage
Katholi, 1978	45 (39)	19 aortic	19 discontinued; resumed post-op day 2	1 hematoma[b]
		26 mitral or combined	26 discontinued; heparin 12 hr post-op; coumadin day 3	1 hematoma
				1 hemorrhage
Tinker, 1978	180 (159)	105 aortic	Variable (average discontinued 1–3 days preop; restart 1–7 days post-op)	7 hemorrhages
		75 mitral, tricuspid, or combined		11 hematomas
Total	279	155 aortic		12 hemorrhages
		114 mitral or combined		2 emboli
				13 hematomas

[a] Data from refs. 269, 271.
[b] Patient received heparin also.

tively (from 3–7 days in most cases) (269–271). Both emboli occurred in one series of 10 patients (269) in whom anticoagulants were discontinued 3–5 days preoperatively. The total duration of anticoagulant cessation and the time of embolization were not reported; the time of death (10 days postoperatively) was reported for one patient. Because of this experience, Katholis (269–270) continued warfarin to within 24 hours of surgery (when its effect was reversed with parenteral vitamin K) and started heparin 12 hours postoperatively in 29 subsequent patients with mitral valve prostheses. None experienced embolic events.

On the 279 patients reported in these three series, about 9% had bleeding complications; 4% hemorrhaged, and 5% had hematomas.

Evaluation

The preoperative evaluation should be conducted as described on pages 115–117, (Table 10.16). Historical or physical examination findings that suggest prosthetic valve malfunction should be sought. The presence of associated cardiac risk factors, (e.g., congestive heart failure, dysrhythmias) should be clearly noted. A baseline prothrombin time, a platelet count, and partial thromboplastin time should be obtained. Echocardiography and/or cardiac catheterization are useful when there is a clinical suspicion of prosthetic valve malfunction.

Management

Noncardiac surgery is generally well tolerated by the patient who has undergone prior cardiac surgery, provided there is no major residual cardiac dysfunction. The management of concomitant cardiovascular diseases is discussed in the relevant sections of this chapter. Factors that impair cardiac performance (p. 91, Table 10.17) should be corrected whenever possible.

Elective noncardiac surgery is usually postponed until 3 months or more after coronary bypass grafting or valve replacement; the data supporting this approach is less firm for valve replacement than for bypass grafting. Emergency or semi-urgent surgery can be undertaken before 6–12 weeks, when the risk of waiting is felt to be greater than the attendant high risk of perioperative morbidity and mortality.

In the absence of definitive data, our management of anticoagulants is based upon the estimated risks of perioperative embolization. A low risk of embolization is considered to be present in patients with aortic valve prostheses. Patients with porcine heterograft valves of any type or atrial fibrillation in the absence of mitral valve disease are considered to be low risk (and often are managed without chronic anticoagulation). An intermediate risk is considered to be present in patients with left ventricular thrombi or atrial fibrillation due to mitral valve disease. A high risk of perioperative embolization is considered to be present in patients with prosthetic, nontissue mitral valves or a history of previous embolic episodes of cardiac origin. Separate protocols are used for anticoagulant management in patients at low versus high risk of perioperative recurrent embolization (Table 10.50). The high-risk protocol is used only when the patient can be closely monitored to ensure that the parameters of anticoagulation remain within the recommended therapeutic range and to detect early signs of hemorrhagic complications.

Prophylaxis for bacterial endocarditis should be administered to patients with prosthetic cardiac valves, including porcine heterografts (see p. 387). The more intensive prophylactic antibiotic regimens should be used in patients with artificial valves because of the high mortality if endocarditis occurs. An aminoglycoside, in addition to penicillin, is therefore administered for routine dental and upper respiratory tract surgery. Antibiotic prophylaxis should not be given in-

Table 10.50. **Management of Anticoagulation during Surgery**

Low or intermediate risk of embolization (see text)

1. Discontinue Coumadin 36–48 hours preoperatively. Daily protime.
2. Aquamephyton (vitamin K_1, phytonadione) 5–10 mg IV, SC, or PO when Coumadin stopped. Repeat 24 hours later if necessary.
3. Prothrombin time should be checked within 12 hours of surgery and should be normal.
4. Coumadin restarted 2–5 days postoperatively (no bleeding or oozing for 24–48 hours and surgeon confident of hematostasis).
5. NPO: For patients unable to take oral medication for longer than 5 days postoperatively (a total of 5–7 days without anticoagulation), intravenous heparin will usually be required, depending on the risk of embolization. Institution of heparin may be delayed to post-op day 3–5.

High risk of embolization (see text)

1. Discontinue Coumadin 18–36 hours preoperatively. Monitor protime every 12–24 hours.
2. Aquamephyton (vitamin K_1, phytonadione) 10–15 mg IV or SC when Coumadin stopped. A second dose will usually be required 12–24 hours later (5–10 mg).
3. Prothrombin time should be checked and normal within 12 hours of surgery.

   Note: If coumadin is stopped more than 36 hours preoperatively, and prothrombin time will be subtherapeutic ($<1.5 \times$ control) for more than 12 hours, administer full-dose heparin. Heparin should be stopped 6–12 hours preoperatively. Both prothombin time and partial thromboplastin time should be checked and normal preoperatively.
4. Heparin administered by continuous intravenous drip is begun 24–72 hours postoperatively (no bleeding or oozing for 12–24 hours and surgeon confident of hemostasis).
5. Coumadin restarted electively when patient stable.

tramuscularly in patients on anticoagulant therapy.

Preoperative digitalization is not routinely required in patients with prior coronary artery bypass or valve surgery. Indications for digitalization are similar in patients with and without prior cardiac surgery (see p. 152).

(see p. 152)

READINGS

1. Goldman L, Caldera DL, Mussbaum SR, et al.: Multifactorial index of cardiac risk in non-cardiac surgical procedures. *N Engl J Med* 297:845–850, 1977.
2. Goldman L, Caldera DL, Southwick FS, et al.: Cardiac risk factors and complications in noncardiac surgery. *Medicine* 57:357–370, 1978.
3. Cooperman M, Pflug B, Martin EW, et al.: Cardiovascular risk factors in patients with peripheral vascular disease. *Surgery* 84:505–509, 1978.
4. Foster ED, Davis KB, Carpenter JA, et al.: Risk of noncardiac operation in patients with defined coronary disease: The coronary artery surgery study (CASS) registry experience. *Ann Thorac Surg* 41:42–50, 1986.
5. Larsen SF, Jacobsen OE, Nielsen H, et al.: Prediction of cardiac risk in non-cardiac surgery. *Europ Heart J* 8:179–185, 1987.
6. Detsky AS, Abrams HB, McLaughlin Jr, et al.: Predicting cardiac complications in patients undergoing non-cardiac surgery. *J Gen Intern Med* 1:211–219, 1986.
7. Mauney FM, Ebert PA, Sabiston DC: Postoperative myocardial infarction: A study of predisposing factors, diagnosis and mortality in a high risk group of surgical patients. *Ann Surg* 172:497–503, 1970.
8. Skinner JF, Pearce ML: Surgical risk in the cardiac patient. *J Chronic Dis* 17:57–72, 1964.
9. Nachlas MM, Abrams SJ, Goldberg MM: The influence of arteriosclerotic heart disease on surgical risk. *Am J Surg* 101:447–455, 1961.
10. Steen PA, Tinker JH, Tarhan S: Myocardial reinfarction after anesthesia and surgery. *JAMA* 239:2566–2570, 1978.
11. Tarhan S, Moffitt EA, Taylor WF, et al.: Myocardial infarction after general anesthesia. *JAMA* 220:1451–1454, 1972.
12. Arkins R, Smessaert AA, Hicks RG: Mortality and morbidity in surgical patients with coronary artery disease. *JAMA* 190:485–488, 1964.
13. Driscoll AC, Hobika JH, Etsten B, et al.: Clinically unrecognized myocardial infarction following surgery. *N Engl J Med* 264:633–639, 1961.
14. Hunter PR, Endrey-Walder P, Bauer GE, et al.: Myocardial infarction following surgical operations. *Br Med J* 4:725–728, 1968.
15. Knapp RB, Topkins MJ Artusio JF: The cerebrovascular accident and coronary occlusion in anesthesia. *JAMA* 182:332–334, 1962.
16. Edwards WH, Mulherin JL, Jr, Walker WE: Vascular reconstructive surgery following myocardial revascularization. *Ann Surg* 187:653–57, 1978.
17. Plumlee JE, Boettner RB: Myocardinal infarction during and following anesthesia and operation. *South Med J* 65:886–889, 1972.
18. Rosen M, Mushin WW, Kilpatrick GS, et al.: Study of myocardial ischaemia in surgical patients. *Br Med J* 2:1414–1420, 1966.
19. Sapala JA, Ponka JL, Duvernoy WFC: Operative and non-operative risks in the cardiac patient. *J Am Geriatr Soc* 223:527–534, 1975.
20. Topkins MJ, Artusio JF: Myocardial infarction and surgery: A five-year study. *Anesth Analg* 43:716–720, 1964.
21. Chamberlain DA, Edmons-Seal J: Effects of surgery under general anesthesia on the electro-

cardiogram in ischaemic heart disease and hypertension. *Br Med J* 2:784–787, 1964.

22. McPhail, N, Menkis A, Shariatmadar A, et al.: Statistical prediction of cardiac risk in patients who undergo vascular surgery. *Can J Surg* 28:404–406, 1985.

23. Detsky AS, Abrams HB, Forbath N, et al.: Cardiac assessment for patients undergoing noncardiac surgery. *Arch Intern Med* 146:2131–2134m, 1986.

24. Nichols KH, Daniels KE: Validation of a cardiac risk factor index for noncardiac surgery in a community osteopathic hospital. *J Am Osteop Assoc* 87:235–239, 1987.

25. Jeffrey CC, Lunsman J, Cullen DJ, et al.: A prospective evaluation of cardiac risk index. *Anesthesiology* 58:462–464, 1983.

26. Zeldin, RA: Assessing cardiac risk in patients who undergo noncardiac surgical procedures. *Can J Surg* 27:402–404, 1984.

27. Waters J, Wilkinson C, Golmon M, et al.: Evaluation of cardiac risk in noncardiac surgical patients. *Anesthesiology* 55:(A)343, 1981.

28. Gerson MC, Jurst JM, Hertzberg VS, et al.: Cardiac prognosis in noncardiac geriatric surgery. *Ann Intern Med* 103:832–837, 1985.

29. Leppo J, Plaja J, Gionet M, et al.: Noninvasive evaluation of cardiac risk before elective vascular surgery. *J Am Coll Cardiol* 9:269–276, 1987.

30. Eagle KA, Singer DE, Brewster DC, et al.: Dipyridamole-thallium scanning in patients undergoing vascular surgery. *JAMA* 257:2185–2189, 1987.

31. Cutler BS, Wheeler HB, Paraskos JA, et al.: Assessment of operative risk with electrocardiographic exercise testing in patients with peripheral vascular disease. *Am J Surg* 137:484–490, 1979.

32. Carliner NH, Fisher ML, Plotnick GD, et al.: Routine preoperative exercise testing in patients undergoing major noncardiac surgery. *Am Cardiol* 56:51–58, 1985.

33. Boucher CA, Brewster DC, Darling RC, et al.: Determination of cardiac risk by dipyridamole-thallium imaging before peripheral vascular surgery. *New Engl J Med* 312:389–394, 1985.

34. McPhail NV, Ruddy TD, Calvin JE, et al.: A comparison of dipyridamole-thallium imaging and exercise testing in the prediction of postoperative cardiac complications in patients requiring arterial reconstruction. *J Vasc Surg* 10:51–56, 1989.

35. Eagle KA, Coley CM, Newell JB, et al.: Combining clinical and thallium data optimizes preoperative assessment of cardiac risk before major vascular surgery. *Ann Intern Med* 110:859–866, 1989.

36. Chin WL, et al.: Failure of dipyridamole-thallium myocardial imagining to detect severe coronary disease. *Cleve Clin J Med* 56:587–589, 1989.

37. Lette J, et al.: Usefulness of the severity and extent of reversible perfusion defects during thallium-dipyridamole imaging for cardiac risk assessment before non-cardiac surgery. *Am J Cardiol* 64:276–281, 1989.

38. Eagle KA, Boucher CA: Cardiac risk of noncardiac surgery (edit). *N Engl J Med* 321:1330–1332, 1989.

39. Homma S, Gilliland Y, Guiney TE, et al.: Safety of intravenous dipyridamole for stress testing with thallium imaging. *Am J Cardiol* 59:152–154, 1987.

40. Cutler BS, Leppo JA: Dipyridamole thallium 201 scintigraphy to detect coronary artery disease before abdominal aortic surgery. *J Vasc Surg* 5:91–100, 1987.

41. Taillefer R, et al.: Thallium-201 myocardial imaging during pharmacologic coronary vasodilation: Comparison of oral and intravenous administration of dipyridamole. *J Am Coll Cardiol* 8:76–83, 1986.

42. Pasternack PF, et al.: The value of radionuclide angiography as a predictor of perioperative myocardial infarction in patients undergoing abdominal aortic aneurysm resection. *J Vasc Surg* 1:320–325, 1984.

43. Kazmers A, Cerqueira MD, Zierler RE: Perioperative and late outcome in patients with left ventricular ejection fraction of 35% or less who require major vascular surgery. *J Vasc Surg* 8:307–315, 1988.

44. Pasternack PF, Imparato AM: Preoperative determination of cardiac risk. *New Engl J Med* 312:1641, 1985.

45. Kazmers A, Cerqueira MD, Zierler RE: The role of preoperative radionuclide left ventricular ejection fraction for risk assessment in carotid surgery. *Arch Surg* 123:416–419, 1988.

46. Goldman L: Assessment of the patient with known or suspected ischaemic heart disease for non-cardiac surgery. *Br J Anaesth* 61:38–43, 1988.

47. Gage AA, et al.: Assessment of cardiac risk in surgical patients. *Arch Surg* 112:1488–1492, 1977.

48. Arous EJ, Bauum PL, Butler BS: The ischaemic exercise test in patients with peripheral vascular disease. *Arch Surg* 119:780–783, 1984.

49. McPhail NN, et al.: The use of preoperative exercise testing to predict cardiac complications after arterial reconstruction. *J Vasc Surg* 7:60–68, 1988.

50. Calvin JE, Kiesser TM, Walley VM, et al.: Cardiac mortality and morbidity after vascular surgery. *Can J Surg* 29:93–97, 1986.

51. Ouyang P, et al.: Frequency and significance of early postoperative silent myocardial ischemia in patients having peripheral vascular surgery. *Am J Cardiol* 64:1113–1116, 1989.

52. Raby KE, et al.: Correlation between preoperative ischemia and major cardiac events after peripheral vascular surgery *N Engl J Med* 321:1296–1300, 1989.

53. Hertzer NR, Beven EG, Young JR, et al.: Coronary artery disease in peripheral vascular patients. *Ann Surg* 199:223–232, 1984.

54. Hertzer NR, Young JR, Beven EG, et al.: Coronary angiography in 506 patients with extracranial cerebrovascular disease. *Arch Intern Med* 145:849–852, 1985.

55. Reul GJ, Cooley DA, Duncan JM, et al.: The effect of coronary bypass on the outcome of

peripheral vascular operations in 1093 patients. *J Vasc Surg* 3:788–798, 1986.

56. Toal KW, Jacocks MA, Elkins RC: Preoperative coronary artery bypass grafting in patients undergoing abdominal aortic reconstruction. *Am J Surg* 148:825–829, 1984.

57. Yeager RA, Weigel RM, Murphy ES, et al.: "Application of clinically valid cardiac risk factors to aortic aneurysm surgery. *Arch Surg* 121:276–281, 1986.

58. Goldman L: Cardiac risks and complications of noncardiac surgery. *Ann Intern Med* 98:504–513, 1983.

59. Brown OW, Hollier LH, Pairolero, et al.: Abdominal aortic aneurysm and coronary artery disease. *Arch Surg* 116:1484–1488, 1988.

60. Rao TLK, Jacobs KH, El-Etr, AA: Reinfarction following anesthesia in patients with myocardial infarction. *Anesthesiology* 59:499–505, 1983.

61. Wells PH, Kaplan JA: Optimal management of patients with ischemic heart disease for noncardiac surgery by complementary anesthesiologist and cardiologist interaction. *Am Ht J* 102:1029–1037, 1981.

62. Rao TLK, El-Etr, AA: Myocardial reinfarction following anesthesia in patients with recent infarction. *Anesth and Anal* 60:2710272, 1981.

63. Blle-Brahe NE, Eickhoff JH: Measurement of central haemodynamic parameters during preoperative exercise testing in patients suspected of arteriosclerotic heart disease. *Acta Chir Scand* 502:38–45, 1980.

63a. Hertzer NR, Young JR, Kramer JR, et al.: Routine coronary angiography prior to elective aortic reconstruction. *Arch Surg* 114:1336–1344, 1979.

64. Morris AL: Guidelines for randomized trials to determine incidence of perioperative myocardial infarction. *Anesthesiology* 61:213, 1984.

65. Goldman L, Caldera DL: Risks of general anesthesia and elective operation in the hypertensive patient. *Anesthesiology* 50:285–292, 1979.

66. Benson H, et al.: The effect of preoperative systemic blood pressure on closed miral valvuloplasty. A study of 1,630 patients with up to 15 year follow-up. *Am Heart J* 75:439–448, 1968.

67. Prys-Roberts C, et al.: Studies of anaesthesia in relation to hypertension: I. Cardiovascular responses of treated and untreated patients. *Br J Anaesth* 43:122–137, 1971.

68. Prys-Roberts C, et al.: Studies of anaesthesia in relation to hypertension: IV. The effects of artificial ventilation on the circulation and pulmonary gas exchanges. *Br J Anaesth* 44:335–348, 1972.

69. Prys-Roberts C: Hypertension and anesthesia—fifty years on. *Anesthesiology* 50:281–282, 1979.

70. Coakley CS, et al.: Circulatory responses during anaesthesia of patients on Rauwolfia therapy. *JAMA* 161:1143–1144, 1956.

71. Smaessaert AA, Hicks RG: Problems caused by Rauwolfia drugs during anesthesia and surgery. *NY St J Med* 61:2399–2403, 1961.

72. Viljocn JF, Kellner GA: Propranolol and cardiac surgery. *J Thorac Cardiovasc Surg* 64:286–830, 1972.

73. Katz RL, et al.: Anesthesia, surgery, and Rauwolfia. 25:142–147, 1964.

74. Munson WM, Jenicek JG: Effects of anesthetic agents on patients receiving reserpine therapy. *Anesthesiology* 23:741–746, 1962.

75. Ominsky AJ, Wollman H: Hazards of general anaesthesia in the reserpinized patient. *Anesthesiology* 30:443–446, 1969.

76. Katz RL: Hazardous effects of drugs in hypertensive patients scheduled for elective surgery. *Cardiovasc Med* 3:1185–1205, 1978.

77. Estaganous, FG: Hypertension in the surgical patient. *Cleve Lin J Med* 56:385–393, 1989.

78. Coltart DJ, et al.: Investigations of the safe withdrawal period for propranolol in patients scheduled for open heart surgery. *Br Heart, J* 37:1228–1234, 1975.

79. Faulkner SL: Time required for complete recovery from chronic propranolol therapy. *N Engl J Med* 289:607–609, 1973.

80. Doudoulas H: Hypersenstivity to adrenergic stimulation after propranolol withdrawal in normal patients. *Ann Int Med* 87:433–436, 1977.

81. Kaplan JA: Propranolol and cardiac surgery: A problem for the anesthesiologist? *Anesth Analg Curr Res* 54:571–577, 1975.

82. Slogoff S: Preoperative propranolol therapy and aortocoronary bypass operation. *JAMA* 240:1487–1490, 1978.

83. Carlops JM: Results of coronary artery surgery in patients receiving propranolol. *J Thorac Cardiovasc Surg* 67:526–529, 1974.

84. Moran JM, et al.: Coronary revascularization in patients receiving propranolol. *CIRC* 49 and 50 (suppl II):II-116–121, 1974.

85. Goldman L: Non-cardiac surgery in patients receiving propranolol. *Arch Int Med* 141:193–196, 1981.

86. Kaplan JA, Dunbab RW: Propranolol and surgical anaesthesia. *Anesth Analg* 55:1–5, 1976.

87. Kopriva CJ, Brown ACD, Pappas G: Hemodynamics during general anaesthesia in patients receiving propranolol. *Anesthesiology* 48:28–33, 1978.

88. Pasternack PF, Imparato AM, Baumann FG, et al.: The hemodynamics of B-blockade in patients undergoing abdominal aortic aneurysm repair. *Circ* 76(Suppl III):III-1III-7, 1987.

89. Prys-Roberts C, et al.: Studies of anaesthesia in relation to hypertension: V. Adrenergic beat-receptor blockade. *Br J Anaesth* 45:671–680, 1973.

90. Prys-Roberts C, Meloche R: Management of anaesthesia in patients with hypertension or ischemic heart disease. *Int Anesth Clin* 18:181–217, 1980.

91. Kaukinen S, et al.: Preoperative and postoperative use of clonidine with neuroleptic anaesthesia. *Acta Anaesth Scand* 23:113–120, 1975.

92. Bruce DL, et al.: Preoperative clonidine withdrawal syndrome. *Anesthesiology* 51:90–92, 1979.

93. Smith NT, et al. (eds.): *Drug Interactions in Anesthesia*. Philadelphia, Lea & Febiger, 1981.

94. Foex R, Prys-Roberts C: Anaesthesia and the hypertensive patient. *Br J Anaesth* 46:575–588, 1974.

95. Dingle HR: Antihypertensive drugs and anaesthesia. *Anaesthesia* 21:151–172, 1966.

96. Kaplan JA, King SB: The precordial electrocardiographic lead (V_5) in patients who have coronary-artery disease. *Anaesthesiology* 45:570–574, 1976.

97. Dalton B: A precordial EKG lead for chest operations. *Anesth Analg* 55:740–741, 1976.

98. Gat JT, Cooperman LH: Hypertension in the immediate postoperative period. *Br J Anaesth* 47:70–74, 1975.

99. Farman JV: The work of a recovery room. *Br J Hosp Med* 19:606–616, 1978.

100. Wycoff CC: Endotracheal intubation: Effects on blood pressure and pulse rate. *Anesthesiology* 21:153–158, 1960.

101. Prys-Roberts C, et al.: Studies of anaesthesia in relation to hypertension: II. Haemodynamic consequences of induction and endotracheal intubation. *Br J Anaesth* 43:531–546, 1971.

102. Takeshimi K, et al.: Cardiovascular response to rapid anaesthesia induction and endotracheal intubation. *Anesth Analg* 43:201–208, 1964.

103. Breslow MJ, Jordan DA, Christopherson R, et al.: Epidural morphine decreases postoperative hypertension by attenuating sympathetic nervous system hyperactivity. *JAMA* 261:3577–3581, 1989.

104. Skydell JL, Machleder HI, Baker JD, et al.: Incidence and mechanism of post-carotid endarterectomy hypertension. *Arch Surg* 122:1153–1155, 1987.

105. Orlowski JP, Vidt DG, Walker S, et al.: The hemodynamic effects of intravenous labetalol for postoperative hypertension. *Cleve Clin J Med* 56:29–34, 1989.

106. Leslie JB, Kalayjian RW, Sirgo MA, et al.: Intravenous labetalol for treatment of postoperative hypertension. *Anesthesiology* 67:413–416, 1987.

107. Adler AG, Leahy JJ, Cressman MD: Management of perioperative hypertension using sublingual nifedipine. *Arch Intern Med* 146:1927–1930, 1986.

108. Wells PH, Hug CC, Kaplan JA: Maintenance of propanolol therapy IV infusion. *Anesthesiology* 53:S128, 1980.

109. Hug CC, McDonald DH, Kaplan JA: Propranolol infusion after abdominal surgery. *JAMA* 249:22, 1983.

110. Smulyan H, Weinberg SE, Howanitz PJ: Continuous propranolol infusion following abdominal surgery. *JAMA* 247:2539–2542, 1982.

111. Salem DN, Chuttani K, Isner JM: Assessment and management of cardiac disease in the surgical patient. *Curr Prob in Cardiol* 14:167–224, 1989.

112. Magram, M., unpublished.

113. Dripps RD, et al. (eds): *Introduction to Anaesthesia, The Principles of Safe Practice.* Philadelphia, WB Saunders, 1977, pp 409–426; 460–461.

114. Churchill-Davidson HC (ed): *A Practice of Anaesthesia.* Philadelphia, WB Saunders, 1978, pp 594–6077.

115. Hardy JD (ed): *Rhoads Textbooks of Surgery* Philadelphia, JB Lippincott, 1977, pp 67–69.

116. Von Knorring J: Postoperative myocardial infarction: A prospective study in a risk group of surgical patients. *Surgery* 90:55–60, 1981.

117. Rose SD, Corman LC, Mason DT: Cardiac risk factors in patients undergoing noncardiac surgery. *Med Clin North Am* 63:1271–1288, 1979.

118. Lowenstein E, Yusuf S, Teplick RS: Perioperative myocardial reinfarction. *Anesthesiology* 59:493–494, 1983.

119. Slogoff S, Keats AS: Does perioperative myocardial ischemia lead to postoperative myocardial infarction. *Anesthiology* 62:107–114, 1985.

120. Prys-Roberts C, Meloche R, Foex P: Studies of anaesthesia in relation to hypertension: I. Cardiovascular responses of treated and untreated patients. *Br J Anaesth* 43:122–137, 1971.

121. Foster ED, Olsson CA, Rutenburg AM et al.: Mechanical circulatory assistance with intra-aortic balloon counterpulsation for major abdominal surgery. *Ann Surg* 183:73–76, 1976.

122. Feruglio G, Bellet S, Stone H: Postoperative myocardiac infarction. *Arch Int Med* 102:345–353, 1958.

123. Wasserman F, Bellet S, Saicheck RP: Postoperative myocardial infarction report of twenty-five cases. *N Engl J Med* 252:967–974, 1955.

124. Becker RC, Underwood DA: Myocardiac infarction in patients undergoing noncardiac surgery. *Cleve Clin J Med* 54:25–28, 1987.

125. Cattolica EV: Effect of transurethral surgery upon the serum enzyme creatinine phosphokipase *J Urol* 106:262–266, 1971.

126. Dixon SH, Fuchs JCA, Ebert PA: Changes in serum creatinine phosphokinase activity. *Arch Surg* 103:66–68, 1971.

127. Ayres PR, Willard TB: Serum glutamic oxalacetic transaminase levels in 266 surgical patients. *Ann Intern Med* 52:1279–1288, 1960.

128. Righetti A, O'Rourke RA, Schelbert H: et al.: Usefulness of preoperative and postoperative Tc-99m (Sn)-pyrophosphate scans in patients with ischemic and valvular heart disease. *Am J Cardiol* 39:43–49, 1977.

129. Boncheck LI, Olinger GN: Intra-aortic balloon counterpulsation for cardiac support during noncardiac operations. *J Thorac Cardiovasc Surg* 78:147–149, 1979.

130. Coriat P, Daloz M, Bousseau D, et al.: Prevention of intraoperative myocardial ischemia during noncardiac surgery with intravenous nitroglycerin. *Anesthesiology* 61:193–196, 1984.

131. Cohen JL, Wender R, Maginot A, et al.: Hemodynamic monitoring of patients undergoing abdominal aortic surgery. *Am J Surg* 146:174–177, 1983.

132. Frishman WH, Murthy VS, Strom JA: Ultrashort-acting B-adrenergic blockers. *Med Clin North Am* 72:359–372, 1988.

133. Gray RJ, Bateman TM, Czer LSC, et al.: Comparison of esmolol and nitroprusside for acute post-cardiac surgical hypertension. *Am J Cardiol* 59:887–891, 1987.

134. Kelley JL, Campbell DA, Brandt RL: The recognition of myocardiac infarction in the early postoperative period. *Arch Surg* 94:673–683, 1967.

135. Miller MG, Hall SV: Intra-aortic balloon counterpulsation in a high-risk cardiac patient undergoing emergency gastrectomy. *Anesthesiology* 42:103–105, 1975.

136. Moffih EA: Anesthesia for patients early after infarction. *Anesth Analg* 55:640–642, 1976.

137. Dripps RD, Cannard TH, Strong MJ: Anesthesia in the patient with cardiovascular disease, in Conn HL, Horowitz O (eds): *Cardiac and Vascular Diseases* 1971, pp 1433–1449.

138. Kaplan JA, Dunbar RW: Anesthesia for noncardiac surgery in patients with cardiac disease, in *Cardiovascular Anesthesia*. pp 377–389.

139. Etsten B, Proger S: Operative risk in patients with coronary heart disease. *JAMA* 159:845–848, 1955.

140. Siegel AJ, Dawson DM: Peripheral source of MB band of creatinine kinase in alcoholic rhabdomyolysis non-specificity of MB isoenzyme for myocardinal injury in undiluted serum samples. *JAMA* 224:580–582, 1980.

141. Kirkpatrick JR, Heibrunn A, Sankaran S: Cardiac arrhythmias: An early sign of sepsis. *Am Surg* 39:380–382, 1973.

142. Weathers LW, Paine R: The risk of surgery in cardiac patients. *Intern Med* 2:57–66, 1981.

143. Fraser JG, Ramachandran PR, Davis HS: Anesthesia and recent myocardinal infarction. *JAMA* 199:96–98, 1967.

144. Baker HW, Grismer JT, Wise RA: Risk of urgent surgery in presence of myocardial infarction and angina pectoris. *Arch Surg* 65:448–456, 1952.

146. Hannigan CA, Wroblewski F., Lewis WH, et al.: Major surgery in patients with healed myocardial infarction. *Am J Med Surg* 222:628–639, 1957.

147. Lochhead RP, Coakley CS, Evans JM: The risk of major surgery in patients with coronary artery disease. *Am J Med Sci* 227:624–627, 1954.

148. Morrison DR: The risk of surgery in heart disease. *Surgery* 23:561–570, 1948.

149. Ohler RL, Dana JB: Influence of heart disease on surgical risk. *JAMA* 162:278–880, 1956.

150. Parsons WH, Whitaker HT, Hinton JK: Major surgery in patients 70 years of age and over: An analysis of 146 operations on 135 patients. *Ann Surg* 143:845–854, 1956.

151. Lawhorne TW, Davis JL, Smith GW: General surgical complications after cardiac surgery. *Am J Surg* 136:254–256, 1978.

152. Cooperman LH, Price HL: Pulmonary edema in the operative and postoperative period: A review of 40 cases. *Ann Surg* 172:883–891, 1970.

153. Morrison DR: The risk of surgery in heart disease. *Surgery* 23:561–570, 1948.

154. Cooperman M, et al.: Cardiovascular risk factors in patients with peripheral vascular disease. *Surgery* 84:505–509, 1978.

155. Finkbeiner JA, Wroblewski F, LaDue JS: The effect of chronic auricular fibrillation on the operative risk. *Am J Med Sci* 227:535–543, 1954.

156. Vanik PE, Davis HS: Cardiac arrhythmias during halothane anesthesia. *Anesth Analg* 47:299–307, 1968.

157. Goldman L: Supraventricular tachyarrhythmias in hospitalized adults after surgery: Clinical correlates in patients over 40 years of age after major non-cardiac surgery. *Chest* 73:450–454, 1978.

158. Katz RL, Bigger JT: Cardiac arrhythmias during anesthesia and operation. *Anesthesiology* 33:193–213, 1970.

159. Bertrand CA, Steiner VN, Jameson G, Lopez M: Disturbances of cardiac rhythm during anesthesia and surgery. *JAMA* 216:1615–1617, 1971.

160. Kuner J, Enescu V, Utsu F, Boszormenyi E, Berstein H, Corday E: Cardiac arrhythmias during anaesthesia. *Dis Chest* 52:580–587, 1967.

161. Krosnick A, Wasseiman F: Cardiac arrhythmias in the older age group following thoracic surgery. *Am J Med Sci* 230:541–550, 1955.

162. Dodd RB, Sims WA, Bone DJ: Cardiac arrhythmias observed during anesthesia and surgery. *Surgery* 51:440–447, 1962.

163. Alexander JP: Dysrhythmia and oral surgery. *Br J Anaesth* 43:773–778, 1971.

164. Popper RW, et al.: Arrhythmias after cardiac surgery: I. Uncomplicated atrial septal defect. *Am Heart J* 64:455–461, 1962.

165. Rogers WR, Wroblewski F, LaDue JS: Supraventricular tachycardia complicating surgical procedures. *Circulation* 7:192–199, 1953.

166. Reinikainen M, Pontimen P: On cardiac arrhythmias during anesthesia and surgery. *Acta Med Scand* 180 (suppl 457):1–66, 19666.

167. Hughes CL, et al.: Cardac arrhythmias during oral surgery with local anesthesia. *J Am Dent Assoc* 73;1095–1102, 1966.

168. Bird CG, et al.: Cardiac arrhythmias during thyroid surgery. *Anesth* 24:180–189, 1969.

169. Tyras DH, et al.: Supraventricular tachyarrhythmias after myocardial revascularization: A randomized trial of prophylactic digitalization. *J Thorac Cardiovasc Surg* 77:310–314, 1979.

170. Stougard J: Cardiac arrhythmias following thoracotomy. *Thorax* 24:568–572, 1969.

171. Beck-Nielsen J: Atrial fibrillation following thoractomy for noncardiac diseases, in particular cancer of the lung. *Acta Med Scand* 193:425–429, 1973.

172. Mowry FM, Reynolds EW Jr: Cardiac disturbances complicating resectional surgery of the lung. *Ann Int Med* 61:688–695, 1964.

173. Ghosh P, Pakrashi BC: Cardiac dysrhythmias after thoracotomy. *Br Heart J* 34:374–376, 1972.

174. Cohen MG, Pastor BH: Delayed arrhythmias following non-cardiac thoracic surgery. *Dis Chest* 32:435–440, 1957.

175. Cerney CI: The prophylaxis of cardiac arrhythmias complicating pulmonary surgery. *J Thorac Surg* 34:105–110, 1957.

176. Massie E, Vallie AR: Cardiac arrhythmias complicating total pneumonectomy. *Ann Int Med* 26:231–239, 1947.

177. Bailey CC, Betts RH: Cardiac arrhythmias following pneumonectomy. *N Engl J Med* 229:356–359, 1943.
178. Currens JH, White PD, Churchill ED: Cardiac arrhythmias following thoracic surgery. *N Engl J Med* 229:369–364, 1943.
179. Rose M, Glassman E, Spencer FC: Arrhythmias following cardiac surgery: Relation to serum digoxin levels. *Am Heart J* 89:288–294, 1975.
180. Fisch C, Oehler RC, Miller JR, Redish CH: Cardiac arrhythmias during oral surgery with halothane-nitrous oxide-oxygen anesthesia. *JAMA* 208:1839–1842, 1969.
181. Dripp RD, Lamont A, Echenoff JE: The role of anesthesia in surgical mortality. *JAMA* 178:261–266, 1961.
182. Taylor G, Larson CP Jr, Prestwich R: Unexpected cardiac arrest during anesthesia and surgery. *JAMA* 236:2758–2760, 1976.
183. Pierce JA: Cardiac arrests and deaths associated with anesthesia. *Anesth Anal* 45:407–413, 1966.
184. McClure JN, Skardiasis GM, Brown JM: Cardiac arrest in the operating area. *Am Surg* 38:241–246, 1972.
185. Bomar WE Jr, Thompson NR, Ashmore JD Jr: Preoperative factors in cardiac arrest. *JAMA* 172:41–43, 1960.
186. Stephen CR: Cardiac arrest is on the decline. *Ann Surg* 155:345–352, 1962.
187. Stephenson HE Jr, Reid LC, Hinton JW: Some common denominators in 1,200 cases of cardiac arrest. *Ann Surg* 137:731–744, 1953.
188. Wisoff BG, Hartstein ML, Aintablian A, Hamby PI: Risk of coronary surgery. *J Thorac Cardivasc Surg* 69:669–673, 1975.
189. Kulbertus HE: The magnitude of risk of developing complete heart block with LAD-RBBB. *Am Heart J* 86:278–280, 1973.
190. Dhingra RC, et al.: Significance of left axis deviation in patients with chronic left bundle branch block. *Am J Cardiol* 42:551–556, 1978.
191. Dhingra RC, et al.: Chronic right bundle branch block and left posterior hemiblock: Clinical, electrophysiologic and prognostic observations. *Am J Cardiol* 36:867–872, 1975.
192. McAnulty JH, et al.: A prospective study of sudden death in high risk bundle branch block. *N Engl J Med* 299:209–215, 1978.
193. Dhingra RC, et al.: Syncope in patients with chronic bifascicular block: Significance, causative mechanisms and clinical implications. *Ann Int Med* 81:302–306, 1974.
194. Kastor JA: Cardiac electrophysiology: Hemiblocks and stopped hearts. *N Engl J Med* 299:249–251, 1978.
195. Ventkataraman K, et al.: Indications for prophylactic preoperative insertion of pacemakers in patients with right bundle branch block and left anterior hemiblock. *Chest* 68:501–506, 1975.
196. Rooney SM, et al.: Relationship of right bundle-branch block and marked left axis deviation to complete heart block during general anesthesia. *Anesthesiology* 44:64–66, 1976.
197. Pastore JO, et al.: The risk of advanced heart block in surgical patients with right bundle branch block and left axis deviation. *Circulation* 57:677–680, 1978.
198. Berg GR, Kotler MN: The significance of bilateral bundle branch block in the preoperative patient: A retrospective electrocardiographic and clinical study in 30 patients. *Chest* 59:62–67, 1971.
199. Kunstadt D, et al.: Bifascicular block: A clinical and electrophysiologic study. *Am Heart J* 86:173–181, 1973.
200. Gertler MM, et al.: Cardiovascular evaluation in surgery: I. Operative risk in cancer patients with bundle branch block. *Surg Gynecol Obstet* 99:441–450, 1954.
201. Bellocci F, et al.: The risk of cardiac complications in surgical patients with bifascicular block. *Chest* 77:343–348, 1980.
202. Siegman-Igra Y, et al.: Intraventricular conduction disturbances: A review of prevalence, etiology, and progression for ten years within a stable population of Israeli adult males. *Am Heart J* 96:669–679, 1978.
203. Ostrander LD Jr: Left axis deviation: Prevalence, associated conditions, and prognosis: An epidemiologic study. *Ann Int Med* 75:23–28, 1971.
204. Averill KH, Lamb LE: Electrocardiographic findings in 67,375 asymptomatic subjects: I. Incidence of abnormalities. *Am J of Cardiol* 6:76–83, 1960.
205. Manning GW: An electrocardiographic study of 17,000 fit, young Royal Canadian Air Force Aircrew Applicants. *Am J Cardiol* 6:70–75, 1960.
206. Hurst JW: *Cardiac Pacing and Cardioversion.* Philadelphia, Charles Press, 1967, p 7.
207. Narula OS: Atrioventricular block, in Narula OS (ed): *Cardiac Arrhythmias: Electrophysiology, Diagnosis and Management.* Baltimore, Williams & Wilkins, 1979, pp 85–113.
208. Johanson BW: Complete heart block: A clinical, hemodynamic, and pharmacological study in patients with and withoiut an artificial pacemaker: IV. Prognostic aspects of complete heart block. *Acta Med Scand* 180 (suppl 451):33–50, 1966.
210. Ohm OJ, Breivik K. Patients with high-grade atrioventricular block treated and not treated with a pacemaker. *Acta Med Scand* 203:521–528, 1978.
211. Atkins JM, et al.: Ventricular conduction blocks and sudden death in acute myocardial infarction: Potential indications for pacing. *N Engl J Med* 288:281–284, 1973.
212. Vandam LD, McLemore GA Jr: Circulatory arrest in patients with complete heart block during anesthesia and surgery. *Ann Int Med* 47:518–532, 1957.
213. Meredith J, Pruitt RD: Cardiac arrhythmia (part 5). Disturbances in cardiac conduction and their management. *Circulation* 47:1098–1107, 1973.
214. Gilchrist AJ: Clinical aspects of high grade block. *Scott Med J* 3:53–75, 1958.
215. Donoso E, et al.: Unusual forms of second-

degree atrioventricular block, including Mobitz Type II block, associated with the Morgagni-Adams-Stokes syndrome. *Am Heart J* 67:150–157, 1964.

216. Wolfe MA, Braunwald E: General anesthesia and non-cardiac surgery in patients with heart disease, in Braunwald E (ed): *Heart Disease: A Textbook of Cardiovascular Medicine.* 1980, pp 1911–1922.

217. Logue RB, Kaplan JA, et al.: Medical management in noncardiac surgery, in Hurst JW, et al. (eds): *The Heart.* 1978, pp 1762–1777.

218. Grogler FM, et al.: Complications of permanent transvenous cardiac pacing. *J Thorac Cardiovasc Surg* 69:895–904, 1975.

219. Escher DJW: Types of pacemakers and their complications. *Circulation* 47:1119–1131, 1973.

220. Campo IN, et al.: Complications of pacing by prevenous subclavian semifloating electrodes including two extraluminal insertions. *Am J Cardiovasc* 26:627, 1970.

221. Simon AB: Perioperative management of the pacemaker patient. *Anesthesiology* 46:127–131. 1977.

222. Dorney ER: The use of pacemakers in the treatment of cardiac arrhythmias, in Hurst JW, et al (eds): *The Heart.* New York: McGraw-Hill, 1978, p 698.

223. Scott DL: Cardiac pacemakers as an anesthetic problem. *Anaesthesia* 25:87–104, 1970.

224. Kaiser GC, et al.: Implantable pacemakers in heart block: Tolerance of elective noncardiac operations. *Arch Surg* 95:351–354, 1967.

225. Wynands JE: Anesthesia for patients with heart block and artificial cardiac pacemakers. *Anesth Analg* 55:626–632, 1976.

226. Fein RL: Transurethral electrocautery procedures in patients with cardiac pacemakers. *JAMA* 202:119–103, 1967.

227. Waljszczuk WJ, et al.: Deactivation of a demand pacemaker by transurethral cautery. *N Engl Med* 280:34–35, 1969.

228. Leiner SM: Suppression of a demand pacemaker by transurethral electrocautery. *Anesth Analg* 52:703–706, 1973.

229. Kohler FP, MacKinney CC: Cardiac pacemakers in electrosurgery. *JAMA* 193:199, 1965.

230. Furman, S.: *A Practice of Cardiac Pacing.* McKisco, N.Y.: Futura, 1986, pp 457–58.

231. Hawthorne JW, et al.: In Thalen JH, Hawthorne JW (eds): *To Pace or Not to Pace: Controversial Subjects on Cardiac Pacing.* Martinus Nijhoff Medical Division, 1978.

232. AHA Committee Report. Prevention of bacterial endocarditis. *Circulation* 70:1123A–1127A, 1984.

233. Wolf WA, Braunwald E: General anesthesia and non-cardiac surgery in patients with heart disease, in Braunwald E (ed): *Heart Disease: A Textbook of Cardiovascular Medicine.* Philadelphia, WB Saunders, 1980, pp 1911–1922.

234. Logue RB, Kaplan JA: Medical management in non-cardiac surgery, in Hurst JW, et al (eds): *The Heart.* New York: McGraw-Hill 1978, pp 1762–1799.

235. Deutsch S, Dalen JE: Indications for prophylactic digitalization. *Anesthesiology* 30:648–656, 1969.

236. Selzer A, et al.: Case against routine use of digitalis in patients undergoing cardiac surgery. *JAMA* 195:141–145, 1966.

237. Selzer A, Cohn KE: Some thoughts concerning the prophylactic use of digitalis. *Am J Cardiol* 26:214–216, 1970.

238. Mason DT, Braunwald E: Studies on digitalis: IX. Effects of ouabain on the non-failing human heart. *J Clin Invest* 42:1105–111, 1963.

239. Braunwald E, et al.: Studies on digitalis: IV. Observations in man on the effects of digitalis preparations on the contractility of the non-failing heart and on total vascular resistgance. *J Clin Invest* 40:52–59, 1961.

240. Goldberg AH, et al.: The effect of digoxin pretreatment on heart contractile force during thiopental infusion in dogs. *Anesthesiology* 22:974–976, 1961.

241. Goldberg AH, et al.: The value of prophylactic digitalization in halothane anesthesia. *Anesthesiology* 23:207–212, 1962.

242. Shimosato S, Epstein B: performance of digitalized hearts during halothane anesthesia. *Anesthesiology* 24:41–50, 1963.

243. Clowes GHA Jr, Del Guercio LE: Circulatory response to trauma of surgical operations. *Metabolism* 9:67–81, 1959.

244. Clowes GHA Jr, et al.: Circulatory response to the trauma of surgery and its relationship to chemical hemostasis. *Circulation* 22:734, 1960.

245. Boyd AD: Estimation of cardiac output soon after intracardiac surgery with cardiopulmonary bypass. *Ann Surg* 150:613–626, 1959.

246. Selzer A, Walter RM: Adequacy of preoperative digitalis therapy in controlling ventricular rate in postoperative atrial fibrillation. *Circulation* 34:119–122, 1966.

247. Wheat MW, Burford TH: Digitalis in surgery: Extension of classical indications. *J Thorac Cardiovasc Surg* 41:162–168, 1961.

248. Johnson LW, et al.: Prophylactic digitalization for coronary bypass surgery. *Circulation* 53:819–822, 1976.

249. Tyras DH, et al.: Supraventricular tachyarrhythmias after myocardial revascularization: A randomized trial of prophylactic digitalization. *J Thorac Cardiovasc Surg* 77:312–314, 1979.

250. Shields, Ujiki GT: Digitalization for prevention of arrhythmias following pulmonary surgery. *Surg Gynecol Obstet* 126:743–746, 1968.

251. McCord BL: The digitalization of elderly patients with cardiovascular disease requiring colectomy. *J Kans Med Soc* 68:295–299, 1967.

252. O'Kane H, et al.: Prophylactic digitalization in aortocoronary bypass patients. *Circulation* 45–46 (suppl): II-199, 1972.

253. Burman, SO: Digitalis and thoracic surgery. *J Thorac Cardiovasc Surg* 70:874–881, 1975.

254. Juler GL, et al.: Complications of prophylactic digitalization in thoracic surgical patients. *J Thorac Cardiovasc Surg* 58:352–360, 1969.

255. Pintor PP, Magri G: Digitalis and mitral surgery. *Cardiology* 55:34–40, 1970.

256. Morrison J, Killip T: Serum digitalis and arrhythmia in patients undergoing cardiopulmonary bypass. *Circulation* 47:341–352, 1973.

257. Owen RAC, Murphy AR: Surgery in old age. *Br Med J* 2:186, 1952.

258. Lown B, et al.: Cardioversion and digitalis drugs: Changed threshold to electric shock in digitalized animals. *Circ Res.* 17:519–531, 1965.

259. Ten Eick RE, et al.: Post-countershock arrhythmias in untreated and digitalized dogs. *Circ Res* 21:375–390, 1967.

260. O'Keefe JH, Shub C, Rettke SR: Risk of noncardiac surgical procedures in patients with aortic stenosis. *Mayo Clin Proc* 64:400–405, 1989.

261. Thompson RC, Liberthson RR, Lowenstein E: Perioperative anesthetic risk of noncardiac surgery in hypertrophic obstructive cardiomyopathy. *JAMA* 254:2419–2421, 1985.

262. Fowler NO: Physiology of cardiac tamponade and pulsus paradoxus: II. Physiological, circulatory, and pharmacological responses in cardiac tamponade. *Mod Concept Cardiovasc Dis* 47:115–118, 1978.

263. Reddy PS, et al.: Cardiac tamponade: Hemodynamic observations in man. *Circulation* 58:265–272, 1978.

264. Crawford ES, Morris GC, Howell JF, et al.: Operative risk in patients with previous coronary artery bypass. *Ann Thorac Surg* 26:215–221, 1978.

265. Scher KS, Tice DA: Operative risk in patients with previous coronary artery bypass. *Arch Surg* 111:807–809, 1976.

266. Majar LJ, Steen PA, Tinker JH, et al.: Perioperative myocardial infarction in patients with coronary artery disease with and without aorta-coronary artery bypass grafts. *J Thorac Cardiovasc Surg* 76:533–537, 1978.

267. McCollum CH, Garcia-Rinaldi R, Graham JM, et al.: Myocardial revascularization prior to subsequent major surgery in patients with coronary artery disease. *Surgery* 81:302–304, 1977.

268. Lucas A, Max MH: Emergency laparotomy immediately after coronary bypass. *JAMA* 244:1829–1831, 1980.

269. Katholi RE, Nolan SP, McGuire LB: Living with prosthetic heart valves subsequent noncardiac operations and the risk of thromboembolism or hemorrhage. *Am Heart J* 92:162–167, 1976.

270. Katholi RE, Nolan SP, McGuire LB: The management of anticoagulation during noncardiac operations in patients with prosthetic heart valves. *Am Heart J* 96:163–165, 1978.

271. Tinker JH, Tarhan S: Discontinuing anticoagulant therapy in surgical patients with cardiac valve prostheses observations in 180 operations. *JAMA* 239:738–739, 1978.

272. Ruby ST, Whittemore AD, Couch NP, et al.: Coronary artery disease in patients requiring abdominal aortic aneurysm repair. *Ann Surg* 201:758–764, 1985.

273. Acinapura AJ, Rose DM, Kramer MD, et al.: Role of coronary angiography and coronary artery bypass surgery prior to abdominal aortic aneurysmectomy. *J Cardiovasc Surg* 28:552–557, 1987.

274. Cruchley PM, Kaplan JA, Hug CC, et al.: Noncardiac surgery in patients with prior myocardial revascularization. *Can Anaesth Soc J* 30:629–634, 1983.

275. Cheanvechai C, et al.: Triple bypass graft for the treatment of severe triple coronary vessel disease. *Ann Thorac Surg* 17:545–554, 1974.

276. Gray TC, et al. (eds): *General Anesthesia.* Woburn, Massachusetts, Butterworths, 1980, pp 1075–76.

277. Stratmann HG, Mark AL, Walter KE, et al.: Preoperative evaluation of cardiac risk by means of atrial pacing and thallium 201 scintigraphy. *J Vasc Surg* 10:385–391, 1989.

278. Roy WL, Edelist G, Gilbert B: Myocardial ischemia during non-cardiac surgical procedures in patients with coronary-artery disease. *Anesthesiology* 51:393–397, 1979.

11

Renal, Fluid and Electrolyte, and Acid-Base Disorders

Paul E. Turer and Gary R. Briefel

Disturbances of body fluid composition or renal function are commonly encountered by the internist consulting on surgical patients. The actual incidence of many electrolyte disorders and their effects on surgical morbidity can only be estimated, because of insufficient data. In general, renal-electrolyte disorders in surgical patients occur in complex settings and have a significant associated morbidity.

Fluid, electrolyte and acid-base disturbances in surgical patients are often multifactorial in origin. They are often as likely to arise from therapeutic maneuvers (nasogastric suction, fluid therapy) as from the underlying surgical problem. In addition, the body's metabolic and endocrinologic response to surgery and trauma further predispose the patient to the development of fluid and electrolyte abnormalities.

The majority of these disturbances of body fluid composition occur in patients with anatomically normal kidneys. However, the incidence of fluid and electrolyte problems increases as renal function declines. Even patients with mild renal impairment are likely to decompensate under the stress of surgery and trauma.

Acute renal failure following surgery or trauma is one of the most difficult complications to manage, and has a high mortality. Although the morbidity of acute renal failure has been modified by dialysis, the best hope in reducing the mortality of acute renal failure lies in its

prevention. The recognition and treatment of factors predisposing to the development of acute renal failure is therefore of paramount importance.

PATIENTS WITH NORMAL RENAL FUNCTION: PREOPERATIVE EVALUATION AND MANAGEMENT

Epidemiology

Although on admission the majority of surgical patients have normal renal function and no significant disturbances of body fluid composition, it is important to be alert for the development of abnormalities, which could complicate the postoperative course. Fluid, electrolyte, and acid-base disorders contribute to the risks of anesthesia, whereas the development of acute renal failure in the surgical setting is associated with a mortality rate of 50% or greater. The chances of developing renal-electrolyte disorders are roughly proportional to the underlying surgical illness and the nature of the operative procedure in patients with normal renal function preoperatively (see "High-Risk Surgery" under "Special Considerations," p. 176). The incidence of such disturbances is also higher in patients with predisposing medical illnesses such as diabetes, congestive heart failure, and cirrhosis. The factors most clearly predisposing to the development of acute renal failure are listed in Table 11.1.

Hou (1) prospectively studied 2262 consecutive hospital admissions to general

Table 11.1.   Risk Factors for Postoperative Renal Failure

1. Volume depletion
2. Hypotension
3. Sepsis
4. Nephrotoxins
   a. Drugs (aminoglycosides)
   b. Radiocontrast materials
   c. Hemoglobinuria
   d. Myoglobinuria
5. High-risk surgical procedures (see p. 176)
6. Preexisting renal insufficiency
7. Advanced age
8. Congestive heart failure

medical and surgical services. The overall incidence of acute renal failure was 4.9%. The incidence of acute renal failure was even higher (14.4%) in those patients whose admission serum creatinine was greater than 1.2 mg/dl. Decreased renal perfusion (42%) (associated with both prerenal states and acute tubular necrosis), and postoperative acute renal failure (18%) were the most common causes. Iatrogenic factors accounted for 55% of the episodes of acquired renal insufficiency, while in 8% of the cases, no definite cause could be found.

Shusterman (2) found the incidence of acute renal failure in a large teaching hospital to be 2%. The odds ratio for the development of acute renal failure in surgical patients was increased to 9.0, 3.0, 4.3, and 1.8 for those with volume depletion, aminoglycoside use, congestive heart failure, and radiocontrast exposure respectively. The risk of dying for all patients with acute renal failure was increased six-fold as compared to patients without renal failure.

Shires (3) has found the risk of acute renal failure following elective surgery to be less than 1%. Emergency or other high-risk surgical procedures (Table 11.2) are associated with much higher incidence of ARF (5–50%) and mortality (80–90%).

Adequate maintenance of intravascular volume has been clearly shown in both clinical and animal studies to be essential in the prevention of acute renal failure.

Besides resulting in pre-renal azotemia, volume depletion appears to potentiate nephrotoxic insults of all types. Hypotension, whether due to fluid or blood losses, third spacing, sepsis, or myocardial dysfunction, is one of the most common causes of acute tubular necrosis (ATN) in the surgical patient. It is difficult, however, in any given patient to correlate the degree and duration of hypotension with the development of acute renal failure. In one study (1) hypotension was documented in only 52% of the episodes of acute postoperative renal failure. Despite the presence of edema, patients with congestive heart failure, nephrotic syndrome, and cirrhosis have decreased effective circulating volumes and may be excessively prone to hypotension from diuretics, sepsis, bleeding, and antihypertensive drugs. Sepsis, with or without hypotension or documented bacteremia, is believed to be a frequent cause of acute renal failure in surgical patients. Intra-abdominal infections with gram-negative organisms are the most common cause of sepsis in these patients and often result in a non-oliguric renal failure. Visceral abscess of the lungs, abdomen, or sinuses has also been reported to cause acute renal failure from

Table 11.2.   Incidence of Renal Insufficiency in Various Clinical Settings[a]

Clinical Setting	% Mild Acute Renal Failure (Scr <3 mg/dl)	% Severe Acute Renal Failure (Scr >3 mg/dl)
Elective surgery	1	<1
Admission to general medical/surgical service	4	1
Aminoglycoside administration	5–20	1–2
Open heart surgery	5–30	2–5
Abdominal aortic aneurysm resection		
Elective	5–10	2–5
Emergency	30–50	15–25
Severe trauma	10–20	1–5

[a] Adapted from Anderson and Schrier (13).

an immune complex-mediated proliferative glomerulonephritis (4–6). Nephrotoxic renal injury is another of the common causes of acute renal failure in surgical patients. A wide variety of drugs have toxic effects on the kidney, ranging from impaired tubular functions to interstitial nephritis and acute tubular necrosis (7). Aminoglycoside antibiotics are among some of the most frequent offenders, producing nephrotoxicity in 10–25% of patients, even when drug levels are within therapeutic concentrations (8). Radiocontrast materials appear to be nephrotoxic, particularly in diabetics, elderly patients (age >60), those with preexisting renal disease, multiple myeloma, or volume depletion (9).

The precise incidence of radiocontrast-induced acute renal failure is difficult to estimate from the literature. Overall, the incidence of reported renal dysfunction following radiocontrast administration is generally between 0–12%. Van Zee (10) reviewed retrospectively the charts of 377 patients and found a >1 mg/dl increase in serum creatinine following intravenous pyelography in 1.4, 9.2, and 39% of all cases when the initial serum creatinine was less than 1.5, 1.5–4.5, and >4.5 mg/dl, respectively. In high-risk patients, such as nondiabetic azotemic patients with initial serum creatinine >4.5 mg/dl, 31% (5/16) developed further renal dysfunction. Harkonen and Kjellstrand found a 76% (22/29) incidence of exacerbation of renal failure in diabetics whose initial serum creatinine was greater than 2 mg/dl (11). In a prospective study, D'Elia et al. found the incidence of acute renal failure following nonrenal angiography to be 33% in patients with a baseline creatinine of greater than 1.5 mg/dl (mean 2.3 mg/dl) (12).

Newer, non-ionic radiocontrast materials are quite expensive, and although it was hoped that they were less nephrotoxic than ionic agents, a recent prospective randomized study in 443 patients undergoing cardiac catherization was un-able to demonstrate a difference in the incidence of nephrotoxicity between patients receiving nonionic and ionic contrast agents (12A). Clinically, radiocontrast-induced renal failure is often mild and generally characterized by oliguria developing within the first 48 hours and lasting an average of 2–4 days. Serum creatinine usually peaks within a week of exposure and returns to baseline in over 75% of cases.

Hemoglobinuria is more likely to be seen following cardiopulmonary bypass surgery than after mismatched blood transfusions. Myoglobinuria, on the other hand, is commonly seen in surgical patients and should be considered in the clinical situations listed in Table 11.3.

The difficulty in successfully managing the complicated surgical patient arises from the fact that more than one of these risk factors are usually present.

Evaluation

In order to most efficiently utilize all the available data, the use of a flowsheet, which should include sequential mea-

Table 11.3. Select Causes of Myoglobinuria in the Surgical Setting

1. Excessive muscular activity
   a. Seizures
   b. Agitated delirium, restraints
   c. High-voltage electric shock
2. Trauma
   a. Fallen weights, auto accident
   b. Compression by body in prolonged coma
3. Ischemic
   a. Arterial occlusion
   b. Compression and anterior tibial syndrome
4. Metabolic
   a. Hypokalemia
   b. Hypophosphatemia
5. Drugs
   a. Alcohol
   b. Narcotics (heroin)
   c. Succinylcholine
   d. Amphetamines
6. Infection (influenza)
7. Heat cramps, malignant hyperthermia, burns
8. Idiopathic

surements of weight, blood pressure, intake and output, serum and urine chemistries, drugs, and other diagnostic or therapeutic interventions is recommended.

History

The history serves to recognize surgically unrelated disorders (diabetes, cirrhosis) or clinical manifestations of the present illness (vomiting, diarrhea), which

Table 11.4. Factors Responsible for Volume Depletion

I. Decreased intake
  A. NPO during diagnostic procedures
  B. Defective thirst mechanism
  C. Lack of access to food/H_2O
  D. Anorexia
II. Excessive loss
  A. Gastrointestinal losses
    1. Vomiting
    2. Diarrhea
    3. Fistula or tube drainage
    4. Enemas (cleansing and barium), cathartics
    5. Bleeding
  B. Renal losses
    1. Diuretics
    2. Osmotic diuresis (radiocontrast dyes, high-protein tube feeding, mannitol, glycerol, glucose)
    3. Salt-wasting nephropathies
    4. Adrenal insufficiency
    5. Diabetes insipidus
      a. Central
      b. Nephrogenic
  C. Skin losses
    1. Excessive sweating
    2. Burns
    3. Extensive skin lesions
III. Third space sequestration
  A. Peritonitis
  B. Intestinal obstruction
  C. Pancreatitis
  D. Crush injuries
  E. Skeletal fractures
  F. Burns
  G. Sepsis
  H. Sites of surgical trauma including wounds (retroperitoneal)
  I. Bleeding
  J. Venous obstruction
    1. Mesenteric venous obstruction
    2. Acute ileofemoral thrombophlebitis

predispose to renal dysfunction or fluid and electrolyte abnormalities. The list of conditions leading to intravascular volume depletion is extensive and is presented in Table 11.4. The history should also include an inventory of all drugs used, both in the past or present, which might have a bearing on renal-electrolyte problems (Table 11.5).

Table 11.5. Drug-related Renal Syndromes Encountered in Surgical Patients

I. Renal dysfunction
  A. Acute renal failure
    Analgesics (aspirin, non-steroidal)
    Antibiotics (aminoglycosides, cephalosporins, polymixin, tetracyclines)
    Antifungal agents (amphotericin B)
    Dextran
    Radiocontrast materials
    Anesthetics (methoxyflurane, enthrane)
  B. Interstitial nephritis
    Analgesics (aspirin, non-steroidals, phenacetin)
    Antibiotics (penicillins, cephalosporins, sulfonamides)
    Furosemide
  C. Papillary necrosis
    Analgesics (aspirin, phenacetin)
  D. Obstructive uropathy
    Intrarenal: chemotherapy for hematologic malignancy-high-dose methotrexate (hyperuricuria)
    Extrarenal
      Methysergide
      Anticholinergics
      Morphine
  E. Increased BUN (without change in GFR)
    Tetracyclines
    Glucocorticoids
II. Fluid disorders
  A. Volume depletion
    Diuretics (thiazides, furosemide, mannitol)
    Cathartics
    Emetics
  B. Nephrogenic diabetes insipidus
    Lithium
    Demeclocyline
    Methoxyflurane, enthrane
III. Electrolyte disorders
  A. Drug-induced hyponatremia
    Chlorpropramide
    Thiazides
    Vincristine
    Cyclophosphamide

(Table continues next page)

Table 11.5. *Continued*

  B. Hypokalemia
   Diuretics
   Gentamycin
   Carbenicillin
   Ticarcillin
  C. Hyperkalemia
   K^+-sparing diuretics
   Non-steroidals
   ϵ-Aminocaproic acid
   Heparin
   ACE inhibitors
  D. Hypomagnesemia
   Gentamycin
   Cisplatin
IV. Acid-base disorders
  A. Renal tubular acidosis
   Amphotericin B
   Acetazolamide
  B. Metabolic alkalosis
   Carbenicillin
   Penicillin G
  C. Respiratory acidosis
   Sedatives
   Narcotics
   Barbiturates
   Muscle paralyzers
   Anesthetics
V. Electrolyte content of common drugs
  A. Sodium
   Ampicillin (3 meq/gm)
   Penicillin G (1.7 meq/million units)
   Cephalothin (2.5 meq/gm)
   Carbenicillin (4.7 meq/gm)
   Ticarcillin (5.2 meq/gm)
   Kayexelate (65 meq/16 gm)
   Fleets phosphosoda (24 meq/15 ml)
  B. Potassium
   Penicillin G (1.7 meq/million units)
   K phosphate (4.4 meq/ml)
   Neutra phosphates (0.019 meq/ml)
  C. Magnesium
   Cathartics
   Antacids

Physical Exam

The physical examination should emphasize the clinical assessment of the extracellular and intravascular volume status. An orthostatic fall in the blood pressure, nondistended neck veins, and a resting tachycardia in the supine position when not due to other causes are associated with a significant ($\geq$1 liter) deficit in intravascular volume. The "classical" signs of volume depletion, such as decreased skin turgor, soft eyeballs, and dry tongue, are of minimal clinical value since they only appear in advanced cases and may be misleading in elderly, cachectic, or mouth-breathing patients. Peripheral and sacral edema, when not due to local causes, always implies excess total body sodium and extracellular fluid volume. Intravascular volume, on the other hand, may be normal, increased, or decreased in patients with edema. Euvolemia is a diagnosis of exclusion and is made in the absence of evidence for volume overload or depletion (Fig. 11.1). The physical exam also serves to detect evidence of urinary tract obstruction by percussing for a distended bladder, palpating for hydronephrotic kidneys, and performing rectal and pelvic exams.

Reliance on any single measurement or observation in the history or physical may be misleading when trying to assess volume status. In addition, orthopedic patients in traction or critically ill surgical patients often present special problems in the assessment of intravascular volume because their conditions preclude adequate testing for orthostasis.

LABORATORY

The minimal renal laboratory evaluation in the seemingly uncomplicated patient should include measurement of the serum sodium, potassium, chloride, CO_2 content, urea nitrogen, creatinine, glucose, and urinalysis with specific gravity. As will be emphasized several times throughout this chapter, urine output alone is not always a good reflection of renal function.

The key to the prevention of postoperative ARF lies in identifying, correcting, or avoiding the risk factors listed in Table 11.1. Assuring sufficient volume and tissue perfusion is of the utmost importance. In the stable patient not receiving diuretics undergoing elective surgery a urine output of 40–50 cc per hour is generally a reflection of an adequate volume status. If any doubt exists preoperatively about

Figure 11.1.   Summary of the Clinical Assessment of Extracellular Fluid Volume.

Volume depletion (low-body sodium)	Interstitial depletion: poor skin turgor, dry skin and mucous membranes Intravascular depletion: orthostasis, azotemia, oliguria, flat neck veins, negative fluid balance, $\downarrow$ weight, $U_{Na} < 20$ meq/L
Hypervolemia (high-body sodium)	Interstitial excess: peripheral and sacral edema Intravascular excess: pulmonary congestion/edema, distended neck veins
Euvolemia (normal-body sodium)	Diagnosis of exclusion, i.e., absence of signs of volume overload or depletion

the patient's intravascular volume status, one of two possible courses may be taken. In the young patient without significant medical problems who is not obviously volume-overloaded, a fluid challenge with normal saline, blood, or colloid may be attempted. The patient's physical exam should be followed closely for signs of volume excess. In more severely ill patients, particularly those with edema, third-space losses, or underlying heart disease, determination of intravascular volume status is more difficult and the use of a central line or, preferably, a Swan-Ganz catheter may be required. Preoperative fluid therapy should be individualized and may include the use of saline, blood, or albumin. The use of mannitol or furosemide in the intraoperative period will be discussed in the section on high-risk surgery.

When it is necessary to use radiocontrast materials diagnostically in the preoperative patient, the patient should be well-hydrated and surgery deferred if possible until the dye is cleared from the vascular system. Most dyes act as osmotic diuretics and so a careful watch of intravascular volume should be continued for up to 24 hours after the radiographic procedures. In patients who are particularly prone to develop acute renal failure following the use of radiocontrast material, the necessary information should be obtained by other means, if possible.

The use of nephrotoxic agents should be avoided or carefully controlled. Methoxyflurane or enthrane should not be used as anesthesia in patients with preexisting renal dysfunction. Minimizing the risk of antibiotic nephrotoxicity involves using the least toxic antibiotic consistent with the clinical situation and avoiding the use of other concomitant nephrotoxic agents. Serum drug levels should be monitored and drug dosage should be adjusted appropriately to the level of renal function. Serum creatinine should be monitored at least every 2 days during the course of nephrotoxic antibiotics and for at least 1 week afterward because ATN may develop several days after the drug has been discontinued. Patients with the greatest risk of aminoglycoside nephrotoxicity are those with preexisting renal disease, advanced age, and those receiving prolonged courses (9–10 days) of therapy. Loop diuretics, methoxyflurane, and possibly the cephalosoporins potentiate aminoglycoside nephrotoxicity.

Hypotension in the preoperative patient should be corrected by treating the underlying source whenever possible. When hypotension is refractory, dopamine in low to moderate dosages is preferable to more selective alpha-adrenergic agents, which further compromise renal blood flow. Adequate volume should be maintained during the intraoperative and postoperative periods. In the uncomplicated patient with normal renal function, monitoring of urine volume will suffice as a reflection of adequate hydration. A more unstable patient may require monitoring with a Swan-Ganz catheter. Management of electrolyte disorders is discussed on pages 197–230.

Postoperative Problems

EPIDEMIOLOGY

The metabolic and hormonal responses to trauma and surgery are intimately related to postoperative disorders of fluid and electrolyte balance (Table 11.6). Both the magnitude and the character of the trauma, as well as the preoperative condition of the patient, will influence the patient's response to surgical stress. Increased secretion of catecholamines, ACTH, aldosterone, and ADH are seen in the postoperative state and usually persist for 2–4 days in uncomplicated cases.

ADH release during the immediate postoperative period is unresponsive to the usual osmotic regulation. Volume depletion, morphine, and pain may further contribute to enhanced ADH secretion. The excess secretion of ADH and aldosterone cause enhanced sodium and water reabsorption, resulting in oliguria. Urinary electrolytes during this period in uncomplicated cases will show a low urinary sodium (U_{Na}) and increased urinary potassium (U_K) (70–90 meq of K^+ per day), which may result in negative potassium balance for 3–6 days postoperatively. Adequate pre- and intraoperative volume replacement will tend to minimize these changes. Increased endogenous water production is the other major alteration seen postoperatively and might result in water intoxication if not taken into account when writing fluid orders.

Table 11.6.   Metabolic Responses to Surgery and Trauma

Response	Effect
↑ Cathecholamines	Hypertension, hyperglycemia, tachycardia
↑ ACTH-cortisol	Hyperglycemia, catabolism
↑ Aldosterone	Salt retention, K^+ wasting, alkalosis
↑ ADH	Water retention
Catabolism	Negative nitrogen balance, K^+ wasting
	↑ Endogenous water production

Evaluation and Management.   See section on fluid and electrolyte disorders.

Special Considerations

HIGH-RISK SURGERY

Epidemiology

The incidence of acute renal failure following most elective surgical procedures is 1% or less. Surgical procedures associated with a higher risk of developing acute renal failure include: cardiopulmonary bypass surgery; operations on the aorta and renal vessels, particularly aneurysectomy, and major gastrointestinal operations, especially when complicated by infection, hemorrhage or biliary tract obstruction (13–20). Women undergoing surgery following third trimester accidents such as abruptio placenta, are also at high risk. A prospective study of acute renal failure following cardiac surgery at Stanford (21) found prolonged duration of cardiopulmonary bypass, preoperative left ventricular dysfunction, and the need for intra-aortic balloon pumping postoperatively to be the best predictors of postoperative renal dysfunction (prerenal azotemia) and acute renal failure. Additional risk factors identified included greater age, active bacterial endocarditis or a history, or prior cardiac surgery. Mean arterial pressure during cardiopulmonary bypass and the duration of aortic cross-clamping was not significantly different in the groups with renal dysfunction or acute renal failure as compared to the control group who had a normal postoperative course. This study also found that postoperative depression of myocardial function characterized by a low cardiac output and elevated pulmonary capillary wedge pressure accompanied by renal hypoperfusion (↓ GFR, fractional excretion of sodium < 1%) was present in all patients who developed postoperative renal dysfunction or acute renal failure. However, hemodynamic function and GFR were similar in the groups with postoperative renal dysfunction (prerenal azotemia) and acute renal failure. It is suggested that the progression to acute renal failure required the superimposition of additional renal insults including: sepsis, nephrotoxic antibiotics, hypotension, hemorrhage, prolonged low cardiac output state, or withdrawal of mechanical or pharmacological circulatory support. Table 11.2 reviews the incidence of acute renal failure following high-risk surgical procedures. The mortality rate for patients with postoperative acute renal failure as a group is 50–70%. The mortality rate is even greater in the small subgroup requiring dialysis, which may range between 60–98% (14, 16, 18).

Evaluation

This is similar to the evaluation outlined earlier for patients with normal renal function. Since maintenance of intravascular volume assumes even greater significance in these patients, we recommend the use of a Swan-Ganz catheter. Even if the preoperative patient is judged to be euvolemic on clinical grounds, redistribution of volume or third space losses during surgery, and the effects of anesthesia on peripheral resistance will require continued readjustment of fluid intraoperatively.

In assessing the patient in the immediate postoperative period, the development of a mannitol or furosemide-induced diuresis may be deceiving since urine output and glomerular filtration rate are not always well correlated. Non-oliguric renal failure is common in these patients and will be missed unless careful monitoring of serum creatinine is performed on a daily basis. In addition, if the patient is not monitored carefully, continued diuresis could lead to further volume depletion.

Management

Surgery, whenever possible, should be delayed until the risk factors listed earlier have been controlled. Although pri-

marily a surgical decision, intraoperative fluid management should also be of interest to the consulting medical physician. The type and amount of fluids administered during surgery that are effective in preventing postoperative acute renal failure have not been established by rigorous studies.

Animal experiments indicate some protection is offered by volume expansion or mannitol-induced diuresis prior to the renal insult. Mannitol and furosemide have also been used to reverse acute renal failure immediately following the presumed renal injury with variable success (22–25). Whether there is a beneficial effect beyond that achieved by maintaining intravascular volume with saline, plasma, or blood is disputed (20, 26–30). Since neither mannitol nor diuretics augment intravascular volume, the primary form of pre- and intraoperative management should be the use of volume expanders.

Urinary Tract Infections

EPIDEMIOLOGY

Up to 10% of hospitalized patients have a community-acquired urinary tract infection (UTI) on admission, while another 10% will develop a UTI in the hospital. Pregnant women, diabetics, and patients with reduced host defenses are even more susceptible. The highest prevalence of UTIs are found in patients with congenital renal diseases (57%), hydronephrosis or nephrolithiasis (85%), and indwelling open drainage urinary catheters (98%) (31).

Between 70–80% of all hospital-acquired UTIs are related to urinary catheterization (32). Most of these patients are asymptomatic, and a proportion will clear their infections spontaneously upon removal of the catheter.

UTIs account for 35–60% of all nosocomial infections (32). Of patients with gram-negative sepsis, 20–30% have the urinary tract as a source. Sepsis is often associated with urologic abnormalities or follows instrumentation. Gram-negative sepsis is also an important predisposing cause of ARF. The mortality rate of gram-negative sepsis arising from the urinary tract is 15% (33).

Escherichia coli is still the most common infecting organism, even in hospitalized patients. The incidence of *Pseudomonas, Proteus, Klebsiella,* and other gram-negative and positive UTIs is higher in hospitalized patients or those with urologic abnormalities.

EVALUATION

The admission evaluation should include a routine urinalysis. If pyuria is found, a urine culture should be obtained. Pyuria may be found in the absence of infection or occasionally may not be seen when the infected kidney is completely obstructed. The clean catch method is the preferred means of obtaining a urine specimen, but many ill or immobile patients will require straight catheterization.

MANAGEMENT

The following therapeutic guidelines should apply to most patients. Acute, uncomplicated infections or relapses in females should be treated. In the elderly patient with frequent relapses who is asymptomatic, the risk of therapy often outweighs the benefits (34). Male or female patients with complicated infections (i.e., with foreign bodies such as stones, catheters, or anatomical abnormalities) should only be treated when blood or tissue invasion in suspected. Routine or prolonged treatment with broad-spectrum antibiotics in such cases will only lead to the development of resistant organisms.

When catheters are used, they must be left in place for the least amount of time as possible. Strict antiseptic insertion and maintenance will help reduce the infection rate. Closed bag drainage (40% infection rate at 2 weeks) should be used. If indicated, 0.25% acetic acid or neosporin-polymixin irrigation can be used as a prophylactic measure against local infection, but does not offer greater protection than a meticulously maintained closed drainage system.

It is rarely necessary to postpone nonurologic surgery due to an asymptomatic UTI. Antibiotic treatment should be started preoperatively. Patients with bacteriuria who require instrumentation or urologic surgery should be treated to reduce the incidence of bacteremia following such procedures. Prophylactic therapy is also recommended for patients prior to urologic surgery who have valvular heart disease or prosthetic devices. The long-term success of treatment for patients with anatomical abnormalities of the GU tract depends on surgical correction of the defect.

Elective surgery may need to be postponed for a variable period following symptomatic urinary infection, from a few days for uncomplicated lower tract infections to 1–3 weeks after pyelonephritis with sepsis.

Living Related Renal Transplant Donor Evaluation

EPIDEMIOLOGY

In hospital centers performing living related donor (LRD) kidney transplants, the internist may be asked to partake in the medical evaluation of the potential donor. The role of the "independent" internist is to examine the donor for problems that would preclude the patient from donation. There are three general categories of diseases that might adversely affect the donor's ability to give a kidney. The first category are diseases that could damage the donor's remaining kidney (diabetes, hypertension, nephrolithiasis); the second includes diseases that might be transmitted to the recipient (HBsAg-positive hepatitis, active syphilis, positive HIV, malignancy; and the final group are diseases that increase the risk of surgery in general (coronary artery, pulmonary, liver diseases).

The incidence of renal abnormalities in

family members (potential donors) of patients on dialysis appears to be increased. In a series reported by Spanos (35), of 209 potential donors (relatives of patients with hereditary renal diseases were excluded), 10% had significant bacteriuria, 5% had diastolic hypertension, 20% had abnormal IVPs, and 4% had major abnormalities of their renal arteriograms. Of the original 209, 40 (19%) were excluded as donors on the basis of one or more of these abnormalities.

The use of family members as donors for patients with hereditary forms of renal disease is controversial. Some centers simply restrict transplantation in such instances to cadaveric sources. Other centers, because the the superior graft survival of LRD compared to cadaveric transplants (75% vs. 50% 2-year graft survival) will evaluate and employ family members as donors.

EVALUATION

Potential donors are selected after establishment of histocompatibility and the exclusion of obvious physical or psychological abnormalities. The selected donor is then generally admitted for more extensive medical, psychological, and urological evaluation. A summary of the entire donor evaluation is presented in Table 11.7.

When the LRD for a patient with a hereditary form of renal disease is being considered, more extensive evaluations, including renal biopsy, are often necessary. For example, in Alport's disease, the earliest manifestations are seen in the glomerulus or tubules when examined by election microscopy. Milutinovic (36) found that young siblings of patients with polycystic kidney disease may have normal urograms, glomerular filtration rates, renal blood flow, ammonia production, and concentrating ability, and yet have tubular dilatation seen on renal biopsy. The evaluation of the diabetic's family members is made more difficult by the complex nature of the genetic component. Even

Table 11.7. **Living Related Transplant Donor Evaluation**

1. Tissue typing
   ABO blood groups
   HLA typing, mixed lymphocyte culture, leukocyte cross-match (DR typing)
2. Psychological screening
3. History and physical
4. Repeat blood pressure determinations, urinalysis, urine culture
5. BUN, creatinine, creatinine clearance, IVP
6. Fasting blood sugar, liver functions, uric acid, calcium, phosphorus, CBC, prothrombin time, partial thromboplastin time, HAA, STS, HIV
7. Chest radiograph, ECG
8. Aortogram

HLA-identical siblings of a diabetic patient may never develop glucose intolerance. If a relative of a diabetic patient is being considered, the minimal evaluation of the potential donor should include a fasting glucose and oral glucose tolerance test. Some centers advocate the use of cortisone or intravenous glucose tolerance tests as well.

MANAGEMENT

A listing of donor complications is found in Table 11.8. Long-term follow-up of large numbers of donors has not revealed any change in life expectancy and renal function returns to 70–80% of the preoperative level within a few months. There has been recent concern that the adaptive changes that occur in the remaining donor kidney (hyperfiltration) may eventually result in damage to the organ. Several long-term series of donors examined to date show only a slight increase in albuminuria and blood pressure without significant decline in glomerular filtration rates.

THE EVALUATION AND MANAGEMENT OF THE SURGICAL PATIENT WITH ACUTE RENAL FAILURE

Epidemiology

More than 50% of the cases of acute renal failure follow either surgery or

Table 11.8.   Postoperative Complications in Living Related Transplant Donors

Group Characteristics	Boston[a] (N = 300)	Colorado[b] (N = 238)	Virginia[c] (N = 120)	Wisconsin[d] (N = 66)	Total (N = 724)
	1954–1973	1964–1969	1966–1972	1966–1973	
Donor age (yr)	12–80	18–57	22–59	21–63	12–80
Percentage of potential donors rejected	23		66		
Overall complication rate (%)	28.3	47	21	34.8	33.8
Complications					
Wound infections	33	4	3		40 (5.5%)
Pneumonia	5				5 (0.7%)
Atelectasis/fever/pneumonia	29	33	5	2	69 (9.5%)
Pleural effusion		12		1	13 (1.8%)
Pneumothorax		26	3		29 (4%)
Pulmonary embolus				2	2 (0.3%)
Acute renal failure	1	1	1		3 (0.4%)
Gastric distention or intestinal ileus		4	3		7 (1.0%)
UGI bleed	1				1 (0.1%)
Hepatitis	2	4			6 (0.8%)
Serum	1				
Anesthesia-related	1	4			
Positive urine culture	39	24		15	78 (10.8%)
Persistent bacteriuria			3	2	5 (0.7%)
Transient hematuria		3			3 (0.4%)
Urinary retention		7			7 (1.0%)
Deep venous thrombosis		3		2	5 (0.7%)
Postaortogram thrombosis			1		1 (0.1%)
Phlebitis	3				3 (0.4%)
Transfusion requirement			3		3 (0.4%)
Transient hypertension	1	10			11 (1.5%)
Minor cardiac arrhythmias	3				3 (0.4%)
Psychiatric problems	21				21 (2.9%)
Transient nerve palsy		4			4 (0.5%)
Prolonged incisional pain		3			3 (0.4%)
Incisional hernia	1		3	2	6 (0.8%)
Mortality (in hospital)	0	0	1	1	2 (0.3%)
Myocardial infarct			1		
Pulmonary embolus				1	

[a] *Surg Gynecol Obstet* 139:894, 1974.
[b] *Arch Surg* 101:226, 1970.
[c] *J Urol* 110:158, 1973.
[d] *J Urol* 111:745, 1974.

trauma. The incidence of acute renal dysfunction ranges from 1% in the general surgical patient to 25% in certain high-risk cases (Table 11.2). Dialysis is required in 30–50% of acute renal failure cases, and mortality averages 50–70%, but may exceed 90% following cardiopulmonary bypass surgery or repair of ruptured aortic aneurysms.

Acute renal failure is a general term encompassing a wide variety of disorders resulting in a rapid, but usually reversible, impairment of kidney function. For clinical purposes, an acute and progressive increase in blood urea nitrogen or serum creatinine above the normal range (or baseline value in a patient with preexisting renal insufficiency) is sufficient for the diagnosis of acute renal failure. The quantity of urine is not always helpful in diagnosis since only 50–70% of cases are oliguric. Reliance solely on urine output as a marker of renal function, therefore, may cause undue delay in making the diagnosis. Common examples of non-oliguric renal failure include: partial obstruction, hypercalcemic nephropathy, and aminoglycoside nephrotoxicity.

Oliguria is defined as a urine output of less than 400 ml/day in a patient with previously normal renal function. This volume represents the minimum urine output required to excrete the average daily solute load. Anuria is defined as a urine volume of less than 50 ml/day. Anuria should always suggest the possibility of obstruction, but other causes include cortical necrosis, acute glomerulonephritis, and bilateral renal artery occlusion. Acute tubular necrosis may on occasion be associated with anuria. Alternating anuria and polyuria, especially with a normal urine sediment, may also be a clue to the presence of obstruction.

Dividing acute renal failure into prerenal, postrenal and intrinsic categories is useful since it provides a framework for the diagnostic classification. Oliguria in the postoperative period, even when associated with mild increments in the serum creatinine or urea nitrogen, is often due to prerenal causes, and does not necessarily imply actual kidney malfunction. Oliguria may result from normal physiological responses occurring postoperatively, such as the increase in ADH secretion, or most commonly, from depletion of intravascular volume. Diminished effective circulatory volume may be due to actual fluid losses or related to cardiac dysfunction.

Postrenal causes account for the minority of acute renal failure cases, but should never be overlooked since they are generally reversible. Bladder outlet obstruction is common in the surgical patient who is often receiving narcotics, or recovering from the effects of anesthesia. Obstruction should be suspected in patients with a history of nephrolithiasis, abdominal or pelvic surgery, rectal or pelvic neoplasms, or prostatism (37, 38). Rupture of the bladder may be seen following up to 15% of pelvic fractures (39).

Although there are a variety of causes of intrinsic acute renal failure, the one most commonly seen in the postoperative or trauma patient is acute tubular necrosis. This is by no means the only etiology, and certain others deserve special mention. Acute drug-induced nephrotoxicity is now being recognized more frequently. Acute interstitial nephritis often develops following the use of drugs such as the penicillins (ampicillin, methicillin), nonsteroidal anti-inflammatory agents, and diuretics. In addition to acute renal failure, the patient with acute interstitial nephritis may also have a fever, rash, eosinophilia, or pyuria (with eosinophils). Patients with bilateral renal artery stenosis treated with ACE inhibitors may develop a reversible form of renal insufficiency due to impaired autoregulation of renal blood flow (40). Pyogenic visceral abscesses have also been associated with acute renal failure due to immune complex-mediated glomerulonephritis (4–6), even in patients without documented bacteremia. The glomerular nature of the lesion is suggested by the presence of hematuria, hypertension, and pulmonary edema. In one study, cryoglobulins were detected frequently, although serum complement was only depressed in 4/11 (35% patients). Chronic renal failure or death is common if diagnosis or therapy is delayed. Early treatment often results in complete resolution. Cholesterol embolization to the kidneys arising either spontaneously or more commonly following insertion of radiographic catheters or aortic surgery is an uncommon cause of renal failure in patients with extensive atheromatous involvement of the aorta. The presence of ischemic toes or livido reticularis should suggest this diagnosis.

Acute tubular necrosis, sometimes called vasomotor nephropathy, is the most common cause of intrinsic acute renal failure in surgical patients. The pathogenesis of this disorder is complex and not totally understood. Hemodynamic or nephrotoxic insults are the usual initiating events (Table 11.9). The maintaining factors are postulated to include persistent renal vasoconstriction, tubular obstruction, decreased glomerular permeability, and back leak of filtrate across damaged tubules.

The clinical course of acute tubular necrosis is generally divided into an oliguric and diuretic phase. The duration of the oliguric phase averages between 10–14 days with a range of a few hours to over a month. However, many patients never have a period of oliguria, or it is of such short duration that it is missed. Complete clinical recovery occurs in the majority of cases, even in patients with prolonged oliguria.

In the functionally anephric patient with uncomplicated acute renal failure, the blood urea nitrogen usually increases by 20–40 mg/dl per day and the serum creatinine by 1 mg/dl per day. In more seriously ill patients, hypercatabolism is reflected by: increases of BUN of greater than 40 mg/dl per day or creatinine greater than 1 mg/dl per day; rapid onset of hyperkalemia; severe metabolic acidosis; a

Table 11.9. Causes of Acute Renal Failure

I. Prerenal
  A. Hypotension
  B. Volume depletion, including peripheral pooling 2° sepsis, acidosis
  C. Ineffective cardiac function
    1. Congestive heart failure
    2. Tamponade
    3. Pulmonary embolism
    4. Cor pulmonale
II. Renal
  A. Toxins
    1. Exogenous: antibiotics, contrast media, anesthetics
    2. Endogenous: myoglobin and hemoglobin
  B. Arterial: emboli, thrombus, dissecting aneurysm, malignant hypertension
  C. Veins: thrombosis, vena caval obstruction
  D. Glomerulus: glomerulonephritis, vasculitis
  E. Tubule: ATN (ischemic and/or nephrotoxic)
  F. Interstitial: drug hypersensitivity, metabolic nephropathy, infection
III. Postrenal
  A. Urethral obstruction
  B. Bladder
    1. Outlet obstruction (BPH, bladder cancer, drugs)
    2. Ruptured bladder
  C. Bilateral urethral obstruction
    1. Intraureteral (uric acid, blood clots, pyogenic debris, stone, edema, necrotizing papillitis)
    2. Extraureteral
      a. Tumor: cervix, prostate, colon, endometriosis
      b. Periureteral fibrosis
      c. Accidental surgical ligature

uric acid of greater than 15 mg/dl; and hyperphosphatemia of 8–10 mg/dl or more, often in association with severe hypocalemia.

Mortality during the oliguric phase is related to hyperkalemia, fluid overload, acidosis, bleeding, or infection (41–44). During the diuretic phase, the BUN and creatinine may continue to rise for several days despite increasing urine output. Once established, the diuresis should proceed smoothly with a gradual and persistent improvement in renal function. A second period of oliguria is associated with a poor prognosis. The recovery phase generally last 2–4 weeks.

The mortality rate for postoperative or post-traumatic acute renal failure approaches 60%. Cioffi et al. (45) analyzed the factors that predicted unfavorable outcomes in a group of 65 patients who developed postoperative acute renal failure requiring hemodialysis. They identified cardiac failure, multisystem organ failure, number of blood transfusions, type of surgery, age, severity of injury, creatinine prior to first dialysis, and interval from acute renal failure to first dialysis as factors that predicted a higher mortality. Only the latter two factors could be modified by the clinician. Other investigators have found that preexisting renal dysfunction also correlated with an increased mortality.

Complications relating to the underlying surgical problems are the most important causes of death. In one autopsy series, the primary underlying disease or its extrarenal complications were considered the main cause of death in 92% of all fatal cases of postoperative acute renal failure (46). Sepsis occurs with a frequency of between 50 and 80% and accounts for about 33% of the deaths. Gastrointestinal bleeding occurs in up to 40% of cases, with a mortality rate of approximately 25%. Infectious complications are particularly common in cases of acute renal failure following trauma or major gastrointestinal operations. The most frequent sites of infection include the lungs, urine, wounds, peritoneum, intravenous sites, and gastrointestinal tract. Other factors associated with a poor prognosis include: advanced age, jaundice, and requirement for a mechanical ventilator. Non-oliguric acute renal failure in some series is associated with a reduced need for dialysis and a better prognosis. In surgical patients, however, non-oliguric renal failure carries a mortality rate of 40%.

Although most patients recover from acute tubular necrosis, up to 40 or 50% have reduced glomerular filtration rates and impaired abilities to either concentrate or acidify their urine. Younger patients tend to have faster and more complete recoveries than elderly patients or those with preexisting mild renal insufficiency (47). In one large series, however 10% of patients were left with severe chronic renal failure (48).

Efforts to reduce the unacceptably high mortality figures in postoperative ARF center about three objectives: *(a)* reversal of early or established ARF, *(b)* more aggressive dialysis schedules, *(c)* improved nutrition. A number of pharmacological maneuvers to restore GFR have been attempted to correct the presumed pathophysiological states resulting in ARF. None of these treatments have unequivocally been shown to be of benefit. Of these various therapies, infusions of saline, mannitol, or furosemide are the most commonly used in the clinical setting. When used judiciously, these treatments are relatively safe. Complications tend to arise when employed in an inappropriate setting or when the desire to achieve a diuresis leads to overly aggressive treatment. Both saline or mannitol infusions can result in pulmonary edema. In addition, too much mannitol can produce hyperosmolality and pseudohyponatremia. Mannitol and furosemide can both result in a vigorous diuresis, which if not appropriately replaced, can lead to worsening renal failure. The combination of volume depletion and furosemide also can potentiate the nephrotoxicity of other drugs. If any of these therapies are to have any chance of success, they must be used early in the course of ARF. Even when a diuresis is achieved by one of these methods, it is not always associated with an improvement in glomerular filtration rate. A larger urine output may make subsequent management easier, however. Whether these maneuvers in fact convert oliguric to non-oliguric renal failure remains to be evaluated by prospective studies (22). Brown et al. have recently shown in a randomized, prospective study involving 58 surgical and trauma patients with ATN that high-dose furosemide (3 g/ day) did not affect the duration of renal failure, the number of dialyses, or mortality (23).

When patients fail to respond to volume replacement and loop diuretics, low dose dopamine, administered at a rate of 2–5 mcg/kg/minute, may result in a significant increase in urine output (49).

Studies by Conger (50), Teschan (51), Fischer (52), and Kleinknecht (53) suggest that early or "prophylactic" dialysis results in a lower mortality rate and a decreased incidence of complications than dialysis performed for specific uremic manifestations. In Kleinknecht's study, mortality in surgical patients with ARF was reduced from 54 to 42%. Mortality due to gastrointestinal bleeding fell from 17 to 6%, but the frequency of septic deaths was unaffected. Other studies using early and frequent dialysis have not shown a similar impact on mortality rates. Nevertheless, it is generally conceded that aggressive dialysis facilitates the management of these patients.

Hypercatabolism, negative nitrogen balance, and weight loss contribute to the morbidity and mortality of postoperative and post-trauma patients with acute renal failure.

Dudrick (54) has shown that an intravenous solution of hypertonic glucose and L-essential amino acids given to patients with postoperative renal failure cause a reduction in BUN, and an amelioration of hyperphosphatemia, hypercalcemia, and acidosis. Dialysis requirements were simultaneously reduced. Abel (55), in a prospective, double-blind study, gave "renal failure fluid" (hypertonic glucose and essential amino acids) to one group of patients with acute renal failure and hypertonic glucose alone to another group. Seventy-five percent of those receiving renal failure fluid survived, as compared to only 56% of those receiving glucose alone. The need for dialysis was not affected by the use of hyperalimentation, nor did hyperalimentation affect the incidence of pneumonia, sepsis, or gastrointestinal bleeding. Baek et al. (56) in a similar study showed a reduction in mortality rate from 70% in the glucose-treated group to 46% in the amino acid plus glucose group. Although urea nitrogen levels were not reduced in this study, hyperkalemia was seen less frequently. In contrast, the renal group at Guy's Hospital was unable to reduce mortality (62%), as compared to their earlier experience, even with intensive dialysis combined with high-protein, high-calorie feedings (57). Since intravenous hyperalimentation is associated with a significant incidence of septic problems, volume overload or iatrogenic electrolyte abnormalities, it should be reserved for those unable to take an oral diet.

Evaluation

The presence of acute renal failure may be suggested by the development of oliguria or an actual rise in blood urea nitrogen (BUN) or creatinine. The evaluation proceeds by excluding prerenal and postrenal causes and then matching the clinical and laboratory findings with the diagnosis of intrinsic renal disease.

Prerenal azotemia is evaluated via the bedside determination of intravascular volume status, as previously described, comparison of weights, input and outputs, Swan-Ganz or central venous monitoring, laboratory analysis of blood and urine chemistries, and, possibly, a diagnostic trial of volume expanders. Prerenal azotemia is ultimately a retrospective diagnosis whereby normal function should return to normal within 72 hours after correction of volume depletion, hypotension or congestive heart failure in a patient with previously normal renal function.

The possibility of bladder outlet obstruction is evaluated by the physical examination, including a rectal and pelvic examination, and catherization of the bladder (or checking the patency of the catheter if one is already in place). Whenever the diagnosis of upper tract obstruction is seriously considered, one of several imaging techniques is essential (see below).

Once pre- and postrenal possibilities have been ruled out, a long list of causes of intrinsic acute renal failure must be considered. The diagnosis is often made by reviewing the immediate past history and finding factors predisposing to acute renal failure. Unfortunately, surgical patients are frequently exposed to numerous nephrotoxic agents and events; often no single cause can be identified. Obviously, this should not detract from the diagnosis since periods of hypotension may be minimal or missed entirely and exposure to nephrotoxins may be brief but sufficient to be harmful.

The urinalysis, although at times very helpful, is usually nonspecific. It may be entirely normal or show finely granular casts in prerenal azotemia. In obstructive uropathy, the findings may include hematuria, pyuria, or be normal. Hematuria, with or without red cell casts, may also be seen in acute glomerulonephritis or vasculitis. Calcium oxalate crystals or urate crystals suggest the diagnosis of methoxyflurane toxicity or uric acid nephropathy, respectively. The urinalysis in acute tubular necrosis may be normal, show a few red cells, or have the characteristic findings of many granular, pigmented casts associated with renal tubular epithelial cells. Pyuria with a high percentage of eosinophils is seen in some cases of acute interstitial nephritis. When a urine positive for blood by dipstick does not show red blood cells on microscopic examination, the diagnosis of myoglobinuria (or hemoglobinuria) should be strongly considered. The urine also often shows pigmented granular casts in myoglobinuric acute renal failure.

The diagnosis of myoglobinuria can be more firmly established by the finding on blood analysis of a rapidly rising or markedly elevated creatinine, potassium, uric acid, phosphate and creatinine phosphokinase (CPK). A definitive diagnosis depends on finding myoglobin in the urine.

One form or another of renal imaging techniques is usually obtained depending on the clinical circumstances. The simplest of these is the KUB, which might reveal kidney size, stones, or a distended bladder. Renal sonography is also simple and non-invasive, and is usually reliable in ruling out the presence of obstruction without the need for radiocontrast materials. If hydronephrosis is detected by sonography, one option is to proceed directly to percutaneous antegrade pyelography and placement of a nephrostomy tube. CT scans (with or without contrast) or cystoscopy with retrograde urography would also be appropriate. Intravenous urography is less commonly used today in the evaluation of acute renal failure due to the risk of radiocontrast-induced nephrotoxicity.

In addition to providing evidence of the presence of obstruction, the appearance of the urogram may also suggest an alternative etiology. The nephrogram phase, which results in opacification of the renal substance, is due to the appearance and concentration of filtered contrast materials in the tubules. In normal subjects, the nephrogram is most dense at the end of injection and quickly disappears as the blood level falls. The pyelographic phase commences with the appearance of the dye in the pelvocalyceal system. In extrarenal obstruction, the nephrogram phase is delayed, but becomes increasingly dense with time. The pyelogram phase is also delayed. Dilation of the collecting system proximal to the obstruction may be visible. In uncomplicated acute tubular necrosis, an immediate dense nephrogram appears, which persists for up to 24 hours or more. The collecting system often is not visualized. Suppurative pyelonephritis, like some cases of chronic renal failure, may give a similar pattern. Advanced renal disease typically gives an immediate but faint nephrogram with a prolonged disappearance time.

Chemical analysis of the urine may be very helpful in making the differential diagnosis of acute renal failure, although it is most useful in differentiating pre-

Table 11.10.   Urinary Diagnostic Indices in Acute Renal Failure

	Prerenal Azotemia	Oliguria ARF	Non-oliguric ARF	Acute Obstruction	Acute Glomerulonephritis	Renal Vascular Occlusion
BUN/creatinine	>20:1	<20:1	<20:1	<20:1	<20:1	<20:1
(U/P) urea	>8	<3	<8	<12	>8	<8
(U/P) creatinine	>40	<20	<20	<20	>40	<20
$(U/P)_{Osm}$	>1.5	1–1.5	1–1.5	1–1.5	>1.2	1–1.5
U_{Osm}	>500	<350	<350	<400	>350	<350 (variable)
U_{Na}	<20	>40	>40[a]	>20	<20	≤30
RFI	<1	>1	>1[a]	>1	<1	<1
FE_{Na}	<1	>1	>1[a]	>1	<1	<1
U/A	Normal	Renal tubular cells or casts, pigmented brown casts	Same as oliguric ARF	Normal or crystals or pyuria	Proteinuria RBC casts	Hematuria pyuria Proteinuria Cholesterol
Urine volume	<400 cc/day	<400 cc/day	>600 cc/day	Anuria or anuria-polyuria	<400 cc/day	Anuria-oliguria
Radiology	Not diagnostic	Not diagnostic, immediate dense, persistent nephrogram	Not diagnostic	Required for diagnosis. Delayed, but increasing nephrogram and delayed pyelogram evidence of obstruction		Renal scan or arteriogram or venogram for diagnosis
Sonography	Normal renal size	Normal renal size	Normal renal size	Dilated calyces		Normal renal size

[a] Tend to be lower on average than oliguric ARF.

renal azotemia from oliguric acute tubular necrosis (58, 59). Interpretation of these results presupposes: (a) previously normal renal function, and (b) that diuretics or other therapeutic maneuvers have not been recently administered. The most commonly obtained measurements include the specific gravity, osmolality, urea, sodium, and creatinine concentrations. The urine osmolality is a more accurate indication of urinary concentration than the specific gravity, since urinary proteins or radiographic dyes do not interfere with its measurement.

In prerenal azotemia, one expects to find an elevated specific gravity (>1.015), a urine osmolality greater than 500 mOsm/kg of H_2O, and a urine sodium concentration below 20 meq/L. The urine in oliguric acute tubular necrosis usually has an os-

molality less than 350 mOsm/kg of H_2O, a specific gravity of 1.010, and a urine sodium concentration of 40 meq/L or above. In those patients with oliguria whose urinary chemistries fall between these limits, the fractional excretion of sodium (FE_{Na})* or the renal failure index (RFI)† are more reliable in separating prerenal causes from acute tubular necrosis (Table 11.10).

Formerly, a fractional excretion of sodium or renal failure index of <1 was consistent with prerenal azotemia and >1 with acute tubular necrosis. Now many

$$*FE_{Na} = \frac{U/P\ (Na)}{U/P\ (creatinine)} \times 100\%$$

$$\dagger RFI = \frac{U\ (Na)}{U/P\ (creatinine)}$$

Table 11.11.   Low Fractional Excretion of Sodium in ARF

1. Radiocontrast-induced ARF
2. Pigment nephropathy (myoglobin, hemoglobin)
3. Sepsis
4. Burns
5. Interstitial nephritis
6. Hepatorenal syndrome
7. Acute glomerulonephritis
8. Early obstructive uropathy
9. Nonoliguric ATN (10–15%)
10. Renal allograft rejection
11. Drugs (Captopril, nonsteroidal anti-inflammatory agents)
12. Postcardiac surgery

exceptions of both oliguric and non-oliguric acute renal failure have been described with low FE_{Na} (<1%) (55) (Table 11.11). The fractional excretion of sodium may be elevated in patients receiving diuretics, in those with chronic renal failure, or during postobstructive diuresis, and, therefore, is of less value in these situations.

Low urinary sodiums may be observed in acute tubular necrosis if a profound stimulus for sodium reabsorption exists such as is seen in terminal hepatic failure, shock, or severe cardiac failure. Nonoliguric renal failure is also associated with a lower urinary sodium concentration than the oliguric form. In acute glomerulonephritis or vasculitis, the urinary sodium concentration and fractional excretion of sodium also tend to be low. The urinary diagnostic indices in early acute obstructive nephropathy may be similar to those of prerenal azotemia, but with time resemble those of ATN. Urinary indices must be interpreted by taking the entire clinical picture into account. They are best utilized either to confirm a clinical impression or to question a diagnosis if markedly different from expected.

Management

Certain aspects of management differ depending on whether acute renal failure occurs in the pre- or postoperative state (60). Preoperatively, it is advisable to postpone non-urgent surgery to allow time for establishing a diagnosis and assessing the effects of therapy. It is usually possible to arrive at a reasonable diagnosis within 24–48 hours.

Elective surgery should be delayed until renal function has returned to baseline. When surgery is more urgent, fluid and electrolyte disturbances should be managed as outlined in the section on fluid, electrolyte, and acid-base disorders. If renal function is severely compromised, dialysis may be necessary.

Since oliguria in the surgical patient is commonly secondary to intravascular volume depletion, an attempt at volume expansion should be considered if signs of overload are absent. A Swan-Ganz catheter should be used when a fluid challenge is considered dangerous in the presence of cardiopulmonary diseases. A wedge pressure that continues to rise above optimal filling pressures (15–18 mm Hg) with no increment in cardiac or urine output is evidence against volume depletion as the cause of oliguria. If the patient's clinical condition allows a fluid challenge without the aid of a Swan-Ganz catheter, 500 ml of normal saline may be given every 30–60 minutes, reassessing frequently for signs of fluid overload. If euvolemia is achieved without improvement in urine output, mannitol or furosemide may be tried.

Mannitol is given as 12.5–25 grams over 10 minutes (50–100 cc of 25% solution). Furosemide may be given in increasing doses up to a maximum of between 240 and 480 mg. Continued administration of furosemide when no effect is evident is likely to result in ototoxicity, particularly if the patient is also receiving aminoglycoside antibiotics. If urine output does not increase following loop diuretics, then dopamine may be infused at a rate of 2–5 mcg/kg/min. A review of other pharmacological maneuvers in ARF has been compiled by Tiller and Mudge (25).

Close attention must be paid to writing fluid orders since the kidney in ARF is unable to compensate. The daily fluid requirements should replace insensible losses (~400 cc/day) plus measurable losses (over the previous 24 hours) from the urine, GI tract, and wounds, as well as estimated third-space losses. Insensible water losses are increased with fever (13% per degree centigrade) and hyperventilation. Insensible losses via the lungs are nil in patients on mechanical ventilators. It should be recalled that hypercatabolic states result in an increased endogenous water of oxidation which tends to decrease net insensible losses.

Progressive weight gain is common in the first 36–48 hours postoperatively, as fluids are administered to compensate for fluid sequestration into surgical third-spaces that accompany burns, inflammation, and soft-tissue trauma. Estimation of third-space requirements are based on hemodynamic measurements such as blood pressure and pulmonary wedge pressure. Fluid loss to surgical third-space is frequently rich in protein (30–50 gm per liter) and may need to be replaced by infusion of albumin or plasmanate. Resorption of third-space fluids should be anticipated after 36–48 hours and intravenous fluids reduced to prevent volume overload. Following this period, the semi-starved, catabolic, postsurgical patient with acute renal failure should be expected to lose 0.3–0.5 kg of weight per day.

Excessive sodium intake during the oliguric period will lead to volume expansion and possibly to congestive heart failure or hypertension; whereas insufficient sodium replacement, particularly during the diuretic phase, may result in hypotension and volume depletion. Daily sodium needs are assessed by following the daily weight and clinical determinations of intravascular volume. It is useful to measure the exact electrolyte content of all available fluids to accurately replace fluid losses. Once volume is replaced, it is general practice to begin water restriction in order to prevent the development of dilutional hyponatremia. Replacement of insensible losses in the euvolemic patient should be sufficient to maintain intravascular volume.

Unless significant hypokalemia is present in the oliguric patient, potassium intake should be restricted to about 20 meq per day. To this amount may be added ongoing potassium losses, which can be quantitated. Special care should be taken to avoid hidden sources of potassium such as antibiotics and certain forms of phosphate supplements. Other measures that may be taken to avoid hyperkalemia include the prompt treatment of infection, debridement of necrotic tissue, providing nonprotein calories in the form of glucose or fat, drainage of accumulated blood, avoiding the use of old, whole, banked blood, and cleaning out the gastrointestinal tract following bleeding. Frequent serum potassium determinations are indicated in patients taking digoxin or the with internal bleeding or severe catabolic states. Patients prone either to hypo- or hyperkalemia should have frequent ECG monitoring. When hyperalimentation is combined with diuretic therapy in acute renal failure, hypokalemia may occur due to intracellular shifts of potassium.

Hypocalcemia is common and due to hyperphosphatemia, decreased renal production of the active form of vitamin D, and resistance to the skeletal effects of parathyroid hormone. Unless the patient becomes symptomatic or the serum calcium falls below 6 mg/dl, calcium supplementation is generally not recommended for patients with acute renal failure. Often, hypocalcemia can be improved by controlling hyperphosphatemia through the administration of phosphate binders, such as aluminum hydroxide or aluminum carbonate. Hypercalcemia may occur particularly during the diuretic phase of acute tubular necrosis secondary to rhabdomyolysis. Hyperuricemia, unless thought to be involved in the etiology of ARF, or if present in a patient with gout, need not be treated.

Proper nutrition plays an important role in the management of postoperative patients with acute renal failure. Protein-calorie malnutrition may lead to increased acidosis, azotemia, hyperphosphatemia, impaired wound healing, and decreased resistance to infection. Dialysis, particularly via the peritoneal route, may also result in further losses of amino acids, proteins, and water-soluble vitamins. In the noncatabolic patient with a functioning gastrointestinal tract, therapy should include moderate dietary protein restriction, a high calorie intake provided by carbohydrates and fats, and supplementation of essential amino acids. A packet of Amin Aid dissolved in 250 cc of water provides 680 kcal, the minimum adult requirement of amino acids, plus histidine. It can be given by mouth or via a nasogastric tube (starting at 20 ml/hr, then increasing to 50–75 ml/hr over the next 2–3 days). Since most of the essential amino acids are absorbed in the proximal intestine, they can even be used in patients with enterocutaneous fistulas.

Hyperalimentation should be considered in the severely stressed surgical patient, particularly following extensive trauma or when prolonged gastrointestinal dysfunction is anticipated. The volume of fluid needed to administer the 30–50 kcal/kg body weight per day required to prevent protein catabolism in the postoperative surgical patient is often considerable. In this subset of patients, however, it is probably better to combine aggressive hyperalimentation with early dialysis to avoid the debilitating effects of unbalanced metabolism. However, in these situations, an experienced hyperalimentation team is mandatory in order to avoid infections, hyperosmolality, and various disorders of electrolytes and mineral balance.

Although the data are somewhat conflicting, the use of early or prophylactic dialysis is desirable. Even if it does not reduce mortality, it allows for more leeway in the use of hyperalimentation or drug therapy. Dialysis may be performed on a daily or every other day basis. A creatinine value which should not be exceeded has not been established, but would reasonably be between 5 and 10 mg/dl.

It is difficult to define precise guidelines governing the timing of dialysis with respect to surgery in the patient with preoperative acute renal failure (61). When surgery is necessary prior to recovery of renal function, it is recommended to dialyze the patient if: fluid, electrolyte or acid-base disturbances are present and unresponsive to conservative management; depressed mental status, uremic bleeding, or pericarditis are present; or if progression of renal insufficiency is such that the need for dialysis would be likely within 24 hours postoperatively. For a given level of serum creatinine, one would be more aggressive in performing dialysis preoperatively in the patient with multiple metabolic derangements or about to undergo major surgery than in the patient with less extensive abnormalities.

The hypercatabolic patient with acute renal failure secondary to multiple trauma or abdominal catastrophe should receive hemodialysis since even continuous peritoneal dialysis is often unable to correct the severe metabolic disorders seen in such patients. Hemodialysis is more efficient and, therefore, more effective than peritoneal dialysis in correcting metabolic abnormalities in the catabolic patient. Its disadvantages result from the need for anticoagulation, greater hemodynamic stresses, and requirement for vascular access. A peritoneal catheter may be placed during abdominal surgery if the need for dialysis is anticipated in the immediate future (62). Peritoneal dialysis is simpler and more widely available but may be complicated by atelectasis, pneumonia, hyperglycemia, and peritonitis. It is preferred in patients with an unstable cardiovascular status, and with head injuries or bleeding since systemic heparinization is unnecessary. Antibiotics may be added to the dialysis solution in the presence of intra-abdominal infection. Recent abdominal surgery or the presence of vascular grafts are relative contraindications to peritoneal dialysis, but, if needed, the catheter should be placed under direct vision rather than by the percutaneous route. Peritoneal lavage has not been shown to benefit patients with severe acute pancreatitis (63).

Continuous arteriovenous hemofiltration (61) (CAVH) is a new extracorporeal therapy (64–65) whereby fluid, electrolytes and small- to medium-sized solutes can be removed by ultrafiltration continuously for days or weeks at a time. Its principle advantage lies in its ability to correct or prevent hypervolemia in hypotensive, hemodynamically unstable patients. It is important to realize that a fixed urine output of 1–2 liters per day may not be adequate to prevent hypervolemia in a patient with postoperative ARF receiving hyperalimentation, pressors and multiple medications. Such patients frequently receive 3–5 liters of fluid per day. CAVH, if started early when the creatinine is relatively low (~3.0 mg/dl), may offer the potential to decrease the mortality in postoperative ARF (2, 65) by allowing full nutritional support and positive energy balance.

Strict attention to all other aspects of therapy, including prevention or prompt treatment of infection, gastrointestinal bleeding, and appropriate tailoring of drug therapy are also important in the care of the patient with postoperative acute renal failure.

THE EVALUATION AND MANAGEMENT OF PATIENTS WITH CHRONIC RENAL FAILURE

Epidemiology

Operations commonly performed in patients with renal failure include: vascular access procedures, parathyroidectomy, pericardiectomy, nephrectomy, and renal transplantation. In patients with mild to moderate renal insufficiency, although fluid and electrolyte disturbances are common, the most serious complication is the superimposition of acute renal failure. Uremic patients also have impairments of wound healing, hemostasis, and immunity. Nevertheless, recent experience dictates that even major surgery can be performed on dialyzed patients with relative safety (66–68). The mortality rate in a series reported by Brenowitz (69), encompassing 31 hemodialysis patients undergoing 40 elective and 9 emergency operations, was 4%. Although intraoperative complications, such as bleeding, directly attributable to uremia were unusual, postoperative problems developed in more than 60% of their patients. Hemodialysis within 24 hours was required in 63%, mainly for treatment of hyperkalemia. The development of postoperative hyperkalemia seemed to be related to the use of blood transfusions rather than the preoperative potassium level. Fistula thrombosis, pneumonia (primarily with gram-negative organisms), and wound infections were relatively common. Also noted were hypotensive episodes not related to fluid losses. Others have also reported an increased incidence of wound dehiscence.

Evaluation

In patients with chronic renal failure of an established etiology, the diagnostic process should be directed at establishing the degree of impairment and documenting the existence of uremic abnormalities (70–73). Part of this evaluation should include a search for conditions that might aggravate existing renal failure such as volume depletion or the use of nephrotoxic drugs. When renal insufficiency is newly discovered, elective surgery should be postponed and the patient evaluated to establish the etiology. The severity of renal impairment should be determined by measurement of serum creatinine and a timed creatinine clearance.

In general, serum electrolyte concentrations are only mildly affected until late in the course of renal failure. Hyponatremia usually results from the administration of hypotonic fluids. The presence of hyperkalemia is often precipitated by volume depletion, catabolic states, acidosis, and excess potassium administration. The development of hyperkalemia should also suggest gastrointestinal bleeding or internal hemorrhage. Most patients with renal failure maintain a serum bicarbonate of ≥15 meq/L. A further reduction in bicarbonate levels should suggest the presence of a superimposed acidosis. If hypermagnesemia is found, all medications should be examined for hidden sources of magnesium such as may be contained in many of the commonly used antacids.

The evaluation of the azotemic patient's volume status is made on the basis of the physical examination, changes in body weight, urine output, or possibly by invasive monitoring. This will usually provide sufficient information as to the status of intravascular volume in patients with mild renal insufficiency. In more advanced cases, in patients who might not tolerate fluid challenges, or in those patients who are expected to have large volume losses or shifts during surgery, the use of a Swan-Ganz catheter is appropriate. Since the usual criteria of volume depletion applied to the urinary electrolytes presuppose normal kidney function, the use of urinary indices such as the sodium concentration osmolality or fractional excretion of sodium are of lesser value in the patient with established renal disorders.

The presence of a generalized bleeding diathesis should not be attributed to uremia unless other commonly encountered causes, such as disseminated intravascular coagulation, can be ruled out. Finding a normal bleeding time makes it unlikely that uremia is contributing to the bleeding problem.

Management

The most clearly defined risk in patients with abnormal kidney function is the development of superimposed acute renal failure. Therefore, a major focus in the preoperative management is to obtain optimal renal perfusion (74). The goals of fluid therapy should be to replenish prior volume deficits are assessed by clinical and laboratory means, the replacement of ongoing losses, and provision for daily metabolic needs. As renal function declines, it becomes more critical for the components of the fluid therapy to reflect the actual losses. This is best accomplished by measuring the volume and electrolyte contents of urine or other body fluids being lost externally.

There are many other details of management that require special attention in patients with chronic renal failure. Adequate nutrition is important in alleviating uremic symptoms and in ensuring proper wound healing in the postoperative period. The type of dietary management depends chiefly on the degree of renal insufficiency. In general, only those patients with advanced renal insufficiency (creatinine clearance of less than 30 ml/min) have significant biochemical abnormalities or clinical manifestations warranting specific dietary therapy. Many patients with a diagnosis of renal disease are reflexively placed on "renal failure" diets, which are often interpreted to mean severe salt and protein restriction. Such a diet may lead to volume depletion and negative protein balance. The role of protein restriction to prevent the progression of renal insufficiency is currently a subject of intense investigation; however, most patients with mild to moderate renal insufficiency do not require protein restriction to relieve symptoms of the uremic syndrome. In more advanced cases, a 40–60 gram protein diet may be useful.

When protein restriction is necessary, particularly when reduced to less than 40 grams per day, essential amino acids or high biologic value proteins must be provided, along with an adequate caloric intake (2000–3000 cal/day) in the form of carbohydrates and fats to prevent negative nitrogen balance. Most often, dialyzed patients are not protein-restricted. Those patients with moderate to advanced renal insufficiency do best on a 4–6 gram salt diet unless they have edema, congestive heart failure, or hypertension, at which time either a loop diuretic, such as furosemide, can be added or salt intake restricted further. Patients who cannot be fed should be hyperalimented prior to and after major surgery. The development of prerenal azotemia indicates that salt and volume restriction is too severe for any given patient.

Potassium restriction in the stable patient is generally not necessary as long as urine output is adequate. Care must be taken, however, to avoid potassium-sparing diuretics or potassium-containing drugs, such as most phosphate supplements, some penicillin preparations, or salt substitutes. ACE inhibitors may also precipitate hyperkalemia in patients with renal insufficiency. Most patients will not require water restriction unless hyponatremia develops. Keeping a patient NPO without an intravenous (IV) line in place may predispose to volume depletion in patients with fixed salt losses.

Hypertension is often present in patients with renal failure and should be controlled throughout the surgical period. Oral medications should be continued up to the evening prior to surgery. Short-acting drugs, such as parenteral hydralizine, may be required to maintain normotension until oral intake is resumed. Patients with stable, minimal elevations of blood pressure may do well without parenteral supplementation. Congestive heart failure, when related to volume overload, should be treated with salt restriction, afterload reduction, or diuretics rather than digitalis. Volume overload should be corrected, if possible, prior to surgery. However, some degree of edema is preferable to volume depletion.

The chronic anemia present in most patients with renal failure is well tolerated, and attempts to transfuse preoperatively in most instances are unwarranted (69). Exceptions include patients with a hematocrit of less than 20%, patients with coronary artery disease and a hematocrit less than 25%, or patients in whom large intraoperative blood losses are anticipated. In most series, patients with stable hematocrits of between 20 and 30% tolerated surgery well without transfusions. Reasons not to transfuse include the precipitation of volume overload or hyperkalemia. Frozen, washed, or leukocyte-poor, packed red blood cells should be used to avoid large potassium loads and sensitization of potential transplant recipients. Blood should be given in advance of the final preoperative dialysis when possible in order for excess potassium to be removed.

The use of prophylactic antibiotics is generally discouraged (70). In one series, they did not prevent postoperative pneumonia although the incidence of wound infections was slightly reduced (69). Prophylactic dialysis in patients with borderline renal function has not been shown to affect morbidity or mortality and should not be performed in the absence of specific indications such as medically unresponsive fluid overload, uremia, or pericarditis. One should anticipate, however, that the additional metabolic stress of surgery may require the use of postoperative dialysis. Surgery in these patients, therefore, should only be performed in hospitals with dialysis capabilities.

Dialysis in the chronically dialyzed patient is generally performed 24 hours in advance of elective surgery in order to improve electrolytes and platelet function (75). Even a brief 2–3 hour dialysis prior to emergency surgery is useful in correcting preoperative electrolyte disturbances. Dialysis can be performed using either regional heparinization (heparin is neutralized by the infusion of protamine after leaving the dialyzer) or "low-dose" heparin infusions. Patients with chronic Tenckhoff catheters for peritoneal dialysis can continue to use their catheters postop, in most cases.

Intraoperative management should include the careful infusion of potassium-free fluids, as well as the replacement of any fluid or blood losses. There is no convincing evidence to support the use of intraoperative mannitol or furosemide in the prevention of postoperative acute renal failure in patients with prior renal disease. Careful positioning of the fistula arm and the avoidance of hypotension are helpful in reducing the incidence of vascular access thrombosis. Frequent monitoring of the ECG and blood chemistries in prolonged operations is necessary for the early detection of electrolyte disturbances. Due to the prolonged effects of neuromuscular relaxants and CNS depressants in the uremic patient, extubation should not be rushed and should only be performed in the presence of the anesthetist. Reintubation in the postoperative period is an all too common but usually avoidable occurrence. During the immediate postoperative period, serum electrolytes should be obtained every 6 to 12 hours in the seriously ill patient. Hourly urine outputs should be recorded as well as daily weight. Because even regional or minimal heparinization may increase the rate of hematoma formation, dialysis is usually delayed for at least 24–48 hours, if possible. Administration of Kayexalate enemas (when not contraindicated) and the careful administration of fluids often keeps patients in electrolyte balance.

Sutures are often left in place for several additional days due to the uremic patient's impaired wound-healing. Respiratory therapy is an important part of the postoperative management in reducing the incidence of pneumonia. Removal of indwelling Foley catheters and central or peripheral IV lines as soon as possible should help reduce the incidence of infection.

Platelet dysfunction, secondary to uremia, often contributes to prolonged bleeding from the gastrointestinal tract or at wound sites. When dialysis fails to improve hemostasis, cryoprecipitate (10 bags) or DDAVP (0.3 micrograms/kg in 50 ml normal saline intravenous over 30 minutes) may be useful in reducing an abnormal bleeding time (67A, 76). Both result only in transient improvement in the bleeding time, with the beneficial effect over by 18 and 8 hours respectively. Cryoprecipitate has a peak effect around 10 hours, while the peak effect with DDAVP is between 1–4 hours. These agents may be useful prophylactically in uremic patients with prolonged bleeding times about to undergo procedures likely to be complicated by bleeding, such as renal or lung biopsy.

Special Considerations

DRUG THERAPY IN THE AZOTEMIC PATIENT

Epidemiology

The frequency of adverse drug reactions is increased to 25% in the azotemic patient, as compared to 9% in patients with normal renal function (78). Drug side effects in patients with reduced GFR can be divided into two subgroups: those which adversely affect kidney function, and those which lead to systemic reactions. Drug nephrotoxicity can be induced by: direct tubular damage (aminoglycoside antibiotics), interstitial nephritis (methicillin), glomerulonephritis (penicillamine), alterations in renal blood flow (ACE inhibitors, non-steroidals) or by intrarenal crystal deposition (methoxyflurane) (7). Systemic effects may be related to abnormally high drug levels (furosemide otoxicity) or increased sensitivity in uremia (CNS depression with narcotics).

Abnormalities of drug metabolism with renal failure include prolonged half-life of renally excreted drugs or active metabolites, alterations in bioavailability, volume of distribution, or protein binding. Decreased absorption of orally administered drugs may occur with nausea, vomiting, or by competition from phosphate binding gels.

Evaluation

It is incumbent on the physician to properly adjust the dosage or frequency of renally-excreted drugs in the presence of abnormal kidney function. Quantitation of both renal and hepatic function is crucial in selecting the proper drug dosage. Elderly patients, even though they have "normal" serum creatinine concentrations, have an age-related decrease in glomerular filtration rate and, therefore, should be treated as carefully as patients with kidney failure.

Management

Alterations to compensate for renal dysfunction include a reduction of dosage or a lengthening of the interval between administrations. In either situation, a normal loading dose should be given to achieve immediate effective levels. Monitoring of the patient should include measurement of blood levels (peak and trough) and observing the patient carefully for side effects. Excellent reviews are available providing complete prescribing information for most drugs in patients with renal insufficiency (79, 80). This section will deal only with those drugs likely to be used in the perioperative period.

Non-narcotic Analgesics

The use of aspirin is generally avoided since it aggravates platelet dysfunction. Nonsteroidal analgesics may be used although moderate reduction in dosage may be required. However, nonsteroidals are known to produce reversible decreases in glomerular filtration rate, particularly in the presence of volume depletion, and have occasionally been implicated in the development of acute interstitial nephritis.

Narcotics

Most of the narcotics including codeine, meperidine, morphine, and pentazocine are hepatically metabolized, but doses may have to be reduced because uremic patients tend to be sensitive to their CNS-depressant effects. Prolonged usage of meperidine has been reported to cause twitching and seizures due to retention of metabolites (81).

Barbiturates, Sedatives, and Hypnotics

Short-acting hepatically metabolized barbiturates, such as pentobarbitol, are preferred over phenobarbitol. Barbiturates are best avoided altogether since they affect the metabolism and alter the protein binding of many drugs. Diazepam is a better alternative when sedation or tranquilization is necessary. Flurazepam is an effective and relatively safe form of sleeping medication.

Anesthetics

Most of the commonly used inhalational agents, such as cyclopropane and halothane, can be used for major surgery in patients with renal failure. Methoxyflurane and enthrane are nephrotoxic and should not be used in patients with chronic renal failure. Succinylcholine may be used as a muscle relaxant; however, it is known to cause an increase in serum potassium. Intravenous and spinal anesthesia should be used whenever deemed appropriate.

Diuretics

The thiazide diuretics should not be used with the onset of moderate renal insufficiency (GFR less than 30 ml/min) since they lose their effectiveness and also reduce renal blood flow. Potassium sparing diuretics (spironolactone, triamterene, or amiloride) are contraindicated in patients with chronic renal insufficiency due to their potassium-retaining effects. Furosemide continues to be effective even in advanced renal insufficiency although higher dosages must be used. The use of prolonged, high-dose, and particularly intravenous furosemide may be complicated by the development of ototoxicity. Ethacrynic acid is also effective in advanced renal failure but has a higher incidence of ototoxicity than furosemide. Metolazone acts synergistically with the loop diuretics, and is effective even in advanced renal failure.

Antihypertensives

Most antihypertensive drugs are administered in the usual dosage. Guanethidine lowers renal blood flow and should be avoided. Intravenous nitroprusside can be used for control of malignant hypertension in patients with mild renal failure but duration of therapy should be brief (<12–24 hours) and levels of its toxic metabolite, thiocyanate, need to be monitored. Nitroprusside should be avoided in moderate to severe renal failure or in combined renal-hepatic diseases because of the risk of cyanide toxicity. Beta-blockers, such as propranolol, may be used in the usual dose. The dosage of some newer beta-blockers (e.g., atenolol, nadolol) should be reduced, since they are excreted by the kidney. Although serum creatinine and creatinine clearance remain virtually unaltered with propranolol, a recent report revealed a significant decrease in inulin clearance (82).

Cardiac Drugs

The digoxin maintenance dose should be reduced in patients with renal insufficiency. The loading dose remains unchanged. Since digoxin drug dosages in renal insufficiency are only approximated by nomograms, digoxin levels need to be monitored. Additional digoxin need not be administered following dialysis. Digitoxin may be used in place of digoxin since it is mostly metabolized in the liver. Extra care must be exerted in any patient receiving digitalis to maintain normal potassium balance. Quinidine and lidocaine require no dose modifications in renal failure. The active metabolite of procainamide, N-acetylprocainamide, accumulates in renal insufficiency. Therefore, levels of both the parent drug and its metabolite must be measured in assessing procainamide therapy.

Antibiotics

Since excretion of penicillin G and most semisynthetic penicillins is by the kidney, large doses should be reduced in moderate to severe renal failure (83). An exception is nafcillin, which does not require dose reduction due to hepatic metabolism. Significant amounts of sodium are given with large doses of sodium penicillin (1.7 meq Na^+/million units) and carbenicillin (4.7 meq/gm). Potassium penicillin G contains 1.7 meq K^+/million units.

The aminoglycosides are potentially nephrotoxic and can produce vestibular and auditory problems as well. They are filtered by the glomerulus and concentrated in the proximal tubule. Early manifestations of aminoglycoside toxicity include concentrating defects, enzymuria, and proteinuria. There is some evidence that tobramycin may be less nephrotoxic than other aminoglycosides (8).

Strict attention to adjusting drug dosages by means of nomograms and monitoring of drug levels is essential in avoiding toxicity. Serum creatinine should be measured every 1–2 days in patients receiving aminoglycoside, since monitoring urine volume alone is not a reliable index of renal function in these patients as they often develop a nonoliguric form of acute renal failure. It should also be noted that the onset of renal failure can be delayed for up to 1 week following discontinuation of the antibiotic.

Significant drug toxicity can occur even when drug levels are in the therapeutic range in the presence of renal insufficiency, volume depletion, metabolic acidosis, or when other nephrotoxic agents are being used simultaneously.

Except for cephaloridine, most of the cephalosporins, including cefamandole and cefazolin, are not highly nephrotoxic. Drug dosage must be reduced in renal insufficiency, however, for some of the second or third generation cephalosporins. Cephalosporins are thought to be nephrotoxic when used in conjunction with aminoglycosides, particularly in volume-depleted patients.

Tetracycline derivatives should be avoided since they increase BUN and potentiate acidosis. Neither chloramphenicol or clindamycin require alteration of dosage in renal failure unless hepatic insufficiency coexists. Vancomycin can be used for treating staphylococcal infections in penicillin-allergic patients, but requires reduced dosage. One gram given intravenously will last approximately 7 days in the patient without significant renal function; however, monitoring of vancomycin blood levels is advisable.

Anticoagulants

Both heparin and coumadin are given in the usual dosage. Both drugs, however, may potentiate uremic bleeding disorders.

Anticonvulsants

Although the half-life of phenytoin (Dilantin) is decreased in renal failure, the usual dose tends to be effective. This is due both to the accumulation of active metabolites and reduced protein binding. It is recommended that phenytoin be administered in divided doses in renal failure patients, to avoid excessively high peak levels.

Antacids

Surgical patients often receive large doses of antacids for therapy or prophylaxis of gastrointestinal bleeding. Since magnesium excretion is impaired in renal insufficiency, the use of magnesium-containing antacids is not recommended. Aluminum-containing antacids may be used, but frequent monitoring of serum phosphate is necessary to avoid hypophosphatemia. The dose of cimetidine should be reduced to 300 mg b.i.d. and rantidine to 150 mg q.i.d. in patients with significant renal insufficiency. Cimetidine has been reported to cause an increase in serum creatinine in patients with normal renal function. This phenomena does not appear to be progressive and reverses once therapy has been discontinued (84). There is an increased incidence of central nervous system symptoms, such as agitation, confusion, and coma in patients with renal insufficiency receiving cimetidine, particularly if they are elderly.

SURGERY IN THE RENAL TRANSPLANT RECIPIENT

Epidemiology

Renal transplant recipients are more likely to be operated on than patients in the general population. Most of their complications requiring surgical solutions derive from the transplant itself or to problems related to their prior uremic state. Operations directly related to the transplanted kidney include: drainage of hematomas, lymphoceles, and wound abscesses, as well as urological procedures such as repair of leaking ureters or bladder. Surgical procedures related to immunosuppression include operations to correct steroid-induced gastrointestinal bleeding and orthopedic procedures for aseptic necrosis. Parathyroidectomy may be necessary for persistent hypercalcemia related to the prior development of secondary hyperparathyroidism. Since no direct comparisons between transplant recipients, uremics, and normal patients have been performed, the effect of a renal transplant on surgical morbidity and mortality is unclear. It is evident, however, that these patients are predisposed to unique complications arising out of their prior uremic state or from transplant immunosuppression.

Combining the results of two recent series of renal transplant recipients from Britain and the United States, 106 of 280 patients required additional surgery, excluding transplant nephrectomy (85, 86) (Table 11.12). In the U.S. series, 32% of the patients requiring additional surgery had multiple procedures. The majority of

Table 11.12.   Surgical Experience in Two Groups of Renal Transplant Recipients

	Leapman et al. (United States) Numbers (%)	Bakkaloglu et al. (Britain) Numbers (%)
Transplant recipients	162	118
Transplants performed	202	132
Patients operated	67 (41)	39 (33)
Elective procedures	62 (60)	30 (46)
Emergency procedures	41 (40)	35 (54)
Mortality	20 (30)	0
Acute renal failure	1 (0.02)	0

procedures were related directly to the transplant itself or to the complications of immunosuppression. The British group routinely treated their patients with 100 mg of hydrocortisone for 4 days, whereas the U.S. group did not augment the dose of steroids. Neither group reported complications attributable to hypoadrenalism. Only one patient in the combined series who already had severely compromised renal function showed any further deterioration. Although the British reported a 0% mortality rate, 20 patients died in the U.S. group's experience at an average of 2 months (1 day to 1 year) following surgery. The majority of deaths were related to sepsis. Urologic surgery tended to carry the poorest prognosis.

Management

Although many patients with successful transplants have "normal" creatinine levels, it is unusual for the creatinine clearance to exceed 70 ml/min. Therefore, all the precautions outlined in the management section of patients with chronic renal insufficiency should be observed. The tailoring of drug dosages and maintenance of adequate volume are of particular importance. Antibiotics should only be used when specifically indicated and should be based on gram stain or culture results. Indwelling lines should be changed frequently or removed if possible. Additional steroid may be required at the time of surgery to prevent manifestations of adrenal insufficiency.

FLUID, ELECTROLYTE, AND ACID-BASE DISTURBANCES IN THE PRE- AND POSTOPERATIVE PATIENT

Fluid, electrolyte, and acid-base disturbances in surgical patients have several unique features as compared to those seen in their medical counterparts. Firstly, disturbances of body composition tend to be more complex and severe, largely due to the nature of surgical disorders and their therapies (87). For example, burns, major trauma, and GI disorders such as intestinal obstruction result in fluid, electrolyte, and acid-base problems, which may be further complicated by the use of potent diuretics, nasogastric suction, or bowel diversion. In addition, the postoperative state itself has the potential for inducing changes in body fluid composition or renal function (88).

The second important consideration is the effect of body fluid disturbances on the proposed anesthesia and surgery. Since fluid and electrolyte disturbances often alter cardiovascular or neuromuscular function, they increase the risk of intraoperative hypotension, life-threatening arrhythmias, and influence the need for postoperative ventilatory assistance. Table 11.13 summarizes the clinical significance of fluid and electrolyte abnormalities in surgical patients and provides rational recommendations for their management with specific reference to the preoperative patients.

Hyponatremia

EPIDEMIOLOGY

Hyponatremia is among the most commonly encountered electrolyte disturbances in surgical patients. The pathophysiology of hyponatremia is relatively uncomplicated. It must either develop from an intake of water exceeding the ability of the kidney to excrete it, or the loss of

Table 11.13. Preoperative Disorders of Fluid, Electrolyte, and Acid-Base Balance and Their Management

Conditions	Clinical Significance	Recommendation
I. Volume disorders		
A. Hypovolemia	Predisposes to hypotension, renal failure	Restore volume to normal
B. Hypervolemia	Predisposes to intraoperative pulmonary edema with hypoxemia and acidosis	Restore volume to normal
II. Electrolyte disorders		
A. Sodium	Often associated with abnormalities of intravascular volume	Assess volume status and restore to normal
		Serum sodium concentration should be between 135–145 meq/L prior to elective surgery, but may be between 130–150 meq/L for emergency surgery
1. Hyponatremia	Produces cellular edema Often associated with dilution or volume depletion	Water restriction (intraoperatively)
2. Hypernatremia	Most have both water and salt depletion	Correct both water and salt depletion
B. Potassium	Associated with arrhythmias, muscle weakness, and ileus	Serum potassium should be between 3.5–5.0 meq/L before elective surgery and 3.0–5.5 meq/L for emergency surgery
1. Hypokalemia	Potentiates digitalis toxicity	Oral replacement preferred
2. Hyperkalemia	Succinylcholine may further aggravate hyperkalemia in burn or trauma patients	Maintain ventilation intraoperatively
	Acidosis and transfusions may result in worsening of hyperkalemia	Monitor electrolytes and ECG See text for discussion of management
C. Calcium		
1. Hypocalcemia	Produces tetany, seizures, and change in mental status Rapid correction of acidosis may precipitate tetany Potentiates neuromuscular effects of hyperkalemia	Postpone surgery if serum calcium is less than 7.5 mg/dl, even if patient is asymptomatic
2. Hypercalcemia	Frequently associated with volume depletion Potentiates digitalis toxicity Predisposes to pancreatitis, renal failure, nephrolithiasis, arrhythmia, and changes in mental status	May operate in asymptomatic patients with mild hypercalcemia (less than 12 mg/dl) if volume depletion and immobilization avoided Postpone surgery with calcium greater than 12 mg/dl
D. Phosphorus		
1. Hypophosphatemia	When severe (less than 1 mg/dl), may lead to respiratory failure, seizures, coma, cardiomyopathy, and increased affinity of hemoglobin for oxygen	Serum phosphorus of less than 1.5 mg/dl should be corrected preoperatively
2. Hyperphosphatemia	Clinical manifestations secondary to hypocalcemia or metastatic calcification	Not an indication by itself to postpone surgery

Table 11.13. *Continued*

Conditions	Clinical Significance	Recommendation
E. Magnesium		
1. Hypomagnesemia	Hypokalemia and hypocalcemia frequently coexist	Postpone surgery if serum magnesium less than 1 meq/L
	Potentiates digitalis toxicity	
	Causes arrhythmia, seizures	
2. Hypermagnesemia	Causes depressed mental status, respiratory muscle paralysis, conduction disturbances	Postpone surgery if level exceeds 5 meg/L
III. Acid-base disorders		
A. Metabolic acidosis	Severe acidosis results in decreased cardiac output, unresponsiveness to catecholamines, arrhythmias	Correct acidosis if pH is less than 7.25 or bicarbonate is less than 16 meq/L preoperatively
	Reduced buffering capacity results in diminished ability to buffer further acid challenges	Maintain appropriate degree of hyperventilation intraoperatively
	Failure to maintain compensatory hyperventilation under anesthesia results in worsening acidosis, hyperkalemia, and arrhythmias	Correct volume abnormalities
		Follow serum potassium closely
	Often associated with volume depletion	
B. Metabolic alkalosis	Frequently associated with volume depletion and hypokalemia	Correct volume depletion with normal saline
	May contribute to arrhythmias, shift of hemoglobin dissociation curve to left	Correct coexisting hypokalemia
	Compensatory hypoventilation may interfere with weaning postoperative patients from mechanical ventilators	
C. Respiratory acidosis	Risk factor for postoperative respiratory failure	Delay elective surgery until underlying cause corrected
	Predisposes to hyperkalemia	
D. Respiratory alkalosis	Results in lowered serum bicarbonate and diminishes body capacity to buffer acid challenge	Search for underlying cause
	Associated with hypokalemia	

salt from the body. Salt loss may lead to volume depletion, which stimulates thirst, ADH secretion, and increased proximal sodium reabsorption, resulting in increased water intake and retention. Thus, as can be seen in Figure 11.2, water retention is the usual final common pathway leading to the development of hyponatremia. It follows, therefore, that hypo-osmolality, under most circumstances, does not occur without water intake. The water intake that results in hyponatremia is often low in absolute terms, but excessive relative to the volume of free water that can be excreted. Hidden sources of water in surgical patients include the increased water of oxidation in catabolic patients, dextrose and water used as a vehicle for

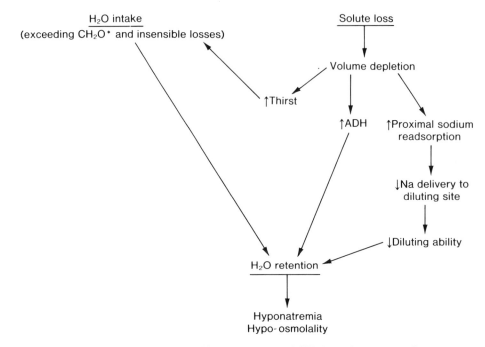

Figure 11.2. Pathophysiology of hyponatremia. *CH_2O = free water clearance.

drug administration (50–100 cc per dose), heparinized solutions used to maintain the patency of arterial lines and Swan-Ganz catheters, and decreased insensible water losses via the lungs in patients on mechanical ventilators.

Hyponatremia is almost always secondary to physiologically induced impairment of renal dilution rather than a primary disturbance in ADH secretion. The majority of conditions producing a low-serum sodium are associated with a low-serum osmolality as well. Hypo-osmolality results in the intracellular movement of water and cellular edema, which is responsible for the clinical manifestations of hyponatremia. Hyponatremia may occasionally be associated with a normal or increased effective serum osmolality and is commonly referred to as "pseudohyponatremia." Pseudohyponatremia may be associated with either no fluid shifts (hyperproteinemia, hyperlipidemia) or intracellular dehydration (hyperglycemia, mannitol administration).

Effective serum osmolality may be cal-

culated from the following formula: effective serum osmolality $= 2\ (Na^+) + glucose/18 + mannitol/18$. The BUN is excluded from the calculation because it does not cause osmotically induced water redistribution. The normal range for effective osmolality is between 280–290 mOsm/kg of H_2O. Serum osmolality may also be measured directly by freezing point depression.

Serum osmolality is regulated chiefly by the hypothalamic-pituitary axis via the action of ADH on the kidney, and by the control of thirst. The body defends itself against hypo-osmolality by inhibiting thirst and ADH secretion, thereby decreasing water intake and producing a dilute urine. A maximally dilute urine for clinical purposes is one with an osmolality of less than 100 mOsm/kg of H_2O. The expression "free water clearance" (C_{H_2O}) represents the quantity of solute-free water excreted during the process of urinary dilution.

ADH secretion is normally determined by changes in the serum osmolality. However, several other important stimuli also affect its release. Chief among these non-osmotic stimuli is a perceived decrease in circulatory volume such as occurs with hemorrhage, isotonic fluid losses, congestive heart failure, or other edematous states. When hypovolemia is severe, the volume stimulus will predominate, resulting in persistent ADH secretion despite a low serum osmolality. Additionally, the increased proximal sodium reabsorption due to volume depletion with decreased sodium delivery to the diluting sites impairs urinary dilution and also contributes to water retention. Emotion, pain, certain drugs (morphine, barbiturates, anesthetics), and the metabolic response to surgery further enhance the stimulus of ADH secretion in the postoperative patient.

As a general rule, hyponatremia can only be maintained if there is a defect in free water excretion, since the normal kidney can excrete 15–20 liters per day of solute-free water. Free water clearance will be diminished by those conditions which lead to either a decreased generation of free water at the diluting site in the ascending limb of Henle or enhanced permeability of the collecting ducts to water as summarized in Table 11.14. Persistent secretion of ADH in response to non-osmotic stimuli is the most common cause for the diminished free water clearance found in hyponatremic patients.

Table 11.14.   Factors Diminishing Free H$_2$O Excretion

I. Decreased generation of free water at diluting site
  A. Decreased Na$^+$ and H$_2$O delivery to diluting site
    1. Renal failure ($\downarrow$ GFR)
    2. Effective volume depletion
  B. Decreased Na$^+$ and Cl$^-$ reabsorption at diluting site
    1. Diuretics
II. Enhanced H$_2$O permeability of collecting ducts
  A. Presence of ADH
  B. Cortisol deficiency (primary or secondary)

Administration of hypotonic fluids in the presence of non-osmotic stimulated secretion of ADH is responsible for the common occurrence of hyponatremia in postoperative patients. Chung (89) prospectively studied 1088 operative procedures and found a 4.4% incidence of postoperative hyponatremia. Euvolemic hyponatremia (42%) was the most common cause of postoperative hyponatremia. Edematous states (21%), hyperglycemia (21%), hypovolemia (8%), and renal failure (8%) accounted for the rest. Postoperative hyponatremia was generally mild (P$_{Na}$ > 125 meq/L) and developed in the first 24 hours. Normovolemic hyponatremia usually resolved by the end of the first week, while edematous patients tended to remain hyponatremic for a longer period of time. Hyponatremia did not affect surgical mortality. Hyponatremia may occasionally be associated with convulsions, respiratory arrest, and permanent brain damage after elective surgery (90). Most of the patients with this syndrome (90) were females, with postoperative syndrome of inappropriate secretion of ADH (SIADH) who received excessive hypotonic fluids without frequent monitoring of electrolytes.

SIGNS AND SYMPTOMS

The symptoms of hyponatremia are nonspecific and generally involve the central nervous system (disorientation, anorexia, nausea) or musculoskeletal (cramps) systems. Many patients remain asymptomatic. Physical findings are also nonspecific and may involve temperature regulation (hypothermia) or neurological function (altered mental status, seizures, pathological reflexes, Cheyne-Stokes respiration, pseudobulbar palsy, and, rarely, focal deficits). The severity of neurological symptoms depends on both the absolute level of serum sodium, as well as the rate of change. Signs and symptoms are usually mild or absent when serum sodium concentration is greater than 120 meq/L, variably present between 110–120 meq/L, and usually severe when less than 110 meq/L. An acute fall in serum sodium produces more severe symptoms than a gradual decline for any given serum sodium. Truly asymptomatic patients with very low-serum sodium concentrations should suggest the possibility of pseudo-hyponatremia.

DIAGNOSIS

Diagnosing the cause of hyponatremia is best approached by making a clinical assessment of the intravascular volume status as previously described (91). Recall that the serum concentration does not correlate with total body sodium stores or the volume of the intravascular or extracellular spaces. The history should be reviewed for sources of solute or water loss or gain, intravenous therapy, and medications. Laboratory determinations of serum sodium, potassium, chloride, bicarbonate, urea nitrogen, creatinine, glucose, uric acid, osmolality, and urine sodium (U_{Na}), and osmolality (U_{Osm}) should be obtained prior to therapy. Once pseudo-hyponatremia has been excluded, correct determination of volume status based on the complete clinical picture will limit the diagnostic considerations in each category as listed in Table 11.15. When doubt exists whether the patient is hypo- or euvolemic, a cautious fluid challenge with normal saline will usually solve the problem. The approach to hyponatremia is summarized in Figure 11.3.

In surgical patients, certain electrolyte patterns will help pinpoint the etiology of the hyponatremia. When metabolic acidosis is associated with a normal- or low-serum potassium, diarrhea or fistula drainage may be the source of electrolyte loss. A high bicarbonate due to metabolic alkalosis associated with normal- or low-serum potassium should suggest nasogastric suction or diuretic use. A BUN less than 10 mg/dl is found so infrequently in adults without liver disease or starvation

Table 11.15. Differential Diagnosis of Hyponatremia

I. Pseudohyponatremia
  A. Isotonic
    1. Hyperproteinemia
      a. Multiple myeloma
      b. Macroglobulinemia
    2. Hyperlipidemia
  B. Hypertonic
    1. Hyperglycemia
    2. Mannitol
    3. Glycerol
II. Hypovolemic hyponatremia
  A. Renal loss
    1. Diuretics[a]
    2. Adrenal insufficiency
    3. Salt-losing renal disease (medullary cystic disease, postobstructive diuresis, diuretic phase ATN)
    4. RTA with bicarbonaturia
  B. Extrarenal
    1. GI loss (vomiting, diarrhea) with hypotonic replacement[a]
    2. Third space (pancreatitis, burns, muscle trauma)[a]
    3. Skin (excess sweating with hypotonic replacement)
III. Euvolemic hyponatremia
  A. SIADH
  B. Psychogenic polydipsia
  C. Hypothyroidism
  D. Glucocorticoid deficiency
  E. Reset osmostat
  F. Drugs (thiazides, chlorpropamide, morphine, barbiturates, antipsychotics, acetaminophen, isoproteronol, indomethacin, cyclophosphamide)[a]
  G. Pain[a]
  H. Emotion
  I. Salt loss with hypotonic replacement resulting in euvolemia[a]
IV. Hypervolemic hyponatremia (edema)
  A. CHF[a]
  B. Cirrhosis[a]
  C. Nephrotic syndrome
  D. Renal failure[a]

[a] Common in surgical patients.

that when present in a hyponatremic patient, it should suggest the syndrome of inappropriate ADH secretion (SIADH). The combination of hyponatremia and hypouricemia should also make one think of SIADH. Psychogenic polydipsia or liver disease may also result in the combination of hyponatremia and hypouricemia.

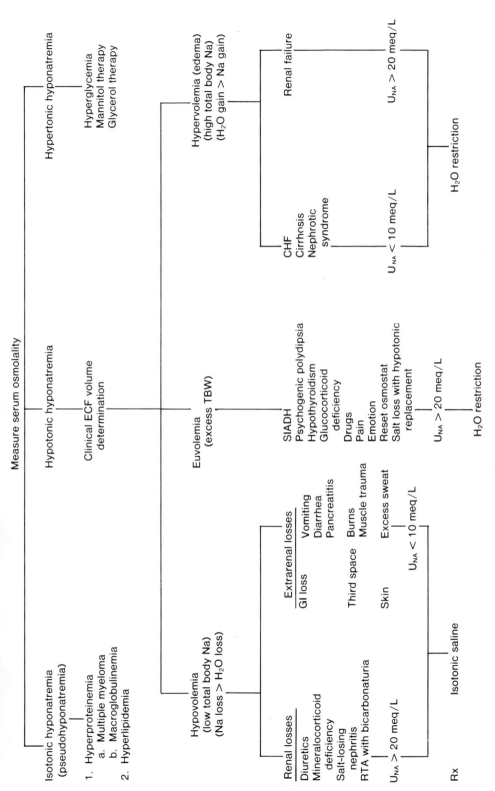

Figure 11.3. Clinical approach to hyponatremia.

Extracellular volume depletion, on the other hand, can result in increased urate reabsorption and hyperuricemia. Determination of the urinary sodium concentration (U_{Na}) is useful in supplementing the clinical determination of intravascular volume. This is because the urinary sodium is mainly determined by the effective circulating volume. Diagnostic use of urinary sodium is valid if renal tubular function is normal. Volume depletion with a low urinary sodium suggests an extra-renal cause of hypovolemia. A high urinary sodium in a volume-depleted patient suggests renal salt loss as a cause. Urinary sodium concentration in the hyponatremic patient who is euvolemic is variable and dependent on dietary salt intake. The urinary osmolality is only moderately helpful in the diagnosis of hyponatremia since renal free water excretion is impaired in most hyponatremic conditions. This diminished free water excretion is associated with an impairment in the ability of the kidneys to maximally dilute the urine ($U_{Osm} < 100$ mOsm/kg of H_2O). Urinary osmolality in most hyponatremic disorders will be hypertonic to plasma but may be isotonic or mildly hypotonic ($U_{Osm} = 150–250$ mOsm/kg of H_2O) and does not necessarily imply the presence of SIADH. Patients with psychogenic polydipsia or essential hyponatremia are the major exceptions where U_{Osm} may be maximally dilute despite the presence of hyponatremia.

The syndrome of inappropriate ADH has five principle features: *(a)* hyponatremia with hypoosmolality; *(b)* $U_{Na} > 20$ meq/L; *(c)* absence of clinical evidence of volume depletion; *(d)* U_{Osm} less than maximally dilute; and *(e)* normal cardiac, renal, adrenal, and thyroid function. A water load test (20 ml/kg of body weight given over 15–20 min) is not needed if all the cardinal features are present. A normal person will excrete 80% or more of the ingested water within 4 hours and lower his urine osmolality to less than 100 mOsm/kg of H_2O (see also p. 299).

Edematous patients usually do not have serum sodium concentrations less than 125 meq/L until end-stage hepatic or cardiac dysfunction occurs. Values for serum sodium below this level with less severe disease may be due to superimposed problems such as diuretics, vomiting, or compulsive water drinking.

MANAGEMENT

Treatment of hyponatremia depends on the underlying cause, the level and duration of hyponatremia, and the presence or absence of symptoms. Arieff's study showed a 50% mortality in acute hyponatremia of less than 12 hours duration with only a 12% mortality in chronic symptomatic patients (92). None of the deaths in the chronic symptomatic group were directly related to hyponatremia per se. Chronic asymptomatic hyponatremia was associated with a 0% mortality.

The treatment of hyponatremia begins with the correct assessment of the patient's volume status. The goal of therapy is to correct both the hyponatremia and any underlying causes.

Hypovolemic hyponatremia is treated with normal saline. In this situation, correction of the hyponatremia results from: *(a)* sodium retention and *(b)* increased free water excretion resulting from decreased ADH secretion secondary to volume repletion. In hemodynamically stable patients with severe or symptomatic hyponatremia, hypertonic saline may occasionally be used. In this situation, calculation of the sodium deficit is estimated by the following equation:

$$\text{Sodium deficit} = 0.6 \times \text{body weight (kg)} \times (\text{desired serum [Na]-actual serum [Na]})$$

Three percent hypertonic saline contains 514 meq of sodium per liter and infusing 70 meq per hour will raise the serum sodium concentration approximately 2 meq/L/hr in a 70 kg person with normal total body water.

Hyponatremia in edematous patients with congestive heart failure, cirrhosis, or nephrotic syndrome is treated with sodium and water restriction. Loop diuretics may sometimes be useful in this situation due to their ability to decrease urine-concentrating ability, resulting in an increased free water clearance.

Hyponatremia in euvolemic patients is treated by water restriction and correction of underlying causes (hypothyroidism, glucocorticoid deficiency, drugs, pain, or conditions associated with SIADH). Severe (serum sodium <110–115 meq/L) or symptomatic (seizures, coma) should be treated with hypertonic saline and furosemide. The rationale behind using hypertonic saline plus furosemide is to quantitatively replace diuretic induced electrolyte losses (Na+, K+). This results in the net excretion of free water. Urinary and serum electrolytes should be monitored frequently, initially every 2 hours, to assure proper corrections and prevent hypokalemia. This is most safely performed in an intensive care unit. The volume of excess free water that needs to be excreted to correct hyponatremia in a patient with SIADH is given by the following formula:

$$H_2O \text{ EXCESS} = .6 \times \text{body weight (kg)} \times \left[1 - \frac{P_{Na} \text{ actual}}{140} \right]$$

The recommended rate of correction of severe hyponatremia is still controversial. The controversy centers around whether severe hyponatremia per se or its overly rapid correction leads to central pontine myelinolysis, a rare disorder characterized by quadriplegia, impaired swallowing and pseudobulbar signs. At the present time, most experts would recommend increasing the serum sodium by 2 meq/L/hr until the serum sodium reaches 120–125 meq/L. This should be followed by water restriction to allow evaporative and urinary losses to restore the sodium level to normal over the ensuing days.

Hypernatremia

PHYSIOLOGY

Hypernatremia most often develops as a result of excess water (hypotonic fluid) losses or inadequate water replacement of normal losses. Only rarely is it due primarily to the gain of excess sodium. Excess water may be lost via the kidneys, gastrointestinal tract, or as insensible losses through the skin and lungs. The presence of a tracheostomy promotes pulmonary water loss up to 1–1.5 liters/day if continuous humidification of the air is not used. Fever and burns also result in increased insensible water loss.

Most patients with hypernatremia have a combined water and sodium loss with the water loss exceeding that of sodium. The greater the degree of sodium loss, the more likely one encounters signs of volume depletion. Such losses occur with an osmotic diuresis from glucose, mannitol, or urea. High protein intake from tube feedings may result in an osmotic diuresis from urea production. Excess sweating may also result in hypotonic fluid losses. Loss of gastrointestinal secretions results in isotonic volume depletion, and hypernatremia results only if water intake is less than normal. Iatrogenic hypernatremia associated with sodium depletion may occur in patients receiving diuretics if water intake is inadequate.

Pure water loss from central or nephrogenic diabetes insipidus is not commonly encountered in the general surgical setting. Approximately 50% of the cases of central diabetes insipidus are idiopathic, the remainder are due mostly to head trauma, hypoxic encephalopathy, hypophysectomy, and neoplasms. Acquired nephrogenic diabetes insipidus may occur with electrolyte abnormalities (hypercalcemia, hypokalemia) and with interstitial forms of renal disease. Certain drugs (lithium carbonate, demeclocycline, enthrane, methoxyflurane, and amphotericin) may also produce nephrogenic diabetes insipidus.

Hypernatremia due to sodium excess is much less frequently seen. The most common cause is the administration of sodium bicarbonate during cardiac arrests or for therapy of severe metabolic acidosis.

The development of hypernatremia is most likely to occur when access to water is limited. This commonly will occur in the hospitalized patient who is debilitated or confined to bed by intravenous lines, catheters, or casts.

Hypernatremia is always associated with hyperosmolality and intracellular volume depletion. Intravascular volume, on the other hand, may be high, low, or normal. The degree of cellular shrinkage is dependent on the degree as well as the rate of development of hypernatremia. In the chronic states of hypernatremia, intracellular water loss is minimized by the creation of "idiogenic" osmoles, which tend to restore intracellular volume.

SIGNS AND SYMPTOMS

Hypernatremia is often asymptomatic and may be first detected with routine electrolyte studies. When present, symptoms of hypernatremia result from intracellular dehydration and include thirst, muscle weakness, and neurological symptoms such as lethargy, stupor, coma, and seizures. Symptoms are related both to the level and the rate of change of the serum sodium concentration. Experimental studies in rabbits showed neurological symptoms developed when plasma osmolality exceeded 350 mOsm/kg of H_2O. Signs of intravascular volume depletion due to pure water loss are not common unless the serum sodium is greater than 170 meq/L since the intravascular volume sustains only 5–8% of any pure water loss. Combined water and salt losses will manifest themselves with hypotension at lower serum sodium levels.

DIAGNOSIS

The diagnostic approach to hypernatremia is based on the determination and interpretation of the urine osmolality (U_{Osm}) as outlined in Figure 11.4. In the presence of an increased serum sodium concentration (serum osmolality greater than 290 mOsm/kg of H_2O), the normal renal response should be a urine osmolality greater than 800 mOsm/kg of H_2O. A urine osmolality less than this in a hypernatremic patient represents a defect in ADH release or effect. Hypernatremia with a urine osmolality greater than 800 mOsm/kg of H_2O suggests that sodium excess, increased insensible losses, or inadequate intake of free water is responsible for the hyperosmolar state.

Patients with central diabetes insipidus or severe nephrogenic diabetes insipidus usually have a urine osmolality less than 300 mOsm/kg of H_2O. When the urine osmolality is between 300–800 mOsm/kg of H_2O, the most likely causes of hypernatremia are partial central diabetes insipidus, complete central diabetes insipidus with volume depletion, acquired nephrogenic diabetes insipidus, or osmotic diuresis. When the diagnosis of diabetes insipidus is entertained, water restriction in conjunction with pitressin administration (water deprivation test) will help establish whether the defect is central or renal in origin (see p. 205). Water deprivation tests should be delayed until after correction of electrolyte abnormalities and after the patient is clinically stable.

Osmotic diuresis may occasionally result in a urine osmolality greater than 800 mOsm/kg of H_2O. Even though the urine has a high osmolality, an osmotic diuresis is characterized by high urine output. Measuring the urinary glucose, urea, mannitol, or sodium concentration will determine which osmole is responsible for the process.

MANAGEMENT

Despite a high-serum sodium concentration, the patient with severe hypovolemia and hypernatremia should be treated with normal saline initially if hemody-

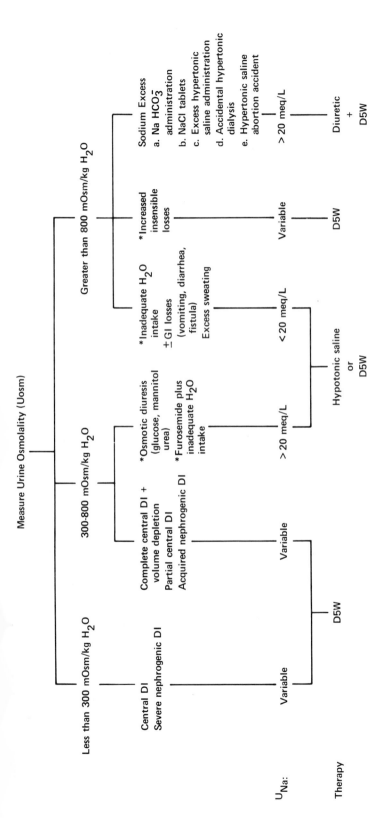

Figure 11.4.   Clinical approach to hypernatremia. DI, diabetes insipidus. *Common in surgical patients.

namically unstable. This is then followed by hypotonic saline or D5W. Hypernatremia due to pure water loss is treated by administering D5W. Hypernatremia associated with sodium excess is treated with diuretics and D5W. An estimate of the free water deficit should be made in all patients with the aid of the following equation:

$$H_2O \text{ deficit} = 0.6 \times \text{body weight (kg)}$$
$$\times \left[1 - \frac{140}{\text{actual serum (Na)}} \right]$$

One-half the calculated deficit should be given in the first 8–12 hours and the remaining deficit corrected over the subsequent 24–48 hours. Maintenance fluids and replacement of ongoing abnormal losses must also be administered simultaneously. In severe symptomatic hypernatremia, serum electrolytes should initially be repeated every 2 hours and less often as the situation improves. The serum sodium should not be corrected more vigorously due to the danger of cerebral edema. Since clinically significant water shifts require a brain-to-plasma osmolality gradient of approximately 30–35 mOsm/kg of H_2O, plasma osmolality should be lowered by more than this in any 4–6 hour period. This corresponds to a maximum reduction of sodium concentration in the first 4–6 hours of 15 meq/L or about 2 meq of sodium per liter per hour.

Patients with complete central diabetes insipidus will also require ADH administration (see "Endocrine Disorders"). Thiazide diuretics may be useful in chronically reducing the urine output of patients with nephrogenic diabetes insipidus by producing contraction of the extracellular fluid volume.

Hypokalemia

EPIDEMIOLOGY

Of the disorders of potassium balance, hypokalemia is seen more frequently than hyperkalemia in surgical patients with normal renal function. The most common conditions predisposing to hypokalemia in these patients include: vomiting, nasogastric suction, inadequate potassium intake, the use of polystyrene sulfonate (Kayexalate), diuretics, and insulin.

PHYSIOLOGY

Potassium homeostasis represents a balance between intake, excretion (renal excretion accounts for 90% of potassium elimination from the body), and transcellular shifts. Decreased intake by itself is rarely the sole cause of potassium depletion but often contributes to the magnitude of the deficit. Tissue injury, acidosis, and catabolism result in the release of potassium from cells that may subsequently be excreted in the urine. Substantial amounts of potassium may be lost in the stool with or without diarrhea. Transcellular shifts affect the concentration but not total body potassium content. Alkalosis results in potassium movement into cells, and acidosis causes potassium to move out of cells. Insulin, and possibly aldosterone, also cause potassium to shift into cells.

When hypokalemia results from extrarenal losses, the renal excretion of potassium falls within 4–10 days to below 20 meq/day, and the spot urinary potassium concentration (U_K) should be less than 10–15 meq/L. Renal potassium wasting (24-hour excretion greater than 20–30 meq) is seen more often as a response to physiological stimuli (alkalosis, hyperaldosteronism) or diuretic use than from primary kidney disease. Hypomagnesemia results in increased potassium excretion by an unknown mechanism. Hypomagnesemia should be suspected in hypokalemic surgical patients receiving gentamicin hyperalimentation or in those suffering from malabsorption.

Hypokalemia produces an increased resting cellular transmembrane potential (hyperpolarization) and results in decreased membrane excitability. This accounts for the clinical manifestations of hypokalemia, which include muscle weakness and cardiac arrhythmias. The effect of any given decrease in serum potassium is augmented by the rapidity of the fall, hypercalcemia, and alkalosis.

It should be noted that the serum potassium and ECG findings only roughly correlate with total body stores. A deficit of approximately 100–200 meq will lower the serum potassium from 4 to 3 meq/L, and every 1 meq/L fall thereafter reflects another 200–400-meq deficit. Continued loss in excess of 400 meq produces relatively small changes in serum potassium due to the transcellular shift out of cells. Arterial pH and the resultant transcellular potassium shift must also be accounted for in estimating the size of the deficit. Failure to estimate the size of the deficit frequently leads to underreplacement and apparent "refractory" hypokalemia.

SIGNS AND SYMPTOMS

Signs and symptoms of hypokalemia may begin to appear when the serum potassium is less than 3 meq/L but do not occur with frequency until levels fall below 2.7 meq/L. Symptomatic hypokalemia usually represents a total body potassium deficit of at least 200–400 meq. Skeletal muscle findings include cramps, tetany, weakness, and paralysis. Muscle weakness usually affects the lower extremities first, followed by the trunk, upper extremities, and respiratory muscles. Rhabdomyolysis and myoglobinuria may rarely occur. Smooth muscle dysfunction results in paralytic ileus and symptoms of abdominal distention (nausea, vomiting, constipation). Chronic potassium depletion may result in hypotension. Renal abnormalities resulting from potassium depletion include: *(a)* decreased GFR; *(b)* nephrogenic diabetes insipidus; *(c)* increased ammonia production by the renal tubules; *(d)* impaired urinary acidification; and *(e)* increased bicarbonate reabsorption. Encephalopathy may be precipitated by hypokalemia in cirrhotic patients.

The electrocardiographic changes occurring with hypokalemia include flattened or inverted T waves, prominent U waves, and ST changes.

DIAGNOSIS

The causes of hypokalemia are listed in Table 11.16. The etiology of hypokalemia often is obvious from the history. Important historical points include: loss of gastrointestinal fluid (vomiting, diarrhea, fistula, nasogastric suction), drugs, and potassium intake (both oral and IV). The physical exam should emphasize the clinical determination of intravascular volume and blood pressure. If the diagnosis is not obvious after a careful history and physical examination, measurement of simultaneous serum and urinary potassium, serum sodium, bicarbonate, creatinine, and arterial pH is usually very helpful. From a practical standpoint, the approach to hypokalemia (see Fig. 11.5) involves separating gastrointestinal from renal potassium losses. Measurement of arterial pH is helpful since these losses frequently are associated with metabolic alkalosis or acidosis. Measurement of urinary chloride concentration (U_{Cl}) and urinary pH may also be useful in the evaluation of coexisting metabolic alkalosis or renal tubular acidosis, respectively (see p. 230).

Measurement of urinary potassium excretion helps to differentiate renal from gastrointestinal losses. Diuretic therapy may confuse the interpretation of U_K regarding the site of potassium loss. Patients with diuretic-induced potassium deficiency will have a higher U_K while the diuretic is still acting, but will have a low U_K once the diuretic effect has worn off.*

---

*Since sodium depletion may limit urinary potassium excretion, a sodium intake (excretion) of 100–150 meq per day is required to properly interpret urinary potassium concentrations. Otherwise, a low urinary potassium concentration may incorrectly be interpreted as indicating extrarenal losses. Proper interpretation depends upon correlating urinary potassium concentration with 24-hour sodium excretion.

Table 11.16.   Etiology of Hypokalemia

  I. Decreased intake (oral, intravenous), prolonged administration of K^+-free fluids[a]
 II. Transcellular shift into cells
    A. Alkalosis[a]
    B. Hypersecretion of insulin (hyperalimentation)[a]
    C. Treatment of megaloblastic anemia
    D. Hypokalemic periodic paralysis
III. Increased loss
    A. Renal
        1. Associated metabolic alkalosis
            a. Hyperaldosteronism
                (1) Primary
                (2) Secondary (renin mediated)
                    (a) Edematous states (CHF, cirrhosis, nephrotic syndrome)
                    (b) Non-edematous states (Bartter's syndrome, accelerated hypertension, renal vascular hypertension, renin-secreting tumor)
            b. Cushing's syndrome
                (1) Primary adrenal disease
                (2) Secondary to non-endocrine tumor
            c. Drugs
                (1) Diuretics (loop diuretics, thiazides)[a]
                (2) Antibiotics (penicillin, carbenicillin)
                (3) Licorice ingestion
                (4) Alkali loading
        2. Associated with metabolic acidosis
            a. Renal tubular acidosis
            b. Diabetic ketoacidosis
            c. Drugs (amphotericin B, outdated tetracyclines, acetazolamide)
        3. Normal acid-base status
            a. Osmotic diuretics (mannitol, glucose)
            b. Hypomagnesemia
            c. Gentamicin
            d. ? Acute myeloid leukemia
            e. Renal salt wasting
    B. Gastrointestinal losses
        1. Vomiting[a]
        2. Diarrhea[a]
        3. Villous adenoma
        4. Intestinal fistula or tube drainage[a]
        5. Laxative abuse
        6. Ureterosigmoidostomy
        7. Obstructed or long ileal loop[a]
    C. Skin (excess sweat)

---

[a] Common in surgical patients.

Thus, hypokalemia with a low U_K (<10–15 meq/L) suggests: *(a)* the potassium deficiency probably has been present for more than a few days, and *(b)* extrarenal potassium loss is occurring most likely from the gastrointestinal tract, providing there has been no recent diuretic administration, or *(c)* sodium depletion is limiting potassium excretion. Similarly, hypokalemia with a high U_K (>10–15 meq/L) suggests *(a)* renal potassium loss, or *(b)* the potassium deficit has been present for less than 1 week.

MANAGEMENT

Potassium chloride is the usual preparation for correction of potassium deficits.

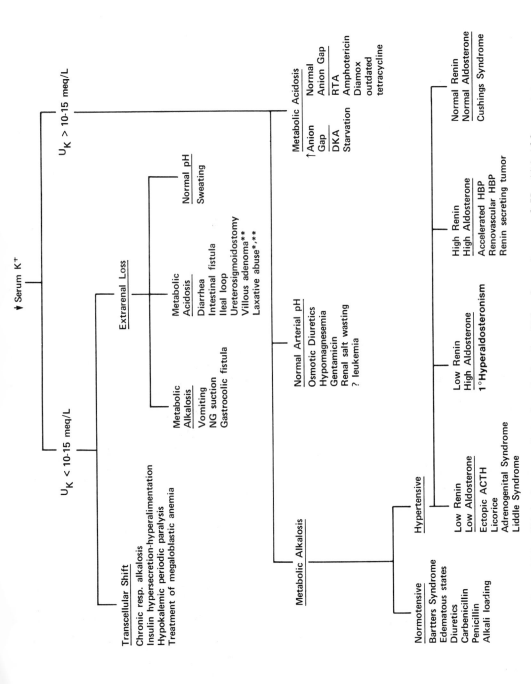

Figure 11.5. Clinical approach to hypokalemia. *May have increased U_k. **Acid-base status actually unpredictable.

The chloride is essential in the correction of any coexisting chloride-sensitive metabolic alkalosis. Beside repairing the deficit, treatment of the underlying disorder to prevent further loss should be initiated when possible. Oral treatment is preferred in mild to moderate hypokalemia, administering 80–120 meq/day (20 meq of K^+ = 15 ml of 10% KCl) in divided doses plus abnormal ongoing losses. Intravenous therapy is indicated when the patient cannot take oral medications or when severe hypokalemia is associated with serious arrhythmias (especially in the presence of digoxin therapy), muscle weakness, respiratory paralysis, rhabdomyolysis or diabetic ketoacidosis. It is best to keep intravenous replacement to less than 100–150 meq/day (or 10 meq/hr) unless life-threatening depletion is present or ongoing losses require larger amounts.

Administration through central lines should be avoided if possible due to the possible danger of transiently high local serum concentrations leading to arrhythmias or cardiac arrest. Up to 10 meq of potassium may be administered intravenously per hour without monitoring. Higher rates of administration require continuous ECG monitoring and frequent serum determinations.

More than 20 meq of potassium per hour intravenously is not recommended. The most difficult clinical situation occurs in patients with renal tubular acidosis or urinary diversion procedures into the colon in which severe hypokalemia is associated with acidosis. In these patients, correction of the acidosis by vigorous bicarbonate therapy without potassium replacement will result in severe life-threatening hypokalemia and respiratory paralysis. Therapy in these patients should include the simultaneous administration of intravenous potassium and sodium bicarbonate.

SPECIAL CONSIDERATIONS

Hypokalemic metabolic alkalosis from vomiting or nasogastric suction requires a few additional comments since this is a common occurrence in the surgical setting. Renal losses represent the major mechanism of potassium depletion in this situation. Factors contributing to kaliuresis include alkalosis, increased aldosterone secretion secondary to volume depletion and increased nonreabsorbable anion (HCO_3^-) delivery to the distal tubule. Loss of potassium contained in gastric secretion (10 meq/L) plays a minor role in determining the size of the deficit. When the total potassium deficit approaches 20% (~700 meq), hydrogen ion is preferentially secreted despite the presence of alkalosis resulting in aciduria. The finding of aciduria in a patient with metabolic alkalosis suggests severe potassium depletion.

Hyperkalemia

EPIDEMIOLOGY

Hyperkalemia in surgical patients is seen most commonly in the setting of acute renal failure. The problem is similar to that occurring in medical patients except for two important considerations. First, hyperkalemia may be more difficult to control in catabolic, postoperative patients due to the increased endogenous potassium load originating from tissue breakdown, acidosis, resorption of blood from the gastrointestinal tract or hematomas, and multiple transfusions of stored whole blood. Secondly, it may not be possible to use potassium exchange resins in patients who have undergone bowel surgery.

PHYSIOLOGY

Renal potassium excretion represents the body's major defense against hyperkalemia. Cellular uptake is of lesser importance. Sustained hyperkalemia rarely develops simply from increased intake (exogenous or endogenous) in patients with normal renal function, although abrupt increases in potassium intake (via intravenous administration) may transiently lead to the development of potentially serious hyperkalemia. Impaired renal potassium excretion is essentially the only cause of chronic hyperkalemia.

Life-threatening hyperkalemia may develop within hours of the onset of acute oliguric renal failure in postoperative, traumatized, or septic patients. Hyperkalemia in acute oliguric renal failure without these complications usually develops more slowly, appearing after 4–5 days. In the non-catabolic, anephric patient, serum potassium should not increase by more than 0.5 meq/L/day. Hyperkalemia may not develop in acute renal failure if urine output is maintained.

Patients with chronic renal insufficiency whose serum creatinine is less than 10 mg/dl or glomerular filtration rate (GFR) greater than 5–10 ml/min generally develop hyperkalemia only with excessive potassium intake (potassium rich foods, salt substitutes), acidosis, volume depletion, or the use of potassium-sparing diuretics.

SIGNS AND SYMPTOMS

The signs and symptoms of hyperkalemia are mainly limited to muscle weakness and abnormalities of cardiac conduction. Paresthesia in the arms and legs is usually the first complaint. Muscle weakness may be seen with serum potassium greater than 8 meq/L and begins in the lower extremities and ascends to the muscles of the trunk and upper extremities. Flaccid paralysis and respiratory arrest may occur.

In general, the cardiographic findings parallel the severity of the hyperkalemia; however, cardiotoxic effects can occur without premonitory clinical signs. The cardiotoxic effects of hyperkalemia are enhanced by the presence of hypocalcemia, hyponatremia, acidosis, and a rapid rise in potassium levels. Acute elevations will produce more marked effects at relatively lower serum potassium levels.

DIAGNOSIS

The differential diagnosis of hyperkalemia is listed in Table 11.17 and the suggested clinical approach to this prob-

Table 11.17. Etiology of Hyperkalemia

I. Factitious
  A. Lab error[a]
  B. Pseudohyperkalemia: *in vitro* hemolysis, improper collection of blood, thrombocytosis, leukocytosis
II. Increased input[a]
  A. Exogenous (oral or IV): KCl, salt substitutes, K^+-containing medications, transfusions of old blood[a]
  B. Endogenous: hemolysis, GI bleeding, rhabdomyolysis[a]
III. Transcellular shift out of cells
  A. Acute acidosis[a]
  B. Drugs: succinylcholine, massive digoxin overdose, arginine HCl
  C. Insulin deficiency
  D. Cellular catabolism: trauma, burns, rhabdomyolysis[a]
  E. Hyperkalemic periodic paralysis
  F. Hyperosmolality (hyperosmotic mannitol or saline infusions)
IV. Decreased renal excretion
  A. Renal failure[a]
    1. Acute
    2. Chronic (GFR < 10 ml/min)
  B. Primary tubular defect in K^+ excretion (SLE, sickle cell disease, postrenal transplantation, amyloidosis)
  C. Impaired renin-angiotensin axis
    1. Primary hypoaldosteronism
    2. Addison's disease
    3. Primary hyporeninism
    4. Tubular unresponsiveness to aldosterone
    5. ACE inhibitors
  D. Volume depletion (inadequate Na delivery to distal tubule)[a]
  E. Drugs inhibiting

$$K^+ \text{ secretion} \nearrow \text{spironolactone}$$
$$\searrow \text{triamterene, amiloride}^a$$

[a]Common in surgical patients.

lem is outlined in Figure 11.6. The history should be reviewed for: *(a)* evidence of renal disease or diabetes mellitus; *(b)* endogenous or exogenous sources of potassium; and *(c)* drugs that interfere with potassium excretion or cause transcellular shifts of potassium out of cells. The physical examination emphasizes the determination of intravascular volume, searching for the stigmata of Addison's disease, and testing muscle strength.

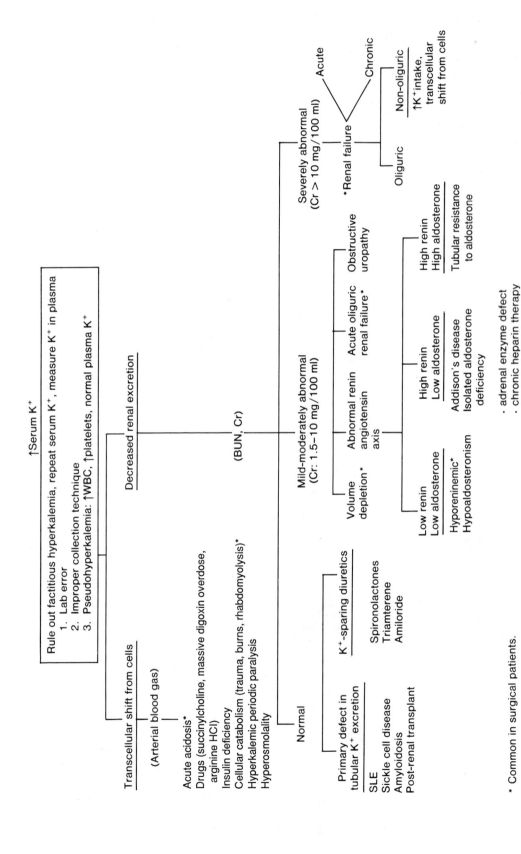

Figure 11.6. Clinical approach to hyperkalemia.

Laboratory determination of sodium, bicarbonate, creatinine, and arterial pH should be obtained.

If an unexpected elevation of potassium is found, immediately a repeat sample should be sent to rule out laboratory error and an electrocardiogram performed. A false elevation of serum potassium may be seen with a hemolyzed blood specimen or when potassium is released from clotted blood with a very high white blood cell (greater than 100,000/mm^3) or platelet count (greater than 1,000,000/mm^3). These latter two rare conditions can be excluded by checking a potassium level in heparinized blood. The difference in potassium concentrations between plasma and serum samples should be less than 0.5 meq/L. The prolonged use of a tourniquet may also falsely elevate the serum potassium. A potassium level of 7 meq/L or greater with a normal electrocardiogram should suggest the presence of pseudohyperkalemia.

After eliminating the above causes of false hyperkalemia, an arterial blood gas should be obtained to evaluate the contribution of acute metabolic or respiratory acidosis to the elevated potassium. Acute acidosis is associated with hyperkalemia.

The medication list should be checked for potassium-containing drugs. In addition to the usual potassium supplements, other drugs such as salt substitutes and phosphate supplements contain large amounts of potassium. Diuretics with potassium-sparing effects should also be sought. ACE inhibitors can also produce hyperkalemia by inhibiting angiotensin production. Impairment of renal function should be looked for next as an explanation of hyperkalemia. Hyperkalemia out of proportion to the degree of renal dysfunction should suggest mineralocorticoid deficiency. Hyporeninemic-hypoaldosteronism is more common than Addison's disease and is commonly found in diabetics or patients with some type of tubulointerstitial renal disease. Hyperchloremic metabolic acidosis may also be present in such patients. This entity can be screened for by measuring stimulated plasma renin activity, aldosterone, and morning plasma cortisol levels (see p. 292).

MANAGEMENT

The aim of management is to correct both hyperkalemia and its underlying cause. The presence of significant electrocardiographic changes due to hyperkalemia is an indication for immediate therapy because the development of fatal cardiac toxicity is often unpredictable. The type of therapy used will depend on the absolute level of serum potassium concentration, how rapidly it is rising, whether the source of potassium can be removed, and most importantly, the type of ECG changes present and the patient's renal function.

In general, a serum potassium concentration between 5.5–6.5 meq/L with only T wave changes may be treated by potassium restriction and potassium exchange resins (Kayexalate). In postoperative patients who are often catabolic, volume-depleted, hemorrhaging, or receiving blood transfusions, therapy may be started even sooner. Under these circumstances, treatment with the above measures may be initiated if the potassium concentration is rising and reaches 5 meq/L.

When the serum potassium concentration is between 6.5–7.0 meq/L, measures which shift potassium into cells should be started. Glucose and insulin infusions will start to have an effect in 10–30 minutes, while sodium bicarbonate administration will have an onset of action in less than an hour. Sodium bicarbonate will be effective, independent of its effect on blood pH.

Serum potassium concentrations greater than 7.0 meq/L and/or ECG changes showing loss of P waves or widening of the QRS complex requires immediate aggressive intervention. Calcium should be given intravenously and is immediately effective in reversing the electrophysiological effects of hyperkalemia. Calcium administration should be immediately followed by infusion of glucose, insulin, and sodium bicarbonate.

None of the treatments which shift potassium into cells reduces total body potassium. An attempt at removing potassium from the body should be initiated as soon as possible. Potassium removal from the body can be achieved by using sodium exchange resins (Kayexalate) or dialysis. Loop diuretics are generally of little value, particularly if renal function is impaired. Dialysis is rarely needed for correction of hyperkalemia alone. It is usually used in patients with severely impaired renal function when volume overload and acidosis coexist. Peritoneal dialysis may not be efficient enough in potassium removal in severely catabolic patients. Hemodialysis, which is much more effective in potassium removal, must then be used. Table 11.18 summarizes the various modalities available to treat hyperkalemia.

The use of succinylcholine should be avoided in the presence of extensive third-degree burns, massive soft tissue injury, or certain neurologic diseases, since this group of patients is exceptionally sensitive to the hyperkalemic effects of this drug.

Hypercalcemia

EPIDEMIOLOGY

Hypercalcemia is most frequently seen in surgical patients being prepared for parathyroidectomy or in patients with malignancy. Hypercalcemia can be worsened by immobilization and volume depletion, both common in surgical patients.

PHYSIOLOGY

Calcium in the extracellular fluid is found in three forms: *(a)* ionized, −50%; *(b)* protein-bound, −40%; and *(c)* non-ionized, ultrafiltrable, −10%. Only the ionized form is biologically active. Albumin is the major serum protein binding calcium. Total serum calcium parallels serum albumin. For each 1 gm/100 ml change in

serum albumin, there is roughly a 0.8-mg/100 ml change in protein bound calcium in the same direction.

Proper blood drawing technique is important when measuring serum calcium. A tourniquet left on for 2–3 minutes may increase the total calcium by 0.5–1.5 mg/100 ml. This results from protein-free fluid leaving the capillaries, resulting in local hyperalbuminemia and increased total serum calcium.

Calcium excretion by the kidney on a normal intake averages between 250–300 mg/24 hours. Calcium absorption parallels sodium reabsorption in the proximal tubule and loop of Henle but not in the distal tubule. This is important clinically because conditions that promote renal sodium reabsorption (volume depletion) will also promote calcium reabsorption. Similarly, volume expansion will result in increased renal excretion of both calcium and sodium. Both PTH and vitamin D result in decreased renal calcium excretion. Cancer-related hypercalcemia may be due to bone destruction from metastasis or the production of bone resorbing tumor products (PTH or PTH "like" substance, prostaglandins, osteoclast activating factor).

SIGNS AND SYMPTOMS

The signs and symptoms of hypercalcemia depend on the rapidity of onset, prior general condition of the patient, and underlying disease (renal CNS). They are summarized in Table 11.19.

DIAGNOSIS

The differential diagnosis of hypercalcemia is listed in Table 11.20. Malignancy (lung, breast, myeloma) and primary hyperparathyroidism account for the vast majority of cases of hypercalcemia. The hypercalcemia of malignancy is generally more severe and more rapid in onset than primary hyperparathyroidism. Chronic hypercalcemia of several years duration, without the appearance of new signs or symptoms, is more likely to be due to

Table 11.18.   Treatment of Hyperkalemia

Mechanism	Administration	Onset	Duration	Comments
I. Antagonism of cardiotoxic effects				
A. Calcium gluconate (10%)	1 amp (10 cc) IV over 2–3 min—may repeat q 5 min × 2 if EKG changes persistent or infusion: 2–3 amps in 1 L D5W	1–5 min	30 min	Contraindicated in patient on digoxin
B. Hypertonic saline (5%)	250 ml IV over 30–60 min	1 hr	1–2 hr	May cause volume overload
II. Enhanced K^+ entry into cells				
A. Glucose and insulin	500 ml D10W over 30 min plus 10 units regular insulin IV or 50 cc of D50 over 5–30 min plus insulin	30–60 min	2–4 hr	Use 1 unit reg. insulin per 5 gm glucose Use D50 when renal failure and volume overload a problem
B. Na HCO_3 (44.5 meq)	1 amp IV over 5 min may repeat q 5–10 min × 2 or 2 amps + 1000 cc D10 + 10 unit insulin infuses over 1–2 hr	30–60 min	1–2 hr	Especially useful when acidosis is present; subsequent doses determined by cause and severity of metabolic acidosis; can produce volume overload
III. K^+ removal from body				
A. K^+ exchange resins (sodium polystyrene sulfonate)	po: 20–50-gm resin + 20 cc 70% sorbitol may repeat q 4 hr for total 4–5 doses enema: 50–100 gm resin + 50 cc 70% sorbitol in 150–200 cc H_2O repeat enema q 2–4 hr as required	1–2 hr	4–6 hr	Sorbitol required to prevent constipation; enema must be retained for 30–60 min to be effective; each enema may decrease serum K^+ by 0.5–1 meq/L; side effects: Na^+ retention, nausea, constipation
B. Dialysis	Peritoneal hemodialysis	Minutes after starting	Few hours after terminating dialysis	Useful for catabolic surgical/trauma patient when G.I. tract cannot be used to accept resins Hemo can remove more K^+ than peritoneal; 25–50 meq K^+/hr *vs.* 10–15 meq K^+/hr

primary hyperparathyroidism than occult malignancy. Primary hyperparathyroidism may coexist with malignancy. Thus, the presence of a known malignancy and hypercalcemia does not necessarily imply a causal relationship. Immobilization should be considered as a cause in bedridden patients with a high rate of bone turnover (children, adolescents, those with Paget's disease). A suggested approach to the work-up of hypercalcemia in outline form is listed in Table 11.21.

Table 11.19.   Signs and Symptoms of Hypercalcemia

A. General: somnolence, lethargy, weakness
B. Gastrointestinal: anorexia, nausea, vomiting, constipation, abdominal pain, peptic ulcer, pancreatitis
C. Renal: polydipsia, polyuria, nephrolithiasis, nephrocalcinosis, renal failure
D. Neurological: stupor, coma, psychotic behavior, visual abnormalities, hyporeflexia, myopathy, occasionally localizing signs, modest increase in CSF protein
E. Cardiac: shortened QT interval, loss of ST segment, and widening of T wave leads to prolonged QT interval with "cove-like" appearance, bradycardia, tachycardia, digitalis sensitivity, arrhythmias, hypertension
F. Skeletal: pain, fractures, skeletal deformities, loss of height
G. Miscellaneous: volume depletion, calcinosis, band keratopathy
H. Signs and symptoms of associated endocrinopathies: Zollinger-Ellison syndrome, pheochromocytoma, medullary carcinoma of thyroid, pituitary and adrenal tumors

Table 11.20.   Differential Diagnosis of Hypercalcemia

I. Lab error[a]
II. Malignancy[a]
III. Primary hyperparathyroidism[a]
   A. Isolated
   B. Part of MEA syndrome
IV. Granulomatous disease
   A. Sarcoidosis
   B. Tuberculosis
V. Ingestions
   A. Milk alkali syndrome
   B. Thiazide diuretics
   C. Vitamins D, A
   D. Calcium supplements
   E. Ca^{2+}-containing antacids (Tums)
   F. Tamoxifen, estrogen, androgen (breast carcinoma)
   G. Lithium
VI. Hyperthyroidism
VII. Renal failure (acute, with rhabdomyolysis, chronic "tertiary" hyperparathyroidism)
VIII. Postrenal transplant
IX. Immobilization[a]
X. Adrenal insufficiency
XI. Hyperglobulinemia (normally ionized Ca^{2+})

[a] Common in surgical patients.

Table 11.21.   Evaluation of Hypercalcemia

I. Initial evaluation
   A. History: ingestions (thiazides, vitamins D, A, Ca^{2+} supplements, Ca^{2+}-containing antacids (Tums)), associated endocrinopathies
   B. Physical exam: volume status, thyroid, evidence of malignancy, stigmata of Addison's disease, or hyperthyroidism
   C. Lab
     1. Blood
       a. Na^+, K^+, Cl^-, HCO_3^-
          (1) Hypernatremia may be present in nephrogenic DI $2°$ ↑ Ca^{2+}
          (2) K^+ (Mg^{+2}) may be ↓ in hypercalcemia of any cause
          (3) HCO_3^- may be low in primary hyperparathyroidism secondary to renal HCO_3 loss; may be ↑ in cancer-related hypercalcemia not mediated by PTH; ? mechanism
       b. BUN/Cr: almost all hypercalcemic patients are volume-depleted; hypercalcemia may cause renal damage
       c. $Ca^{2+} \times 2$: repeat to rule out lab error
       d. $PO_4^{-2} \times 2$
          a. May be low in primary or ectopic hyperparathyroidism
          b. Suspect coexisting primary hyperparathyroidism when low in breast carcinoma
       e. Alkaline phosphatase
          1) May be hepatic or bone origin
          2) Elevated alkaline phosphatase from bone without evidence of osteitis fibrosa on x-rays of bones makes primary hyperparathyroidism less likely
       f. Albumin/globulin
          1) Required to properly interpret serum Ca^{2+}
          2) Initial step in detection of dysproteinemia
       g. Serum protein electrophoresis
          1) Monoclonal spike of myeloma

Table 11.21. *Continued*

2) Diffuse hyperglobulinemia of sarcoid
3) Increased α_2-, β-globulins in hyperparathyroidism

   h. PTH (RIA)
1) COOH-terminal assay is best assay in differential diagnosis of hypercalcemia when primary hyperparathyroidism is a consideration (↑ in 95% of patients with primary hyperparathyroidism)
2) Cancer with ectopic PTH production → PTH C-terminal fragment normal or mildly elevated
3) Low or undetectable with hypercalcemia unrelated to PTH excess

  2. Urine
    a. Urinalysis
1) Hematuria may suggest hypernephroma, renal calculi
    b. 24-hr urinary Ca^{2+}
1) Probably not required if no history of renal calculi
2) Will be low in volume-depleted patients or patients with impaired renal function

  3. X-rays
    a. Chest x-rays: may detect bronchogenic carcinoma, lymphoma, sarcoidosis, resorption of acromioclavicular joints (primary hyperparathyroidism)
    b. Flat plate of abdomen: nephrocalcinosis rare in cancer hypercalcemia and suggests primary hyperparathyroidism
    c. Skull: punched out lesions of myeloma, "salt and pepper" appearance of primary hyperparathyroidism
    d. Hands: subperiosteal reabsorption of primary hyperparathyroidism
    e. X-rays of abnormal areas on bone scan or symptomatic areas

  4. Bone scan: looking for metastatic disease
  5. ECG: look for changes due to hypercalcemia

II. Second order of evaluations
  A. Blood
    1. Thyroid function tests → hyperthyroidism
  B. X-rays
    1. IVP: hypernephroma
    2. No need to do GI series in absence of iron deficiency anemia or positive stool guaiac or symptoms pointing to GI tract since gastrointestinal malignancies are an uncommon cause of hypercalcemia
  C. Biopsy
    1. Bone marrow aspirate and biopsy: myeloma, lymphoma, granuloma, metastatic tumor
    2. Abnormal tissue, including bone

MANAGEMENT

Management of hypercalcemia involves general supportive measures, treatment of hypercalcemia itself, and treatment of the underlying disorder. Serum calciums equal to or greater than 13 mg/dl usually require immediate reduction, even without symptoms, to prevent soft tissue calcification, renal failure, and disturbances of CNS function. Moderate hypercalcemia (serum calciums between 11–13 mg/dl) without symptoms does not require immediate reduction, and the aim is usually to lower serum calcium in 12–24 hours. The presence of coexisting hyperphosphatemia probably warrants prompt treatment at even lower levels of elevation of serum calcium.

Hydration with normal saline (lactated Ringer's solution contains calcium) is the most important initial step in treating the hypercalcemic patient. Most of these patients are already volume-depleted secondary to vomiting, decreased intake, hypercalcemia-induced nephrogenic diabetes insipidus, and sodium diuresis. Only after the patient is well-hydrated and urine output adequate should furosemide be given for its calciuretic effect. It is crucial to maintain intravascular volume for this method to work since hypovolemia leads to increased calcium absorption in the proximal tubule and will decrease calcium excretion. Furosemide should be given intravenously in a dose of 40–80 mg and repeated as needed to maintain the urine output between 200–500 cc/hr. Potassium and magnesium need to be replaced because deficits of these electrolytes are commonly present in hypercalcemic patients of any cause, in addition to their ongoing urinary losses resulting from the vigorous diuresis. Frequent (every 2–4 hr) monitoring of serum and urinary electrolytes will help guide sodium, potassium, and magnesium replacement. A CVP catheter or a Swan-Ganz catheter is indicated in most of these patients to guide fluid therapy. Forced diuresis will not be successful in patients with significant intrinsic renal impairment.

Mithramycin, which acts by inhibiting RNA synthesis necessary for PTH-induced bone resorption, may be given if significant hypercalcemia exists after hydration and furosemide. It may be used regardless of the etiology of hypercalcemia. Glucocorticoids may be effective in hypercalcemia secondary to myeloma, adrenal insufficiency, vitamin D intoxication, sarcoidosis, or tuberculosis. However, its onset of action is delayed about 48–96 hours. Calcitonin is probably never the drug of first choice except in hypercalcemia associated with Paget's disease. Tolerance may develop after hours or days and it is less effective than mithramycin or phosphate in malignancy. Still, since it is such a safe drug, little is lost by using it early in addition to forced diuresis in the treatment of severe hypercalcemia.

Diphosphonates are a class of drugs that inhibit the rate of bone formation and appear to be a promising form of therapy for treatment of hypercalcemia (93). Intravenous phosphate should probably be reserved for situations where other methods fail or are contraindicated since it may lead to soft tissue calcification. However, in severe symptomatic hypercalcemia which does not respond to the above measures, intravenous phosphate will predictably decrease serum calcium within minutes. The maximum decline in serum calcium may be delayed as long as 5 days and some hypocalcemic effect may persist for 5–15 days. It is not necessary to repeat the dose of phosphate within 24 hours, and generally no more than two doses is required. The serum calcium should have reached its nadir and begun to rise before repeating the second dose of phosphate. Significant hyperphosphatemia (5–6 mg/100 ml) is a contraindication to phosphate therapy, as is a rising creatinine or oliguria. Complications (hypotension, hypocalcemia, acute renal failure) from intravenous phosphate therapy have been seen when large doses have been given rapidly (100 mmol over 3–4 hr). Using a smaller dose of intravenous phosphate over a longer period of time (50 mmol over 6–8 hr) and carefully monitoring serum calcium and phosphorus should avoid these complications.

Oral phosphorus (1–3 gm/day) may be used to treat chronic hypercalcemia. The lowest effective dose should be used to keep serum phosphorus <5.5 mg/dl, in order to minimize soft tissue calcification. All oral preparations can cause diarrhea, but hypotension or hypocalcemia does not occur with this route of administration.

Hemodialysis may occasionally be useful when diuresis is not possible or ineffective in patients with renal failure (94). Its hypocalcemic effect is likely to be transient and may sometimes be followed by a rebound hypercalcemia.

Indomethacin (75–150 mg/day) may also be tried in the treatment of chronic hypercalcemia due to cancer. Its effect is related to prostaglandin inhibition. Table 11.22 summarizes drugs useful in the treatment of hypercalcemia.

Hypocalcemia

EPIDEMIOLOGY

Hypocalcemia following thyroidectomy is uncommon but may occur due to the inadvertent removal of the parathyroid glands, infarction of the parathyroid glands due to interference with their blood sup-

Table 11.22.   Drugs Useful in Treatment of Hypercalcemia

Drug	Dose	Adminis-tration Frequency	Route	Onset Hypocalcemic Effect	Complications	Contraindications
Furosemide and saline	40–200 mg	1–2 hr	IV push	Immediate	Hypovolemia; hypokalemia; hypomagnesemia	Impaired renal function; digoxin intoxication
Mithramycin	25 μg/kg	24–48 hr	IV push	24–48 hr	Hemorrhage; hepatocellular necrosis; azotemia, proteinuria	Thrombocytopenia; severe renal dysfunction; severe hepatic dysfunction
Phosphate (50 mmol/L)	1.5 gm	24 hr	IV over 6–8 hr	24 hr	Hypotension; hypocalcemia; soft tissue calcification	Hyperphosphatemia with severe renal impairment
Calcitonin	4–8 MRC U/kg 8 MRC U/kg	12 hr 6 hr	IM, subcut IM, subcut	2–3 hr 2–3 hr	None serious	None except allergy
Steroids (hydrocortisone)	100–150 mg	12 hr	IV	48–96 hr	Hypokalemia; Na retention	GI bleeding; glucose intolerance
Prednisone	40–60 mg	24 hr	P.O.	48–96 hr	Hypokalemia; Na retention	GI bleeding, glucose intolerance

ply, or increased skeletal calcium uptake. Hypocalcemia in this situation usually develops within 24 hours postoperatively. Transient hypocalcemia frequently occurs after removal of parathyroid adenomas due to atrophy of the remaining glands.

Massive and rapid transfusions of citrate-containing blood (5-10 units) may result in hypocalcemia due to calcium binding by citrate. This is more likely to occur in the presence of liver disease where the metabolism of citrate is reduced. Patients with diffuse small bowel disorders and malabsorption may develop hypocalcemia. Subtotal gastrectomy and gastrojejunostomy may also lead to vitamin D deficiency, hypocalcemia, and osteomalacia. Acute hypocalcemia is also seen in patients with hemorrhagic pancreatitis.

Anticonvulsants are capable of producing hypocalcemia due to their stimulatory effect on hepatic microsomes resulting in increased conversion of vitamin D_3 and 25-hydroxyvitamin D_3 to biologically inactive metabolites.

Gentamicin and other aminoglycosides may result in hypocalcemia secondary to excessive urinary losses of magnesium. Hypomagnesemia (<0.8 meq/L) produces hypocalcemia by interfering with parathyroid hormone release and its action on bone. Table 11.23 summarizes the causes of hypocalcemia.

SIGNS AND SYMPTOMS

The important signs and symptoms of hypocalcemia are related to the neuromuscular system and depend on the level of serum calcium, its rate of development, and duration. Clinical manifestations of hypocalcemia include tetany, confusion, stridor, Chvostek's and Trousseau's signs. Other causes of tetany, besides hypocalcemia, are both metabolic and respiratory alkalosis, hypomagnesemia, and acute hyperkalemia.

DIAGNOSIS

The history of hypocalcemia should emphasize: *(a)* previous surgery (thyroidectomy, parathyroidectomy, gastric, or small

Table 11.23. Etiology of Hypocalcemia

I. Hypoalbuminemia (normal ionized Ca^{2+})[a]
  A. Malnutrition
  B. Hepatic cirrhosis
  C. Nephrotic syndrome
II. Hyperphosphatemia
  A. Renal failure (acute and chronic)[a]
  B. Oral or intravenous phosphate infusions
  C. Phosphate-containing enemas
  D. During therapy of leukemia
III. Hypoparathyroidism
  A. Idiopathic
  B. Surgical[a]
IV. Pseudohypoparathyroidism
V. Vitamin D deficiency
  A. Nutritional deficiency[a]
  B. Malabsorption from small bowel disease
VI. Magnesium deficiency[a]
VII. Acute pancreatitis[a]
VIII. Massive transfusion of citrated blood[a]
IX. Drugs
  A. Anticonvulsants (hydantoin, phenobarbitol)
  B. Gentamicin $-2°$ to renal Mg^{2+} loss
  C. Mithramycin
  D. Neomycin
  E. Glucocorticoids
  F. Glucagon
X. Neoplastic disorders
  A. Osteoblastic metastasis (breast, prostate)
XI. Renal tubular acidosis
XII. Healing phase of metabolic bone disease

---

[a] Common in surgical patients.

intestinal resection); *(b)* blood transfusions; *(c)* drugs (anticonvulsants, phosphates, mithramycin, aminoglycosides); *(d)* symptoms suggesting malabsorption; *(e)* alcoholism (magnesium deficiency); and *(f)* renal failure. Initial blood chemistries should include: calcium, phosphate, magnesium, albumin, BUN, creatinine, arterial blood gases, and a parathyroid hormone (PTH) level. Metastatic prostate cancer is the most common cancer-producing hypocalcemia in association with osteoblastic metastasis. Calcification of the basal ganglia on skull x-ray may be visible in hypocalcemic patients with idiopathic hypoparathyroidism. The electrocardiogram may show prolongation of the QT interval due to lengthening of the ST segment. A low albumin will reduce the total calcium without producing clinical effects.

The presence of hyperphosphatemia suggests renal insufficiency, hypoparathyroidism, or phosphate administration as the cause of hypocalcemia. Normal or low serum phosphorus suggests vitamin D deficiency or malabsorption. The serum phosphorus in magnesium deficiency is variable. Serum PTH concentration will be low in hypocalcemia due to hypoparathyroidism and high in vitamin D deficiency, malabsorption, renal failure, or pseudohypoparathyroidism. PTH concentration may be low, normal, or high in hypocalcemia due to magnesium deficiency.

MANAGEMENT

Symptomatic or severe hypocalcemia should be treated with intravenous calcium gluconate. This form is preferred over calcium chloride (which contains four times as much elemental calcium) because it may be less irritating if the solution extravasates. Calcium gluconate should be diluted with at least an equal volume of dextrose or normal saline to reduce any irritation associated with parenteral administration.

Usually two to three ampules of 10% calcium gluconate (1 amp = 10 cc = 5 meq) in 100 cc of D5W administered over a 15-minute period is sufficient to alleviate the effects of symptomatic hypocalcemia. This should be followed by an intravenous drip of calcium prepared by putting 4–6 amps of 10% calcium gluconate in 1000 cc of D5W and titrating the rate to maintain a serum calcium between 8.0–8.5 mg/100 ml. Oral calcium supplements should be started when the clinical signs and symptoms have improved. The rate of administration of calcium gluconate should not exceed 2 ml/min (200 mg of calcium gluconate = 0.92 meq of calcium). The maximum rate of administration should probably be slower (0.5 ml/min) if the patient is receiving digoxin. The serum calcium concentration needs to be monitored closely, and a total dose of 2 grams of calcium gluconate should not be exceeded without repeating the serum calcium. Asymptomatic and chronic hypocalcemia can be treated with oral calcium salts, and/or various forms of vitamin D.

There are several vitamin D preparations from which to choose. Dihydrotachysterol is a synthetic compound that undergoes 25 hydroxylation in the liver to become an analogue of 1–25 dihydroxycholecalciferol. It is three times as potent as vitamin D_2 in raising the serum calcium concentration. It also has a much more rapid onset of action than vitamin D_2, which is a definite advantage in the treatment of postsurgical hypocalcemia. Calcitriol (Rocaltrol) is the synthetically produced active form of vitamin D, 1,25-dihydroxycholecalciferol. Magnesium-containing antacids should not be used concomitantly with calcitriol due to the danger of developing hypermagnesemia.

Patients already on calcium supplements and vitamin D preparations may require surgery. Chronic renal failure patients constitute the majority of such patients encountered clinically. Vitamin D preparations presently in use have relatively long durations of action and can be safely discontinued perioperatively until the patient is able to resume oral intake. The duration of action of some common vitamin D preparations after cessation of therapy are: (a) vitamin D_2 (ergocalciferol): 6–18 weeks; (b) dihydrotachysterol: 1–3 weeks; (c) 25-hydroxy-D_3: 4–12 weeks; and (d) 1,25-dihydroxy-D_3: 3–7 days. Calcitriol is also available as an intravenous injection (Calcijex) and may be useful in surgical patients with advanced renal failure during the perioperative period.

Patients with renal insufficiency can safely have their calcium supplements withheld for several days perioperatively while monitoring the serum calcium concentration and controlling the serum phosphorus. If a patient's condition is such that oral intake or nasogastric administration will not be possible for longer periods, the calcium may be given intravenously. Maintenance intravenous therapy with 200–400 mg of elemental calcium administered continuously over 24 hours should be sufficient in most stable patients. Serum calcium should be followed initially at least daily and intravenous calcium administered if the serum calcium level falls between 8.0–8.5 mg/dl.

Patients deficient in parathyroid hormone or vitamin D should receive maintenance intravenous calcium therapy throughout the intraoperative and postoperative period until oral intake can be resumed. There is usually no need for routine calcium administration in postoperative patients unless a specific indication exists.

Hypomagnesemia

EPIDEMIOLOGY

Hypomagnesemia should be suspected in surgical patients with malabsorption, small bowel disease or resection, prolonged nasogastric suction, diarrhea, hyperalimentation, prolonged aminoglycoside use, hypocalcemia, refractory hypokalemia, refractory arrhythmias, unexplained digoxin toxicity, or a prior history of alcoholism. Magnesium deficiency should always be considered in postoperative surgical patients exhibiting neuromuscular or CNS hyperactivity, especially those with a history of alcoholism. This is especially true if the patient has a nonfunctioning gastrointestinal tract and has been on prolonged parenteral fluid therapy. Magnesium replacement should be routine in these patients. Transient hypomagnesemia on the day after an operation of any type may occur apparently as part of the metabolic response to surgery and does not necessarily indicate magnesium deficiency.

PHYSIOLOGY

Magnesium is predominantly an intracellular cation involved in various membrane and enzymatic functions. Serum magnesium (1.5–2.0 meq/L) does not correlate well with total body content of magnesium. In fact, magnesium deficiency may be present despite the presence of a normal serum magnesium. Renal magnesium excretion is a major determinant of magnesium homeostasis in the body. A transport maximum (Tm) exists for magnesium near its normal serum concentration, so that small increases in serum magnesium above normal quickly result in increased renal excretion. The kidney is also very efficient in conserving magnesium. In the presence of decreased intake or absorption, resulting in magnesium deficiency, renal excretion will decrease to less than 1/meq per day within 7 days. Decreased intake alone is thus a rare cause of magnesium deficiency but may contribute to the magnitude of the magnesium deficit when abnormal losses are occurring.

Hypokalemia and hypocalcemia frequently coexist with hypomagnesemia. Magnesium deficiency results in increased urinary potassium excretion by an unknown mechanism. Magnesium deficiency also results in decreased PTH secretion and effect of PTH on bone.

SIGNS AND SYMPTOMS

Symptomatic hypomagnesemia usually corresponds to a serum magnesium concentration less than 1 meq/L. The clinical manifestations of magnesium deficiency are somewhat difficult to define because other electrolyte abnormalities (hypokalemia, hypocalcemia) frequently coexist. Most of the symptoms of magnesium deficiency relate to neuromuscular function and altered mentation and are summarized in Table 11.24.

DIAGNOSIS

The diagnosis of magnesium deficiency depends on an awareness of those clinical conditions commonly associated with hypomagnesemia and the recognition of the resultant symptoms. The differential diagnosis of hypomagnesemia is listed in Table 11.25. Measurement of a spot urinary magnesium should be obtained in all hypomagnesemic patients when the cause is not obvious. Extrarenal causes of magnesium deficiency will be associated with a urinary magnesium excretion less than 1 meq per day provided the deficit is at least 1 week old. High renal magnesium excretion in the presence of hypomagnesemia implies that renal magnesium loss is at least partly responsible for the magnesium deficit.

Table 11.24. Signs and Symptoms of Hypomagnesemia

General:	Anorexia, nausea, weakness, apathy
Neurologic:	Altered mentation (depression, irritability, psychosis), carpal pedal spasm, tetany, muscular fibrillation, vertigo, ataxia, tremor, Chvostek's sign, Trousseau's sign, hyperreflexia
ECG:	Prolonged QT interval, broadening and decreased amplitude of T waves, ST segment shortening, arrhythmias (supraventricular, ventricular)

MANAGEMENT

Therapy of magnesium deficiency is empirical since it is difficult to estimate the size of the deficit. The amount required is actually larger than the estimated deficit because approximately half of the administered magnesium will be lost in the urine, even in the presence of a severe magnesium deficiency. Fifty per cent magnesium sulfate (1 gm/2 ml of $MgSO_4 = 8$ meq of magnesium) is the preferred form for parenteral therapy. The dose and rate of administration depend upon the clinical situation. In general, for initial treatment of severe deficiency, not more than 100 meq of magnesium should be given in any 12-hour period, and the rate should be slowed to 40–100 meq/day once symptoms subside. The rate of intravenous infusion should not exceed 1 meq/min (0.3 ml of 50% of $MgSO_4$/min). There is little danger of overtreatment in adults with normal renal function due to the large capacity of the kidney to excrete

Table 11.25.   Etiology of Hypomagnesemia

I. Decreased intake
  A. Protein calorie malnutrition (kwashiorkor disease)
  B. Prolonged intravenous therapy without magnesium[a]
  C. Chronic alcoholism[a]
II. Increased loss
  A. Gastrointestinal
    1. Malabsorption
    2. Diarrhea
    3. Excessive use of cathartics
    4. Nasogastric suction[a]
    5. Intestinal or biliary fistula[a]
  B. Renal loss
    1. Diuretic therapy
    2. Diabetic ketoacidosis
    3. Gentamicin toxicity[a]
    4. Chronic ECF volume expansion: SIADH, hyperaldosteronism
    5. Chronic alcoholism
    6. Hypercalcemia
    7. RTA
    8. Hyperthyroidism
    9. Chronic renal failure with Mg^{2+} wasting
    10. Idiopathic renal Mg^{2+} wasting
    11. Diuretic phase of acute renal failure
    12. Bartter's syndrome
    13. Certain renal diseases (hydronephrosis, glomerulonephritis)
    14. Cisplatin
III. Miscellaneous
  A. Acute pancreatitis
  B. Multiple transfusions with citrated blood
  C. Severe burns
  D. Following parathyroidectomy
  E. Hypoparathyroidism

[a] Common in surgical patients.

magnesium. However, in patients with renal insufficiency, the dose needs to be decreased.

Frequent monitoring of serum levels is mandatory. Magnesium should not be given to patients with renal insufficiency unless a magnesium deficit has been documented by serum levels. The patellar reflexes should be checked every several hours when magnesium is given parenterally and administration stopped if these reflexes disappear (Table 11.26). Not greater than 10 cc of 50% $MgSO_4$ is given intramuscularly at a time because of pain at the injection site. Less severe magne-

sium deficits can be replaced with 0.25–0.5 meq of magnesium/kg of body weight/day until serum levels become normal. Magnesium oxide (250–500 mg q.i.d.) can be given orally in patients with chronic hypomagnesemia. At this dose diarrhea usually is not a problem.

Prevention of hypomagnesemia is also important. Patients with gastrointestinal fluid losses or those on prolonged intravenous therapy should receive 10–15 meq of magnesium/day to prevent depletion.

Hypermagnesemia

EPIDEMIOLOGY

Hypermagnesemia is essentially limited to patients who have both renal insufficiency and receive magnesium-containing antacids or cathartics. On the surgical service, this occurs most commonly in patients with acute or chronic renal failure receiving magnesium antacids for gastrointestinal bleeding or via hyperalimentation fluids containing magnesium. Uncommon causes of hypermagnesemia include adrenal insufficiency, hypothroidism, and hypothermia.

SIGNS AND SYMPTOMS

The signs and symptoms of hypermagnesemia result from central and peripheral suppression of neuromuscular transmission. Changes in mental status (drowsiness, coma), decreased deep tendon reflexes, and muscle paralysis may be seen. Reflexes are regularly lost with serum magnesium levels greater than 6–8 meq/L. Respiratory paralysis may be seen with serum magnesium concentrations greater than 10 meq/L. Deep tendon reflexes disappear before respiratory paralysis occurs. Hypotension and ECG changes (prolonged PR and QT intervals, delayed AV and intraventricular conduction, sinus bradycardia, increased sensitivity to vagal stimuli) may occur. Nausea, vomiting, and soft tissue calcification are also sometimes seen. Hypermagnesemia should be suspected in lethargic,

Table 11.26. Treatment of Severe Hypomagnesemia in Adults with Normal Renal Function

Preparation	Route	Dose
50% $MgSO_4$ (8.13 meq Mg^{2+}/gm $MgSO_4$)[a]	IV	Day 1: 12 ml (6 gm = 49 meq Mg^{2+}) in 1 liter of D5W over 3 hr, followed by 10 ml (5 gm = 40 meq Mg^{2+}) in each of two 1-liter bottles of glucose-containing solution over remainder of the first 24 hr Days 2–5: 12 ml (49 meq Mg^{2+}) equally distributed in daily IV fluids
50% $MgSO_4$	IM	Day 1: 4 ml (2 gm = 16.3 meq Mg^{2+}) q2h × 3 doses, then q4h × 4 doses Day 2: 2 ml (8.13 meq Mg^{2+}) q4h × 6 doses Days 3–5: 2 ml (8.13 meq Mg^{2+}) q6h
MgO (magnesium oxide) (50 meq Mg^{2+}/gm MgO)	PO	250 (12.5 meq Mg^{2+}) to 500 mg (25 meq Mg^{2+}) q.i.d.

[a]One gram of hydrated magnesium sulfate ($MgSO_4$ $7H_2O$, MW = 246.5) contains 8.13 meq of elemental magnesium.

renal failure patients with unexplained hypotension and loss of deep tendon reflexes.

DIAGNOSIS

The diagnosis should be suspected in patients with renal insufficiency receiving magnesium-containing compounds and is confirmed by measuring serum magnesium concentration.

MANAGEMENT

Prevention is the key to management in patients with renal insufficiency. A careful review of their medications should verify that they are not receiving any antacid or cathartic that contains magnesium and are not taking similar medication at home without a physician's prescription.

The initial step in the management of magnesium intoxication involves stopping all forms of magnesium administration and giving calcium gluconate intravenously if signs or symptoms of toxicity are present. Calcium antagonizes the effects of magnesium excess, including respiratory depression, hypotension, and cardiac arrhythmias, and represents the treatment of choice in life-threatening hypermagnesemia. Ten to twenty cc's of 10% calcium gluconate administered slowly

intravenously is usually effective. If this is ineffective, or in patients with renal failure, dialysis can decrease serum magnesium to safe levels in 4–6 hours. If renal function is adequate, hydration and furosemide may be tried to enhance magnesium excretion.

Hypophosphatemia

EPIDEMIOLOGY

Of the many causes of phosphorus depletion, only a few result in severe hypophosphatemia (<1mg/dl) (95,96). The most frequent situations predisposing to profound phosphorus depletion in surgical patients include hyperalimentation (without phosphorus supplementation), refeeding of patients with protein-calorie malnutrition, and the recovery phase of severe burns. Hypophosphatemia rarely results from inadequate intake or decreased intestinal absorption except in patients receiving prolonged courses of phosphate-binding antacids (aluminum hydroxide), or alcoholism. Prolonged respiratory alkalosis, diabetic ketoacidosis, and alcohol withdrawal are also associated with severe hypophosphatemia. Modest degrees of hypophosphatemia may be seen in patients following prolonged hypothermia as used in open heart surgery.

PHYSIOLOGY

Since several species of phosphorus are present in the serum (HPO_4^{-2}, $H_2PO_4^{-1}$) and are influenced by pH, it is conventional to express concentration in terms of elemental phosphorus (mg) per 100 dl. Serum phosphorus concentration is not tightly controlled and undergoes diurnal variation. It may vary by 1–2 mg/dl over the course of a day. A fasting concentration must be obtained for proper interpretation.

Intestinal absorption of phosphorus is very efficient and varies inversely with the phosphorus content of the diet (normal range 800–1500 mg/day). The daily phosphorus requirement is 600–1200 mg/day (20–40 mmol/day).

Most of the causes of acute hypophosphatemia are due to shifts of phosphorus into cells. Anything that stimulates glycolysis (acute respiratory alkalosis, glucose and insulin administration, epinephrine) shifts phosphorus intracellurarly and may result in hypophosphatemia. Inhibition of glycolysis (acute acidosis) results in phosphorus leaving the intracellular compartment and hyperphosphatemia. Hyperalimentation without adequate phosphorus supplementation results in intracellular phosphorus sequestration by rapidly dividing cells associated with normal total body stores. The anabolic/diuretic phase of recovery from burns or the provision of a normal amount of calories to patients with protein calorie malnutrition (nutritional recovery syndrome) results in intracellular movement of phosphorus and hypophosphatemia. Patients with burns may also develop hypophosphatemia as a result of urinary losses of phosphorus when retained salt and water are mobilized during the diuretic phase.

Renal phosphorus excretion is the major determinant of phosphorus homeostasis. Volume expansion results in increased renal sodium and phosphate excretion. Metabolic acidosis, magnesium, and potassium depletion also result in increased renal phosphate excretion. Phosphorus depletion in diabetic ketoacidosis results from the combined effects of acidosis and osmotic diuresis, resulting in increased urinary phosphate loss. Phosphorus deficiency in hospitalized alcoholics is multifactorial, relating partly to poor intake, magnesium deficiency, ketoacidosis, and glucose administration.

SIGNS AND SYMPTOMS

Severe hypophosphatemia (<1 mg/dl) can lead to: *(a)* muscle weakness with respiratory failure, or congestive cardiomyopathy; *(b)* neurologic dysfunction (apprehension, confusion, coma, seizures, paresthesia, ataxia, tremors); *(c)* hematologic disorders (hemolytic anemia, decreased phagocytosis, platelet dysfunction; and *(d)* rhabdomyolysis. The diverse consequences of severe hypophosphatemia reflect the important role phosphorus plays in membrane structure and function. More moderate degrees of hypophosphatemia (1.0–2.5 mg/dl) do not usually result in noticeable symptoms. Chronic hypophosphatemia in adults may result in osteomalacia.

DIAGNOSIS

The differential diagnosis of hypophosphatemia is listed in Table 11.27. A high index of suspicion for phosphate depletion should exist for patients who are alcoholics, who are receiving hyperalimentation, or other hypertonic glucose solutions, or who are on phosphate-binding antacids (for chronic renal failure, peptic ulcer disease, or prophylaxis against gastrointestinal bleeding). In addition to the serum phosphorus, an arterial blood gas determination should be made looking for respiratory alkalosis; a urinary phosphorus concentration should be obtained to help determine the site of phosphorus loss. A urine phosphorus concentration of greater than 4 mg/dl suggests renal losses, while less than this suggests extrarenal losses.

Table 11.27.   Etiology of Hypophosphatemia

I. Decreased intake/absorption[a]
  A. Phosphate-binding antacids $(Al(OH_3)_3,$ $Mg(OH)_2)$ with dialysis or phosphate-poor diets[a,b]
  B. Hyperalimentation or prolonged intravenous therapy without[a,b] phosphorus supplementation
II. Transcellular shift into cells
  A. Severe respiratory alkalosis[a,b]
  B. Alcohol withdrawal
  C. Hyperalimentation[a]
  D. Nutritional recovery syndrome[a,b]
  E. Anabolic recovery/diuretic phase after severe burns[a,b]
  F. Recovery phase of diabetic ketoacidosis[a]
  G. Drugs: anabolic steroids
  H. Glucose infusion[b]
  I. Recovery from hypothermia
III. Increased renal PO_4 loss
  A. Primary hyperparathyroidism
  B. Secondary hyperparathyroidism
    1. Vitamin D deficiency (malabsorption)
    2. Chronic metabolic acidosis
  C. Defective renal tubular PO_4 reabsorption
    1. Fanconi syndrome
    2. Vitamin D-resistant rickets
  D. RTA
  E. K^+ depletion
  F. Mg^{2+} depletion

[a] Conditions associated with severe hypophosphatemia (<1 mg/dl).
[b] Common in surgical patients.

MANAGEMENT

Serum phosphorus, like other predominately intracellular ions, may not accurately reflect total body stores. In any hypophosphatemic patient, neither the size of the deficit nor the response to phosphorus therapy can be predicted. Therapy is thus empirical, and close monitoring of the serum phosphorus concentration is required.

The preferable way to prescribe phosphorus therapy is in millimoles for the phosphate ion or in milligrams of elemental phosphorus (rather than meq) since both are independent of pH (1 mg = 0.032 mmol). Tables 11.28 and 11.29 list suggested doses for phosphorus therapy and available preparations (97).

Oral therapy may be used in mild to moderate hypophosphatemia (>1 mg/dl) with an initial daily dose of 1–2 gm of elemental phosphorus. Milk, which contains one gram of inorganic phosphorus per quart, is a good initial therapy. Although oral therapy may produce diarrhea, it is less likely to result in hypocalcemia than intravenous administration.

Intravenous phosphorus therapy is indicated in severe hypophosphatemia (<1 mg/dl), especially if seizures, coma, or respiratory muscle weakness are present. Parenteral therapy is also required in patients who do not tolerate or absorb oral phosphate. Intravenous phosphorus therapy is potentially hazardous. Possible complications include: *(a)* hyperphosphatemia; *(b)* hypocalcemia (calcium supplementation may be required if the patient is already hypocalcemic); *(c)* metastatic

Table 11.28.   Therapeutic Phosphorus Preparations

Preparation	Content			
	Phosphate	Phosphorus	Sodium	Potassium
Oral				
Neutra phos capsule		250 mg/capsule	28.5 meq/capsule	28.5 meq/capsule
Neutra K phos capsule		250 mg/capsule	0 meq/capsule	57 meq/capsule
Phospho soda	4.2 mmol/ml	129 mg/ml	4.8 meq/ml	0 meq/ml
Parenteral				
K phosphate	3.0 mmol/ml	93 mg/ml	0 meq/ml	4.4 meq/ml
Na phosphate	3.0 mmol/ml	93 mg/ml	4.0 meq/ml	0 meq/ml
Neutral Na, K phosphate	0.1 mmol/ml	3.1 mg/ml	0.162 meq/ml	0.019 meq/ml

Table 11.29. Treatment of Severe Hypophosphatemia[a]

Clinical Situation	Initial Dose[b]
Recent uncomplicated hypophosphatemia	2.5 mg of phosphorus/kg body weight (0.08 mmol/kg)
Prolonged multiple causes	5.0 mg phosphorus/kg body weight (0.16 mmol/kg)

[a] Adapted from Lentz RD, et al.: *Ann Intern Med* 89:941, 1978, with permission.

[b] Note:

1. All doses in severe hypophosphatemia should be given intravenously over a 6-hour period. Above doses are for patients with normal renal function.

2. The initial dose should be 25–50% higher if the patient is symptomatic; lower if the patient is hypercalcemic.

3. Maximum dose is 7.5 mg/kg (0.24 mmol/kg) (16.8 mmol = 525 mg for a 70-kg man) over 6 hr.

4. Major complications have been reported in the literature when doses of 50–100 mmol phosphate have been given intravenously in less than 3 hours.

5. Repeat serum phosphorus concentration and reassess clinical situation before repeating phosphorus dose.

6. Conversion factors:
   1 mmol phosphate = 31 mg elemental phosphorus
   0.032 mmol phosphate = 1 mg elemental phosphorus
   0.323 mmol phosphate/L = 1 mg/dl elemental phosphorus
   1 mmol phosphate/L = 3.1 mg/dl elemental phosphorus

quently and therapy started as soon as possible. Since patients likely to develop hypophosphatemia are also prone to develop hypokalemia, part of the potassium deficit may be given as potassium phosphate. Maintenance phosphate requirements are 20–40 mmol/day.

Hyperphosphatemia

EPIDEMIOLOGY

Renal failure (acute or chronic) is the most common cause of hyperphosphatemia encountered in clinical practice (98). Very severe hyperphosphatemia (>10 mg/dl) may be seen in myoglobinuric acute renal failure associated with rhabdomyolysis and following chemotherapy for leukemia and lymphoma.

SIGNS AND SYMPTOMS

The clinical manifestations of hyperphosphatemia are secondary to hypocalcemia and extraskeletal calcification.

DIAGNOSIS

The differential diagnosis of hyperphosphatemia is listed in Table 11.30.

MANAGEMENT

Decreasing the intestinal absorption of phosphate is the major means of treating

calcification; *(d)* hypotension; *(e)* hyperkalemia from potassium salts; and *(f)* dehydration and hypernatremia (due to an osmotic diuresis resulting from the hypertonic nature of parenteral phosphate solutions). Absolute contraindications to intravenous phosphorus therapy include: *(a)* hypercalcemia (unless used for treatment of severe hypercalcemia refractory to conservative measures); and *(b)* conditions associated with rising phosphorus level (oliguria, tissue necrosis). Parenteral phosphorus in an initial dose of 1.0–2 grams per day will correct most cases of severe hypophosphatemia. Serum phosphorus should be monitored fre-

Table 11.30. Etiology of Hyperphosphatemia

I. Administration of phosphate
  A. Oral: Laxatives containing PO_4, K^+ phosphate tablets
  B. Rectal: phosphate enemas
  C. Intravenous phosphate
II. Decreased renal phosphate excretion
  A. Renal failure[a]
    1. Acute
    2. Chronic (GFR < 20–30 ml/min)
  B. Hypoparathyroidism
  C. Pseudohypoparathyroidism
III. Transcellular shift out of cells
  A. Acute acidosis
  B. Treatment of lymphoma/leukemia with chemotherapy
IV. Artifact: in vitro hemolysis

[a] Common cause in surgical patients.

hyperphosphatemia. This is achieved by administering aluminum salts (aluminum hydroxide, aluminum carbonate), which bind the phosphate in the gut, preventing absorption.

ACID-BASE DISORDERS

Epidemiology

Acid-base disturbances are very common in surgical patients. Various circumstances either related to the surgical illness or therapy may both contribute to the development of a primary disturbance in acid-base balance or alter the expected compensation. Table 11.31 summarizes the factors that lead to the production of or affect the response to acid-base disorders in the surgical setting. Due to the complex nature of these problems in the surgical patient, a few principles of acid-base physiology deserve mention.

Physiology

The acidity of the blood may be expressed in terms of either the hydrogen ion concentration [H$^+$] or pH. It follows from the Henderson equation:

$$[H^+] = 24 \frac{pCO_2}{[HCO_3^-]} \qquad (1)$$

that the [H$^+$] is determined by the ratio of pCO$_2$/[HCO$_3$] and not their absolute values alone. This equation may be used to calculate [H$^+$], [HCO$_3^-$] or pCO$_2$ when values for any two of these three terms are known. The [pH$^+$] may also be calculated from the Henderson-Haselbach equation where:

$$pH = 6.1 + \log \frac{[HCO_3^-]}{0.03 \, pCO_2} \qquad (2)$$

If the measured [H$^+$], pH, pCO$_2$, and [HCO$_3^-$] fail to satisfy the Henderson-Haselbach equation, then either there is a laboratory error or the serum electrolytes and arterial blood gases were not drawn simultaneously.

Table 11.31. Conditions Affecting Acid-Base Balance and Factors Contributing to Development of Acid-Base Disorders in Surgical Patients

Primary Acid-Base Disorders	Contributing Factors
Respiratory alkalosis	Overventilation
	Hypoxemia
	Sepsis
	Pain
	Apprehension
	Neurologic damage
	Liver disease
	Pulmonary embolism
Metabolic alkalosis	Vomiting
	NG suction
	Massive blood transfusions
	Excess HCO$_3$ administration
	Steroids
Respiratory acidosis	Drugs (preanesthetic medication, muscle paralyzing drugs)
	Pneumothorax
	Flail chest
Metabolic acidosis	Loss of alkaline GI fluids (biliary, small bowel, pancreas)
	Hypotension (hemorrhage, sepsis)
	Renal failure
	Vasopressor usage without adequate volume repletion
	Starvation ketosis
	Hyperalimentation

Factors Contributing to Impaired Compensation to Acid-Base Disorders in Surgical Patients

Conditions	Interferes with
Thoracic-abdominal operations	Respiratory compensation for metabolic acidosis
Peritonitis	"
COPD	"
CHF	"
Drugs (respiratory depressants)	"
Volume depletion	Renal HCO$_3^-$ excretion for correction of metabolic alkalosis
K$^+$ depletion	
Renal failure	
Hypercapnea	"
Renal failure	Metabolic compensation for respiratory acidosis

Acid-base homeostasis is maintained by three lines of defense: *(a)* body fluid and tissue buffers; *(b)* respiratory excretion or retention of CO_2; and *(c)* renal HCO_3 absorption or excretion. The bicarbonate buffer system is the most clinically important buffer of the extracellular fluid (ECF). Chemical buffering via the bicarbonate system occurs instantaneously. Intracellular buffering with intracellular-extracellular shifts takes 2–4 hours to occur. Respiratory compensation for primary metabolic disturbances in acid-base balance begins within minutes, but may take 12–24 hours for maximum compensation. If the acidosis develops slowly, full compensatory hyperventilation develops simultaneously. Renal compensation requires up to 5 days, but is usually 90% complete within 3 days.

Acid-base disorders are said to be either simple or mixed. A simple acid-base disorder is defined as one primary disorder coupled with its appropriate amount of compensation. Mixed disorders are defined as the presence of two or more primary acid-base disorders.

Before briefly discussing the four simple acid-base disorders, it is important to remember that you cannot diagnose an acid-base disorder by looking at the $[HCO_3^-]$ or pCO_2 alone. The pH, pCO_2 and $[HCO_3^-]$ must be combined with the clinical picture to correctly interpret any set of blood gases. Any increase or decrease in $[HCO_3^-]$ or pCO_2 may be part of the primary disorder or its compensation (as summarized in Table 11.32) (99).

Simple Metabolic Acidosis

EPIDEMIOLOGY

The most common causes of metabolic acidosis in surgical patients are those associated with a high anion gap, and include lactic acidosis, ketoacidosis, and uremic acidosis. Lactic acidosis is usually associated with poor tissue perfusion secondary to low cardiac output, hypotension, or sepsis. The common causes of

Table 11.32. Etiology of Abnormal HCO_3^- or pCO_2 Concentrations

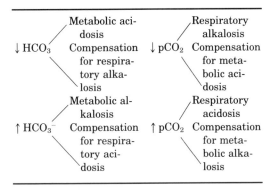

normal anion gap acidosis in surgical patients are loss of bicarbonate from the gastrointestinal tract, early renal failure (creatinine 3–8 mg/dl), and ureteral diversion, particularly when accompanied by obstruction.

Morbidity is more likely to be attributable to the underlying disease (i.e., sepsis) than the acidosis itself. However, severe acidosis, in itself, may be harmful since it results in: direct myocardial depression; unresponsiveness to the effects of catecholamines in maintaining vascular tone, and a decreased threshold for ventricular fibrillation. These manifestations are thought to appear as the pH falls below 7.1–7.2. Elderly patients, or those with cardiovascular disease, are more likely to suffer the consequences of acidosis than young patients.

DIAGNOSIS

The first step in determining the etiology of a metabolic acidosis is the calculation of the anion gap (AG). The anion gap is defined as the difference between the serum sodium concentration and the sum of serum Cl^- and HCO_3^- concentration:

$$AG = Na^+ - (HCO_3^- + Cl^-)$$

The normal range of the anion gap is 8–16 meq/L. This permits all metabolic acidosis to be divided into one of two types

Table 11.33. **Etiology of Metabolic Acidosis**

High Anion Gap	Normal Anion Gap

1. Ketoacidosis[a]
  a. Diabetic
  b. Alcoholic
  c. Starvation
2. Lactic acidosis[a]
3. Renal failure[a]
4. Ingestions
  a. Salicylate
  b. Methanol
  c. Ethylene glycol
  d. Paraldehyde
	Normal to high potassium type
	  1. Early renal failure (Cr = 6–8 mg/100 ml)[a]
	  2. Obstructive uropathy[a]
	  3. Hypoaldosteronism
	    a. Hyporeninemia
	    b. Renal aldosterone resistance
	  4. Dilutional acidosis
	  5. Acidifying agents (HCl, NH_4Cl, arginine HCl, lysine HCl, $CaCl_2$)
	  6. Sulfur toxicity
	  7. Recovery stage of diabetic ketoacidosis
	Low potassium type
	  1. GI HCO_3^- loss[a]
	    a. Diarrhea
	    b. Pancreatic, biliary, small bowel drainage, or external fistula
	    c. Cholestyramine
	  2. Renal tubular acidosis
	    a. Proximal
	    b. Distal
	  3. Carbonic anhydrase inhibitors
	    a. Acetazolamide (Diamox)
	    b. Mafenide (Sulfamylon)
	  4. Posthypocapnic metabolic acidosis
	  5. Ureteral diversions[a]
	    a. Ureterosigmoidostomy
	    b. Ileal ureter
	    c. Obstructed ileal bladder

[a] Common in surgical patients.

(Table 11.33): *(a)* high anion gap metabolic acidosis, or *(b)* normal anion gap (hyperchloremic) metabolic acidosis. The normal anion gap metabolic acidosis may be further subdivided into two groups according to the serum potassium concentration.

The diagnosis of ketoacidosis is established when a strongly positive nitroprusside reaction (Acetest) is found in the serum. Clinical situations associated with tissue hypoxia may give a falsely negative reaction because the Acetest tablet detects only acetoacetate and not beta-hydroxybutyrate, which is predominately formed in such states. Typical uremic acidosis (anion gap) is seen only in advanced renal failure (creatinine clearance less than 25 ml/min). Lactic acidosis is usually a diagnosis of exclusion but may be confirmed by the finding of an elevated serum lactate level.

MANAGEMENT

In either lactic acidosis or ketoacidosis, therapy, to be successful, must be directed at the underlying cause (improving tissue perfusion or the administration of insulin). Often this will result in normalization of pH without additional (bicarbonate) therapy.

Guidelines for the use of sodium bicarbonate in severe metabolic acidosis include: *(a)* a serum pH less than 7.1 (7.2 in the patient with heart disease); *(b)* a serum bicarbonate less than 10 meq/L; or *(c)* the presence of a maximum ventilatory response ($pCO_2 \leqslant 12$ mm Hg). The initial aim of therapy is to increase serum bicarbonate approximately 4–6 meq/L over the first several hours and to a bicarbonate concentration of 14–16 meq/L by 24 hours. Elderly patients with gram-negative sepsis, shock, arrhythmias, and a pH of 7.2 should probably receive bicarbonate, whereas young diabetics with a pH of 7.1 but without hypotension may not require any bicarbonate because treatment with insulin should rapidly improve the acidosis and their cardiovascular systems are more stable.

Serum bicarbonate should be raised to 16–18 meq/L in patients with metabolic acidosis who have lung disease or who are about to receive anesthesia since they are more prone to impairment of their respiratory compensation.

The approximate total amount of bicarbonate that needs to be administered to achieve a desired level can be estimated by the following formula:

$$Bicarbonate\ deficit = weight\ (kg) \times 0.5\ [HCO_3\ desired - HCO_3\ measured]$$

The actual amount required will vary widely because of large differences in the volume of distribution. The actual amount tends to be greater when the acidosis is severe or ongoing and when bicarbonate continues to be lost. Therefore, there is no substitute for frequent measurement of pH and bicarbonate concentration.

Bicarbonate therapy should never be considered lightly. Potential complications include hypokalemia, decreased ionized calcium with tetany, volume overload, hypernatremia, and cerebral acidosis. "Overshoot" alkalosis may occur when the change in bicarbonate is more rapid than the change in pCO_2 or when lactate or the salts of ketoacids are remetabolized to bicarbonate. Volume overload may impair the respiratory compensatory response and result in an actual decline of pH. Diuretics or dialysis may occasionally be needed to handle the excess sodium load resulting from bicarbonate therapy.

In patients with severe acidosis from renal failure accompanied by hypocalcemia, it may be necessary to provide intravenous calcium (20–30 ml of 10% calcium gluconate) to avoid precipitating tetany or convulsions. When severe acidosis and hypokalemia coexist, a large potassium deficit is usually present. In this situation, the pH and potassium deficiency must be corrected simultaneously.

Simple Metabolic Alkalosis

EPIDEMIOLOGY

Metabolic alkalosis in surgical patients most commonly develops from gastric losses of hydrogen through vomiting or gastric suction (100). Alkalosis due to potassium depletion, diuretic use, or posthyperventilation syndrome are also common. Because many of these patients are also volume-depleted, leading to renal retention of bicarbonate, the metabolic alkalosis tends to persist.

Critically ill surgical patients commonly are alkalotic (metabolic and/or respiratory), and mortality has been shown to increase with pH above 7.55 (Table 11.34) (101). Metabolic alkalosis also results in hypoventilation, which may interfere with weaning a patient from mechanical ventilation. Correction of the metabolic alkalosis in patients with mixed respiratory acidosis and metabolic alkalosis has been shown to result in improvement in arterial blood gases and clinical symptoms.

PHYSIOLOGY

Metabolic alkalosis can be divided into two types: chloride-responsive and chloride-resistant. Most of the chloride-responsive forms of metabolic alkalosis are associated with intravascular volume depletion and a low-spot urine chloride concentration ($U_{Cl} < 10$–20 meq/L). The U_{Cl} is more useful than the U_{Na} in assessing effective circulating volume in metabolic alkalosis because sodium may be lost in

Table 11.34.   Acid-Base Disorders in Critically Ill Patients[a]

Frequency of Acid-Base Disorders in Critically Ill Patients

	N = 105 Surgical Patients (Lyons)	N = 1415 Surgical Patients (Wilson)	N = 8209 ABG Determinations in an ICU (Mazzara)
Alkalosis	64%	12.5%	69%
Respiratory	57%	11.0%	46%
Metabolic	13%	1.5%	23%
Acidosis			21.5%
Respiratory			13.4%
Metabolic			8.1%
Normal			8.6%

Mortality Related to pCO_2 or pH in Critically Ill Alkalotic Patients

Mazzara		Wilson[b]	
pCO_2 (mm Hg)	Mortality (%)	pH	Mortality (%)
15	88	7.55–7.56	41
20–25	77	7.57–7.59	47
25–30	73	7.60–7.64	65
35–45	29	7.65–7.7	80

[a] Sources: Mazzara JT, Ayres SM, Grace WJ: Extreme hypocapnea in the critically ill. *Am J Med* 56:450–456, 1974; Wilson RF, et al.: Severe alkalosis in critically ill surgical patients. *Arch Surg* 105:197–203, 1972; Lyons JH, Moore FD: Posttraumatic alkalosis: Incidence and pathophysiology of alkalosis in surgery. *Surgery* 60:93–106, 1966.
[b] Wilson did not find mortality related to pCO_2.

the urine despite the presence of volume depletion if bicarbonaturia is occurring. The U_{Cl} may be high despite intravascular volume depletion in three conditions: *(a)* renal insufficiency; *(b)* severe hypokalemia (potassium < 2 meq/L); and *(c)* acute hypercapnea. Chloride-sensitive metabolic alkalosis can be corrected with chloride administration, either as KCl or NaCl or both.

Chloride-resistant metabolic alkalosis is associated with a high urinary chloride (U_{Cl} > 10–20 meq/L). Most are rare and due to some form of mineralocorticoid ex-

cess. Chloride administration in this group has no effect because they are not chloride (volume) depleted. Table 11.35 lists the differential diagnosis of metabolic alkalosis.

SIGNS AND SYMPTOMS

Severe alkalosis can result in mental confusion, seizures, or coma. The oxyhemoglobin dissociation curve shifts to the left, resulting in impaired oxygen release from hemoglobin. Arrhythmias are much more common in alkalotic patients who may also have coexisting hypokalemia or hypomagnesemia, and who may be receiving digoxin.

DIAGNOSIS

The history and bedside determination of intravascular volume are the keys to the diagnosis of the cause of a metabolic alkalosis. If the etiology is not obvious from the history and physical exam, suspect: *(a)* surreptitious vomiting; *(b)* diuretic ingestion; or *(c)* mineralocorticoid excess. Measurement of U_{Cl} will be helpful in these cases.

MANAGEMENT

Definitive treatment of any metabolic alkalosis involves correction of the underlying cause. Increased renal bicarbonate excretion may be achieved by correcting those conditions responsible for maintaining the metabolic alkalosis ($\downarrow$ECF volume, potassium deficiency, hypercapnea) by elevating the renal bicarbonate threshold. Increase in urinary chloride excretion to 60–100 meq/day implies adequate replacement of chloride stores. If the effective circulating volume cannot be improved (e.g., edematous states), acetazolamide (250–500 mg b.i.d.-q.i.d.) may be tried. This may be very helpful in improving pulmonary function in patients hypoventilating as a response to metabolic alkalosis. The combination of metabolic alkalosis (nasogastric suction) and postoperative renal failure represents a special problem when the alkalosis is se-

Table 11.35.   Etiology of Metabolic Alkalosis

Chloride-responsive ($U_{Cl} < 10$–20 meq/L)	Chloride-resistant ($U_{Cl} > 10$–20 meq/L)
1. Gastrointestinal causes a. Gastric losses (vomiting, nasogastric suction)[a] b. Cl^--losing diarrhea (villous adenoma of colon, congenital Cl^--losing diarrhea) 2. Diuretic administration (late)[a] 3. Posthypercapneic metabolic alkalosis[a] 4. Antibiotics (carbenicillin, penicillin)	1. Hyperaldosteronism 2. Cushing's syndrome 3. Bartter's syndrome 4. Licorice ingestion 5. Severe K^+ depletion 6. Excessively rapid HCO_3^- administration (especially in renal failure) 7. Drugs a. Diuretics (early) b. Exogenous glucocorticoid or mineralocorticoid c. Carbenoxalone

[a] Common in surgical patients.

vere. Volume replacement and NaCl, and KCl administration do not reverse the alkalosis because the kidney cannot excrete the excess bicarbonate that is present. This situation may be treated with the administration of dilute (0.1 N) hydrochloric acid or dialysis with a high chloride-low acetate bath (102,103). Ammonium HCl and arginine HCl are less desirable in patients with renal failure due to the increased nitrogen load. Dilute (0.1 N) HCl contains 100 meq of hydrogen ions per liter and must be administered through a central line to avoid its sclerosing effects. The dose of dilute HCl may be estimated from the following equation:

$$\text{meq acid required} = \text{Wt (kg)} \times 0.5 \times [HCO_3^- \text{ initial-}HCO_3^- \text{ desired}]$$

From this formula, it follows that approximately 5 meq of acid per kg of body weight is required to reduce the serum bicarbonate by 10 meq/L. This 10-meq/L decrease in bicarbonate should be accomplished over 12–24 hours. If the gastric drainage is large, an estimate of ongoing hydrogen ion loss may be obtained by applying the electroneutrality principle to the gastric contents:

$$\text{Ongoing gastric } H^+ \text{ loss (meq/L)} = Cl^+ - (Na^+ + K^+)$$

This ongoing loss of acid should be added to the calculated acid deficit in correcting severe metabolic alkalosis. Cimetidine, which reduces gastric acid secretion, can also be used to minimize hydrogen ion losses.

Treatment of severe chloride-resistant metabolic alkalosis may be achieved with large doses of potassium or acidifying agents. Definitive treatment depends on correcting the underlying disorder.

Simple Respiratory Acidosis

EPIDEMIOLOGY

Acute respiratory acidosis is not an uncommon problem in the postoperative period. Severe COPD is a definite risk factor for the development of postoperative acute respiratory acidosis. Factors contributing to postoperative hypoventilation include: pain from abdominal incisions and abdominal distention limiting diaphragmatic excursion, flail chest, atelectasis, pleural effusions, pneumonia, airway obstruction, and drugs (sedatives, anesthetics, muscle paralyzers).

DIAGNOSIS

The development of postoperative restlessness, hypertension, and tachycardia may be due to respiratory acidosis, hypoxia, or pain and should be evaluated by

Table 11.36.   Causes of Respiratory Acidosis

1. Respiratory center depression
   a. Drugs (general anesthesia, narcotics, sedatives)[a]
   b. CNS lesions (trauma, medullary tumor, vertebral artery occlusion)
   c. Pickwickian syndrome
   d. Increased intracranial pressure
   e. Oxygen therapy in chronic hypercapnea[a]
2. Neuromuscular disorders
   a. Neuropathies (poliomyelitis, Guillain-Barre syndrome, botulism, spinal cord injury)
   b. Myopathies (myasthenia gravis, muscular dystrophy, hypo- and hyperkalemic paralysis)
3. Thoracic cage disorders
   a. Kyphoscoliasis
   b. Flail chest[a]
   c. Alkylosing spondylitis
   d. Pneumothorax[a]
   e. Scleroderma
4. Airway obstruction
   a. Aspiration
   b. Foreign body
   c. Laryngeal edema
5. Pulmonary disease
   a. COPD[a]
   b. Pulmonary edema
   c. Pneumonia
   d. Severe bronchospasm

[a] Common in surgical patients.

obtaining an arterial blood gas. Table 11.36 summarizes the causes of respiratory acidosis.

MANAGEMENT

Treatment involves improving pulmonary ventilation by clearing secretions, bronchodilators, corticosteroids, and possibly intubation.

Simple Respiratory Alkalosis

EPIDEMIOLOGY

Apprehension, pain, and overventilation contribute to the development of respiratory alkalosis. Unexplained respiratory alkalosis may be an important first clue to the presence of sepsis in a surgical patient. On the surgical service, acute respiratory alkalosis is also seen following head trauma, pneumothorax, over-ventilation by a mechanical respirator, and with pulmonary embolism.

SIGNS AND SYMPTOMS

Hypocapnea leads to cerebral vasoconstriction and may further compromise cerebral blood flow in patients with cerebrovascular disease. Cardiac arrhythmias may develop with severe respiratory alkalosis, especially if hypokalemia exists and the patient is receiving digoxin. Table 11.37 summarizes the causes of respiratory alkalosis.

MANAGEMENT

The primary mode of therapy involves correction of the underlying disorder. On occasion, reducing respirations by pharmacological (sedation, muscle paralyzers)

Table 11.37.   Causes of Respiratory Alkalosis

1. Hypoxemia[a]
2. Anxiety[a]
3. Drugs (hormones)
   a. Salicylates
   b. Progesterone (pregnancy)
   c. Epinephrine
4. CNS disorders
   a. Subarachnoid hemorrhage
   b. Meningitis, encephalitis
   c. Head trauma
   d. Cerebrovascular accident
   e. Brain tumor
5. Pulmonary disorders
   a. Pneumothorax[a]
   b. Pulmonary emboli[a]
   c. Early restrictive disorders
   d. Pneumonia[a]
   e. Pulmonary hypertension
   f. Congestive heart failure[a]
6. Hypermetabolic states
   a. Fever[a]
   b. Thyrotoxicosis
   c. Anemia
   d. Delirium tremens
7. Miscellaneous
   a. Gram-negative septicemia[a]
   b. Endotoxemia[a]
   c. Ventilator-induced[a]
   d. Liver disease
   e. Sudden recovery from metabolic acidosis[a]
   f. Severe burns[a]

[a] Common in surgical patients.

or mechanical (increasing dead space) means may be necessary.

Mixed Acid-Base Disorders

EPIDEMIOLOGY

The presence of a mixed acid-base disorder should be suspected when analysis of the arterial blood gas and electrolytes reveals either an inadequate or excessive degree of compensation. Often it will be clinically obvious that several individual processes are occurring simultaneously in a given patient, combining to produce more than one primary acid-base disturbance. For instance, a patient who might be septic (respiratory alkalosis, metabolic acidosis) following surgery for an abdominal abscess and who has a nasogastric tube (metabolic alkalosis) and is on a respira-tor (respiratory acidosis or alkalosis) has several separate processes, each capable of producing abnormalities of acid-base homeostasis. The final pH, in this hypothetical patient, would depend on the relative severity of each of the single disorders.

PHYSIOLOGY

Before one can properly approach mixed disorders, it is necessary to understand the normal patterns of compensation to primary acid-base disturbances. This topic is well reviewed in several articles dealing with mixed disorders (104,105). The expected compensation for each of the primary acid-base disorders can be derived from the acid-base map constructed by Goldberg (106) (Fig. 11.7) or from the formulae summarized in Table 11.38.

ACID-BASE MAP

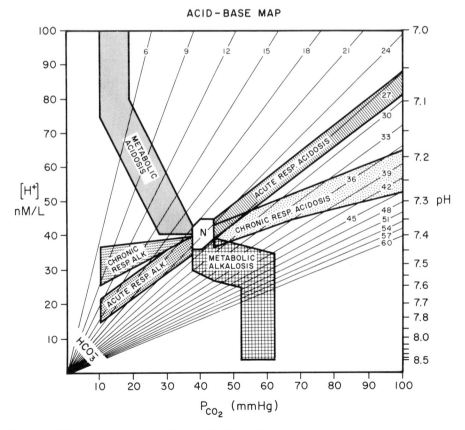

Figure 11.7. Acid-base normogram. (From Goldberg M, et al.: Computer-based instruction and diagnosis of acid-base disorders: A systematic approach. *JAMA* 223:269, 1973. Copyright 1973, American Medical Assn. Used with permission.)

Table 11.38.   Compensation for Acid-Base Disorders

Metabolic acidosis	$pCO_2 = 1.5 \, [HCO_3^-] + 8 \pm 2$ $pCO_2 \downarrow$ by 1–1.3 per meq/L $\downarrow$ HCO_3^-	Measured $pCO_2 >$ expected pCO_2: superimposed primary respiratory acidosis or insufficient time for complete resp. compensation (acidosis < 24 hr) Measured $pCO_2 <$ expected pCO_2: superimposed primary respiratory alkalosis or delayed ventilatory adjustment to sudden increase in plasma HCO_3^-
Metabolic alkalosis	$pCO_2 \uparrow$ by 0.5–0.7 mm Hg per meq/L $\uparrow$ HCO_3^-	Measured $pCO_2 >$ expected pCO_2: suggests superimposed primary respiratory acidosis (resp. compensation may be absent in mild metabolic alkalosis $HCO_3^- < 37$ meq/L) Measured $pCO_2 <$ expected pCO_2: suggests superimposed primary respiratory alkalosis
Acute respiratory acidosis	$HCO_3^- \uparrow$ by 1 meq/L for every 10 mm Hg rise in pCO_2, not increasing more than total of 3–4 meq/L or exceeding a $HCO_3^- = 30$ meq/L $\Delta H^+ = 0.8 \, \Delta pCO_2{}^a$	$HCO_3^- > 30$ meq/L suggests superimposed primary metabolic alkalosis $HCO_3^- < 24$ meq/L suggests superimposed primary metabolic acidosis $\Delta H^+ \neq 0.8 \, \Delta pCO_2$ suggests superimposed metabolic disorder or laboratory error
Chronic respiratory acidosis	$\Delta HCO_3^- = 0.4 \, \Delta pCO_2 \pm 3$ $\Delta H^+ = 0.33 \, \Delta pCO_2$	Measured $HCO_3^- >$ expected HCO_3^- suggests superimposed primary metabolic alkalosis Measured $HCO_3^- <$ expected HCO_3^- suggests superimposed primary metabolic acidosis $\Delta H^+ \neq 0.33 \, \Delta pCO_2$ suggests superimposed metabolic disorder or laboratory error
Acute respiratory alkalosis	$\Delta HCO_3^- = 0.2 \, \Delta pCO_2 \pm 2.5$ (HCO_3^- usually not < 18 meq/L) $\Delta H^+ = 0.8 \, \Delta pCO_2$	Measured $HCO_3^- >$ expected HCO_3^- suggests superimposed primary metabolic alkalosis $HCO_3^- < 18$ meq/L suggests superimposed primary metabolic acidosis $\Delta H^+ \neq 0.8 \, \Delta pCO_2$ suggests superimposed metabolic disorder or laboratory error
Chronic respiratory alkalosis	$\Delta HCO_3^- = 0.5 \, \Delta pCO_2 \pm 2.5$ (HCO_3^- usually not < 15 meq/L) $\Delta H^+ = 0.17 \, \Delta pCO_2$	Measured $HCO_3^- >$ expected HCO_3^- suggests superimposed primary metabolic alkalosis $HCO_3^- < 15$ meq/L suggests superimposed primary metabolic acidosis $\Delta H^+ \neq 0.17 \, \Delta pCO_2$ suggests superimposed metabolic disorder or laboratory error

[a] Δ, change from normal.

Table 11.39.   Diagnostic Approach to Acid-Base Disturbances

I. History
    A. Clinical diagnoses capable of producing acid-base disorders (COPD, renal failure, diabetes mellitus)
    B. Drugs
        1. Diuretics
        2. Steroids
        3. Acidifying/alkalinizing agents
        4. Respiratory stimulants/depressants
        5. Antibiotics
            a. Aminoglycosides ($\rightarrow$renal failure, neuromuscular blockade)
            b. Carbenicillin (metabolic alkalosis)
        6. Toxins (aspirin, methanol, ethylene glycol, paraldehyde)
    C. Therapeutic maneuvers
        1. Mechanical ventilation
        2. Sodium restriction
II. Physical examination
    A. Vital signs: Kussmaul respiration, hypotension$\rightarrow$metabolic acidosis
    B. Fundus: papilledema (CO_2 retention, methanol)
    C. Cyanosis, COPD$\rightarrow$respiratory acidosis
    D. Nasogastric tube$\rightarrow$metabolic alkalosis
    E. Fever$\rightarrow$respiratory alkalosis
III. Laboratory
    A. Routine electrolytes
        1. Na^+
        2. K^+
        3. Cl^-
        4. HCO_3^-
        5. Calculate anion gap: $AG = Na^+ - (Cl^- + HCO_3^-)$
            a. Look for value of anion gap before acid-base disorder developed or factors that may decrease
                its size (i.e., hypoalbuminemia)
    B. Arterial blood gases
    C. Supplementary data
        1. Blood
            a. Glucose
            b. BUN, creatinine
            c. Osmolality
            d. Serum ketones
            e. Toxicology screen (methanol, ethylene glycol, paraldehyde, salicylate)
            f. Lactate level
        2. Urinalysis: glucose/ketones, oxylate (ethylene glycol)
        3. Pulmonary function tests
        4. Blood cultures
IV. Synthesize data
    A. Rule out lab error
    B. Arterial blood gases different from expected
        1. ? Miss something
        2. ? Overemphasis of some process in history
    C. Calculate expected compensation for any primary acid-base disorder present

The more severe the primary acid-base disturbances, the less likely the pH will be normal and the more likely that a normal pH indicates the presence of a mixed acid-base disorder. Compensation does not usually return the pH to normal. Compensation in mild disorders may possibly return the pH to the normal range but not to the initial value.

What appears to be an "inappropriate" degree of compensation may actually be the effect of a separate primary disorder. Even apparently appropriate compensation may represent the chance occurrence

Table 11.40.   Examples of Mixed Acid-Base Disorders

I. Respiratory acidosis + metabolic acidosis
  A. COPD (chronic respiratory acidosis) + septic shock[a]
  B. COPD + severe acute hypoxia ($pO_2 < 30$ mm Hg)[a]
  C. Cardiopulmonary arrest[a]
  D. Acute respiratory failure + renal failure[a]
  E. Pulmonary edema[a]
  F. Metabolic acidosis with inadequate respiratory compensation due to pulmonary disease (COPD, pleural effusion), CHF, severe hypokalemia, severe PO_4 depletion[a]
II. Respiratory acidosis plus metabolic alkalosis
  A. COPD + diuretics/Na restriction/glucocorticoids
  B. ARDS + nasogastric suction[a]
III. Respiratory alkalosis plus metabolic acidosis
  A. Septic shock[a]
  B. Liver disease[a]
    1. Hepatorenal syndrome
    2. Cirrhosis + alcoholic ketoacidosis or RTA
  C. Salicylate intoxication
  D. Severe burns treated with Sulfamylon[a]
  E. Recovery phase of severe metabolic acidosis
  F. Hemodialysis (high mass transfer of acetate)
IV. Respiratory alkalosis plus metabolic alkalosis
  A. CHF + diuretics[a]
  B. Posthypercapneic metabolic alkalosis[a]
  C. Cirrhosis + vomiting[a]
  D. Pregnancy + vomiting/diuretics
  E. Excessive HCO_3^- therapy in metabolic acidosis with persistence of compensatory hyperventilation[a]
  F. Sepsis + massive transfusions or nasogastric suction[a]
  G. Severe hypoxemia + metabolic alkalosis
 V. Acute and chronic respiratory acidosis: COPD with exacerbation (infection, O_2 therapy, sedatives)[a]
VI. Metabolic acidosis plus metabolic alkalosis
  A. Diarrhea + vomiting/nasogastric suction
  B. Renal failure + vomiting/nasogastric suction
  C. Ketoacidosis + vomiting/nasogastric suction
  D. Organic (lactate, ketones) acidosis + "overshoot" metabolic alkalosis from excessive HCO_3^- therapy[a]
VII. Mixed metabolic acidosis
  A. Mixed hyperchloremic and high-anion gap metabolic acidosis
  B. Mixed high-anion gap acidosis
  C. Mixed hyperchloremic acidosis
VIII. Triple disorder
  A. Metabolic acidosis + metabolic alkalosis + respiratory acidosis
  B. Metabolic acidosis + metabolic alkalosis + respiratory alkalosis

---

[a] Common in surgical patients.

of a dual or triple acid-base disorder. The duration of the acid-base disorder must be known to interpret the appropriateness of compensatory mechanisms. Otherwise, insufficient compensation will incorrectly be attributed to a complicating primary disorder rather than simply insufficient time to reach a new steady state of acid-base balance with maximal compensation.

Values falling within the confidence bands for a simple acid-base disorder does not prove that a simple disorder exists; only that the data are consistent with a single disturbance. If a point falls outside a band, the presence of a mixed disorder is suggested. Since there are always several possible explanations for any point on the acid-base map, the correct interpretation can only be made by utilizing the clinical information available. Table 11.38 lists the possible explanations when the actual compensatory response differs from the expected or calculated response.

DIAGNOSIS

A systematic approach to the diagnosis of both simple and mixed acid-base disorders is outlined in Table 11.39 and is largely self-explanatory. The history and physical examination are searched for conditions known to be associated with disorders of acid-base balance. The indicated laboratory data confirms the presence of an acid-base disorder and helps in establishing its etiology. Finally, to decide if a mixed acid-base disorder is present, the expected compensation for any primary acid-base disorder must be compared to the actual compensation. It cannot be overemphasized, however, that only by incorporating the clinical picture, including the estimated duration of the acid-base disturbance, can the blood gases by correctly interpreted in a given patient. The common causes of mixed acid-base disorders are summarized in Table 11.40.

MANAGEMENT

The treatment principles of mixed and simple acid-base disorders are similar. The aim is to restore the pH toward normal and to identify and correct all underlying conditions. If the pH is severely abnormal in a patient with mixed metabolic acidosis and metabolic alkalosis, the predominant disorder should be treated first.

READINGS

1. Hou SH, Bushinsky DA, Wish JB, et al.: Hospital acquired renal insufficiency: a prospective study. *Am J Med* 74:243, 1983.
2. Shusterman N, Strom BL, Thomas MG, et al.: Risk factors and outcome of hospital-acquired acute renal failure: Clinical epidemiologic study. *Am J Med* 83:65, 1987.
3. Shires GT, Carrico CJ: *Renal Responses.* Philadelphia: WB Saunders, 1972.
4. Beaufils M, Morel-Maroger L, Sraer JD, et al.: Acute renal failure of glomerular origin during visceral abscesses. *N Engl J Med* 295:185, 1976.
5. Zappacosta AR, Ashby FL: Gram-negative sepsis with acute renal failure. Occurrence from acute glomerulonephritis. *JAMA* 238:1389, 1977.
6. Spector DA, Millan J, Zauber N, et al.: Glomerulonephritis and staphylococcal aureus infections. *Clin Nephrol* 14:256, 1980.
7. Bennett WM, Plamp C, Porter GA: Drug-related syndromes in clinical nephrology. *Ann Intern Med* 87:982, 1977.
8. Smith CR, Lipsky JJ, Laskin OL, et al.: Double-blind comparison of the nephrotoxicity and auditory toxicity of gentamicin and tobramycin. *N Engl J Med* 320:1106, 1980.
9. Byrd L, Sherman RL: Radiocontrast-induced acute renal failure: A clinical and physiologic review. *Medicine* 58:270, 1979.
10. Van Zee BE, Hoy WE, Talley TE, et al.: Renal injury associated with intravenous pyelography in nondiabetic and diabetic patients. *Ann Intern Med* 89:51, 1978.
11. Harkonen S, Kjellstrand DM: Exacerbation of diabetic renal failure following intravenous pyelography. *Am J Med* 63:939, 1979.
12. D'Elia JA, Gleason RE, Alday M, et al.: Nephrotoxicity from angiographic contrast material: A prospective study. *Am J Med* 72:719, 1983.
12A. Schwab SJ, Hlatky MA, Pieper KS, et al.: Contrast nephrotoxicity: A randomized controlled trial of nonionic and ionic radiographic contrast agent. *New Engl J Med* 320:149, 1989.
13. Anderson RJ, Schrier RW: Clinical spectrum of oliguric and nonoliguric acute renal failure, in Brenner BM, Stein JH (eds): *Contemporary Issues in Nephrology: Acute Renal Failure.* New York, Churchill Livingstone, 1980.
14. Abel RM, Buckley MJ, Austen WG, et al.: Etiology, incidence, and prognosis of renal failure following cardiac operations. *J Thorac Cardiovasc Surg* 71:323, 1976.
15. Abbott WM: Renal failure complicating vascular surgery, in Bernhard VM, Towne JB (eds): *Complications in Vascular Surgery.* New York, Grune & Stratton, 1980.
16. Bhat JG, Gluck MC, Lowenstein V, et al.: Renal failure after open heart surgery. *Ann Intern Med* 84:677, 1976.
17. Casali R, Simmons RL, Najarian JS, et al.: Acute renal insufficiency complicating major cardiovascular surgery. *Ann Surg* 181:370, 1975.
18. McLeish KR, Luft FC, and Kleit SA: Factors affecting prognosis in acute renal failure following cardiac operations. *Surg Gynecol Obstet* 145:28, 1977.
19. Tilney NL, Bailey GL, Morgan AP: Sequential system failure after rupture of abdominal aortic aneurysm. *Ann Surg* 178:117, 1973.
20. Dawson JL: Renal failure in obstructive jaundice: Clinical aspects. *Postgrad Med J* 51:510, 1975.
21. Hilberman M, Myers BD, Carrie BJ, et al.: Acute

renal failure following cardiac surgery. *J Thorac Cardiovasc Surg* 77:880, 1970.

22. Anderson RJ, Linas SL, Berns AS, et al.: Nonoliguric acute renal failure. *N Engl J Med* 296:1134, 1977.

23. Brown CB, Ogg CS, Cameron JS: High dose furosemide in acute renal failure: A controlled trial. *Clin Nephrol* 15:90, 1981.

24. Levinsky NG, Bernard DB, Johnston PA: Enhancement of recovery of acute renal failure: Effects of mannitol and diuretics, in Brenner BM, Stein JH (eds): *Contemporary Issues in Nephrology*. Churchill Livingstone, Inc., 1980.

25. Tiller DJ, Mudge GH: Pharmacologic agents used in the management of acute renal failure. *Kidney Int* 18:700, 1980.

26. Thompson JE, Vollman RW, Austin DJ, et al.: Prevention of hypotensive and renal complications of aortic surgery using balanced salt solution. *Ann Surg* 167:767, 1968.

27. Barry KG, Mazze RI, Schwartz FD: Prevention of surgical oliguria and renal hemodynamic suppression by sustained hydration. *N Engl J Med* 270:1371, 1964.

28. Bismuth H, Kuntziger H, Corlette MD, Cholangitis with acute renal failure: Priorities in therapeutics. *Ann Surg* 181:881, 1975.

29. Shin B, Mackenzie CF, McAsland TC, et al.: Postoperative renal failure in trauma patients. *Anesthesiology* 51:218, 1979.

30. Polk HC, Vargas A: The prevention of postoperative renal failure. *South Med J* 63:1068, 1970.

31. Kunin CM: *Detection, Prevention, and Management of Urinary Tract Infections*. 3rd ed. Philadelphia, Lea and Febiger, 1979.

32. Schaberg DR, Haley RW, Highsmith AK, et al.: Nasocomial bacteriuria: A prospective study of case clustering and antimicrobial resistance. *Ann Intern Med* 93:420, 1980.

33. McHenry MC, Hawk WA, Straffon RA: Gramnegative bacillemia. *Urol Clin N Am* 3:333, 1976.

34. Nicolle LE, Mayhew WJ, Bryan L. A prospective randomized comparison of therapy and no therapy for asymptomatic bacteriuria in institutionalized elderly women. *Am J Med* 83:27, 1987.

35. Spanos PK, Simmons RL, Lampe E, et al.: Complications of related kidney donation. *Surgery* 76:741, 1974.

36. Milutinovic J, Agodoa LCY, Cutler RE, et al.: Autosomal dominant polycystic kidney disease. Early diagnosis and consideration of pathogenesis. *Am J Clin Pathol* 73:740, 1980.

37. Rastogi SP, Reid IS: Bilateral ureteral obstruction following aortic bypass surgery. *Clin Nephrol* 14:250, 1980.

38. Hinman F: Postoperative overdistention of the bladder. *Surg Gynecol Obstet* 142:901, 1976.

39. Mazze RI: Critical care of the patient with acute renal failure. *Anesthesiology* 47:138, 1977.

40. Coulie P, DePlaen JF, Van Ypersele de Strihou C. Captopril induced acute reversible renal failure. *Nephron* 35:108, 1983.

41. Baek SM, Makabali GG, Shoemaker WC: Clinical determinants of survival from postoperative renal failure. *Surg Gynecol Obstet* 140:685, 1975.

42. Milligan SL, Luft FC, McMurray SD, Kleit SA: Intra-abdominal infection and acute renal failure. *Arch Surg* 113:467, 1978.

43. Polk HC, Shields CL: Remote organ failure: A sign of occult intra-abdominal infection. *Surgery* 81:310, 1977.

44. Scott RB, Ogg CS, Cameron JS, et al.: Why the persistently high mortality in acute renal failure? *Lancet* 2:75, 1972.

45. Cioffi WG, Ashikaga T, Gamelli RL; Probability of surviving postoperative acute renal failure. Development of a prognostic index. *Ann Surg* 200:205, 1984.

46. Kornhall S: Acute renal failure in surgical disease with special regard to neglected complications. A retrospective study of 298 cases treated during the period 1960–1968. *Acta Chir Scand (Suppl)* 419:3, 1971.

47. Hall JW, Johnson WJ, Maher FI, et al.: Immediate and long-term prognosis in acute renal failure. *Ann Intern Med* 73:515, 1970.

48. Merino GE, Buselmeier TJ, Kjellstrand CM: Post-operative chronic renal failure: A new syndrome? *Ann Surg* 182:37, 1975.

49. Grazioni G, Cantaluppi A, Casati S, et al.: Dopamine and furosemide in oliguric acute renal failure. *Nephron* 37:39, 1984.

50. Conger JD: A controlled evaluation of prophylactic dialysis in posttraumatic acute renal failure. *J Trauma* 15:1056, 1975.

51. Teschan PE, Baxter CR, O'Brien, TF, et al.: Prophylactic hemodialysis in the treatment of acute renal failure. *Ann Intern Med* 53:992, 1960.

52. Fischer RP, Griffen WO, Reiser M, et al.: Early dialysis in the treatment of acute renal failure. *Surg Gynecol Obstet* 123:1019, 1966.

53. Kleinknecht D, Graneval D: Preventive hemodialysis in acute renal failure. Its effect on mortality and morbidity, in Friedman EA, Eliahou HE (eds): *Proceedings Conference on Acute Renal Failure*. New York, DHEW Publications No. (NIH) 74–608:165, 1973.

54. Dudrick SJ, Steiger E, Long JM: Renal failure in surgical patients. Treatment with intravenous essential amino acids and hypotonic glucose. *Surgery* 68:180, 1970.

55. Abel RM, Beck CH, Abbott WM, et al.: Improved survival from acute renal failure after treatment with intravenous essential L-amino acids and glucose. Results of a prospective, double-blind study. *N Engl J Med* 288:695, 1973.

55A. Zarich Z, Fang L, Diamond JR. Fractional excretion of sodium. Exceptions to its diagnostic value. *Arch Int Med* 145:108, 1985.

56. Baek SM, Makabali GC, Bryan-Brown CW, et al.: The influence of parenteral nutrition on the course of acute renal failure. *Surg Gynecol Obstet* 141:405, 1975.

57. Brown CB, Cameron JS, Ogg CS, et al.: Established acute renal failure following surgical operations, in Friedman EA, Eliahou HE (eds): *Proceedings Conference on Acute Renal Failure*. New York, DHEW Publications No. (NIH) 74–608:187, 1973.

58. Miller TR, Anderson RJ, Linas SL, et al.: Urinary diagnostic indices in acute renal failure. A prospective study. *Ann Intern Med* 89:47, 1978.

59. Miller PD, Krebs RA, Neal BJ, et al.: Polyuric prerenal failure. *Arch Intern Med* 140:907, 1980.

60. Knochel JP: Acute renal failure. *Semin Nephrol* 1:5, 1981.

61. Champion H, Long W, Smith H, et al.: Indications for early hemodialysis in multiple trauma. *Lancet* 1:1125, 1974.

62. Tzamaloukas AH, Garella S, Chazan JA: Peritoneal dialysis for acute renal failure after major abdominal surgery. *Arch Surg* 106:639, 1973.

63. Mayer AD, McMahon MJ, et al.: Controlled clinical trial of peritoneal lavage for the treatment of severe acute pancreatitis. *New Engl J Med* 312:399, 1985.

64. Bosch JP: Continuous arteriovenous hemofiltration (CAVH): Operational characteristics and clinical use. *Nephrology Letter* 3:15, 1986.

65. Bartlett RH, Mault JR, Dechert RE, et al.: Continuous areteriovenous hemofiltration: Improved survival in surgical acute renal failure? *Surgery* 100:400, 1986.

66. Francis GS, Sharma B, Collins AJ, et al.: Coronary-artery surgery in patients with end-stage renal disease. *Ann Intern Med* 92:499, 1980.

67. Lansing AM, Leb DE, Berman LB: Cardiovascular surgery in end-stage renal failure. *JAMA* 204:134, 1968.

68. Haimov M, Glabman S, Schupak E, et al.: General surgery in patients on maintenance hemodialysis. *Ann Surg* 179:863, 1974.

69. Bernowitz JB, Williams CD, Edwards WS: Major surgery in patients with chronic renal failure. *Am J Surg* 134:765, 1977.

70. Burke GE, Gulyassy PF: Surgery in patients with renal disease and related electrolyte disorders. *Med Clin N Am* 63:1191, 1979.

71. Dornfeld L, Narins RG: Pre- and postoperative renal failure. *Urol Clin N Am* 3:363, 1976.

72. Egan JD: How to evaluate the surgical patient with renal disease. *Geriatrics* 32:46, 1977.

73. Herrin JT: Preparation of the renal patient for surgery. *Int Anesthiol Clin* 13:183, 1975.

74. Tasker PR, MacGregor GA, DeWardener HE: Prophylactic use of intravenous saline in patients with chronic renal failure undergoing major surgery. *Lancet* 2:911, 1974.

75. Silberman H: Renal failure and the surgeon. *Surg Gynecol Obstet* 144:775, 1977.

76. Janson PA, Jubilerer SJ, Weinstein MJ, et al.: Treatment of the bleeding tendency in uremia with cryoprecipitate. *N Engl J Med* 303:1318, 1980.

77. Deykin D: Uremic bleeding. *Kidney Int* 24:698, 1983.

78. Smith JW, Seidl LG, Cluff LE: Studies on the epidemiology of adverse drug reactions: V. Clinical factors influencing susceptibility. *Ann Intern Med* 65:629, 1966.

79. Bennett WM, Muther RS, Parker RA, et al.: Drug therapy in renal failure: Dosing guidelines for adults. *Ann Intern Med* 93:62, 1980.

80. Bennett WM, Muther RS, Parker RA, et al.: Drug therapy in renal failure: Dosing guidelines for adults. *Ann Intern Med* 93:286, 1980.

81. Inturrisi CE: Disposition of narcotics in patients with renal failure. *Am J Med* 62:528, 1977.

82. Bauer JH, Brooks CS: The long-term effect of propranolol on renal function. *Am J Med* 66:405, 1979.

83. Bryan CS, and Stone WJ: "Comparably massive" penicillin G therapy in renal failure. *Ann Intern Med* 82:189, 1975.

84. Finkelstein W, Isselbacher K: Cimetidine. *N Engl J Med* 299:992, 1978.

85. Bakkaloglu M, Hamilton NH, Macpherson SG, Briggs JD: Morbidity and mortality in renal transplant patients after incidental surgery. *Br J Surg* 65:228, 1978.

86. Leapman SB, Vidne BA, Butt KM, et al.: Elective and emergency surgery in renal transplant patients. *Ann Surg* 183:266, 1976.

87. Brown RS, Epstein FH: Fluid and electrolyte disorders in urologic patients. *Urol Clin N Am* 3:267, 1976.

88. Orloff MJ, Hutchin P: Fluid and electrolyte response to trauma and surgery, in Kleeman CR, Maxwell MH (eds): *Clinical Disorders of Fluid and Electrolyte Metabolism.* New York, McGraw-Hill, 1972.

89. Chung HM, Kluge R, Schrier RW, et al.: Postoperative hyponatremia. A prospective study. *Arch Int Med* 146:333, 1986.

90. Arieff AI. Hyponatremia, convulsions, respiratory arrest, and permanent brain damage after elective surgery in healthy women. *New Engl J Med* 314:1529, 1986.

91. Berl T, Anderson RJ, McDonald KM, Schrier RW: Clinical disorders of water metabolism. *Kidney Int* 10:117, 1976.

92. Arieff AI, Llach F, Massry SG: Neurological manifestations and morbidity of hyponatremia: Correlation with brain water and electrolytes. *Medicine* 55:121, 1976.

93. Mundy GR, Wilkinson R, Heath DA. Comparative study of available therapy for hypercalcemia of malignancy. *Am J Med* 74:421, 1983.

94. Cardella CJ, Birkin BL, Roscoe M, et al.: Role of dialysis in the treatment of severe hypercalcemia: Report of two cases successfully treated with hemodialysis and review of the literature. *Clin Nephrol* 12:285, 1979.

95. Knochel JP: The pathophysiology and clinical characteristics of severe hypophosphatemia. *Arch Intern Med* 137:203, 1977.

96. Juan D, Elrazak M: Hypophosphatemia in hospitalized patients. *JAMA* 242:163, 1979.

97. Lentz RD, Brown DM, Kjellstrand CM: Treatment of severe hypophosphatemia. *Ann Intern Med* 89:941, 1978.

98. Slatopolsky E, Rutherford WE, Rosenbaum R, et al.: Hyperphosphatemia. *Clin Nephrol* 7:138, 1977.

99. Carroll HJ, Oh MS: *Water, Electrolyte, and Acid-Base Metabolism: Diagnosis and Management.* Philadelphia, JB Lippincott, 1978.

100. Lyons JH, Moore FD: Posttraumatic alkalosis:

Incidence and pathophysiology of alkalosis in surgery. *Surgery* 60:93, 1966.

101. Wilson RF, Gibson D, Percinel AK, et al.: Severe alkalosis in critically ill surgical patients. *Arch Surg* 105:197, 1972.

102. Shavelle HS, Parke R: Postoperative metabolic alkalosis and acute renal failure: Rationale for the use of hydrochloric acid. *Surgery* 78:439, 1975.

103. Swartz RD, Rubin JE, Brown RS, et al.: Correction of postoperative metabolic alkalosis and renal failure by hemodialysis. *Ann Intern Med* 86:52, 1977.

104. McCurdy DK: Mixed metabolic and respiratory acid base disorders. *Chest* 62:355, 1972.

105. Narins RG, Emmett M: Simple and mixed acid base disorders: A practical approach. *Medicine* 59:161, 1980.

106. Goldberg M, Green SB, Moss ML, et al.: Computer-based instruction and diagnosis of acid base disorders: A systematic approach. *JAMA* 223:269, 1973.

107. Bear R, Goldstein M, Phillipson E, et al.: Effect of metabolic alkalosis on respiratory function in patients with chronic obstructive lung disease. *Can Med Assoc J* 22:117, 1977.

12

Gastroenterology

Harold Tucker

Disorders of the digestive system frequently affect the outcome of surgery. The operative risk to the patient may be increased, as in the patient with liver disease, or new complications may occur in the postoperative period, e.g., stress ulcerations. In this section, the relationship between surgery and gastrointestinal diseases will be discussed, with emphasis on the preoperative assessment of these surgical risks in patients with hepatic and peptic ulcer disease, as well as on the management of gastrointestinal-related postsurgical complications.

NUTRITION

Gastrointestinal disorders may result in significant nutritional deficiencies. These deficiencies may result in intravascular volume depletion, electrolyte imbalance, protein loss, and catabolism. Protein malnutrition contributes to poor wound healing and immune incompetence. A detailed discussion of the evaluation of a patient's nutritional status and the management of various nutritional deficiencies is provided in Chapter 5.

LIVER DISEASE

Liver disease may create a variety of problems that can increase the risk of surgery. These problems include: metabolism of anesthetic drugs; coagulation defects; electrolyte disorders; impaired renal function in the presence of severe liver disease; postoperative development of encephalopathy and ascites; increased risk of infection; and potential contamination of surgical personnel and material by hepatitis virus. It is important to recognize

and evaluate these problems early in order to lessen the risk for surgery and to weigh the risk to benefit ratio for a given surgical procedure.

Epidemiology and Pathophysiology

INCIDENCE OF COMPLICATIONS

Although it is generally well-accepted that severe liver disease poses special risks for the surgical patient, the actual frequency of adverse outcome from surgery is not well-documented in the literature.

It has been estimated that 200–300 patients per year will undergo general anesthesia while incubating viral hepatitis (1). There are several reports showing hepatic deterioration following surgery in patients with acute hepatitis. Harville and Summerskill (2) reported from the Mayo Clinic a 9.5% operative mortality in patients with acute viral hepatitis (none in drug-induced hepatitis) and a 12% incidence of serious complications. Dykes (3) and Marx (4) reported a similar deterioration of hepatic function. While these data do not provide an actual incidence, they do suggest that the risk of surgery is significantly increased during acute viral hepatitis.

Increased mortality and morbidity rates may also occur in the setting of alcoholic hepatitis. The incidence of complications for non-shunt surgery for this same class of patients is unknown. The severity of the liver dysfunction may be underestimated as the transaminases are frequently only mildly abnormal. However, as noted previously, the histologic finding of alcoholic hyaline indicates a worse outcome from surgery, with a mortality rate from emergency portacaval shunt surgery of over 80% in one series (5). Postoperative deterioration in hepatic function is generally due to hepatic ischemia caused by anesthesia and intraoperative hypovolemia. Overt signs of hepatic failure may then appear postoperatively. Accumulation of ascites with subsequent abdominal wound dehiscence is a major concern. Variceal bleeding may occur in the postoperative state secondary to increases in portal pressure and overzealous efforts to maintain good intravascular volume. Renal failure may also occur, either as a consequence of the surgery or from the "hepato-renal syndrome" associated with marked deterioration in liver function. Wound infection and increased bleeding may also complicate the recovery period.

Surgery in patients with cirrhosis has been clinically accepted to carry a high risk, whether the surgery is unrelated to or is for complications (e.g., variceal bleeding) of the liver disease. Little literature is available to document the increased risk, to quantify the magnitude of risk; or to determine risk factors identifying subgroups of high-risk patients (5–7).

Gallbladder surgery in the presence of cirrhosis carries about a 21–25% total mortality risk (8–10). The risk rises to 30–83% if the prothrombin time is prolonged. Not all deaths are related to the liver disease; liver disease specific mortality figures are not available. Child's classification or the factors making up this index seem to be predictive of mortality in two small preliminary studies (8–9) (Table 12.1), similar to more extensive studies for mortality for portal shunts (Table 12.2) (11). Whether data for gallbladder surgery, which is liver related, are representative of risks for *unrelated* general surgery in cirrhosis must await studies of patients undergoing other types of surgery, which are not currently available.

Table 12.1. Risk of Biliary Surgery in Cirrhosis: Preliminary Data on Child's Classification (8)*

Child's Classification**	Mortality (%)
A	13%
B	25%
C	50%

*Data from Cryer HM, Howard DA, Garrison RN: Liver cirrhosis and biliary surgery: Assessment of risk. *S Med J* 78:138, 1985.
**See Table 12.2 for explanation of classification.

The high risk of shunt surgery in patients with varices has been documented (11), but the nature of the patient population and surgery probably preclude applying this risk data to other types of surgery.

Laboratory abnormalities of liver function tests will be found in an estimated 0.02 to 3% of surgical patients (see chapter 23). Liver enzyme abnormalities, "unexpected", by history and physical examination, will be found in an estimated 0.03% of surgical patients. The incidence of abnormal liver enzymes not suspected by clinical examination may be higher, depending on whether "trivial" elevations of enzymes (e.g., transaminases 1–10 points above normal) are included and the specificity of the laboratory method. The risk for surgery of these minor elevations of liver enzymes unexpected and unexplained by history and physical examination has not been determined. An estimated one-third of these patients may have incubating, acute liver disease in one-study (12), although clinical experience suggests the risk may be lower.

IDENTIFICATION OF HIGH-RISK PATIENTS

The severity and activity of the liver disease are major determinants of the surgical risk in patients with hepatic dysfunction. Unfortunately, conventional "liver function tests" correlate poorly with the actual degree of liver impairment. The transaminase tests (SGOT and SGPT) are

Table 12.2. Classification of Hepatic Function and Surgical Risk for Portasystemic Shunt[a]

	Class		
	A	B	C
Albumin (gm/100 ml)	>3.5	3.0–3.5	<3.0
Bilirubin	<2.0	2.0–3.0	>3.0
Ascites	None	Easily controlled	Poorly controlled
Encephalopathy	None	Minimal	Moderate to severe
Nutrition	Excellent	Good	"Wasted" to poor
Operative mortality[b]	0–1%	9–10%	>50%

[a] Adapted from Child CG III: *Portal Hypertension,* Philadelphia, WB Saunders, 1974, p. 82.
[b] Mortality rate for portasystemic shunting.

not useful as prognostic indicators, and do not reflect the severity of hepatic pathology. Hypoalbuminemia, however, may indicate chronic liver disease and has been suggested as an indicator of poor surgical risk (13). A useful classification of patients with liver disease was formulated by Child (8,14), combining clinical and biochemical parameters (Table 12.2). Measurements of serum bilirubin and albumin in conjunction with assessment of nutritional status, degree of ascites, and degree of encephalopathy were used to categorize patients. With this classification, the surgical risk for portasystemic shunting could be evaluated for different patients. Class C patients with obvious evidence of severe liver disease had the worst risk, with 53% operative mortality, while class A patients tolerated surgery well. While Child's classification is the most widely used for patients with liver disease undergoing major surgery, modifications have been proposed using other tests to improve on the predictive value of the classification. Pugh (15) adds the prothrombin time, a good test for chronic liver dysfunction, to the parameters measured by Child. Others have evaluated various hemodynamic measurements, including the cardiac index and arteriovenous shunting, and have formulated a survival index for patients undergoing portasystemic shunting procedures (16). There is little evidence that any of these various classifications is superior to the others in predicting survival for major surgery.

A preoperative liver biopsy may also be useful in assessing the severity of the hepatic disease. Differentiation between fatty liver and alcoholic hepatitis, and between chronic-active and chronic-persistent hepatitis is best made by liver biopsy, not by various biochemical tests. Steatosis, or fat accumulation in the liver, disappears rapidly, usually within several weeks, once the patient abstains from alcohol and consumes a nutritious diet. Therefore, the finding of excessive fat in the liver may warrant a delay in surgery for several weeks to allow the liver function to improve. The presence of Mallory bodies on liver biopsies suggests a higher risk. Several studies have demonstrated that patients undergoing portasystemic shunting had a higher mortality if the preoperative liver biopsy demonstrated hyaline necrosis (Mallory bodies) (5,17–19). The mortality for elective portasystemic shunting was 65% for patients with hyaline necrosis compared to only 6% without this histologic abnormality (5). For patients with hyaline necrosis, emergency surgery was associated with an 83% mortality rate compared to only 6% for those without Mallory bodies. However, Rouselot et al. (20) cast some doubt on the value of this histologic finding as they reported only a 15% mortality in patients with hyaline necrosis undergoing shunting procedure. No comparative figures were given for those without hyaline necrosis, however. Finally, the presence of cirrhosis can be readily detected on liver biopsy, even when the biochemical parameters are only minimally abnormal or even normal (21).

PROBLEMS RELATED TO ANESTHESIA

In patients with liver disease, two major issues must be considered in choosing an anesthetic agent: (a) the metabolism and inactivation of the various anesthetic drugs; (b) the effect of these compounds on the liver itself. Due to alterations in metabolism, the dose and type of sedative, analgesic, and anesthetic agent used in the perioperative period need to be monitored closely in the patient with liver disease. Problems with the metabolism of the anesthetic drugs in patients with liver disease include: impaired transformation of anesthetic agents from lipid-soluble compounds to more water soluble ones; hypoproteinemia resulting in decreased binding of drugs; impaired biliary clearance; and decreased enzyme levels to inactivate drugs (e.g., decreased pseudocholinesterase levels needed to metabolize d-tubocurarine). The anesthesiologist must be aware of the extent of liver disease in order to properly administer the various anesthetic agents.

Anesthetic agents may also directly affect liver function. Nearly all anesthetic agents, including those administered via spinal and extradural routes, reduce liver blood flow (LBF), causing a fall in oxygen uptake (22). Normally, LBF is derived from the portal vein (approximately 70%) and from the hepatic artery. In patients with portal hypertension, there is a decrease in the portal vein contribution with an "arterialization" of LBF. Further decreases in LBF may, therefore, result in ischemic injury to the liver with deterioration in liver function postoperatively. Anesthetic agents, hypercarbia, and alpha stimulation can increase the splanch-

nic vascular resistance and thereby reduce liver blood flow. Of the anesthetic agents, methoxyflurane is notable for its vasoconstrictive effects on the hepatic artery. Halothane seems least harmful. The reduction of LBF is perhaps the most important contributing factor to the deterioration of liver function that may occur postoperatively in patients with severe liver disease.

While the choice of anesthetic agent belongs to the anesthesiologist, the internist should recognize that the selection is based on the effect of the various agents on splanchnic blood flow, as well as possible direct hepatotoxic effects. As spinal and extradural anesthesia may also produce similar decreases in splanchnic blood flow, these agents should not be assumed to be safer for the patient with severe liver disease.

COAGULATION DEFECTS

Coagulation defects are present in the cirrhotic patient that may predispose to increased bleeding. The prothrombin time is often prolonged in patients with severe liver disease, reflecting low levels of clotting factors I, II, V, VII, IX, X, XI, and XII, whose production is dependent on normal liver function (22–23). Thrombocytopenia is also common due to hypersplenism, folate deficiency, and alcoholism. These abnormalities need to be identified and corrected prior to surgery.

In the patient with a prolonged prothrombin time, parenteral vitamin K_1 at doses of 10–20 mg per day for 3 consecutive days should be administered. This dose will generally correct the prothrombin time if obstructive jaundice or malabsorption is the cause for the coagulation defect. However, in advanced parenchymal liver disease, with severe depression of the clotting factors, the prothrombin time may remain prolonged. In such cases, fresh frozen plasma should be given preoperatively to correct the coagulation abnormality, and be continued through the operative and postoperative period to prevent bleeding (see Chapter 14). Platelet transfusions are rarely needed as very low platelet counts are unusual and the platelets function normally. When hypersplenism is present (as opposed to primary bone marrow suppression secondary to alcohol or folate deficiency), platelet transfusions are of little value as they will be consumed rapidly by the spleen.

EFFECT OF LIVER DISEASE ON RENAL FUNCTION

The incidence of postoperative renal failure may be increased in patients with marked hyperbilirubinemia. The incidence of this complication is higher than in the anicteric population and is most common in patients with obstructive jaundice (24). Various causes have been suggested including hypoxia; decreased renal blood flow; possible toxic effects from bilirubin (4); and excess endotoxin produced from the patient's own bowel flora (25).

It has been suggested but not proven that the risk of renal failure can be reduced by inducing a diuresis before surgery and maintaining it through the immediate postoperative period (26). Mannitol has been recommended for its ability to increase intravascular volume and promote an osmotic diuresis. However, careful monitoring of intravascular volume and electrolytes is essential.

Diuretic-induced hypovolemia may result in hypotension during surgery with its consequent deleterious effect on the liver. Hypokalemia may similarly result from a brisk diuresis and may precipitate hepatic encephalopathy. Other measures that have been recommended to prevent postoperative renal failure in patients with hyperbilirubinemia include: volume repletion prior to surgery; selection of anesthetic agents that have least vasoconstrictive effect on renal blood flow; preoperative antibiotics to reduce the bowel flora capable of producing endotoxins; and use of dopamine to dilate splanchnic circulation (28). The efficacy of these various measures has not been proved in preventing postoperative renal failure. Percutaneous catheter biliary drainage can effectively lower bilirubin levels preoperatively, but its value in preventing this complication has yet to be proven.

Preoperative Evaluation

The history should focus on any previous episodes of hepatitis or jaundice, or recent exposure to hepatitis or hepatotoxic agents (e.g., alcohol, drugs, etc.). The physical examination should carefully assess the presence of jaundice or hepatomegaly. Palmar erythema and spider angiomata may suggest chronic liver disease, while the presence of ascites or splenomegaly may signify portal hypertension from cirrhosis.

Routine measurements of SGOT or SGPT levels in asymptomatic patients is generally not indicated as they are of low specificity and therefore not cost-effective (22) (see chapter 23). The prevalence of hepatitis in the asymptomatic patient is also low at 0.25/1000. Transaminase, alkaline phosphatase, and bilirubin levels should be obtained in those cases where the history, physical examination, or routine screening tests suggest liver disease.

Patients with a remote history of jaundice or hepatitis should have transaminases, alkaline phosphatase, bilirubin, prothrombin time, albumin and globulin levels, and a HBsAg screen. If these studies and the physical examination are normal, there is no evidence of any increased risk to the patient from surgery and no further evaluation is needed. If these studies are abnormal, further evaluation should be performed to determine the nature and severity of the hepatitis. When the patient recalls hepatic abnormalities following previous surgery, records must be reviewed to determine the cause. If the anesthetic agent is implicated, then a different agent must be selected.

For the patient with newly discovered hepatomegaly, or with abnormal liver function tests, further investigation into the nature of the hepatic disease is indicated preoperatively. Analysis of the liver function tests generally dictates the direction of the evaluation. Hepatitis, either of infectious or drug etiology, is generally characterized by markedly abnormal transaminases with only a mild elevation in alkaline phosphatase. Further identification of the offending agent should be determined by measuring HBsAg, HBcAb (hepatitis B core antibody), HBsAb (hepatitis B surface antibody), hepatitis A antibody, as well as a detailed history of exposure to potential hepatotoxins (including alcohol and medications). When acute hepatitis is present, surgery should be deferred when possible until the acute illness has resolved. Patients with known chronic hepatitis should be assessed based on clinical and laboratory criteria outlined previously (Table 12.2). Liver biopsy may be needed to determine the etiology of the hepatitis (alcohol vs. viral), to evaluate the severity of the liver disease, and to differentiate chronic persistent from chronic active hepatitis.

In patients with disproportionately high alkaline phosphatase levels in relationship to the transaminase levels, cholestatic liver disease should be suspected. Differentiation between intrahepatic and extrahepatic causes of cholestasis may be possible by clues in the history and physical examination but not generally by analysis of the "liver" chemistry. Recent use of drugs known to induce cholestasis (phenothiazines, estrogen compounds) or the presence of a palpable gallbladder are helpful distinguishing features for intrahepatic and extrahepatic diseases, respectively. The presence of a dilated biliary tract seen on ultrasound examination or computerized tomography (CT) examination of the abdomen is a clear indication of extrahepatic disease, e.g., stones or tumor. Further preoperative delineation of the cause of extrahepatic obstruction can be obtained by endoscopic or transhepatic cholangiography. The over-

all accuracy of ultrasound in distinguishing intrahepatic and extrahepatic cholestasis is 90% (23, 24). Correction of the cause of intrahepatic cholestasis should be achieved prior to elective non-biliary tract surgery as the morbidity and mortality of surgery in such patients may be increased. In patients with extrahepatic obstruction, mortality and morbidity for biliary tract surgery increases with increasing elevations of the bilirubin, particularly with levels greater than 20 mg/100 ml (25).

Common, treatable complications of liver disease, which increase the risk of surgery, should be searched for in all patients with liver disease preoperatively. These complications include encephalopathy, ascites, infection, electrolyte disturbance, gastrointestinal bleeding, infection, malnutrition, abnormal clotting factors and platelets, anemia, and decreased renal function. Medications received by the patient should be reviewed to identify those drugs that are hepatotoxic, will worsen liver function, or produce complications, such as bleeding and encephalopathy (especially, aspirin, sedatives, and pain medications).

In summary, patients undergoing anesthesia and surgery should be screened for liver disease by a careful history and physical examination. When there is evidence to suggest the presence of liver disease, further evaluation is needed. In patients with significant liver disease, either acute or chronic, the morbidity and mortality from surgery appears to be increased. Hepatic deterioration commonly occurs in such patients postoperatively for a variety of reasons, including ischemic injury to the liver secondary to the effects of anesthesia on liver blood flow. Recognition of the severity of the liver disease preoperatively is essential in predicting the risk of surgical procedures and in preventing postoperative complications. Poor prognostic features include: *(a)* ascites; *(b)* encephalopathy; *(c)* poor nutritional status; *(d)* hypoalbuminemia;

(e) hyperbilirubinemia; *(f)* prolonged prothrombin time; *(g)* alcoholic hyaline on liver biopsy.

Management

Patients with known liver disease should be prepared for surgery with attention to specific postoperative complications. Risks of surgery should be well understood by the patient, his family, and the surgeon. The anesthesiologist should be well aware of the patient's hepatic disease. Electrolyte abnormalities and coagulation defects should be corrected preoperatively. Ascites should be well controlled. Infection and gastrointestinal bleeding should be sought and as effectively stabilized as time before surgery allows. Nutritional support will be required in some cases of malnutrition, but will require special solutions to avoid hepatic encephalopathy (see chapter 5). The patient's mental status should be documented preoperatively, so changes that may occur postoperatively can be readily identified. Great care should be given to maintain an adequate intravascular volume, so as to minimize intraoperative hepatic ischemia, while at the same time not excessively increasing portal pressure. Defining the patient's hepatic status preoperatively with attention to potential postoperative complications is the most helpful way to handle these challenging patients.

The decision to proceed with, postpone, or cancel surgery will depend on the type of liver disease and the urgency of the surgery. The severity of the liver disease has a significant but less important impact on the surgical decision. In general, all but emergency, immediately life-saving surgery should be postponed in the presence of acute viral and alcoholic hepatitis. Although data indicate drug-induced hepatitis carries a lesser operative risk (2), this data is based on a small number of patients, and surgery should be postponed for drug hepatitis also. No information exists on the optimal waiting time for elective surgery following acute hepatitis. General clinical guidelines suggest waiting until all clinical and laboratory parameters of hepatitis have normalized for at least 6 weeks, although some authorities would wait longer for up to 6 months. The decision in individual cases must also consider the type, severity of the hepatitis, and the urgency of the surgery.

Surgery needs to be carefully considered in all cases of cirrhosis. Cirrhotic patients in Child's Class A with no ascites, bilirubin less than 2 mg/100 ml, normal albumin, no encephalopathy, and good nutrition seem to carry a lower risk. A normal prothrombin time, stable rather than deteriorating cirrhosis, and lack of superimposed acute liver disease (e.g., alcoholic hepatitis) seem also to lower risk although the latter two clinical factors have not been confirmed statistically. However, even in the presence of all "good" risk factors, the mortality of certain general surgery (e.g., biliary surgery) may be as high as 25%. Therefore, a very careful consideration of the benefit of the surgery to the patient must be made, before deciding to proceed with surgery in the cirrhotic patient; the risk remains significantly elevated even in "good" risk patients.

No firm data exist on the risk of deteriorating liver function, major complications, or death in the patient with no known liver disease who has mildly elevated liver enzymes found unexpectedly on preoperative laboratory testing. Evaluation can often find a cause in patients with substantial elevations (more than 2–3 times normal) of liver enzymes, but often no or an uncertain, etiology can be found in patients with small elevations (data are not available in the literature for this group of patients with mild liver enzyme abnormalities). Patients with unexplained elevations of liver function should have surgery postponed if possible, until the abnormalities can be evaluated (see p. 249).

Repeating the liver enzymes are the

first step in evaluating mild unexpected abnormalities of liver function. Other tests that should be done include a full set of liver enzymes (SGOT, SGPT, alkaline phosphatase), prothrombin time, and albumin, if not done as part of the original blood testing. Often repeat testing will be normal, because of laboratory error or, more commonly, because of the way normal values are set. (Normal values for most screening batteries are based on the 95% percentile, so 1 in 20 normal patients will be abnormal; see chapter 23.) If the remainder of the history, physical, and laboratory evaluation points against the presence of liver disease, often this is as far as the evaluation needs to be taken.

If the repeat liver enzymes remain elevated, they should be evaluated as for the patient with liver disease described above (see p. 249), and surgery postponed. If laboratory testing does not discover an etiology, causes of liver dysfunction to be considered are hidden alcoholism (a very common cause), medications (especially over the counter, such as aspirin), drug abuse, and a mild viral illness. If no cause can be found as is often the case, we recommend postponing surgery and following serial liver enzymes for about 6 weeks before deciding on surgery, as a prudent decision (5). However, we recognize the lack of data, the frequent inconvenience this causes, and that other clinicians will decide to go ahead, especially if the elevations are only a few points, the surgery is minor, and local or regional anesthesia will be used. Firm recommendations on what to do in this situation must await prospective studies of surgical risk, which are not presently available.

Special Considerations

HBsAg CARRIER

The patient who is a chronic carrier of hepatitis B surface antigen (HBsAg) poses the special problem of infecting surgical personnel and of contaminating hospital equipment. Such patients may be entirely asymptomatic with normal liver function or may suffer from chronic hepatitis. For the asymptomatic carrier without evidence of liver disease, there is no increased risk to surgery, nor is there any evidence of activation of the virus by anesthesia (26).

Such patients must be clearly identified and exposure of hospital personnel to the patient's blood products must be minimized whenever possible. All blood specimens from such patients should be clearly labeled as being HBsAg-positive. The number of personnel in the operating room should be kept to a minimum. Persons coming in contact with the patient's blood, via either needle stick or spilling of blood on open cuts, should receive hepatitis B immune globulin (HBIG) (27). Patients with chronic hepatitis associated with HBsAg should be evaluated for severity and activity of liver disease according to the criteria of Childs (14) and Pugh (15) as discussed above.

PANCREATITIS

Epidemiology

It has long been a surgical dictum that surgery should be avoided in the presence of acute pancreatitis. Factors associated with acute pancreatitis that may increase the surgical risk include: preoperative hypovolemia and electrolyte disturbances; technical factors in dealing with peripancreatic tissues that are inflamed, edematous, and highly vascular; potential for introducing infection into the inflamed pancreatic tissue (producing an infected pseudocyst or pancreatic abscess); increased renal and pulmonary complications; and postoperative exacerbation of pancreatitis. Following surgery, it may be difficult to distinguish the consequences of the surgical procedure from the complications of ongoing pancreatitis. Thus, in most cases of acute pancreatitis, surgical exploration may be deleterious and should be avoided.

Evaluation

However, due to the variable clinical presentations of acute pancreatitis, it may be difficult in some cases to establish the diagnosis of acute pancreatitis or to distinguish this condition from other disorders that do require surgical treatment. While acute abdominal pain and hyperamylasemia are the most characteristic features of acute pancreatitis, other conditions may present in a similar fashion, including cholecystitis, choledocholithiasis, and intestinal infarction. In some cases, only serial observations of the clinical course over several hours to days may permit the definitive differentiation among these various pathologic entities.

The laboratory diagnosis of pancreatitis is based on the detection of hyperamylasemia, an increased urinary amylase, or an elevated amylase to creatinine clearance ratio. An elevated amylase value can be found in the majority of patients with acute pancreatitis during the first 48 hours of illness. However, in some patients, particularly in those with multiple previous episodes of pancreatitis, the amylase levels may remain normal. The height of the amylase level does not correlate with the severity of the illness, but values of over 1000 units tend to indicate a surgical cause for the pancreatitis (e.g., stones) (29). Hyperamylasemia is not specific for pancreatitis and may be seen with common duct stones without concomitant pancreatitis, mumps, and penetrating ulcers. Serum lipase is also nonspecific for the pancreas. The serum lipase stays elevated longer than amylase.

An elevated amylase to creatinine clearance ratio has been suggested as being more specific for pancreatitis (30). The ratio is obtained according to the following formula:

$$\frac{\text{Amylase clearance}}{\text{Creatinine clearance}} \%$$

$$= \frac{(\text{urine amylase})}{(\text{serum amylase})} \times \frac{(\text{serum creatinine})}{(\text{urine creatinine})}$$

In pancreatitis, the ratio is three times that of normal. However, the test has been limited by a lack of sensitivity and by confusion over appropriate methodology in measuring amylase levels. Recent evidence also shows a false-elevation in postoperative patients (31). In addition, an elevated ratio can be found in other conditions, such as diabetic ketoacidosis, burns, postcardiac surgery, and perforated duodenal ulcer. Thus, while the test may still be useful in some selected cases, its clinical application has become very limited.

Ultrasonography and CT scan of the abdomen may also be helpful in diagnosing acute pancreatitis by identifying an edematous pancreas or a pancreatic pseudocyst. Sensitivity and specificity of these modalities in the diagnosis of acute pancreatitis remain to be established, but in an individual patient, these modalities may confirm the presence of a diseased pancreas and rule out other potential causes for acute abdominal pain.

Management

In certain circumstances, surgery may be required despite ongoing pancreatitis. Surgical exploration has been advocated: (a) to decompress the biliary tree in patients with impacted common duct stones; (b) to exclude other conditions (infarcted gut, perforated viscus); and (c) to manage the complications of pancreatitis (drainage of pseudocyst or abscess) (32). While it is difficult to assess accurately the relative risk of surgery in the face of acute pancreatitis, sufficient experience with severe complications in such cases has led to the reluctance to operate except for the above indications. Recently, percutaneous, fluoroscopically guided skinny needle-catheter drainage of pancreatic pseudocysts or abscesses has been advocated as, at least, a temporizing measure.

A separate issue is the timing of a cholecystectomy in the patient with suspected gallstone-induced pancreatitis. As noted previously, in the severely ill patient with acute pancreatitis, jaundice, and gallstones, early biliary decompression has been advocated. However, cholecystectomy without common bile duct decompression may not be beneficial during the early course of the pancreatitis. For most patients, the pancreatitis will subside, and the cholecystectomy can be performed on a more elective basis. In the past, it has been recommended that the cholecystectomy be performed after the pancreatic inflammation has subsided, generally at least 6 weeks after the acute episode. However, more recent data have suggested that earlier surgery should be performed. Kelly (33) has demonstrated that the optimal time to operate is during the same hospitalization as the acute episode, usually 5–7 days after resolution of the pancreatitis. Earlier surgery (within 48–72 hours) as suggested by Acosta (34) is associated with a higher mortality and often involves more extensive surgery (sphincterotomy for impacted stones and common duct exploration). In patients who recovered from the acute pancreatitis and were scheduled for elective cholecystectomy 2–6 months later, recurrent gallstone pancreatitis occurred in over 38% prior to the scheduled elective operation, and was associated with a higher mortality than in the group who underwent elective surgery during the same hospitalization. Ranson (35) reported similar results but emphasized that surgery should be deferred until the pancreatitis has resolved. He noted a decrease in mortality from 29 to 1.5% by deferring the surgery until after resolution of the acute process. Thus, in patients with gallstone pancreatitis, surgery should be performed during the initial hospitalization, after the pancreatitis has resolved.

POSTOPERATIVE PANCREATITIS

Epidemiology

Pancreatitis is a serious problem in the postoperative period, with mortality rates of up to 36% and major complications of up to 50% (36). Postoperative pancreatitis is an infrequent problem, with only 22 cases found over an 11-year period from one hospital (36). Most often the pancreatitis follows surgery in the upper abdomen. In a series from the Mayo Clinic, pancreatitis occurred in up to 3% of patients following gastric resection (37).

Evaluation

The diagnosis of pancreatitis is often made only after severe manifestations of the disease are present. Hypotension, oliguria, jaundice, or a mass are frequently present when postoperative pancreatitis is finally diagnosed. Jaundice may be seen in 30% of patients. A prolonged paralytic ileus and hypovolemia should suggest pancreatitis. Hyperamylasemia is often found.

Management

Therapy is aimed at maintaining intravascular volume and electrolyte balance and relief of pain. Anticholinergics and prophylactic antibiotics are of little value. A variety of agents including glucagon, cimetidine, and trasylol have been tried in pancreatitis with little objective data to support their use. Parenteral hyperalimentation should be employed in the severely ill patient with postoperative pancreatitis.

PEPTIC ULCER DISEASE

Epidemiology

A history of peptic ulcer disease can be elicited in 10–12% of the adult population (38). Despite this prevalence, there is little data on its effect on the outcome of non-ulcer surgery. Patients undergoing surgery may have a history of ulcer disease but are now asymptomatic. They may have symptoms without documented ulcer disease, or, they may be on therapy for documented active ulcer disease.

Evaluation

Patients with only a history of ulcer disease in the past who are now asymptomatic and have a normal physical examination (no abdominal tenderness or fecal blood) appear to have no increased risks from surgery compared to the normal population. Theoretically, one might speculate that patients with a history of ulcer disease are more likely to develop exacerbations during the perioperative period. Patients with duodenal ulcer disease hypersecrete acid both basally and following stimulation. Stress has been shown to increase gastric acidity (39) and ulcer symptoms (40). Furthermore, mucosal resistance may be diminished during periods of hypotension and hypoxia during surgery. However, despite these theoretical concerns, there is little evidence to suggest an increased risk of new peptic ulcer formation perioperatively. There is also no evidence for increased risk of stress ulcerations in patients with a previous history of peptic ulcer disease.

Patients who have symptoms of ulcer disease should be evaluated further. Risk factors for peptic ulcer disease include: cigarette smoking, aspirin use, and a family history of peptic ulcer disease. Features in the history that suggest exacerbation of the ulcer condition include: (a) change in the pain-food-relief patterns; (b) change in the daily pattern of pain; (c) nocturnal pain; (d) radiation of the pain to the back; (e) vomiting. While food typically relieves the pain of duodenal ulcer patients, in patients with gastric ulcer disease, the pain may not have a clear relationship to meals or may be exacerbated by eating. Vomiting and weight loss may occur in such patients. On physical examination, epigastric tenderness may be elicited. The stool may be positive for occult blood.

The diagnosis of ulcer disease can be confirmed by x-ray studies or by endoscopy. With newer air contrast techniques, gastritis and drug-induced gastric erosions can be identified (41). Even with these newer techniques, barium studies are less sensitive than endoscopy with an error rate of 6–8% (41–42). Upper endoscopy is generally very well-tolerated, particularly with the newer instruments, and lasts less than 15 minutes. In the preoperative setting, if documentation of an ulcer crater will alter plans for surgery, then endoscopy is recommended due to its increased accuracy.

Management

In patients with documented ulcer craters, it is generally recommended that elective surgery be deferred until the ulcer has healed. This recommendation seems reasonable, although there is little data to support or refute it, and the incidence of ulcer-related complications postoperatively is poorly documented in the literature. The major concern is the risk of precipitating hemorrhage or perforation in the postoperative period. As noted previously, there are theoretical reasons to support these concerns. Thus, the identification of an active ulcer is an accepted indication for delaying elective surgery until healing has occurred. Simple relief of symptoms is not sufficient, as ulcer pain has been shown to correlate poorly with the presence of an ulcer crater (43).

Patients with an active ulcer should be treated intensively for 4–6 weeks prior to surgery. Cigarette smoking and aspirin should be discontinued. The H_2-antagonists (cimetidine, ranitidine, famotidine and nizatidine) or sucralfate should be given for 6 weeks. All of these agents are equally effective and well tolerated. Antacid therapy can also be given in a dose equivalent to 30 cc of a concentrated antacid (such as Mylanta II or Maalox-TC) 1 and 3 hours following meals and at bedtime, but is less well tolerated. Maintenance therapy to decrease ulcer recurrence (e.g., cimetidine 400 mg, ranitidine 150 mg, or famotidine 20 mg at bedtime) should be used until surgery is performed, as the recurrence rate for ulcer disease following the cessation of therapy is over 50% within a 6-month follow-up period (45). With a maintenance dose of cimetidine (400 mg) at bedtime following initial healing of the ulcer, the cumulative recurrence rate is reduced to 17% over a 6-month period (45).

Gastric ulcers are managed in the same way as duodenal ulcers. Gastric ulcers should be followed to complete healing and may require 3 months of medical therapy.

STRESS ULCERS

Epidemiology

Acute stress ulcers or erosions may present with massive gastrointestinal hemorrhage in the postoperative setting. These lesions represent disruptions in the gastric or duodenal mucosa that are rapid in onset and occur in the setting of severe physical stress. Prospective endoscopic studies in high-risk patients (e.g., trauma or burn patients) have identified discrete mucosal changes that occur within the first 24–72 hours in over 75% of these patients (46). However, significant bleeding occurs infrequently from these superficial lesions. The exact incidence of bleeding from stress ulcerations is difficult to determine, but in critically ill patients in an intensive care unit setting, the incidence of bleeding stress ulcers appears to be about 10–20%.

Various factors have been identified that increase the risk of stress ulcers. These risk factors include: (a) respiratory failure; (b) sepsis; (c) jaundice; (d) peritonitis; (e) renal failure; and (f) hypotension. A combination of these factors further increases the risk with an incidence of hemorrhage from stress ulcers of 9% in patients with only one risk factor, 20% with two risk factors, and 40% with three or more risk factors (47).

The pathophysiology of the formation of stress ulcers is uncertain. Ischemic injury to the gastric mucosa, disruption of the mucosal barrier, and impaired energy metabolism of the gastric mucosal cells have all been suggested as pathophysiologic mechanisms in stress ulcer formation.

Evaluation

Clinically, stress ulcers present with painless bleeding. The bleeding may be slow and occult, resulting in a gradual decline in hematocrit or may present with massive exsanguinating hemorrhage. The clinical picture correlates with the pathologic findings of varying degrees of penetration of the stress ulcers through the mucosa and into larger submucosal vessels.

Endoscopy provides the best method for establishing the correct diagnosis. During endoscopy, multiple superficial lesions may be seen, occurring most often in the proximal portion of the stomach. Selective angiography may also be used to identify an actively bleeding mucosal lesion. Barium studies are of little diagnostic value in this setting.

Management

Primary therapy should be aimed at the prevention of stress ulcer formation. Critically ill patients should be given prophylactic therapy. Intensive antacids appear to be the most effective preventive therapy. Hastings et al. (48) reported in a randomized prospective study of 100 critically ill (but not all postoperative) patients that hourly antacid therapy titrated to maintain gastric pH greater than 3.5 reduced the frequency of bleeding from 25 to 4%. H_2-antagonists have also been found to be effective in reducing the incidence of acute mucosal bleeding (49). However, in comparing intensive antacids (titrated to maintain intragastric pH greater than 3.5) to cimetidine (dose of 1200–2400 mg per day), Priebe et al. (50) found antacid prophylaxis superior. No patient in the antacid treated group bled, while 18% on cimetidine had documented bleeding. These results may be due to the breakthrough in acid secretion between bolus doses of the H_2-antagonists. Continuous infusion of cimetidine or ranitidine, or use of famotidine with its longer duration of acid inhibition, may prove to be highly successful, well tolerated and easy to administer.*

Other drugs have also been found to be effective in the prophylaxis of stress ulcers. Sucralfate has been as effective as the H_2-antagonists in several small studies (51–52). Significant bleeding did occur however in a small percentage of patients. Misoprostil, a prostaglandin analog, has been very effective in early studies.* Diarrhea has been a troublesome side effect, however.

While H_2-antagonists and antacids have proved very useful in stress ulcer prevention, patients given these drugs while in the intensive care unit (ICU) on respirators appear to be at increased risk of aspiration pneumonia (51–52). This appears particularly true for the antacid group. Whether this problem is related to acid inhibition promoting gastric-esophageal-pharyngeal bacterial colonization remains to be definitively proven. Use of sucralfate does not appear to be associated with this problem (51–52).

Data on combining cimetidine with antacids or sucralfate are not yet available.

Based on these studies, it is recommended that critically ill patients be given some form of stress ulcer prophylaxis. If a nasogastric tube is needed postoperatively, the administration of sucralfate seems most appropriate. When no nasogastric tube is present, infusion of an H_2-antagonist sufficient to maintain intragastric pH greater than 4.0 is recommended. Alternatively, a minimum of 30 cc of a high potency antacid may be administered hourly to maintain intragastric pH greater than 3.5.

Once bleeding has occurred from stress ulcers, conventional supportive therapy is needed. Curtis (53) has suggested that antacid therapy titrated to control intragastric pH at greater than 7 is effective in controlling active bleeding. When bleeding continues despite these measures, vasopressin infusion may be utilized. Selective intra-arterial infusion of vasopressin can control acute gastric mucosal hemorrhage in over 80% of patients (54). Complications of vasopressin include myocardial, mesenteric and systemic vasoconstriction, as well as water overload from its antidiuretic effect. Intravenous vasopressin for mucosal hemorrhage has not been well-studied, but may be initiated at the same dose prior to angiography. Surgery for stress ulceration carries a high mortality, and often requires extensive gastric resection. Surgery is reserved for severe bleeding refractory to medical therapy.

GASTROESOPHAGEAL REFLUX

Gastroesophageal reflux may be exacerbated by surgery due to the abdominal distension associated with an ileus and prolonged nasogastric intubation. A preoperative history of significant reflux, particularly if associated with a history of esophageal ulcerations or bleeding, should prompt the recommendation of intensive antireflux therapy during the postoperative period. The head of the bed should be elevated and the nasogastric tube removed as soon as possible. H_2-antagonists can be used intravenously to decrease the acidity and volume of gastric contents. Alternatively, antacids can be administered to patients with intact gastrointestinal tracts. In addition, metoclopramide can also be used intravenously at a dose of 10 mg every 6 hours to accelerate gastric emptying of acid and to improve lower esophageal sphincter tone. Drugs that weaken the lower esophageal sphincter (e.g., anticholinergics) should be avoided.

---

*This is not an FDA approved use or mode of administration for this drug.

INFLAMMATORY BOWEL DISEASE

There is little evidence that extraintestinal surgery is associated with any increased risk of exacerbation in the patient with inflammatory bowel disease (ulcerative colitis and Crohn's disease). In some patients, stressful events frequently produce increased symptoms, but this reaction is highly variable and unpredictable even in the same patient. Patients should be watched carefully for exacerbations and should they result, then specific therapy should be instituted. There is little data to support "prophylactic" increases in steroids or in other therapeutic agents prior to surgery. Patients with inflammatory bowel disease on chronic steroid therapy will require extra steroid coverage for stress during the immediate operative and postoperative period (see Chapter 13).

POSTOPERATIVE JAUNDICE AND LIVER DYSFUNCTION

Epidemiology and Pathophysiology

Jaundice is an infrequent complication of surgery. While many factors relating to surgery may impair hepatic function, hyperbilirubinemia greater than 2 mg/dl suggests severe derangement. The incidence of this complication varies with the type of surgery, the occurrence of intraoperative hypotension, the use of various drugs (including anesthetic agents), and the patient's underlying preoperative liver function. Evans et al. (55) found in a prospective study that mild jaundice (bilirubin less than 4 mg/100 ml) occurred in 17% and severe jaundice (bilirubin greater than 4 mg/100 ml) occurred in 4% of patients undergoing major surgery. Open heart surgery for valvular heart disease was accompanied by jaundice in 8% of patients (56). Jaundice was reported in 2% of patients who were in shock during surgery (57). The incidence of postoperative jaundice following elective abdominal surgery, however, is less than 1% (58). The most common causes of massive hepatic necrosis in the postoperative period are shock, overwhelming infection, preexisting liver disease, and anesthetic hepatitis (4).

The causes of postoperative jaundice can be classified into three pathophysiological mechanisms (Table 12.3): *(a)* overproduction of bilirubin; *(b)* hepatocellular dysfunction; and *(c)* extrahepatic obstruction. Establishment of the etiology of jaundice is important as some causes require surgical intervention, others may require specific medical measures (e.g., withdrawal of drugs), while other conditions resolve spontaneously. In some cases, clear delineation of the specific cause is impossible, but understanding of the underlying mechanisms provides for a rational approach to such patients.

As in any case of jaundice, the mechanism is suggested by the relative elevation in the level of unconjugated and

Table 12.3. Classification of Postoperative Jaundice*[a]*

I. Increased pigment load
   A. Hemolysis
   B. Transfusions
   C. Resorption of hematomas or hemoperitoneum
II. Impaired hepatocellular function
   A. Hepatitis-like picture
      1. Viral hepatitis
      2. Drug and anesthetic-induced hepatitis
      3. Ischemia
      4. Sepsis
      5. Post-pump syndrome
   B. Cholestatic picture
      1. "Benign" intrahepatic cholestasis
      2. Drug-induced cholestasis
      3. Sepsis
   C. Fatty liver and cirrhosis following intestinal bypass surgery
   D. Hepatic resection
   E. Hepatic transplantation and rejection
III. Extra-hepatic obstruction
   A. Choledocholithiasis
   B. Bile duct injury
   C. Pancreatitis
   D. Cholecystitis

[a] Adapted slightly from LaMont J, Isselbacher K: Postoperative jaundice. *N Engl J Med* 288:305, 1973, with permission.

conjugated bilirubin, and the relative rise in serum transaminase and alkaline phosphatase.

As listed in Table 12.3, hemolysis and reabsorption of blood can result in an overproduction of bilirubin pigment, causing "unconjugated" jaundice. Associated laboratory abnormalities include an elevated reticulocyte count and LDH level, and a depressed haptoglobin.

When primarily conjugated hyperbilirubinemia is present, differentiation must be made between hepatic parenchymal disease and extrahepatic obstruction. Hepatocellular dysfunction can present as either a hepatitis-like pattern or as cholestasis. The latter can resemble extrahepatic obstruction on liver function testing. Specific examples of causes of postoperative jaundice will be described below.

OVERPRODUCTION OF BILIRUBIN PIGMENT

The liver is responsible for handling about 250–500 mg of bilirubin per day that is produced by the destruction of senescent erythrocytes. The liver is able to increase by several-fold its capacity to handle excess bilirubin loads. However, when liver function is impaired or when erythrocyte breakdown is rapid and massive, the hepatic capacity can be overwhelmed and jaundice ensues. Hypoxia, hypotension, and sepsis may impair the hepatic ability to handle bilirubin. Massive hemolysis, resorption of blood products from hematomas or from a hemoperitoneum, and transfusion of stored blood may contribute to excessive pigment load that can overwhelm the impaired hepatic reserve.

Hemolysis is a rare cause of postoperative jaundice. When jaundice is due to hemolysis postoperatively, common causes are transfusions, and defects such as glucose-6 phosphate dehydrogenase (G-6-P-D) deficiency or sickle cell anemia. Drugs, such as aspirin or sulphonamides, may induce hemolysis in patients with G-6-P-D deficiency. Sickle cell hemolytic episodes may be precipitated by surgery if associated with hypoxia or infection. At times, these hemolytic episodes may present with severe abdominal pain and fever-mimicking cholecystitis. Detection of elevated unconjugated bilirubin levels suggests the presence of hemolysis as the cause for jaundice.

Transfusion of blood is another cause of increased pigment load. It is estimated that 10% of the red blood cells in a unit of stored blood will undergo hemolysis within the first 24 hours of transfusion, accounting for an extra 250 mg of bilirubin (59). While the normal liver can easily handle this load even after multiple transfusions, jaundice frequently occurs post-transfusion in the patient with preexisting liver disease. Thus, in patients undergoing portacaval shunting for bleeding esophageal varices, bilirubin elevation is frequently noted, in part due to the multiple transfusions. In such patients with preexisting hepatocellular disease, the hyperbilirubinemia is of both the conjugated and unconjugated forms.

Finally, reabsorption of blood from bleeding sites may also cause excessive bilirubin production. Hematomas, gastrointestinal bleeding, and bleeding into the peritoneum may result in resorption of hemoglobin from the breakdown of red cells. Jaundice in these situations usually occurs only when parenchymal liver disease is also present (60).

HEPATOCELLULAR DYSFUNCTION

Hepatocellular dysfunction is the most common cause of postoperative jaundice. The liver may be injured by a variety of factors during surgery, including drugs, hypoxia, decreased liver blood flow, and sepsis. The clinical picture may be one of hepatitis or cholestasis. A few conditions may produce a mixed picture.

Hepatitis-like Patterns

Hepatitis can be produced by anesthetic compounds, drugs, infections, and ischemia (Table 12.3). The clinical, biochemical, and histologic picture for these various conditions may be similar.

Halothane-induced liver injury is infrequent but serious. Similar hepatitis has been reported for enflurane, but is rare (63). Carney and Van Dyke (61) reviewed five retrospective studies and noted an incidence of hepatitis in one in 2,500 patients receiving this drug, and fatal liver failure occurring in 1/11,000. The national Halothane study (62) found an incidence of fatal liver injury secondary to halothane in one case per 36,000. The etiology of the liver damage is believed to be a hypersensitivity reaction (64). Repeated exposures, particularly within a short interval, and obesity appear to be major risk factors for severe liver injury.

Clinically, halothane hepatitis presents with fever and leukocytosis occurring 2–3 days postoperatively. Jaundice usually occurs within 3–10 days. Jaundice occurring more than 3 weeks postoperatively is rarely due to halothane exposure. A history of multiple exposures can be obtained in 75–90% of patients (65, 66).

Marked elevations of bilirubin (greater than 10 mg/100 ml) and prolongation of the prothrombin time are the most reliable biochemical indicators of a poor prognosis. Eosinophilia may occur but its absence does not exclude halothane as a cause for the liver injury.

Histologically, the picture is one of acute hepatocellular necrosis. Fatty infiltration and eosinophils are occasionally found. In severe cases, massive necrosis may be seen and cirrhosis may occur following repeated exposures (67).

In the majority of cases, complete recovery occurs. However, the mortality rate is approximately 20%, with a wide range in the severity of the acute illness (68). Chronic hepatitis is generally not a consequence of an isolated episode of halothane hepatitis. In a patient with a history of halothane hepatitis, repeated use of this anesthetic agent is contraindicated. However, there is no evidence of increased risk from halothane in patients with preexisting liver injury. Treatment is supportive; corticosteroids are of no value.

Methyoxyflurane hepatitis may be caused by a methoxyflurane, a halogenated anesthetic agent structurally related to halothane. Its clinical picture is similar to halothane-induced hepatitis. Cross-sensitivation to halothane has been reported (69). Non-oliguric renal failure may also occur in combination with hepatic injury or as a separate entity.

Drugs commonly administered in the perioperative period are capable of causing liver damage. Drug-induced hepatitis may present with a hepatitis-like pattern, with a cholestatic pattern, or with a mixed reaction (Table 12.4). Isoniazid, methyldopa, and tetracycline are examples of drugs that may produce a hepatitis-like pattern. Careful scrutiny of the medication chart is necessary to identify exposure to potential hepatic toxins. With removal of the offending agent, the hepatitis rapidly resolves. Rechallenge is generally unnecessary and may be hazardous. Liver biopsy generally is not revealing as it rarely demonstrates features specific for drug-induced injury. The finding of peripheral eosinophilia or excessive eosinophilic infiltration in the portal area or in the hepatic parenchyma strongly suggests drug-induced hepatitis. Drugs, excluding halothane, were believed to be the cause of liver failure in 8% of patients in one retrospective study of postoperative hepatic failure (62).

Ischemic hepatitis with ischemic injury to the liver is an infrequent cause of postoperative jaundice, but may play a significant role in hepatic deterioration postoperatively in patients with preexisting severe liver disease. Patients with cirrhosis or active hepatitis tolerate hypotension poorly. In patients with normal hepatic architecture, significant hepatic injury usually occurs only following prolonged hypotension, as in shock secondary to trauma or following a cardiac arrest. In such cases, marked elevations in

Table 12.4. Drug-induced Liver Injury

Histologic Classification	Hepatocellular Necrosis	Cholestasis	Mixed (Hepatocellular Necrosis and Cholestasis)	Fat
Biochemical features				
SGOT, SGPT	↑↑ (often >10-fold)	↑	↑	Slightly ↑
Alkaline phosphatase	↑ (<3 fold)	↑↑ (>4 fold)	↑	Normal to ↑ slightly
Examples	Halothane, enflurane, methoxyflurane Isoniazid, Dilantin Tetracycline, methyldopa	Chlorpromazine Oral contraceptives Erythromycin estolate Amitriptyline Chlorpropramide Anabolic steroids	Sulfonamides Phenylbutazone Thiouracil	Tetracycline Methotrexate

transaminases and jaundice occur in the first week postoperatively. The transaminase values may range from 100 units to several thousand units, and the bilirubin may rise to 20 mg/100 ml (59). Other factors, such as transfusions, infections, and passive congestion of the liver from heart failure, may also play a role in promoting the hepatic injury. In the majority of cases, complete resolution occurs, often with rapid falls in the markedly elevated transaminase levels. Mortality is highest in patients with preceding hepatic disease, especially chronic passive congestion of the liver due to congestive heart failure.

Post-transfusion hepatitis (PTH) is another cause of hepatocyte damage and jaundice in the postoperative patient. Unlike halothane hepatitis, which occurs within 2 weeks of exposure, post-transfusion hepatitis is usually not evident for more than 3 weeks following exposure. As many patients undergoing major surgery receive blood, this diagnosis must be recognized as a potential late complication in the surgical patient.

Post-transfusion hepatitis is now recognized to be caused by a variety of viruses. Initially, hepatitis B virus was believed to be the main cause of PTH. With routine screening of blood for hepatitis B over the past several years, it has become an infrequent cause of PTH, accounting for less than 10% of all cases. However, the incidence of PTH remains high, with a frequency of 7–10% ("non-A, non-B hepatitis") (70).

Hepatitis A virus does not appear to play a role in PTH. In addition, the incubation period for hepatitis A virus (generally 3–4 weeks) is too short for the observed incubation period of most post-transfusion hepatitis (7–8 weeks). Further, hepatitis A is not associated with a chronic carrier state and does not progress to chronic liver disease, two features that characterize post-transfusion hepatitis.

Current evidence suggests the existence of more than one causative agent of PTH, hence, the general term "non-A, non-B" hepatitis. Non-A, non-B hepatitis may be transmitted by blood transfusion but also can be found in families, among drug addicts, and in patients on hemodialysis. Non-A, non-B hepatitis may account for up to 20% of isolated cases of hepatitis worldwide. The mean incubation for transfusion associated non-A, non-B hepatitis is 7–8 weeks, which is intermediate between the incubation period for type A and type B hepatitis.

Clinically, the course of non-A, non-B hepatitis resembles more closely type B hepatitis. Overall, it appears to be less severe of an illness than hepatitis B with lower means of transaminase levels, and with two-thirds of cases being anicteric. However, resolution of the acute illness is often prolonged, with abnormal hepatic enzyme levels persisting for more than 6 months in the majority of patients (71). Chronic hepatitis is common following post-transfusion hepatitis with a frequency of 40–50% in several series (72, 73). The chronic hepatitis morphologically is either chronic-active or chronic-persistent hepatitis. Cirrhosis has also been noted in a small percentage of patients with chronic disease. Overall, the course of the chronic hepatitis appears to be relatively mild with development of cirrhosis occurring in less than 20% of patients, often after 10–20 years of illness. There is no evidence currently to support the use of steroids or immunosuppressive therapy for chronic non-A, non-B hepatitis.

EXTRA-HEPATIC OBSTRUCTION

Biliary duct obstruction may occur postoperatively from a variety of causes and result in jaundice. While this complication is infrequent, it is of significance because surgical intervention may be required. Retained common duct stones may present with jaundice and an elevated alkaline phosphatase and must be differentiated from intrahepatic cholestasis syndromes. Most often, there is pain and fever associated with the extrahepatic blockage, but retained stones should also be suspected in patients with persistent painless jaundice following cholecystectomy. Cholangiography is often necessary to diagnose this problem and may be performed through a T-tube drain (if the common duct has already been explored) or via endoscopic or transhepatic cholangiography. Intravenous cholangiography may be attempted if the bilirubin is less than 2 mg/100 ml. Should retained common duct stones be found, removal is generally indicated. Removal of the common bile duct stones can be achieved by re-

operation, through the T-tube if still present, or following endoscopic sphincterotomy.

Bile duct injury may occur inadvertently following upper abdominal surgery, common duct exploration, or cholecystectomy. Failure to properly identify the common bile duct intraoperatively can result in resection or ligation of the duct, an injury that is often unrecognized during surgery. Jaundice often occurs within 1 week postoperatively and may be associated with cholangitis, bile peritonitis, and abscess formation. Prompt surgical repair is necessary to avoid further hepatic damage. Once injured, the bile duct may become strictured, leading to intermittent cholangitis, jaundice, and biliary cirrhosis if uncorrected.

Postoperative pancreatitis or cholecystitis may also cause postoperative jaundice or abnormal liver function tests. Jaundice may occur in 20–30% of patients with postoperative pancreatitis (see below), secondary to partial bile duct obstruction by the edematous pancreas. Postoperative cholecystitis is an unusual occurrence but may present with right upper quadrant pain and mild hyperbilirubinemia (see below). The pathogenesis of both pancreatitis and cholecystitis in the postoperative patient is unclear. High mortality has been reported in both of these complications.

CHOLESTATIC JAUNDICE (Cholestasis)

Hepatic dysfunction postoperatively may also present with a cholestatic picture, characterized by markedly elevated alkaline phosphatase levels and hyperbilirubinemia. This pattern may occur as part of a benign intrahepatic cholestasis syndrome, secondary to drugs, or in association with sepsis.

Benign postoperative intrahepatic cholestasis is a syndrome described in postoperative patients, characterized by transient cholestatic jaundice. The incidence of this complication is uncertain but may occur in one out of several hundred general surgical patients. Schmid described 11 patients with postoperative cholestasis, which occurred in one hospital during an 8-month interval (74). Typically, the patient had undergone a major operative procedure and had required multiple transfusions. Jaundice was often noted on the first or second postoperative day but may have been delayed up to 10 days following surgery. The hyperbilirubinemia generally peaked about 1 week postoperatively with values of 15–40 mg/100 ml. The alkaline phosphatase was also abnormal, often to markedly elevated values. Transaminases were minimally abnormal. Hepatosplenomegaly and hepatic encephalopathy are not features of this condition. Liver biopsy reveals changes characteristic of cholestasis with bile canalicular dilatation, biliary casts, and bile staining of hepatocytes. Necrosis of liver cells and a prominent inflammatory infiltrate are not usually seen. These features reflect the cholestatic process, but are not specific for this postoperative syndrome as they may also be found in drug-induced cholestasis.

The etiology of this condition is unclear. Common features of patients with this condition include: hypotension, hypoxemia, and multiple blood transfusions. However, as already discussed, these conditions generally do not produce a cholestatic pattern but more often cause hepatocellular necrosis.

The prognosis of this condition is good. Generally, the jaundice subsides within 2–3 weeks. Resolution is complete and chronic liver disease is not associated with this postoperative syndrome. However, benign, transient cholestasis must be differentiated from more serious causes of jaundice and, in particular, extrahepatic causes of jaundice, such as stones or common bile duct injury. Clinically, these conditions may be difficult to distinguish, especially during the first week when bilirubin values are climbing. The development of hepatomegaly, abdominal pain, and fever suggest common bile duct obstruction rather than the syndrome of benign postoperative cholestasis. In doubtful cases, a cholangiogram (either endoscopic retrograde cholangiography or percutaneous transhepatic cholangiography) may be needed to differentiate these conditions.

Drug induced cholestasis is one type of drug-induced liver injury that must always be considered in the postoperative patient. A cholestatic pattern may be seen following use of various drugs, such as chlorpromazine, erythromycin, anabolic steroids, oral hypoglycemic agents, and antithyroid medications. In general, drug-induced cholestatic injury is less likely to produce hepatic failure and has, therefore, a better prognosis than does the acute hepatitis-like syndrome. Rarely, however, a chronic cholestatic picture resembling biliary cirrhosis has been reported to develop following acute injury by drugs.

SEPSIS

Bacterial infections have also been associated with a cholestatic picture. Pneumococcal pneumonia and bacteremia with gram-negative organisms are the infections most commonly associated with the development of jaundice. The hepatic dysfunction is usually mild, with liver function test abnormalities occurring usually 5–12 days after the onset of the infection (59). Often, other factors are also present in the same patient that are capable of causing liver damage, such as drugs and hypotension. The mechanism of this type of injury associated with sepsis is unknown.

Management of Postoperative Hepatic Dysfunction

Postoperative hepatic dysfunction is most often mild, with complete resolution occurring in the majority of cases. In a small percentage of cases, the hepatic injury is extensive and hepatic failure may occur. In patients with preexisting liver diseases, even mild degrees of damage may result in marked deterioration in hepatic function. In general, patients with a hepatitis-like pattern of injury have a higher morbidity and mortality than those who develop a cholestatic pattern postoperatively. In patients who develop hepatic coma, the mortality rate is over 80% (75).

Fulminant hepatic failure may occur as a complication of viral hepatitis or of exposure to hepatotoxic agents. The clinical course is one of rapid deterioration in mental status, progressing from agitation to deep coma often within several days. Serum transaminases are usually markedly elevated, bilirubin values rise progressively, and the prothrombin time becomes markedly prolonged. In patients with preexisting liver disease, hepatic failure may occur more insidiously, but still with a progressive deterioration in mental status and worsening of liver function tests.

Therapy is largely supportive. Early identification of the patient with a severe liver injury and intensive effort to prevent potential complications are important. Therapy should be instituted to reduce blood ammonia levels, and to prevent infection, bleeding, and electrolyte abnormalities. Drugs that may exacerbate the encephalopathy, either by inducing further liver damage or by causing further deterioration in mental status, should be discontinued.

Oral protein intake should be reduced and gastrointestinal bleeding should be treated aggressively. Colonic contents including blood should be evacuated with enemas and laxatives. Lactulose or neomycin should be given to decrease absorption and production of ammonia.

In addition to treating the encephalopathy, efforts should be directed at preventing other complications. Hypoglycemia may occur due to depletion of glycogen stores within the liver and its resultant symptoms may be confused with those of the hepatic encephalopathy. Frequent monitoring of serum glucose levels and appropriate glucose administration are essential. Gastrointestinal bleeding may occur more often from stress ulcers than from variceal hemorrhage in this setting, and prophylactic H_2-antagonists or antacid therapy are indicated. Finally, sepsis should always be suspected.

Ascites may develop in the face of hepatic dysfunction, but other potential causes in the postoperative setting must also be ruled out. A paracentesis should be performed to rule out infections (either due to perforation of a viscus with peritonitis or spontaneous bacterial peritonitis), venous occlusion, pancreatic duct disruption, and metastatic disease.

Variceal hemorrhage is a serious complication of postoperative hepatic dysfunction. Documentation that the bleeding is due to varices is essential as other causes of postoperative gastrointestinal bleeding require different forms of therapy. Gastric lavage, restoration of blood volume, correction of coagulation defects, and prevention of hepatic encephalopathy are all essential features in the management of these patients. Injection sclerotherapy is the preferred method to arrest acute variceal bleeding. In addition, vasopressin could be infused either intravenously or intra-arterially (into the superior mesenteric artery) to decrease portal pressure and control the variceal hemorrhage. Both methods are equally effective with similar degrees of toxicity (76). The dose usually needed ranges from 0.2–0.4 units per minute. Balloon tamponade of the varices may also be used effectively to control the hemorrhage, but this requires greater expertise in placing the tube and maintaining its proper position. In patients who fail vasopressin infusion, balloon tamponade may prove beneficial. Emergency portacaval shunting for uncontrollable variceal hemorrhage carries a high mortality but can effectively stop bleeding.

POSTOPERATIVE CHOLECYSTITIS

Acute cholecystitis is an infrequent postoperative complication that often presents as a diagnostic dilemma. The acute attack may develop following any form of surgery, not necessarily following abdominal operations. The episode may occur within several days of the initial operation, but more often is delayed up to 4 weeks postoperatively.

Clinically, the patient presents with fever, right upper quadrant pain, and tenderness. Mild liver function test abnormalities may occur with mild hyperbilirubinemia. With this presentation in a postoperative setting, the condition is easily confused with a subhepatic abscess or hepatic dysfunction. Radionuclear biliary scanning may demonstrate occlusion of the cystic duct, but false positive and false negative scans are frequent in this setting. In some patients, surgical exploration is needed before the diagnosis is actually established, as many of the usual preoperative tests may be normal or difficult to perform. Pathologically, acute cholecystitis is found but stones are absent in as many as 50% of cases. Common bile duct obstruction is generally not observed. The mechanism for this acalculous cholecystitis is unclear, but a similar phenomenon has been observed in trauma patients. Gangrene of the gallbladder occurs in one-third of patients. The mortality rate is reported to be as high as 20% (77–78).

POSTCHOLECYSTECTOMY SYNDROME

Pathophysiology and Epidemiology

The term "postcholecystectomy syndrome" has been applied to a heterogeneous group of disorders and symptoms that are present following cholecystectomy. The term is a confusing one, as it implies some causal relationship between the cholecystectomy and the symptoms, a relationship that in fact does not exist in most cases. Indeed, in many cases the symptoms were present prior to the operation and were often the indication for the cholecystectomy. Categorizing such patients as having the postcholecystectomy syndrome seems only to confuse the

issue and obscure the correct diagnosis. Nonetheless, the internist is often referred such patients with the working diagnosis of postcholecystectomy syndrome and an appropriate understanding of this entity is therefore needed.

The main symptoms of this syndrome are abdominal pain and dyspepsia. The pain may be severe and in some cases strongly suggests biliary colic. Dyspeptic symptoms include vague abdominal discomfort following a meal, food intolerance, and gaseousness. Alteration in bowel habits are also reported with both diarrhea and constipation occurring. The incidence of these complaints following cholecystectomy ranges from 25–40% in various series (79). In the majority of cases the symptoms are mild, but in about 5%, severe symptoms, particularly pain, persist. There appears to be a good correlation between the degree of scarring of the gallbladder and the complete relief of symptoms with a cholecystectomy. Most patients with postcholecystectomy syndrome have a thin-walled unscarred gallbladder found at the time of surgery. The condition is more common in females.

The causes for the postcholecystectomy syndrome are varied and include: *(a)* biliary tract disease: retained common duct stones, common bile duct strictures, stenosis of the sphincter of Oddi, and cystic duct remnant; *(b)* extra-biliary tract disease: the irritable bowel syndrome, gastritis, gastroesophageal reflux, peptic ulcer disease, and pancreatitis; and *(c)* functional disorders: biliary dyskinesia. In over 50% of cases, demonstrable organic pathology, such as stones or gastritis, can be found in patients with postcholecystectomy syndrome (79). Disturbances in the bile duct motor function (biliary dyskinesia) is suspected in others.

Persistent biliary tract disease must always be investigated in patients with the postcholecystectomy syndrome. Retained stones occur in about 40% of patients with postcholecystectomy syndrome following cholecystectomy.

The cystic duct remnant has often been blamed for persistent syndromes following cholecystectomy. Potentially, a long cystic duct may provide a nidus for stone formation and be the cause for recurrent common bile duct stones. However, in many asymptomatic patients, a cystic duct remnant can be identified and, thus, its causal relationship in the symptomatic patient is unclear.

Other gastrointestinal disorders that may cause the patient's symptoms should be carefully considered. Gastritis may often cause many of the same complaints and can be diagnosed by gastroscopy. The irritable bowel syndrome may be characterized by intermittent, sometimes severe pain and may be overlooked in a patient with gallstones. In some cases, the irritable bowel syndrome symptoms are exacerbated following cholecystectomy.

In about 50% of cases of postcholecystectomy syndrome, no organic pathology is found (80), and the diagnosis of biliary dyskinesia is considered. This syndrome refers to a disturbance in the motility of the biliary ducts, either in the speed of evacuation of the biliary tree, in the function of the sphincter of Oddi, or in the coordination of activity of the various segments of the bile ducts and the sphincter.

Evaluation

Most commonly, patients with biliary dyskinesia present with recurrent biliary-like colic, often postprandially. Nausea and vomiting are common. Fever, chills, and jaundice are generally absent. The condition is more common in females between 20–50 years of age.

Currently, this diagnosis is generally made by exclusion of other causes of the postcholecystectomy syndrome. Careful evaluation of the biliary tract must be performed to rule out small stones or strictures. Liver function studies should be normal even during an attack of pain. Other disorders, such as gastroesophageal reflux and the irritable bowel syndrome, are to be ruled out as noted earlier.

Endoscopic manometry of the sphincter of Oddi has recently become available and has demonstrated alteration in distal bile duct peristalsis and the response of the sphincter to various physiologic and pharmacologic stimuli in patients with the postcholecystectomy syndrome. As this procedure becomes more standardized and available, it may become the procedure of choice in diagnosing this condition.

POSTGASTRECTOMY SYNDROME

Following ulcer surgery, a wide variety of problems may develop. These complications may occur after any form of ulcer surgery and do not necessarily depend on the amount of gastric resection. A significant contributing role in the development of the postgastrectomy syndrome appears to be the performance of a truncal vagotomy. As a result, newer operations are designed to reduce the extent of the vagotomy. About 10% of patients will suffer from chronic sequelae directly related to the altered anatomy and physiology in the postgastrectomy state.

Postcibal Problems: Abdominal Pain, Bilious Vomiting, Early Satiety, and the Dumping Syndrome

In the postgastrectomy state, a wide variety of symptoms may develop in response to eating a normal meal. The most common complaints include early satiety, postprandial vomiting, and epigastric pain. The incidence of these symptoms is from 20–60% in various series and occurs following simple drainage procedures, as well as following more extensive gastric resection. The exact mechanism for these meal-related symptoms is not known, but a variety of alterations in normal physiology can be documented in these patients.

It has been suggested that the postcibal complications are related to the abnormal entry of fluid into the small intestine. The timing of the postprandial symptoms is similar to the timing of the transit of solutions from the stomach into the intestines, usually within the first 30 minutes following a meal. Experimentally, distension of the proximal small bowel may reproduce many of these same symptoms. Vagotomy has been shown to inhibit the fundic relaxation that occurs with swallowing of food. Thus, as the stomach fails to distend, liquids in particular are emptied into the small bowel more rapidly, resulting in the distension of the intestine, as well as the rapid delivery of hypertonic contents.

These complaints may be associated with vasomotor phenomena, such as lightheadedness, diaphoresis, and postural hypotension. The combination of these postprandial complaints and these vasomotor symptoms is commonly referred to as "the dumping syndrome." Current concepts of the pathophysiology of the dumping syndrome deal with the effect of various hormones (serotonin, gastric inhibitory peptide), which can induce similar vasomotor phenomena in experimental situations. Release of these hormones may be induced by intestinal distension and/or the influx of hypertonic solutions into the jejunum.

Therapy for this condition is directed toward slowing the gastric emptying, avoiding hypertonic solutions, and overdistension of the intestine. Frequent small feedings that are high in protein and low in carbohydrate have been recommended. Importantly, liquids, which may accelerate gastric emptying, should be avoided while eating a solid meal. Lying down after a meal may also be beneficial as it slows down gastric emptying and may reduce the intensity of vasomotor symptoms.

The epigastric pain and vomiting may be due to a variety of disorders, including distension of the stomach or small bowel, afferent loop obstruction, gastric outlet obstruction, recurrent ulcerations, and reflux gastritis. In some cases, these symptoms subside over a period of time or with alteration in dietary intake. In other cases, revisional surgery is required.

Partial afferent loop obstruction is an unusual complication that results in postprandial abdominal pain and bilious vomiting. The pain occurs with distension of the afferent limb by pancreatic and biliary secretions that are stimulated following a meal. The vomiting is typically bilious and contains little if any food. The diagnosis is made by the radiographic demonstration of a dilated afferent limb that is slow to empty. Endoscopy may document the inability to pass the endoscope into the afferent loop or demonstrate retention of copious volumes of biliary secretions within the obstructed limb. When the diagnosis is established, surgical revision is necessary.

Gastric outlet obstruction, on the other hand, is generally associated with vomiting of large amounts of retained or undigested food. Barium studies will generally demonstrate the gastric obstruction with retention of the barium. Causes for such obstruction include scarring or surgical deformity at the anastomosis, as well as recurrent ulcerations.

Anastomotic ulcers must always be considered as a cause for post-prandial pain and vomiting. These ulcers generally occur around the intestinal side of the anastomosis and most commonly present with epigastric pain. The pain is no longer relieved by food as is common in duodenal ulcer disease but may actually be aggravated by meals. Conventional barium studies may fail to disclose the anastomotic ulcer in as many as 50% of cases (81). Air-contrast barium studies and endoscopy are more sensitive in the detection of these lesions.

Bile gastritis (also termed alkaline or reflux gastritis) is a poorly defined entity that may cause abdominal pain and bilious vomiting. With loss or bypass of the pyloric sphincter, bile is now able to reflux freely into the stomach. Experimentally, chronic bile perfusion of the gastric mucosa can result in acute and probably chronic gastritis. The reflux of bile into the postsurgical stomach, and the finding of perianastomotic gastritis are common. Unfortunately, the correlation between the severity of the symptoms and the severity of the gross and microscopic appearance of the gastritis is poor. When the gastritis is endoscopically and histologically severe, and no other cause for the symptoms is evident, the diagnosis of bile gastritis is usually made.

Therapy for this condition, however, is extremely difficult. There is no medical therapy of proven value or efficacy. Since the pathogenesis of the bile gastritis is believed to be the combined actions of bile and acid on the gastric mucosa, medical therapy has been aimed at either binding the bile (cholestyramine) or reducing the acid present. However, studies have failed to show any benefit from such therapy (82).

Surgical diversion of the bile flow away from the stomach appears to be the most successful approach to ameliorating the patient's symptoms. Formation of a Roux-en-Y anastomosis has achieved very good results in a number of reports. Conversion of a vagotomy and pyloroplasty to a Billroth II or of a Billroth II to a Billroth I has been of little value.

Diarrhea

Chronic diarrhea is common following ulcer surgery and occurs in 10–40% of patients. It appears to be a less common complication following parietal cell vagotomy. While some surgeons claim that the severity and prevalence of the diarrhea decreases with time, in the prospective VA Study (83), there was no difference in the diarrhea at 2 and 5 years postoperatively. Multiple etiologies have been implicated in postgastrectomy diarrhea and in some patients, several factors may be working in concert. Causes for this type of diarrhea include: (a) rapid intestinal transit; (b) rapid gastric emptying; (c) lac-

tose intolerance; (d) increase in fecal bile acid; (e) malabsorption; (f) gastrocolic fistula; (g) Zollinger-Ellison syndrome; and (h) inadvertent gastroileal anastomosis.

The evaluation of the patient with postgastrectomy diarrhea follows the same guidelines as the evaluation of any patient with chronic diarrhea. Significantly, one must differentiate problems of absorption from problems related to mechanical and motility factors. Thus, fecal collections for volume and fat content are important, with greater than 10–12% fecal fat excretion indicating significant malabsorption. Barium studies should be performed to review the anatomy and to provide a crude estimate of motility pattern.

Excess fecal bile acids have been implicated in a number of studies in patients with postgastrectomy or postvagotomy diarrhea (84). Many such patients respond to the empiric use of the bile salt-binding resin, cholestyramine. Lactose intolerance is a common cause of diarrhea in the postgastrectomy setting. Patients with borderline levels of the intestinal enzyme, lactase, may become symptomatic with the rapid delivery of a lactose load that overwhelms the enzymatic capacity to metabolize the sugar. Thus, lactose-restricted diets are advocated in many such patients.

Significant malabsorption occurs rarely in the postgastrectomy state. Causes for malabsorption include poor mixing of food with pancreatic and biliary secretions, rapid transit, bacterial overgrowth in the afferent loop, and latent celiac disease being unmasked by ulcer surgery. When greater than 12% of ingested fat is excreted in the stool, evaluation for these causes of malabsorption should be performed. A small bowel biopsy will generally be needed to rule out celiac disease. A bile salt breath test or all three parts of the Shilling test may be useful in documenting bacterial overgrowth.

In still other patients, rapid transit will be seen on the barium study, and some patients complain of a prominent postprandial urge to defecate. In such patients unresponsive to either cholestyramine- or a lactose-restricted diet, antidiarrheal medications such as diphenoxylate or loperamide may be useful.

Weight Loss

Weight loss is a significant problem following ulcer surgery. A 10% reduction in preoperative body weight may occur after any standard ulcer operation, and is not necessarily related to the extent of the gastric resection. The most common cause for weight loss is a reduction in caloric intake. Often, the patient avoids eating because of postprandial symptoms such as early satiety, dumping syndrome, diarrhea, and abdominal pain. Treatment of these postprandial symptoms as noted above may improve caloric intake. Encouraging the patient to consume small feedings and even to supplement their intake with high caloric additives may be helpful.

Anemia

The gradual development of mild anemia (hemoglobin values of 10–12 g/ml) is common following ulcer surgery. This complication appears to occur somewhat more frequently after gastrojejunostomy than after other operations. Most frequently, this anemia is due to iron deficiency. Iron absorption is commonly decreased in these patients due to bypass of the duodenum. In addition, the decreased food intake and the lack of gastric acidity may play some role in decreasing the amount of iron available for absorption. In addition, reflux gastritis and stomal ulcerations may cause bleeding, thus accounting for iron deficiency.

A macrocytic anemia may also develop due to B_{12} or folate deficiency. B_{12} deficiency develops in less than 10% of postgastrectomy patients due to either loss of intrinsic factor secretion by the stomach or due to bacterial overgrowth. Folic acid deficiency may also develop in the setting of bacterial overgrowth. As with iron deficiency anemia, this anemia is generally mild, and in patients with severe anemia or precipitous falls in hemoglobin levels, other causes should be considered.

Postoperative Recurrent Ulcer

Recurrent ulceration following ulcer surgery is an infrequent but significant problem. The frequency with which these anastomotic or marginal ulcers develop varies with the type of ulcer surgery performed, with less than a 1% recurrence rate after vagotomy and gastric resection, and a 6–8% rate after vagotomy plus pyloroplasty.

It is too early to determine the recurrence rate after parietal cell vagotomy performed in this country, as the incidence of recurrent ulceration varies widely with the experience of the surgeon. These recurrent ulcers occur most commonly on the intestinal side of the anastomosis.

Clinically, these ulcers present with abdominal pain, bleeding, and, often, weight loss. The pain may be continuous and is often located in the epigastric area. The pain from these ulcers may not be relieved by meals. Vomiting and weight loss are common, and bleeding occurs in two-thirds of patients. Occasionally, the recurrent ulcer may penetrate into the colon forming a gastrojejunal-colonic fistula, which can present dramatically with feculent vomiting.

The diagnosis is best made by endoscopy or air-contrast upper gastrointestinal series. A conventional barium study may miss these lesions in 50% of cases.

The most common cause for recurrent ulcerations is inadequate initial surgery—either incomplete vagotomy or inadequate gastric resection. Other causes include Zollinger-Ellison syndrome, retained antrum, possibly hyperparathyroidism, and ulcerogenic drugs. Thus, evaluation of these patients should include several fasting serum gastrin determinations to rule out the Zollinger-Ellison syndrome and retained antrum. In both these conditions, the gastrin level is markedly elevated. These latter disorders can be differentiated by performing a secretin stimulation test. After injection of secretin, in normal patients and in patients with the retained antrum, basal gastrin levels decline over the first 30–45 minutes. However, in patients with the Zollinger-Ellison syndrome, gastrin levels paradoxically rise.

A gastric analysis is sometimes helpful to document the level of acid secretion. However, it is often technically difficult to perform in the postgastrectomy patient as there is often mixing of gastric secretions with bile and difficulty in maintaining the position of the tube within the stomach. While in the Zollinger-Ellison (Z-E) syndrome there is marked basal hypersecretion, there is significant overlap with non-Z-E duodenal ulcer patients. The insulin-hypoglycemia gastric analysis (Hollander test) is of controversial value.

Both medical and surgical therapy are useful in the treatment of these recurrent ulcers. H$_2$-antagonists have been shown to be effective in the healing of these postoperative recurrences. The duration of therapy and the role of maintenance cimetidine in preventing further recurrences has not been fully evaluated. Antacid therapy alone has not been very successful in managing these patients.

For patients who fail to heal on medical therapy or who develop a serious complication from the recurrence, such as bleeding or fistula formation, surgical therapy is required. In general, a repeat vagotomy with more extensive gastric resection is required, with lesser operations resulting in a high frequency of a second recurrence. In some patients with an initial adequate gastric resection, a repeat abdominal or even a thoracic vagotomy only may be needed.

MANAGEMENT OF THE OSTOMATE

Proper management of the ostomate (the preferred term for a person with an ostomy) begins with a preoperative preparation of the patient and his family. During this preoperative period, the patient should be encouraged to express his fears and concerns about being an ostomate. Certain aspects should be emphasized to the patient: (a) modern appliances are easy to use and keep the patient clean; (b) no one will be able to detect that the patient is wearing an appliance under clothing; (c) there is no problem with foul odor; (d) physical activity, including swimming, sports, and dancing, are not limited by having an ostomy; (e) sexual function depends on the results of the surgery but may remain normal with an ostomy.

An enterostomal therapist (nurse specially trained in the management of ostomies and ostomates) should also visit the patient preoperatively. The therapist will mark the proper location for the ostomy, depending on the patient's posture, skin crease lines, and location of the incision. The therapist is also very helpful in providing information and counseling to the patient. A visit from a member of the local chapter of the United Ostomy Association is also very helpful in allowing the patient to overcome his/her misconceptions about life with an ostomy.

Ileostomy

An ileostomy and colostomy have differing features. Conventional ileostomies require that the patient continuously wear an appliance or pouch to retain the frequent discharge of ileal effluent. This pouch adheres to the skin by an adhesive that provides a water tight seal. This pouch can be emptied into a toilet by unclipping the bottom end of the pouch several times per day. The ileal discharge is watery and odorless. In some patients, a continent ileostomy is performed by creating a reservoir pouch in the abdomen from loops of small bowel, allowing the patient to be free of an outer appliance. The patient can drain this intestinal pouch several times per day by inserting a catheter through a nipple-like opening on the abdominal wall into the pouch. The choice of which type of ileostomy to be performed depends on the patient's illness (Crohn's of the ileum is a contraindication), the experience of the surgeon, and the desires of the patient.

Colostomy

Most permanent colostomies are sigmoid colostomies (following resection of rectal carcinoma). As only the rectum is removed, the patient's preoperative bowel function will generally persist following surgery. Thus, patients who are "regular by the clock" with their bowel habits will continue the same pattern even with a colostomy and can develop control of the evacuation by the use of irrigation enemas. As a result, some colostomates will only need to wear a small gauze pad instead of a pouch, while others still prefer the security of the pouch. Similarly, those patients with eratic bowel habits preoperatively will continue to have unpredictable bowel movements through the ostomy. In these patients, continence between irrigations is very difficult and the appliance will generally need to be worn.

When the colostomy is performed proximal to the splenic flexure, the discharge is looser and contains greater liquid content. This type of colostomy is generally only temporary to relieve obstructions or to permit healing of a diverticular abscess. This type of colostomy is less desirable since evacuation is very frequent and cannot be controlled by irrigation, and the discharge is malodorous due to colonic bacterial action. Also, these ostomies are often placed above the belt line, making it difficult to wear an appliance. A permanent ileostomy is preferable to this type of "wet" colostomy.

While in the hospital, the patient and a member of his family should learn about the management of the ostomy and the appliance and should become comfortable with its use. The physician should also feel comfortable with inspecting the stoma periodically and being sure that the patient is managing the appliance properly. At times, skin breakdown may be a problem. Hypersensitivity to adhesives or to the pouch may occur. Skin problems occur more frequently among the ileostomates. Skin irritation can be treated with a cortisone spray (e.g., Kenalog) and an antifungal powder (e.g., Mycostatin). Ointments and creams are to be avoided as they interfere with adhesion of the appliance.

Occasionally, odor is a problem, more often in the colostomate than in the ileostomate. Dietary factors may be important and certain foods such as onions, eggs, and oils should be eliminated in such cases. Malabsorption from small bowel disease may also produce malodorous discharge. A variety of deodorants are available and can be placed into the pouch (examples include Ostoban powder, Nilodor, and Banish). Proper cleansing and drying of the appliance between uses is also important in preventing colonization with odor-forming bacteria. Sudden onset of problems with excessive gas or odor should suggest the possibility of partial bowel obstruction.

Leakage rarely occurs with modern appliances under usual circumstances. Occasionally, if the stoma is placed poorly or is very large (as in some loop colostomies) so that an appliance cannot be properly sealed around the stoma, then leakage will be a problem. For this reason, preoperative marking of the proper location for the stoma by the enterostomal therapist is important. In addition, significant weight gain postoperatively or pregnancy may alter the abdominal configuration necessitating refitting of the appliance. The stoma can be expected to retract during the first few months postoperatively and monitoring of the amount of protrusion of the stoma is important. A stoma that is flush with the abdominal wall will create problems with leakage and frequently result in skin breakdown.

Significant problems related to the stoma include obstruction, prolapse, and retraction. Obstruction of the stoma may result from volvulus, herniation, or adhesions. Herniation can be suspected by the presence of a large parastomal bulge. Crampy abdominal pains, distension, vomiting, and diarrheal discharge suggest the presence of obstruction. The stoma may retract, or loops of bowel may prolapse through the stomal opening in the abdominal wall. These problems are seen more frequently with ileostomies; they usually require surgical consultation and correction.

Many patients note periodic changes in consistency and color of the ostomy discharge, often related to dietary factors. At first, the patient may be alarmed by these changes and seek medical attention. The patient should be reassured that these occurrences are normal. Dietary restrictions are, in general, minimal, with recommendations to avoid odor-producing foods and, particularly in the ileostomy patient, to increase water and salt intake during the hot summer months.

The psychological and sexual adjustments may be more troublesome for some patients than the medical aspects of the ostomy. In some patients, particularly women, there is a loss of self-esteem and sense of physical attractiveness. In other cases, the spouse may openly express rejection at the thought of dealing with an ostomy. These adjustment problems are often ignored during the early postoperative period, but the physician should discuss these matters openly with the patient and his family. Attendance at local ostomy chapter meetings may be beneficial to the couple experiencing these adjustment problems.

Sexual dysfunction may occur secondary to neurologic impairment, depression with loss of libido, inhibition because of the stoma (either embarrassment or concern of damage to the stoma), and occasionally due to rejection by the spouse. Impotence is common after colostomies performed for rectal carcinoma, occurring in up to 50% of such cases. Impotence following ileostomy is unusual. The physician should inquire about these potential problems.

Supportive therapy, involvement in a local ostomy chapter, and when appropriate, psychiatric therapy can all be very beneficial to the ostomate in coping with these problems.

READINGS

1. Dykes MHM, Bunker JP: Hepatotoxicity and anesthetics. *Pharmacol Physicians* 4:1, 1970.
2. Harville D, Summerskill W: Surgery in acute hepatitis. Causes and effects. *JAMA* 184:275, 1963.
3. Dykes MHM, Walzer SG: Preoperative and postoperative hepatic dysfunction. *Surg Gynecol Obstet* 124:747, 1967.
4. Marx G, Nagayoshi M, Shoukas J, et al.: Unsuspected infectious hepatitis in surgical patients. *JAMA* 205:793, 1968.
5. Mikkelsen W: Therapeutic portacaval shunt. Preliminary data on controlled trial and morbid effects of acute hyaline necrosis. *Arch Surg* 108:302, 1974.
5a. Friedman LS, Maddrey WC: Surgery in the patient with liver disease. *Med Clin N Am* 71:453, 1987.
6. Aranha GV, Greenlee, HB: Intra-abdominal surgery in patients with advanced cirrhosis. *Arch Surg* 121:275–277, 1986.
7. Garrison RN, et al.: Clarification of risk factors for abdominal operations in patients with hepatic cirrhosis. *Ann Surg* 199:648–655, 1984.
8. Cryer HM, Howard DA, Garrison, RN: Liver cirrhosis and biliary surgery: Assessment of risk. *S Med J* 78:138, 1985.
9. Aranha GV, Sontag SJ, Greenlee HB, Cholecystectomy in cirrhotic patients: A formidable operation. *Am J Surg* 143:55, 1982.
10. Schwartz EI: Biliary tract surgery and cirrhosis: A critical combination. *Surgery* 90:577, 1981.
11. Resnick RH, et al.: A controlled study of the therapeutic portacaval shunt. *Gastroenterology* 67:843, 1974.
12. Schemel WH: Unexpected hepatic dysfunction found by multiple laboratory screening. *Anesth Analg* 55:810, 1976.
13. Burnstein CL: Relationship between hypoproteinemia and toxicity of anesthetic agents. *Anesth Analg* 27:287, 1948.

14. Child CG: The liver and portal hypertension, in Child CG (ed): *Major Problems in Clinical Surgery*. WB Saunders, Philadelphia, 1964, vol 1.
15. Pugh RHN, et al.: Transection of the esophagus for bleeding varices. *Br J Surg* 60:646, 1973.
16. Siegel J, Williams J: A computer-based index for prediction of operative survival in patients with cirrhosis and portal hypertension. *Ann Surg* 169:191, 1969.
17. Mikkelsen WP, Kern WH: The influence of acute hyaline necrosis on survival after emergency and elective portacaval shunting. *Major Prob Clin Surg* 14:233, 1974.
18. Kern W, Mikkelsen W, Turrill F: The significance of hyaline necrosis in liver biopsies. *Surg Gynecol Obstet* 129:749, 1969.
19. Mikkelsen W, Turrill F, Kern W: Acute hyaline necrosis of the liver. A surgical trap. *Am J Surg* 116:266, 1968.
20. Rouselot LM, et al.: Prognostic value of liver biopsy in the electively shunted patient. *Gastroenterology* 64:165, 1973.
21. Abdi W, Millan J, Mezey E: Sampling variability on percutaneous liver biopsy. *Arch Intern Med* 139:667, 1979.
22. Strunin L: Preoperative assessment of the patient with liver dysfunction. *Br J Anaesth* 50:25, 1978.
22a. Robbins J, Mushlin A: Preoperative evaluation of the healthy patient. *Med Clin N Am* 63:1145, 1979.
23. Losowsky M, Simmons A, Mitoszeloski K: Coagulation abnormalities in liver disease. *Postgrad Med* 53:117–152, 1973.
23a. Malini S, Sabel J: Ultrasonography in obstructive jaundice. *Radiology* 123:429, 1977.
24. Dawson JL: The incidence of postoperative renal failure in obstructive jaundice. *Br J Surg* 52:613, 1965.
24a. Neiman HL, Mintzer RA: Accuracy of biliary duct ultrasound: Comparison with cholangiography. *Am J Roentgenol* 129:979, 1977.
25. Baum M, Sterling G, Dawson JL: Further study into obstructive jaundice and ischemic renal damage, *Br Med J* 2:229–231, 1969.
25a. Brausch J, Gray B: Considerations that lower pancreatoduodenectomy mortality. *Am J Surg* 133:480, 1977.
26. Bailey M: Endotoxin, bile salts, and renal function in obstructive jaundice. *Br J Surg* 63:774, 1976.
26a. Dykes MHM: Is halothane hepatitis chronic active hepatitis. *Anesthesiology* 46:233, 1975.
27. Dawson JL: Postoperative renal function in obstructive jaundice: Effect of mannitol diuresis. *Br Med J* 1:82, 1965.
27a. Center for Disease Control: Immune serum globulin for protection against viral hepatitis. *Ann Intern Med* 77:427, 1972.
28. Siefkin A, Bolt R: Preoperative evaluation of the patient with gastrointestinal or liver disease. *Med Clin N Am* 63:1309, 1979.
28a. McSherry CK, Glenn F: The incidence and causes of death following surgery for nonmalignant bilitary tract disease. *Ann Surg* 191:271, 1980.
29. Scholhamer C, Spiro H: The first attack of acute pancreatitis: A clinical study. *J Clin Gastroenterol* 1:325, 1979.
30. Warshaw AL, Fuller AF: Specificity of increased renal clearance of amylase in diagnosis of acute pancreatitis, *N Engl J Med* 292:325, 1975.
31. Gross JB, Levitt MD: Postoperative elevation of amylase-creatinine clearance ratio in patient without pancreatitis. *Gastroenterology* 77:497–499, 1979.
32. Babb R: The role of surgery in acute pancreatitis. *Am J Digest Dis* 21:672, 1976.
33. Kelly T: Gallstone pancreatitis: The timing of surgery. *Surgery* 88:345, 1980.
34. Acosta JM, Rossi R, Galli OMR, et al.: Early surgery for acute gallstone pancreatitis: Evaluation of a systematic approach. *Surgery* 83:367, 1978.
35. Ranson JC: The timing of biliary surgery in acute pancreatitis. *Ann Surg* 189:654, 1979.
36. Peterson L, Collins J, Wilson R: Acute pancreatitis occurring after operation. *Surg Gynecol Obstet* 127:23, 1968.
37. Malgaleda J, Go VL, Remine WH, et al.: Postsurgical complications involving the pancreas. *Clin Gastroenterol* 8:455, 1979.
38. Sturdevant R, Walsh JH: Duodenal ulcer, Ch. 49, in Sleisenger M, Fordtran J (eds): *Gastrointestinal Disease*. Philadelphia, WB Saunders, 1978.
39. Mahl GF: Anxiety, HCl secretion, and peptic ulcer etiology. *Psychosom Med* 12:158, 1950.
40. Davies DT, Wilson ATM: Observations on the life history of chronic peptic ulcer. *Lancet* 2:1353, 1937.
41. Laufer I: Assessment of the accuracy of double contrast gastroduodenal radiology. *Gastroenterology* 71:874, 1976.
42. Laufer I, Mullens JE, Hamilton J: The diagnostic accuracy of barium studies of the stomach and duodenum: Correlation with endoscopy. *Radiology* 115:569, 1975.
43. Ippoliti A, Peterson W: The pharmacology peptic ulcer disease. *Clin Gastroenterol* 8:53, 1979.
44. Binder HJ, Coico A, Crossley RJ, et al: Cimetidine in the treatment of duodenal ulcer. A multicenter double-blind study. *Gastroenterology* 74:380, 1978.
45. Bodemar G, Walan A: Maintenance treatment of recurrent peptic ulcer by Cimetidine. *Lancet* 1:403, 1978.
46. Czaja A, McAlhany JC, Pruitt BA Jr: Acute gastroduodenal disease after thermal injury. An endoscopic evaluation of incidence and natural history. *N Engl J Med* 291:925, 1974.
47. Fromm D: Stress ulcer. *Hosp Med* 62:58, 1978.
48. Hastings P, Skillman J, Bushnell L, et al.: Antacid titration in the prevention of acute gastrointestinal bleeding: A controlled randomized trial in 100 critically ill patients. *N Engl J Med* 298:1041, 1978.
49. MacDougall BRD, Bailey RJ, Williams R: H$_2$ receptor antagonists and antacids in the prevention of acute gatrointestinal hemorrhage in fulminant hepatic failure. *Lancet* 1:617, 1977.
50. Priebe H, et al.: Antacid versus cimetidine in

preventing acute gastrointestinal bleeding: A randomized trial in 75 critically ill patients. *N Engl J Med* 302:426, 1980.

51. Tryba M: Side effects of stress bleeding prophylaxis. *Am J Med* 86(S6A) 85, 1989.

52. Laggner, AN, Lenz K, Base W, et al.: Prevention of upper gastrointestinal bleeding in long–term ventilated patients. *Am J Med* 86(S6A):81–84, 1989.

53. Curtis L, et al.: Evaluation of the effectiveness of controlled pH in the management of massive upper gastrointestinal bleeding. *Am J Surg* 125:474, 1973.

54. Athanasoulis C, Baum S, Waltman AC, et al.: Control of acute gastric mucosal hemorrhage with intraarterial infusion of posterior pituitary extract. *N Engl J Med* 290:597, 1974.

55. Evans C, Evans M, Pollock AV: The incidence and causes of postoperative jaundice. *Br J Anesth* 46:520, 1974.

56. Sanderson RG, Ellison JH, Benson JA, et al.: Jaundice following open heart surgery. *Ann Surg* 165:217, 1967.

57. Nunes G, Blaisdill FW, Margaretten W: Mechanism of hepatic dysfunction following shock and trauma. *Arch Surg* 100:546, 1970.

58. Dawson B, et al.: Hepatic function tests: Postoperative changes with halothane or diethyl ether anesthesia. *Mayo Clin Proc* 41:599, 1966.

59. LaMont JT, Isselbacher K: Postoperative jaundice. *N Engl J Med* 288:305, 1973.

60. Kantrowitz PA, Jones WA, Greenberger NJ, et al.: Severe postoperative hyperbilirubinemia simulating obstructive jaundice. *N Engl J Med* 280:591, 1967.

61. Carney FMT, Van Dyke RA: Halothane hepatitis: A critical review. *Anesth Analg* 51:135, 1972.

62. Summary of the National Halothane Survey. *JAMA* 197:775, 1966.

63. Lewis JH, Zimmerman HJ, Ishak KG, et al.: Enflurane hepatotoxicity. *Ann Int Med* 98:984, 1983.

64. Brown BR: Halothane hepatitis revisited. *New Eng J Med* 313:1347, 1985.

65. Trey C, et al.: Fulminant hepatic failure. *N Engl J Med* 279:798, 1968.

66. Moult PJA, Sherlock S: Halothane-related hepatitis. *Q J Med* 44:99, 1975.

67. Klatskin G, Kimberg D: Recurrent hepatitis attributable to halothane sensitization in anesthetist. *N Engl J Med* 280:515, 1969.

68. Sherloc S: Halothane hepatitis. *Gut* 12:324, 1971.

69. Joshi PA, Conn H: The syndrome of methoxyflourane-associated hepatitis. *Ann Intern Med* 80:395, 1974.

70. Alter HJ, et al.: Post-transfusion hepatitis after exclusion of commercial and hepatitis B antigen-positive donor. *Ann Intern Med* 77:691, 1972.

71. Koretz R, Stone O, Gitnick G: The long-term course of non-A, non-B posttransfusion hepatitis. *Gastroenterology* 79:893, 1980.

72. Berman M, et al.: The chronic sequelae of non-A, non-B hepatitis. *Ann Intern Med* 91:1979.

73. Rekele J, Radeker AG: Chronic liver disease after acute non-A, non-B viral hepatitis. *Gastroenterology* 77:1200, 1979.

74. Schmid M, et al.: Benign postoperative intrahepatic cholestasis. *N Engl J Med* 272:545, 1965.

75. Scharschmidt B: Approach to management of fulminant hepatic failure. *Med Clin N Am* 59:927, 1975.

76. Chojkier M, et al.: A controlled comparison of continuous intraarterial and intravenous infusions of vasopressin in hemorrhage from esophageal varices. *Gastroenterology* 77:540, 1979.

77. Howard RJ, DeLaney JP: Postoperative cholecystitis. *Am J Digest Dis* 17:213, 1972.

78. Ottinger LW: Acute cholecystitis as a postoperative complication. *Ann Surg* 184:162–165, 1976.

79. Bodvall B: The postcholecystectomy syndrome. *Clin Gastroenterol* 2:103, 1973.

80. Tondelli P, Gyr K, Stalder GA, Allgower M: The biliary tract: Post-cholecystectomy syndromes. *Clin Gastroenterol* 8:487, 1979.

81. Wychulis AR, Priestley JT, Foulk WT: A study of 360 patients with gastrojejunal ulcerations. *Surg Gynecol Obstet* 122:89, 1966.

82. Meshkinpour H, Elashoff J, Stewart H, Sturdevant RAL: Effects of cholestyramine on the symptoms of reflux gastritis. *Gastroenterology* 73:441, 1977.

83. Postlethwait RW: Five-year follow-up results of operations for duodenal ulcer. *Surg Gynecol Obstet* 137:387, 1973.

84. Allan JG, Gerskowitch VP, Russell RI: The role of bile acids in the pathogenesis of postvagotomy diarrhea. *Br J Surg* 61:516, 1974.

13

Endocrine Disorders

Thomas J. McGlynn, Jr. and Richard J. Simons

DIABETES MELLITUS

Overview

Medical consultants should review and reinforce long-term diabetic care, evaluate complications, and manage perioperative intermediary metabolism and postoperative complications. They should prepare patients for surgery through a series of office visits when possible. Elective surgery should be scheduled once diabetic care is optimized.

Epidemiology and Pathophysiology of Perioperative Care

Six million patients in the United States, 2–5% of the population, are diabetic. With appropriate management, the perioperative mortality of these patients is 2%, comparable to the mortality of nondiabetics. Atherosclerotic vascular disease accounts for approximately 30% and infections 20% of the perioperative mortality. Infections account for two-thirds of postoperative complications. Serious derangements of intermediary metabolism are less common. Hypoglycemia, often in the 4th to 6th postoperative day, occurs in 10% of the insulin-dependent patients. Preoperative assessments and perioperative management focus on cardiovascular and infectious complications, end-organ complications, and intermediary metabolism.

Increased platelet aggregation, poor tissue oxygenation, lowered red cell 2, 3-diphosphoglycerate levels, and high glycosylated hemoglobin levels may contribute to the pathophysiology of perioperative diabetic vascular complications (1,2). Diabetics may be vulnerable to infections because the insulin-deficient or hyperglycemic states can inhibit antibody formation, granulocyte chemotaxis or phagocytosis and lymphocyte responsiveness. Physiologic aberrations within the urinary tract may predispose the diabetic to microbial invasion and infection.

Surgery promotes catecholamine release, gluconeogenesis, and lipolysis, but inhibits insulin release and muscle glucose utilization. Glucagon and growth hormone release also increase blood glucose and ketone body formation. A spectrum of disorders, ranging from mild hyperglycemia and electrolyte imbalance to ketoacidosis and hyperosmolar coma may follow. Infections, medications, or anesthetic agents can further aggravate derangements of intermediary metabolism.

Preoperative Assessment of Long-term Care and Complications

Hospitalization provides an opportunity to enhance long-term management of chronic disorders. The patient's current level of glucose control should be measured by collecting fingerstick blood glucose samples, a 14-hour fasting triglyceride, cholesterol, and HDL profile before elective surgery (not during high stress), and a glycosylated hemoglobin level. These values should be compared to current standards for control (3), (Table 13.1). In conjunction with nursing staff and a dietician, the adequacy of the patient's diet, exercise regimen, compliance, overall educational status and motivation should be assessed. Long-term management ini-

Table 13.1. Perioperative Diabetic Care Flow Sheet

Long-term care assessments
Adequacy of control: Assessed through plasma samples

	Normal	Acceptable	Fair	Poor
Fasting glucose (mg/dl)	115	140	200	>200
Postprandial glucose	140	175	235	>235
Glycosylated hemoglobin (%)	6	8	10	>10
Cholesterol (mg/dl)	200	225	250	>250
Triglycerides (mg/dl)	150	175	200	>200

*From Rifkin, H (ed): Management of Type II Diabetes Mellitus. In *The Physician's Guide to Type II Diabetes (NIDDM)*. New York, American Diabetes Association, 1984. Reproduced with permission from the American Diabetes Association, Inc.
Assess diabetes education, diet education, exercise program, overall program compliance and motivation.
Assess blood pressure control, eye care needs, daily foot care, and the presence of kidney disease.
Assess cardiovascular status and evaluate EKG (test autonomic response).
Initiate 4 measures (text) to minimize infection.

Management of intermediary metabolism
All patients:
—Monitor preprandial and before bed fingerstick glucose.
—Provide 100cc 5% D&W/hour intravenously until oral intake is resumed.
Diet and oral hypoglycemic controlled patients:
—Discontinue oral agents and monitor.
—Establish a sliding scale of subcutaneous regular insulin if needed.
Insulin dependent patients:
—Give one-half to two-thirds of daily dose as intermediate-acting insulin on morning of surgery.
—For minor procedures, resume diet and give remainder of insulin dose in recovery room.
—Reduce or eliminate daily dose of AM short acting insulin and give additional (sliding scale) regular insulin as needed.
Poorly controlled, insulin-dependent patients:
—Mix 50 units of regular insulin in 500 cc of saline.
—Administer a constant infusion of 1–5 units/hour until glucose is 250 mg/dl, then reduce or discontinue infusion.
—Administer fluids as clinically indicated.

tiatives that can be pursued during recovery should be identified. The efforts of the patient's primary physician should be extended through educational programs (4,5).

The impact of active disease complications on any rehabilitation program should be considered. Hypertension should be tightly controlled since it significantly influences the rate of progression of both retinal and renal complications. Although thiazide diuretics may aggravate glucose intolerance and beta-blockers may blunt the clinical manifestations of hypoglycemia and insulin secretion, both groups of drugs can be used as first-line agents. Captopril must be given with care in the presence of renal disease (6).

Patients with early funduscopic changes, any visual impairment or eye symptoms should be referred to an ophthalmologist. Early intervention with laser therapy preserves vision. Early retinal changes are difficult to see on routine funduscopic examination.

Patient education about daily foot care is underemphasized even though it clearly decreases morbidity. The principles of care should be reviewed with all patients. Emphasize proper shoe wear, daily foot and shoe inspection, proper washing, moistening and oiling of feet, callus and toe nail management. Inspect the skin of the feet and lower limbs, palpate pulses and test sensation. The latter is often well preserved even in the presence of advanced neuropathic disease when tested with crude vibration sense and pin prick methods. Dry, scaly and fissured skin requires daily moistening and oiling of the feet. The daily application of topical antifungal agents (e.g., Clotrimazole) to the entire foot effectively treats associated dermatophyte infections. Other skin care recommendations may include the appropriate use of "eggcrate" mattresses, sheepskins, heel booties, and the avoidance of compressive stockings in patients with advanced arterial disease.

Local measures (cleansing, betadine wash, wet-to-dry dressings, filing of calluses, avoidance of undue pressure, and optimal daily foot care) often suffice for uncomplicated superficial ulcerations. Complicated, deep and infected ulcerations may require intravenous antibiotic therapy and plethysmography to demonstrate arterial adequacy for healing. The mixed flora often isolated from deep tissue infections frequently respond to a third-generation cephalosporin, such as Cefoxitin. Aminoglycosides should be avoided when possible because of renal toxicity related to cumulative dose. In the presence of advanced diabetic osteodystrophy with ulcerations and tissue necrosis, underlying bony autolysis cannot be accurately evaluated for the presence of osteomyelitis through the use of bone scans. Bone biopsy and culture (with antibiotic therapy and management based on culture results) are probably indicated more often than they are currently used. In the absence of strong evidence for osteomyelitis, judicious local measures over an extended period are often effective (7,8)

Immediate Perioperative Management

The choice of anesthetic belongs to the anesthesiologist. No agent is categorically contraindicated. Because diabetics suffer more frequent and/or severe cardiovascular complications at a younger age than nondiabetics, an in-depth cardiovascular examination and review is always in order. Patients with advanced disease and multiple end-organ complications may suffer from autonomic insufficiency, which occasionally predisposes them to an acute respiratory and cardiac arrest in the recovery period. At-risk patients should be fully awake before leaving the intensive observation of the recovery room. At-risk patients can be identified by the advanced state of their clinical disease and with a bedside EKG test. Upon deep inspiration, normal patients demonstrate a difference of greater than 15 beats per minute between the maximal and minimal heart rate. Patients with significant autonomic insufficiency display a beat-to-beat variation of less than 5 (9).

Four measures to minimize infections include: (a) avoiding the use of urinary catheters for convenience, (b) looking for white cells in the urinalysis (>2–3/hpf), culturing and treating infections when pyuria is present, (c) frequently examining the legs and feet and emphasizing good feet and skin care and (d) maintaining the patient's blood glucose below 250mg/ml. This level is an arbitrary upper level of optimum glucose control, which is selected because white cell dysfunction and other physiologic derangements (osmotic diuresis) frequently become significant at this level. When a significant infection develops, antibiotic selection should consider *staphylococcus,* a common pathogen in this setting (10).

A serum creatinine level should be obtained to assess renal status. The electrolytes of patients with advanced or chronic disease should be measured, looking for evidence of low-renin hypoaldosteronism (hyperkalemia, hyperchloremia, mild acidosis).

Intermediary Metabolism

The blood glucose should be maintained between 150–250 mg/100 ml throughout the perioperative period. These levels minimize the risks of hypoglycemia and physiologic dysfunction. No data to date provide evidence that tighter control is more effective. The blood glucose should be monitored using bedside finger-stick techniques (Autolet and Chemstrip bG, Dextrometer [Ames]), four times daily, before each meal and at bedtime (11).

Diabetics **treated with weight control, exercise, and diet** are simply followed with four times daily glucose assessments and proper diet. Patients who take **oral hypoglycemic agents** are treated in the same manner. Appropriate for the duration of action of each drug (tolbutamide, 6–12 hr; acetohexamide, 12–24 hr; tolazamide, 16–24 hr; glipizide, 24 hr; glyburide, 24hr; chlorpropamide, 24–36 hr), oral agents should be discontinued prior to surgery. If glucose control is mildly suboptimal (200–350mg/100ml), patients are started on small subcutaneous doses of monocomponent regular insulin (Novo or Iletin) to minimize the risks of antibody formation. Individual doses, usually 2–5 units, are based on preprandial and before bed blood glucose values (12).

If time permits and a patient cannot be properly controlled by diet, weight loss and full dose oral agents, **initiate insulin** as an outpatient or inpatient, depending on the patient's reliability, educational resources, personal support and clinical status. Begin with small doses of preprandial regular insulin and monitor the patient's glucose reponse. Once a total requirement of regular insulin (at least 20 units per day) has been established, give half the daily requirement of insulin as a morning dose of intermediate-acting insulin. Titrate the optimum control of fasting, preprandial and before bed glucose levels, using increasing morning doses of intermediate-acting insulin and decreasing doses of preprandial regular insulin. It is often most effective to first optimize control of fasting levels and then evening glucose levels. Split doses (AM and PM intermediate insulin, with or without regular insulin) may be necessary to optimize control (13–14).

All patients receive 50–100 grams of glucose per 24 hours to prevent periop-erative **starvation ketosis.** This is provided parenterally as 5% D&W and is started the morning of surgery. Postoperative ketonuria, without associated ketonemia or a change of blood pH, occurs if daily caloric requirements are not met. Intra- and postoperative hyperglycemia reflects glucose infusion rates, glucose underutilization due to insulin deficiency and overall hydration status. Surgery scheduled in the early AM facilitates management.

The eight **principles of perioperative insulin management** are: (a) on the day of surgery, give a morning dose of intermediate-acting insulin, which is about one-half to two-thirds of the patient's established daily requirement; (b) anticipate that this dose will be inadequate and monitor the patient's response and overall condition (check intraoperative glucose if procedure lasts more than 2 hours); (c) begin parenteral carbohydrate (5% D&W, 100 cc/hr) the morning of surgery and continue throughout surgery and postoperative recovery; (d) for minor procedures, give the remainder of the patient's insulin in the recovery room, once the patient is awake and ready to eat; (e) for major procedures and extended recovery, continue carbohydrate supplements and give small doses of subcutaneous regular insulin with individual doses based on preprandial and before bed blood glucose levels (or every 6 hour samples) during early recovery; (f) return the patient to a full presurgery dose of insulin once he is able to resume full oral intake; (g) continue monitoring the patient throughout the recovery period; (h) closely monitor patients who use **constant subcutaneous insulin infusion pumps** because they rapidly become ketotic within an hour of discontinuing the pump infusion. They must be started immediately on a low-dose intravenous insulin infusion.

Low-dose insulin infusions provide the most efficient option if small additional subcutaneous doses of regular insulin are inadequate or time is at a premium. Several clinical studies have shown that low-dose constant infusions of regular insulin (or intermittent intramuscular insulin) are effective for perioperative and operative glucose control (1–2 U/hr) and during severe ketoacidosis (5–10 U/hr) (15).

Six physiologic **principles of low-dose insulin** infusion therapy provide a basis for therapeutic advantages: *(a)* a loading bolus of about 10 units effectively saturates available insulin receptors, even in severe ketoacidosis; *(b)* the activity half-life of intravenous insulin is about 5 minutes, and excess doses are harmlessly metabolized; *(c)* an optimum decrease of glucose (50–75 mg/100 ml/hour) can be anticipated and monitored with bedside techniques during therapy; *(d)* therapy can be adjusted or terminated within minutes; *(e)* patients can be protected from hypoglycemia with an infusion of 5% (incomplete protection) or 10% D&W during therapy when the glucose falls below 250 mg/100 ml; *(f)* adherence of small quantities of insulin to infusion systems is not clinically significant.

For **poorly controlled patients (glucose 300–500 mg/100ml) who need prompt surgery**, administer 5 units of regular insulin intravenously as a loading dose. Add 50 units of regular insulin to 500 cc of normal saline, and flush the system with about 50 cc to saturate the insulin binders in the system. Infuse 1–5 units of insulin each hour (10–50 cc/hr of the above solution) until the blood glucose is 250 mg/ml. At that point, decrease the infusion rate to 1–2 units of insulin per hour (10–20 cc of solution), and begin a separate infusion of 5% D&W at a rate of 100 cc per hour. When the glucose is less than 150 mg/100 ml, stop the infusion of insulin and monitor the blood glucose to assure continued control. Additional fluid requirements are determined by clinical parameters (blood pressure, pulse, etc.).

Ketoacidosis

Two aspects of ketoacidosis present diagnostic challenges. Patients with acute, severe ketoacidosis commonly develop nausea, vomiting, and gastric dilatation. In addition, some patients develop severe **abdominal pain, distention, and guarding**, often associated with **hyperamylasemia** of salivary and pancreatic origin with altered amylase clearance. When attempting to distiguish patients with primary ketoacidosis from those with surgically correctable conditions that precipitate ketoacidosis, keep several principles in mind.

The nausea and vomiting asssociated with ketoacidosis almost always precedes the onset of **abdominal pain.** Many acute abdominal catastrophies are characterized by the onset of abdominal pain, followed by other symptoms. Abdominal pain due to ketoacidosis usually occurs in younger patients with severe acidosis. If the patient is older than 40 years of age and the bicarbonate value is in excess of 10meq/L, a specific underlying cause of the abdominal pain other than ketoacidosis should be sought. Persistent abdominal pain beyond the first few hours of treatment for ketoacidosis suggests a cause for the pain other than the ketoacidosis. **Hyperamylasemia** due to ketoacidosis occurs with 60% of ketoacidosis patients, often in the presence of profound hyperglycemia (glucose values of 500 mg/100 ml). Peak values of greater than 1000 Samoji units may occur after therapy has begun. Be conservative about making the diagnosis of pancreatitis in the presence of ketoacidosis (16–20).

In the presence of an **anion gap acidosis**, measure the arterial pH, blood ketone and lactate levels and serum creatinine. A combination of renal tubular acidosis due to dehydration, lactic acidosis due to shock, and ketoacidosis due to insulin deficiency may be factors in the acidosis of some patients. To treat ketoacidosis, correct three deficits: insulin deficiency, volume deficiency, and electrolyte imbalances. Anticipate two early complications (hypoglycemia and hypokalemia) and one uncommon late problem (disequilibrium syndrome). Therapeutic goals are efficiently and conveniently achieved through constant infusion of low-dose insulin. Other less convenient regimens (subcutaneous and intramuscular regimens) can be equally effective in experienced hands.

Saturate insulin receptors with a **loading intravenous bolus** of 10 units of regular insulin. Begin the **continuous infusion** with 2–8 units of regular insulin per hour (20–80 cc of 50 units of insulin in 500 cc of saline). As little as 2.4 units per hour produces plasma insulin levels of 100 uU/ml, which are well within the effective therapeutic range. The rate of glucose fall in the first hour may exceed 75–100 mg/100 ml per hour due to the combined effects of insulin and of fluids. Subsequent hourly rates of fall are rather predictable. The patient can be rebolused and insulin and fluid infusion rates adjusted if optimum rates of glucose fall are not achieved. Continue an effective infusion rate until the glucose is 250 mg/100 ml. At that point, begin 5 or 10% D&W at a rate of 100 cc per hour, and adjust the insulin infusion rate to 1–2 units/hour, adequate to maintain a glucose of 150–200 mg/100 ml. An alternative is to discontinue the insulin infusion once the glucose is below 250 mg/100 ml and begin small doses of subcutaneous insulin, as needed.

Ketosis (bicarbonate less than 20) may persist up to 9 hours despite correction of hyperglycemia. This indicates a continued need for liberal fluid infusion to decrease catecholamine production, which drives ketosis and a need for intracellular insulin to shut off lipolysis, which leads to ketosis. In this circumstance, continue the infusion of 1–2 units of insulin per hour and 5% D&W at a minimum rate of 100 cc/hour until the bicarbonate is above 20.

Serious **electrolyte and fluid deficiencies** are always present in ketoacidosis. The osmotic diuresis induced by glycosuria is roughly equivalent to half normal saline with 35–63 meq of potassium per liter. The volume of fluid required by individual patients varies widely but averages 3–4 liters during the first 6 hours of therapy and 6–8 liters over the first 24 hours. Fluid therapy is initiated through an individual line to which the insulin infusion solution is piggybacked. Begin with normal saline at an infusion rate of 1000–250 cc/hour. The rate and volume of the remainder of each patient's therapy is based on the patient's volume status, observed ability to tolerate rapid infusion rates and electrolyte status. A common error among inexperienced staff is to undertreat with fluids for fear of precipitating congestive failure.

To **estimate electrolyte needs**, remember that each 100 mg/100 ml of glucose above normal displaces approximately 2 meq of sodium. Thus, a patient with a glucose of 600 mg/100 ml and a sodium of 128 meq/L is about equally sodium and water deficient. The patient's serum sodium of 128 meq/L is equivalent to 138 meq/L. A patient with the same glucose level but a sodium of 118 meq/L is severely sodium and fluid deficient. The latter patient will require more normal saline than the former patient. Hyperlipidemia can spuriously lower the serum sodium value through displacement. Lactescent serum suggests this possibility.

Low-dose insulin regimens may reduce the risks of **hypokalemia.** Immediately treat the hypokalemia of patients who present in ketoacidosis with a potassium of 3.5 meq/L or less, once an adequate urine output (40 cc/hour) has been established. For patients above this level, treatment is not necessary until potassium falls below these levels. Measure serum electrolyes and glucose every 1–2 hours. Potassium replacement can be added to intravenous fluids as KCl or a combination of KCl and K_2PO_4. The total potassium needs of patients varies from 0–300 meq or more over the first 24 hours (average need 10–20 meq/hr). K_2PO_4 can replace **depleted phosphate stores** of seriously ill patients and significantly improve the patient's response. This therapy should be offered to all patients with low phosphate levels and those who are doing poorly because intracellular PO_4 depletion is not always reflected by a decreased serum level (21).

The most recent formal clinical evaluations of **bicarbonate** therapy suggest that this therapy adds little, even in the presence of severe acidosis (pH less than 7.1) (22). Nonetheless, one or two ampules (44 meq/ampule) can be given intravenously to patients with a pH of 7.1 or lower.

Cerebral disequilibrium occurs relatively late in the course of ketoacidosis when glucose levels are falling, bicarbonate levels are improving, and the patient is in satisfactory electrolyte balance. Patients may develop stupor, coma, and an areflexic state, which may be followed by death. The syndrome seems related to the development of cerebral edema from overly aggressive use of sodium bicarbonate or the overly rapid correction of electrolyte abnormalities. Cerebral fluid acidosis may persist and results in an ionic imbalance, which induces cerebral edema. Treatment consists of corticosteroids (8 mg of dexamethasone intravenously) and an osmotic diuretic (23).

Hyperosmolar Coma

Ten percent of severe intermediary metabolism disorders are due to hyperosmolar coma. It is most common among older, type II diabetics, many of whom were previously undiagnosed or had been treated with oral hypoglycemic agents. Progressive hyperglycemia and dehydration are initiated by many factors, including drugs (diazoxide, corticosteroids, immunosuppressive agents, diuretics, dilantin, propranolol, parenteral hyperalimentation), and stress (dialysis, anesthesia, pneumonia, cerebral vascular accidents, pancreatitis, etc). Mortality has been as high as 40% in some patient populations.

The insidious onset of symptoms and signs over a period of days to weeks (average, 12 days) belies the serious nature of this disorder. Early manifestations of the hyperosmolar state are nonspecific and include irritability, weakness, polyuria, vomiting, and polydypsia. All of these findings are often attributed to other factors present in the average surgical population. Therapy usually requires about 8 hours and fluid requirements average about 8 liters. Fluids are initiated with 0.45% sodium chloride and followed by normal saline, as plasma osmolarity and sodium values decline. A low-dose infusion of regular insulin (2–3 units/hour) often suffices, and total insulin requirements are often surprisingly small (12–25 units) (24).

HYPERTHYROIDISM

Epidemiology

It is well established that the risk of surgery in the untreated thyrotoxic patient is substantial. The major concern is the precipitation of thyroid storm, a life-threatening clinical syndrome characterized by hypermetabolism and/or adrenergic excess. In the past, the most common precipitant of thyroid storm was surgery—thyroidectomy for Graves' disease on an inadequately prepared patient (25). A wide spectrum of both major and minor surgical and obstetrical procedures has been reported to precipitate thyroid storm, including dental extraction, abdominal surgery, childbirth, and cesarean section. With the advent of more efficacious antithyroid drugs, improved preparation of patients prior to surgery, and readily available measurement of thyroid function, perioperative thyrotoxic storm should be a rare occurrence today.

Preoperative Assessment

The best treatment for surgically induced thyroid storm is prevention through the preoperative recognition of hyperthyroidism. Symptoms of thyroid hormone excess—palpitations, heat intolerance, weight loss without anorexia, tremor, menstrual irregularity or amenorrhea and muscular weakness—should be sought. A more subtle presentation of hyperthyroidism is seen in elderly patients with so-called "apathetic" hyperthyroidism. Many clinicians are under the mistaken impression that hyperthyroidism is uncommon in the elderly. In fact, studies have shown **a seven-fold greater prevalence of the disease in older age groups** (26–28). Originally coined more than a half century ago, apathetic hyperthyroidism is the term used to describe patients who show "nonactivation" rather than the usual hyperkinesis of the typical young hyperthyroid patient. In such patients, many of the expected signs and symptoms are not present and cardiac findings tend to predominate. Thus, this form of hyperthyroidism is more likely to be missed in a preoperative evaluation. Occult hyperthyroidism should be suspected in any elderly patient who presents with unexplained tachycardia, atrial fibrillation or arrhythmias, or weight loss. If the consultant elicits signs or symptoms suggestive of hyperthyroidism in a patient scheduled for an elective procedure, surgery should be delayed until the patient's thyroid status is clarified. Measurements of thyroxine (T_4) and the T_3 resin uptake test should be obtained on all patients with suspected hyperthyroidism. In a patient in whom there is a high clinical index of suspicion in the face of a normal T_4 and free thyroid index, a T_3 RIA may be helpful in detecting the rare patient with T_3-thyrotoxicosis. Occasionally, a TRH stimulation test may be needed to confirm the diagnosis when routine tests of thyroid function are not definitive.

The three major classes of agents used in the treatment of hyperthyroidism include the thioamides (propylthiouracil and methimazole), iodides, and the beta-adrenergic antagonists. The thioamides block thyroid peroxidase and thus inhibit thyroid hormone biosynthesis. This inhibitory effect on thyroid hormone synthesis may be found within one hour of administration of these agents. Both drugs have weak immunosuppressive effects. Agranulocytosis is the most feared complication, which occurs in less than 0.2% of patients. Routine blood counts are of no use in predicting this complication. The half-life of propylthiouracil is 1–2 hours, whereas methimazole is 4–8 hours. The usual dosage for propylthiouracil is 300–900 mg/day in 3 divided doses. Methimazole can be given as a single daily dose, ranging from 30–90 mg/day. Dosage should be titrated to achieve and maintain biochemical and clinical euthyroidism.

Iodide is a potent and prompt inhibitor of thyroid hormone release. It is the most effective agent for lowering thyroid hormone acutely and this is useful in patients who need rapid correction of the hyperthyroid state. Because iodide interferes with thyroid hormone synthesis and reduces the vascularity of the overactive thyroid gland, it is an ideal agent for the preoperative preparation of the hyperthyroid patient. The dose and route of administration is discussed below.

Beta-adrenergic blocking agents are usually employed in the treatment of the patient with thyrotoxicosis. The time-honored beta blocker, propanolol, is effective in abolishing many of the hyperdynamic signs and symptoms of thyrotoxicosis. It is postulated that hyperthyroid subjects exhibit an extreme sensitivity to the action of catecholamines. One must use great caution in administering propanolol to patients with a history of bronchospasm or congestive heart failure. On the other hand, propanolol may be helpful in the treatment of congestive heart failure when tachycardia is a major contributing factor.

For elective surgery, even minor procedures, the patient should be rendered euthyroid prior to the operation. Propylthiouracil has been the mainstay of therapy. However, compared with propylthiouracil, methimazole is cheaper, can be given as a single daily dose, and is associated with less major toxicity (29). Although euthyroid levels of thyroid hormone can be achieved in 2–3 weeks, surgery is usually postponed from 1–3 months to ensure reversal of the effects of hyperthyroidism.

If a patient with untreated or partially treated hyperthyroidism requires emergency surgery, it is necessary to treat that individual with propanolol and iodides prior to induction of anesthesia. Intravenous preparations of both propanolol and iodide can be used as discussed below. These patients require careful management in the postoperative period in terms of fluid and hemodynamic status. Antithyroid drugs (propylthiouracil or methimazole) should be initiated as soon as the patient is able to take oral or NG fluids.

If a subtotal thyroidectomy is deemed necessary, the patient should be prepared for surgery with propanolol. In many elective cases, this agent has been used successfully as the sole preparatory medication. However, in some patients, propanolol alone is insufficient preparation for thyroid surgery. Feed and colleagues (30) have recommended that therapy be initiated with propanolol, but that daily doses of potassium iodide (60 mg every 8 hours) be added, beginning 10 days before surgery. The combination of potassium iodide and propanolol has been very effective in preparing such patients for surgery. Elective surgery for previously hyperthyroid patients who have been in clinical and laboratory remission off of medications for 3 or more months carries little or no added risk.

With the appropriate preoperative evaluation and care, thyroid storm will be averted in the vast majority of patients. However, the internist who provides a consultative service to the surgeon should be prepared to treat this condition since it can arise unexpectedly following any surgical procedure.

Postoperative Management: Thyroid Storm

The clinical presentation of thyroid storm can be quite variable, ranging in severity from a febrile reaction following subtotal thyroidectomy to hypotension, coma, and even death. Criteria for thyroid storm are varied due to the fact that there is no defined point at which severe thyrotoxicosis becomes thyroid storm. Although multiple systems can be affected, the cardiac, central nervous, and gastrointestinal systems predominate. Arrhythmias and hypotension are common. High-output congestive heart failure may be present even in the absence of underlying heart disease. Tremor and agitation are the most common neurologic manifestations, although overt psychosis, stupor, and even coma have been observed. The gastrointestinal symptoms include diarrhea, jaundice, vomiting, and occasionally abdominal pain. Finally, fever—regarded by most as a sine qua non—may be mistaken for infection and may be as high as 106°F.

Surgery frequently precipitates thyroid storm and its recognition by the consultant demands immediate action (Table 13.2) The therapy of thyroid storm has five goals: (a) identification and treatment of the precipitating cause, (b) blockade of thyroid hormone production, (c) blockade of the release of thyroid hormone, (d) blockade of excess beta-adrenergic stimulation, and (e) general supportive measures.

General supportive measures include the replacement of fluid and electrolytes and control of hyperthermia. Aspirin should be avoided since it may further increase the patient's metabolic rate by displacing thyroid hormone from its binding proteins. Hypothermic blankets, fans, and ice packs may be used to control fever.

Congestive heart failure may require the use of oxygen and diuretics. Antibiotics should be administered in the presence of established infection. Most au-

Table 13.2. Role of Surgery on Precipitating Thyroid Storm

Study	(Hyperthyroid Patients) or Procedures in Hyperthyroid Patients	% Thyroid Storm Due to Surgery	% Hyperthyroid Patients Undergoing Surgery Developing Storm
McArthur (1974)	1383	25/36 (69%)	36/1383 (2.6%)
Waldstein (1960)	(20)	4/21 (19%)	
Maftaferri (1969)	(20)	7/22 (32%)	
Nelson (1967)	(2329)	2/21 (9.5%)	

thorities agree on the use of **adrenal steroids** since there may be a relatively inadequate adrenal reserve. Hydrocortisone 300 mg/day is usually sufficient.

Antithyroidal drugs should be given in high doses. Propylthiouracil is the drug of choice since, in addition to its action in the thyroid gland of inhibiting thyroid hormone synthesis, it also appears to inhibit the extrathyroidal conversion of thyroxine to triiodothyronine (T_3), usually resulting in a significant reduction in serum T_3 within 24 hours. Methimazole probably does not possess this latter action and should not be used for thyroid storm. Treatment with propylthiouracil should be initiated with a loading dose of 600–1000 mg orally or by nasogastric tube. After the loading dose, patients are usually maintained on 100–300 mg every 8 hours.

The administration of iodide should be delayed for at least 1–2 hours after propylthiouracil is administered to avoid any thyroidal accumulation of iodide that could, at a later time, be utilized for the synthesis of more thyroid hormone. Iodide is given orally in the form of a Lugol's solution, at a dose of up to 30 drops per day. Alternatively, sodium iodide, 1–2 gm intravenously over 24 hours, can be given. The iodide is usually continued for 7–10 days.

Unless there is an absolute contraindication, all patients with thyroid storm should receive a beta-adrenergic blocking agent. Propranolol has been shown to have a peripheral inhibitory effect on the con-version of T_4 to T_3 and is considered the agent of choice. Propranolol quickly controls the cardiac and psychomotor manifestations of thyrotoxicosis. The dosage of propranolol must be individualized. Therapy is usually initiated with 20–40 mg orally given every 6 hours or with 2–10 mg intravenously by slow infusion not to exceed 1 mg per minute. The dosage should be increased depending on the clinical response, with the resting pulse being the best indicator of the adequacy of beta blockade. Fever, restlessness, and tremor usually respond promptly. The total daily dose of propranolol may range from 40–1280 mg.

Even with the therapeutic modalities mentioned above and summarized in Table 13.3, thyroid storm still carries significant morbidity and mortality. Prevention through early recognition of impending thyroid storm remains the most important aspect of treatment.

HYPOTHYROIDISM

Surgical Risk

Surgery in the patient with untreated hypothyroidism carries the risk of several potential complications. These patients may manifest extreme sensitivity to sedatives and anesthetic agents, resulting in prolonged unconsciousness following the administration of seemingly normal doses. Induction of anesthesia in the hypothyroid patient has resulted in hypotension, cardiac arrest, and myxedema coma. The risks of anesthesia and surgery include

Table 13.3. Management of Thyroid Storm

I. Treatment of precipitating cause (sepsis, diabetes, etc.)
II. Blockade of thyroid hormone production
    1. Propylthiouracil (600–1000 mg p.o. or by nasogastric tube as loading dose, then 100–300 mg every 8 hours).
III. Blockage of thyroid hormone release
    1. Lugol's solution (30 drops/day p.o.) or sodium iodide, 1 gm intravenously every 8–12 hr). Note: Iodide should be started after propylthiouracil and continued for 7–10 days.
IV. Beta-Adrenergic blockade
    1. Propranolol (initially, 20–40 mg p.o. every 6 hr or 2–10 mg by slow intravenous infusion every 6 hr).
    Note: Dosage should be titrated to achieve a resting pulse <90.
V. General supportive measures
    1. Hydrocortisone (200–500 mg daily parenterally).
    2. Control fever with fans, hypothermic blankets, or acetaminophen. Avoid aspirin.
    3. Fluid and electrolyte replacement.

hypoventilation, cardiopulmonary arrest, hyponatremia, and precipitation of congestive heart failure.

Hypothyroid patients have a reduced maximal breathing capacity, diminished carbon monoxide diffusion capacity, and a reduction in hypoxic ventilatory drive. Alveolar hypoventilation is especially common in the obese hypothyroid. These abnormalities in pulmonary function can all be corrected with thyroid hormone replacement.

Left ventricular dysfunction has been documented in patients with severe hypothyroidism. Also, electrocardiographic abnormalities including flat or inverted T-waves, sinus bradycardia, and low voltage are common. Occasionally, the presenting manifestation of hypothyroidism is congestive heart failure associated with bradycardia and pericardial effusion. Such effusions are not hemodynamically significant, tamponade rarely occurs, and they resolve with thyroid replacement. However, in the stressed hypothyroid patient, **congestive heart failure may develop rapidly and respond poorly to conventional therapy.**

Patients with hypothyroidism have impaired ability to excrete a free water load. This abnormality, which is corrected by giving replacement doses of thyroid hormone, is probably caused by inappropriate secretion of antidiuretic hormone (ADH). Such patients are at risk for significant iatrogenic hyponatremia.

Several recent studies have attempted to better define the surgical risk for untreated hypothyroid patients. Ladenson et al. (42) performed a retrospective controlled analysis, comparing the relative frequencies of perioperative complications in hypothyroid and control patients undergoing surgery with general anesthesia. Most of the hypothyroid patients were judged to have clinically mild or moderate hypothyroidism (serum thyroxine level 2.4 ± 1.2 ug/ml, mean ± SD). The hypothyroid patients had a statistically greater incidence of intraoperative hypotension, heart failure, gastrointestinal and neuropsychiatric complications. There were no differences in perioperative blood loss, duration of hospitalization, or prevalences of perioperative arrhythmia, hypothermia, hyponatremia, delayed anesthetic recovery, abnormal tissue integrity, impaired wound healing, pulmonary complications, or death. In another study by Drucker and Burrow, ten patients with untreated mild to moderate hypothyroidism undergoing cardiac surgery with cardiopulmonary bypass were compared to a control group of 30 patients (43). There was no difference in the number of postoperative complications nor length of hospital stay. Furthermore, no problems were encountered with discontinuation of cardiopulmonary bypass or reversal of hypothyroidism. Caution should be exercised, however, in extrapolating these results to patients with severe or profound hypothyroidism.

Preoperative Evaluation and Diagnosis

The diagnosis of hypothyroidism can be easily missed. Its clinical onset is usually insidious and its manifestations protean. Associated signs and symptoms are often ascribed to debilitation caused by surgical or other medical illnesses. Common complaints include lethargy, weakness, dyspnea, fatigue, cold intolerance, and weight gain with little or no change in appetite. Distension, flatulence, and constipation dominate the gastrointestinal complaints, while arthritis and carpal tunnel syndrome are the most common musculoskeletal problems. The neuropsychiatric manifestations include memory loss, dementia, cerebellar ataxia, and myxedema coma. Bradycardia, hypothermia, brittle hair, dry skin, and slow relaxation of deep tendon reflexes are common physical findings. Laboratory clues include a normochromic, normocytic anemia, hypercholesterolemia, elevation of muscle enzymes (CPK), and hyponatremia.

The diagnosis of hypothyroidism is confirmed with the measurement of thyroid function tests. A low T_4 in combination with an elevated TSH is diagnostic of primary hypothyroidism. Variations in thyroid binding protein concentrations secondary to drugs or disease states may result in high or low T_4 values. (The T_4 by radioimmunoassay measures both protein-bound and free thyroxine.) The free T_4 index, derived from the T_4 and T_3 resin uptake test, remains the most popular clinical method for assessing abnormalities in serum protein binding of thyroid hormone.

The clinician must be aware that in severely ill patients even the free T_4 index may not accurately reflect thyroid status. Despite a low T_4, and borderline or low free T_4 index, most of these patients are thought to be clinically euthyroid and comprise the **"euthyroid sick syndrome"**. A recent study supports the theory that the low thyroxine state of severe illness is at least partially related to suppression of thyrotropin secretion (44). At the present time, most authorities do not recommend thyroid replacement in patients with the euthyroid sick syndrome.

The differentiation between primary hypothyroidism and secondary hypothyroidism can be made by measuring the plasma level of thyroid-stimulating hormone (TSH) and response to thyrotropin-releasing hormone (TRH). Sparse or absent pubic and axillary hair, absence of a palpable thyroid gland, and thin, finely wrinkled, pale skin suggest the possibility of secondary hypothyroidism.

A past history of treatment of hyperthyroidism by thyroidectomy or with radioactive iodine should raise the possibility of thyroid deficiency. Lithium blocks the release of thyroid hormone. Long-term treatment of psychiatric patients with lithium has been reported to result in a 3–4% incidence of hypothyroidism. It has also been observed that patients with Graves' disease who are euthyroid after treatment are particularly sensitive to the blocking effect of lithium. Iodine also inhibits thyroid hormone release and if administered in a sufficient dose can occasionally cause hypothyroidism. This most commonly occurs in patients with pulmonary disease who are given potassium iodide for chronic obstructive airway disease. In a series of over 2000 patients treated with potassium iodide, Bernecker (45) reported that hypothyroidism developed in 0.2% when the dose was 5–7 gm of iodine per day, and 2.9% if the dose was 20–30 gm per day. However, with the introduction of more effective agents for the treatment of asthma, such high doses of iodide are rarely employed today. Patients with Hashimoto's thyroiditis and treated Graves' disease seem to be particularly sensitive to iodine, and doses as low as 0.5 gm per day can induce hypothyroidism. Amiodarone, an antiarrhythmic agent used in the treatment of refractory ventricular tachycardia, may result in hypothyroidism with a characteristic laboratory profile: T_4 levels are high, T_3 levels are low, and the TSH is elevated. Other substances which may sometimes cause goiter and, rarely, hypothyroidism include: p-aminosalicylic acid, aminoglutethimide, and phenylbutazone. Post-radiation hypothyroidism may also occur in patients treated for neoplastic processes involving the neck or superior mediastinum.

Hashimoto's thyroiditis (or autoimmune thyroiditis) is the most common spontaneous form of hypothyroidism. It is characterized by the presence of circulating antithyroid antibodies and a firm, rubbery thyroid gland. Antibodies specific to gastric parietal cells, adrenal cortex, ovary, testis, pancreatic islets, and pituitary lactotrophs have also been detected and may result in polyendocrine syndromes, in which the patient may manifest more than one endocrine deficiency. The presence of vitiligo may be a clue to the polyendocrine deficiency syndrome. One must be particularly alert to the coexistence of thyroid and adrenal insufficiency. These patients should be carefully examined for postural changes in blood pressure and for evidence of hyperpigmentation, especially in old scars and in the palmar creases.

Perioperative Management

Because of the multiple abnormal physiologic responses discussed above, the risk of surgery can be considerable in the patient with severe hypothyroidism. Therefore, in the patient with profound hypothyroidism, elective surgery should be postponed until the patient is treated with thyroid hormone and rendered clinically euthyroid. It may take 2–3 months or longer in order to achieve optimal replacement, especially in older patients or patients with cardiac disease, since rapid replacement can precipitate angina or even myocardial infarction. The patient with subclinical or mild hypothyroidism may be cleared for surgery. However, close follow-up of these patients in the postoperative period is essential with anticipatory planning for the potential complications discussed above.

If an untreated or inadequately treated hypothyroid patient requires emergency surgery, the anesthesiologist must be informed. Lower anesthetic doses are usually required and recovery from anesthesia will generally be prolonged. Assisted ventilation will probably be required not only during anesthesia but also in the postoperative period for up to 2–3 days. The indiscriminate use of sedatives and narcotics in these patients is to be avoided. **Sudden respiratory arrest** has been reported in postoperative hypothyroid patients. In addition, because these patients have an impaired ability to handle a free water load, particular attention must be paid to fluid and electrolyte management to prevent hyponatremia and congestive heart failure from overhydration.

The ultimate expression of severe hypothyroidism is **myxedema coma.** Although it can occur at any age, it is most commonly seen in elderly hypothyroid women who develop myxedema coma in the winter months following some stressful event, with pneumonia leading the list. The typical signs of infection including fever, tachycardia, sweating, and leukocytosis may be blunted, however, because of the hypothyroid state. Other intercurrent medical illnesses, including myocardial infarction and congestive heart failure, can also precipitate myxedema coma. Occasionally, a surgical procedure is the precipitating cause. These individuals usually have a long antecedent history of symptoms suggestive of hypothyroidism, and the physical examination will provide corroborative findings. At least 80% of these patients are hypothermic and, in fact, a normal body temperature is suggestive of an intercurrent infection.

Myxedema coma is usually associated with hypoventilation and carbon dioxide retention with a variable degree of respiratory acidosis. (Carbon dioxide narcosis is reported to be the predominant factor in at least one-third of patients.) Hypoglycemia can occur in both primary and secondary hypothyroidism, although it is more common in the latter. Hyponatremia, cerebral hypoxia from decreased cardiac output and decreased cerebral perfusion, hypothermia, intercurrent infection and the thyroid hormone deficiency itself can all contribute to this neurologic state.

Myxedema coma is a medical emergency. Therapy must be instituted promptly, often before laboratory confirmation of the hypothyroid state is obtained. General guidelines for the treatment of myxedema coma are outlined in Table 13.4. Replacement of thyroid hormone is the single most specific aspect of therapy in the treatment of myxedema coma. There was a tendency in the past to administer thyroxine in small doses because of the fear of precipitating coronary ischemia. However, it has been sug-

gested that therapeutic failures in myxedema coma may have been secondary to inadequate administration of thyroxine. The current recommendation is to administer 400–500 μg of thyroxine as a slow bolus intravenous injection. With this approach, there is a rapid normalization of circulating thyroid hormone levels, such that by 24 hours the TSH has decreased and serum T_4 levels are within the normal range.

There are a number of other general principles regarding the management of these patients, which should be emphasized. Although most of these individuals are hypothermic, attempts at rewarming should be discouraged since it inappropriately increases body metabolism and oxygen consumption. Since the laboratory distinction between primary and secondary hypothyroidism could require several days, myxedematous patients should be given **parenteral glucocorticoids.** Also, even in myxedema due to primary hypothyroidism, the ACTH response to stress is impaired.

If the patient is hypotensive, the blood pressure usually responds to thyroid hormone and volume replacement. Vasopressors should be used with caution since serious cardiac arrhythmias may occur when they are given together with large doses of thyroid hormone. Dosages of digitalis should be reduced, since even normal serum levels of digoxin can be associated with digitalis intoxication.

Table 13.4.   Treatment of Myxedema Coma

I. General supportive measures
  1. Maintain a patent airway and adequate ventilation.
  2. Rewarming hypothermic patients is unnecessary.
  3. Careful monitoring of fluid and electrolytes to prevent volume overload and hyponatremia.
  4. Hydrocortisone (100 mg q 8 hr) for at least a week. The dose can be tapered in the second week.
II. Treatment of metabolic complications
  1. Hypoglycemia
  2. Hyponatremia
III. Treatment of precipitating cause
  1. Careful evaluation for a source of infection or other intercurrent medical illness.
IV. Thyroid hormone replacement
  1. Thyroxine (500–1000 μg) by slow intravenous infusion followed by 50–100 μg per day.

ADRENAL GLAND

Overview

Acute perioperative adrenal insufficiency is uncommon. Patients present with nonspecific symptoms, and adrenal insufficiency must be considered in certain clinical situations. At-risk patients can be easily tested or given prophylactic corticosteroids. Treatment consists of hydrocortisone and fluid and electrolyte replacement.

Epidemiology and Pathophysiology

Acute primary or secondary adrenal insufficiency occurs among less than 0.001% of all surgical patients. Occasionally, patients with acute insufficiency are admitted for acute surgery because of high fever and intense abdominal pain, prominent symptoms in one-third of adrenal crises. More commonly, the use of corticosteroids is missed during the admission history or preoperative prophylaxis is overlooked. Borderline compensated patients can survive surgery without prophylaxis only to decompensate during a later stress. Associated medical conditions can produce a crisis: metastatic cancer or lymphoma to the adrenal glands, thyroid administration in pituitary insufficient patients, heparin administration with spontaneous adrenal hemmorrhage, high-dose medroxyprogesterone therapy for breast carcinoma, high-dose ketoconazole therapy, or rifampin therapy in adrenal insufficient patients.

Symptoms, signs and laboratory abnormalities of postoperative adrenal insufficiency are often attributed to other causes. The characteristic spectrum of findings rarely develops. Hypotension and shock can be the first and only symptoms. Some patients present with nonspecific central nervous system changes or a high fever (39.2 C, 103 F). Common symptoms of nausea and vomiting are frequently attributed to other causes. Less than half of the patients present with classic laboratory findings of hyponatremia, hyperkalemia, acidosis, eosinophilia, hypoglycemia and prerenal azotemia. Skin hyperpigmentation occurs only with primary adrenal insufficiency. It is often subtle and confined to skin creases and knuckles.

Patients at Risk for Adrenal Cortical Suppression

Hypothalmic-pituitary-adrenal (HPA) suppression varies with the **type of steroid** administered, the **dose schedule and route** of administration, the **total daily dose** and the **duration of therapy.** Long-acting corticosteroids with a 48 hour or longer effect (betamehasone, dexamethasone, triamcinolone) suppress the HPA more effectively than shorter acting agents with a 24–36 hour effect (cortisol, cortisone, prednisone, prednisolone, methylprednisolone). A small evening dose of a corticosteroid disrupts the normal diurnal variation of HPA function. Inhaled agents cause HPA suppression only after prolonged administration of doses in excess of those which are recommended. Intramuscular injections of long-acting agents carry a risk of HPA suppression. Infrequent intra-articular injections are not associated with a significant risk.

Single, small oral AM doses of short acting agents (less than 7.5 mg of prednisone/day) generally do not suppress HPA function. However, prolonged use of daily subphysiologic doses (e.g., prednisone 5 mg/day for a year or more) can cause some changes in HPA responsiveness. Some practitioners provide prophylaxis during surgery for patients who receive long-term, daily, physiologic doses of corticosteroids. **Alternate day therapy** with short-acting agents, given once in the AM every other day, does not cause HPA suppression, even when large alternate day doses are used for years. **ACTH therapy** in general does not suppress HPA function, although some feel these patients should receive prophylaxis. Routine applications of **topical agents** do not present a risk. Long-term applications of fluorinated compounds over large skin areas is occasionally associated with adrenal suppression.

Patients with chronic disorders that wax and wane often receive intermittent high-dose daily therapy, which puts them at uncertain risk for perioperative HPA suppression. The relationship between the duration of therapy and HPA function has been incompletely defined. The higher the daily dose, the longer and more recent the exposure, the more likely suppression will occur. One week of high-dose therapy (20 mg of prednisone daily) produces an abnormal response to ACTH stimulation. Patients treated within a year with high-dose regimens for a week or longer are at some risk of HPA insufficiency. The precise risk is indeterminate. It is relative to the total daily dose, the duration of therapy, and the time interval between surgery and the withdrawal of corticosteroid therapy. Immediately after extended (1 year), high dose (>20mg prednisone/day) corticosteroid therapy withdrawal, the pituitary and adrenal response to stress can be deficient for about 1 month. During the following 2–5 months, patients recover pituitary responsiveness. The adrenal response can require another 1–3 months to fully recover. Most patients recover completely after 9 months, a few take longer. After adrenal surgery for adrenal hyperfunction, the remaining gland frequently requires more than a year to achieve normal HPA responsiveness. Table 13.5 summarizes recommendations for perioperative corticosteroid coverage and management of adrenal issues (54, 55). A precise definition of the smallest doses and the minimum duration of therapy associated with adrenal suppression, and the duration of HPA function suppression after therapy is discontinued, cannot be ascertained from available data.

The **Cortrosyn stimulation test** quickly identifies those with deficient HPA

Table 13.5. Adrenal Insufficiency and Surgery

Symptoms and Signs

Consider acute insufficiency in any at-risk patient with unexplained shock, hypotension, mental changes, fever, abdominal pain, hypoglycemia or failure to thrive.

At risk patients

Risk of hypothalamic/pituitary/adrenal (HPA) suppression is relative to: total daily dose, duration of therapy, time interval between corticosteroid withdrawal and surgery. Consider HPA suppression when patients receive:

— >20 mg of prednisone per day, for one week, within one year.

—7.5–10 mg of prednisone per day, for one month within one year.

—5 mg of prednisone per day for one year or longer.

—recurrent intramuscular or "Depot" therapy within one year.

—all other oral regimens that are taken longer than a week, other than single, AM doses of short-acting corticosteroids.

Test, prophylax, or monitor with care when HPA status is uncertain.

HPA testing

Administer 25 units of Cortrosyn intramuscularly.

Measure baseline, one-half hour, and one-hour serum cortisol.

Axis is adequate if either post injection cortisol is above 20 μg/dl.

Prophylaxis

Major surgery—Give hydrocortisone hemisuccinate, 100 mg intravenous bolus every 6–8 hours for 72 hours. Begin with preoperative medication.

Minor surgery—Provide same regimen for 24 hours.

Minor procedure or stress—Administer hydrocortisone hemisuccinate, 100 mg intramuscularly in a single dose before procedure.

Acute Crisis

Draw serum cortisol, electrolytes, BUN, glucose, creatinine.

Administer hydrocortisone hemisuccinate 100 mg intravenous bolus stat, then every 6–8 hours until stable. Then, taper dose.

Administer 1000 cc 5% dextrose and normal saline in first hour, additional fluids according to clinical parameters.

After tapering intravenous corticosteroids, begin hydrocortisone acetate 25 mg in the AM and 12.5 in the PM. If patient has primary insufficiency, Florinef 0.05 or 0.1 mg is often necessary.

Watch for late hypokalemia, treat with intravenous and oral potassium supplements.

---

function. This is done by obtaining a baseline cortisol level and administering 25 units of synthetic ACTH, (Cortrosyn, cosyntropin) and measuring the serum cortisol at one-half and one hour after injection. A peak level of 20 µg/dl or more (550 mmol/liter) provides a single criteria adequate to exclude adrenal insufficiency. There is a marked interdependence of basal cortisol concentration, peak and increases in the levels of cortisol. Additional testing is necessary to confirm the presence of new insufficiency but retesting with Cortrosyn does not increase test sensitivity or specificity (58).

Knowledge of the **adrenal response to surgery** in normal patients provides guidelines for use of perioperative corticosteroids. Plumpton's and other studies of the response of normal adrenal glands to major surgical stress reveals that normal adrenals will secrete a maximum amount of corticosteroids equivalent to 300–400 mg of hydrocortisone daily on the day of surgery and for the next 48 hours in the immediate postoperative period (59, 60). Secretion then falls sharply and returns toward normal over 24 hours once the immediate stress is over. Elaborate postoperative tapering of corticosteroids is not needed unless stress is protracted by complications.

When in doubt about HPA function, the practitioner has three options: (a) to test HPA function, (b) to withhold steroids and be prepared to provide replacement with the occurrence of any symptoms suggesting adrenal insufficiency, and (c) to provide prophylaxis. The latter simply provides exogenous corticosteroids in lieu of the patient's normal adrenal reponse to surgical stress. For **major surgery,** give 100 mg of hydrocortisone hemisuccinate or phosphate as an intravenous bolus every 6–8 hours, beginning at the time of preoperative medication and continuing for 72 hours. Hydrocortisone hemisuccinate or phosphate is water soluble, and immediately provides adequate physiologic replacement, as well as a simple but entirely effective regimen. For **minor surgery** (herniorraphy), provide 24-hour coverage only (100 mg of intravenous hydrocortisone every 6–8 hours). For **short procedures,** (endoscopy, dental work) give 100 mg of hydrocortisone hemisuccinate intramuscularly prior to the procedure.

Treatment of Acute Adrenal Crisis

Measure the serum cortisol, electrolytes, glucose, BUN and creatinine as therapy is initiated. A serum cortisol value of greater than 22 µg/dL in the presence of severe stress (high fever, hypotension) is consistent with normal adrenal-pituitary responsiveness. Values below this level warrant additional study for adrenal insufficiency. Immediately administer a water-soluble glucocorticoid, hydrocortisone phosphate or hemisuccinate, 100 mg (or 1.5 mg/kg) intravenously and then every 6 hours. Initial fluid therapy for primary insufficiency (cortisol and mineral-corticoids) consists of 1000 ml of 5% dextrose and normal saline over the first hour. Administer high volumes of similar fluids at the same or higher rates until hypotension is reversed. Most primary adrenal insufficiency patients are 20% volume depleted and require 3–4 liters over several hours.

Patients with the more common secondary insufficiency require less vigorous fluid therapy since they retain mineralocorticoid function. They are primarily cortisol deficient. Delerium, fever, and hypotension are due to coritsol deficiency. Hyperkalemia and prerenal azotemia are uncommon. When diarrhea, nausea and vomiting are present, a substantial absolute deficiency in whole body sodium may be present. Continue fluid therapy based on clinical parameters (blood pressure, pulse, etc.). Watch for late hypokalemia during recovery. Add 20–40 meq of potassium to each liter of fluid replacement. Oral supplements can also be prescribed.

Taper corticosteroids over 48 hours or

longer if necessary. Begin 25 mg in the AM and 12.5 mg in the PM of oral cortisone acetate (equivalent of 7.5 mg of Prednisone). Monitor the patient's response and dose adequacy. Most patients with primary insufficiency require mineralocorticoid supplements (Florinef 0.05–0.10 mg daily) when given less than 50 mg of cortisone each day. Upon discharge, prescribe a medic alert tag and an emergency corticosteroid kit (hydrocortisone Mix-o-vial).

SELECTIVE ALDOSTERONE DEFICIENCY

Epidemiology and Pathophysiology

Selective aldosterone deficiency commonly occurs among patients with renal insufficiency (70% of patients) and advanced diabetes mellitus (50%) or among patients using prostaglandin inhibitors or captopril. The identifying characteristic of this relatively infrequent but potentially lethal syndrome is persistent hyperkalemia. **Hyperkalemia, hyperchloremia, and metabolic acidosis** are present in half of the patients. The syndrome is further characterized by low stimulated-renin and plasma aldosterone values with preserved ability to acidify urine in the presence of acidosis, hyperkalemia with low fractional potassium excretion, and decreased ammonium excretion (63).

Three out of four patients are asymptomatic. The remainder present with weakness or arrhythmias. With dehydration, deteriorating renal function, or the use of spironolactone, dangerous hyperkalemia and acidosis can quickly develop.

A similar syndrome, **hyperkalemic distal renal tubular acidosis** is associated with obstructive uropathy, amiloride or hydrochloride therapy, and sickle cell hemoglobinopathy. These patients have impaired distal tubular function and also demonstrate an inability to secrete hydrogen and potassium and lower their urinary pH below 5.5 in the presence of acidosis and hyperkalemia. A **combined syndrome** can be encountered in association with obstructive uropathy or lead nephropathy (66).

Diagnosis

Four criteria must be met to establish the diagnosis: *(a)* eliminate other causes of hyperkalemia and acidosis, *(b)* document a low or low-normal baseline renin and aldosterone levels, *(c)* document a blunted response of renin and aldosterone to stimulation, and *(d)* document the absence of renal tubular acidosis.

Eliminate common causes of hyperkalemia or acidemia with simple observations and tests. Elevated serum potassium due to exogenous intake (diet, salt substitutes, low sodium diets, potassium-sparing diuretics) and endogenous causes of hyperkalemia (gastrointestinal bleeding, hemolysis, catabolic states, crush injuries) are eliminated through the patient interview and physical examination. Pseudohyperkalemia and laboratory error due to in vitro hemolysis, thrombocytosis, or leukocytosis are eliminated by simultaneously measured serum and plasma potassium concentrations, which agree within 0.2 meq/L and a normal peripheral smear. Dehydration and associated diminished sodium delivery to the distal tubules does not account for hyperkalemia unless the urinary sodium secretion has also fallen to 10–20 meq/day. Chronic renal failure alone does not cause hyperkalemia until the glomerular filtration rate is only 10–15 ml/min. Common alternative explanations of acidemia are excluded by measuring serum lactate levels, ketones, electrolytes and arterial blood gas levels when the clinical situation warrants.

The next group of considerations include selective aldosterone deficiency, adrenal insufficiency and hyperkalemic distal renal tubular acidosis. Hyperkalemic, hyperchloremic acidosis occurs in six situations: Addison's disease, renal tubular acidosis, exogenous potassium administration, use of potassium-sparing diuretics and prostaglandin inhibitors, obstructive uropathy and selective aldosterone deficiency. The Cortrosyn stimulation test quickly identifies adrenal insufficient patients; the history eliminates other conditions.

Confirm the presence of **low or low-normal renin and aldosterone** levels in selective aldosterone deficiency with basal serum measurements. After rendering the patient normokalemic, stimulate the plasm renin and aldosterone reponse with volume contraction and again assay the serum levels. The normal serum response (increased levels) will be blunted. Give the patient three 40-mg doses of oral furosemide, one dose each at 6 PM, midnight and 6 AM. Measure serum renin, aldosterone and potassium values at 9 AM. Interpret the patient's values relative to the patient's serum potassium value. Further confirmation of a defect within the adrenal gland can be obtained by infusing ACTH or angiotensin and demonstrating a subnormal response in aldosterone secretion (67; see summary Table 13.6).

Renal tubular dysfunction is suggested by impaired potassium excretion (persistent hyperkalemia) in the presence of a functional renin-aldosterone axis. Demonstrate the **absence of distal renal tubular acidosis** by showing that the patient can decrease the urine pH below 5.5. Give the patient 1 mg of oral fludrocortisone acetate the night before. On the morning of study, infuse 500 ml of a 4% solution of sodium sulfate over 45–60 minutes. Measure the pH of urine samples obtained at 60, 120, 180, and 240 minutes (67).

Treatment of Selective Aldosterone Deficiency

Fludrocortisone acetate (Florinef), 0.1–0.4 mg orally each day corrects hyperkalemia. Many patients are elderly and vulnerable to the complications of sodium and fluid retention. Benefits of therapy

Table 13.6.   Selective Aldosterone Deficiency

Symptoms and Signs
Persistent hyperkalemia, weakness, arrythmias
Diagnosis
Eliminate common causes of hyperkalemia
Low or low-normal baseline serum renin and aldosterone levels
Blunted renin/aldosterone response to furosemide-induced volume contraction
RTA eliminated when patient lowers urinary pH after sodium sulfate infusion following oral fludrocortisone acetate
Treatment
Avoid potassium supplement.
Administer fludrocortisone acetate 0.1 mg to 0.4 mg daily if needed.
Administer potassium wasting diuretics, bicarbonate or potassium-binding resins if needed.

must outweigh risks. Alternative measures include **potassium wasting diuretics,** as well as sodium **bicarbonate** therapy which will help correct the hyperkalemia and acidosis. **Sodium-potassium exchange resins** (sodium polysterene sulfonate) can be used in appropriate situations. Patients with mild hyperkalemia (5.0–5.6 meq/L) often require no therapy. Avoid volume contraction and drugs which impair renal potassium excretion.

PRIMARY HYPERALDOSTERONISM

Epidemiology

In 1955, Conn described a patient with hypertension, hypokalemia, and neuromuscular symptoms who was found to have an aldosterone-producing adenoma of the adrenal cortex (69). Removal of the tumor reverses the clinical and biochemical abnormalities. Since the original description of primary hyperaldosteronism, this disorder has been studied extensively, and presently four subsets of this entity are recognized. Yet, primary hyperaldosteronism is an uncommon cause of hypertension with a prevalence among unselected hypertensives of less than 1%. Despite its rarity, the consulting internist must be familiar with this disorder, for it represents one of the potentially curable forms of hypertension. Effective consultation in this area requires consideration of the following questions: Which patients should be suspect for primary hyperaldosteronism? What are the appropriate screening tests? How should patients be evaluated definitively for this syndrome? And, finally, how should patients with suspected primary hyperaldosteronism be managed during the perioperative period?

Diagnosis

The consultant should consider this entity in all hypertensive patients with spontaneous hypokalemia. The hypertension may be mild, moderate or severe. Symptoms reflect the hypokalemia and include muscle weakness, polyuria, nocturia, paresthesia, tetany, and muscle paralysis. Headache is often a predominant feature. Some patients have no symptoms and may present with an incidental finding of hypokalemia. It should be kept in mind, however, that approximately 20% of patients with primary hyperaldosteronism have serum potassium values >3.5 meq/liter (70). Many of these patients with normokalemia develop problematic hypokalemia when treated with diuretics, which should alert the consultant to a possible hyperaldosterone state. On the other hand, a serum potassium level of 4.0 meq/L or greater (in the absence of potassium supplementation or aldosterone antagonists) makes the diagnosis of hyperaldosteronism extremely unlikely (72).

Once primary hyperaldosteronism is suspected, further laboratory steps are necessary in pursuing this diagnosis. Although the medical literature contains many seemingly different methods designed for the assessment of primary hyperaldosteronism, it is less confusing if one recalls that despite subtle differences among the various protocols, they are all designed to bring out the two biochemical

Table 13.7. Outpatient Screening Method for Primary Hyperaldosteronism*

1. Discontinue all antihypertensive agents 3 weeks prior to evaluation and maintain the patient on a regular diet without sodium restriction.
2. Have the patient report to an appropriate outpatient procedure room at 9:00 AM, having had nothing to eat or drink since 10:00 PM the previous night.
3. Insert a heparin lock and obtain blood for plasma electrolytes.
4. Administer furosemide, 40 mg intravenously, through the heparin lock. The patient remains in bed for 1 hour and is then free to walk about for 2 hours, at the end of which time blood is drawn for measurement of plasma renin activity.
5. The patient is given lunch between 12:00 and 12:30, and 0.9% NaCl (2 L) is infused intravenously (heparin lock) over 3.5–4 hours, with the patient recumbent. When the infusion is complete, at about 4:00 PM, blood is drawn for measurement of plasma aldosterone and the patient discharged.

*As modified from Streeten et al.: Reliability of screening methods for the diagnosis of primary aldosteronism. Am J Med 67:403–413, 1979.

hallmarks of primary hyperaldosteronism. Namely, patients with this disorder fail to increase their plasma renin activity in response to a variety of stimuli (furosemide, Na depletion, upright posture), and they fail to suppress their plasma or urinary aldosterone in response to salt loading or following mineralocorticoid administration. Streeten et al. have described a sensitive and convenient 8-hour outpatient protocol for assessing the plasma renin response to furosemide stimulation and plasma aldosterone response to saline infusion (71). Their protocol is reproduced in Table 13.7. In their experience, further evaluation was indicated if: (a) the plasma aldosterone concentration after saline infusion was above 8.0 ng/ml/hr, or (b) the plasma potassium concentration at 9:00 AM was 3.5 meq/L or below, or (c) the plasma renin activity after naturesis and standing for 2 hours was less than 1.7 ng/ml/hr.

Lyons and colleagues have recently described a simple test utilizing the converting enzyme inhibitor, **captopril** (73). In their protocol, a single 25 mg dose of captopril is administered orally while the patient is in a seated position. Blood samples are obtained just prior to and 2 hrs after the captopril is given for measurement of aldosterone and renin. In their original study, a plasma aldosterone concentration above 15 ng/dl (measured after captopril administration) or aldosterone to renin ratio greater than 50 showed high specificity for the diagnosis of primary hyperaldosteronism. The rationale for this test is based on the assumption that in normotensive or essential hypertensive patients, captopril will decrease angiotensin II and aldosterone production and increase renin release by inhibiting negative feedback. However, in patients with primary hyperaldosteronism, the production of aldosterone is autonomous and thus captopril should have little if any effect on aldosterone secretion or renin production. The captopril test probably needs further evaluation over time before its value is known. The authors emphasize the relative safety, convenience, and low cost of this test compared to those which involve the administration of large volumes of saline.

For the definitive diagnosis, we have found the method of Weinberger to be sensitive and convenient, requiring a 3-day hospitalization (72). An outline of this protocol is given in Table 13.8.

After the biochemical diagnosis of primary hyperaldosteronism has been established, it is of considerable clinical importance to determine which of the two principal forms of primary aldosterone excess is present. Not only is the pathogenesis distinct, but treatment is different: adrenal surgery is indicated for patients with an adrenal tumor, whereas medical therapy with spironolactone is the treatment of choice for bilateral adrenal hyperplasia or idiopathic hyperaldosteronism. In Bravo's study, severe, persistent hypokalemia, increased plasma 18-hydroxycorticosterone values, and an

Table 13.8.   Protocol for Establishing the Biochemical Diagnosis of Primary Aldosteronism*

1. Withdraw antihypertensive agents at least 2 weeks before study. If necessary, attempt to normalize the serum potassium with supplements.
2. Day 1: Draw baseline plasma renin and aldosterone (upright) at 0800 hr, and begin an intravenous saline infusion (0.9%, 2 L/4 hr). Repeat the plasma renin activity and plasma aldosterone (supine) at 1200 hr.
3. Day 2: Maintain the patient on a 10 meq sodium diet, and start furosemide, 40 mg p.o. at 1000, 1400, and 1800 hr.
4. Day 3: After 2 hours of ambulation, repeat the plasma renin activity (upright).

*Adapted from Weinberger *et al.*: Primary aldosteronism—diagnosis, localization, and treatment. *Ann Intern Med* 90:386–395, 1979.

anomalous postural decrease in plasma aldosterone concentration were the best predictors for adenoma (70). Methods to localize the site of an adenoma include selective adrenal vein catheterization for measurement of aldosterone concentration, contrast venography and examination of glands by scintillation scanning, computed tomography, or ultrasound. No single localizing technique is infallible.

Preoperative Management

For the patient who is hypertensive and hypokalemic, and no cause for the hypokalemia is apparent (i.e., diuretics, vomiting, diarrhea, laxative abuse, licorice ingestion, or intestinal fistula), elective surgery should be postponed and further investigation as outlined above should be undertaken. If the patient's surgery cannot be delayed, it is necessary to correct the hypokalemia before induction of anesthesia. It is important to recall that since most of the total body potassium is intracellular, a slightly depressed potassium level may require several hundred milliequivalents to normalize. The patient's blood pressure should also be controlled by conventional means prior to surgery. Unlike patients with pheochromocytoma, undiagnosed primary hyperaldosteronism does not appear to impose excessive perioperative risks as long as the blood pressure is reasonably controlled and the hypokalemia corrected. Abrupt hypotension after removal of the adrenal tumor is unlikely to occur and, in fact, several weeks are often required to demonstrate an antihypertensive effect from the surgery.

Finally, for the hypokalemic, hypertensive patient who has been receiving a diuretic, interpretation of renin and aldosterone levels can be very difficult. Diuretics stimulate both renin and aldosterone release, while hypokalemia tends to inhibit aldosterone release. If the diagnosis of primary hyperaldosteronism is suspect in such a patient, the diuretic should be withdrawn while maintaining the patient on a normal or even high sodium intake. After a period of at least one week, a 24-hour urine sample for measurement of sodium and potassium should be obtained. If the patient remains hypokalemic and the urine has at least 100 meq of sodium and less than 30 meq of potassium, it is most likely that diuretics are the cause of the hypokalemia. However, if the 24-hour urinary potassium is greater than 30 meq and the patient remains hypokalemic, further investigation for primary hyperaldosteronism is indicated as previously discussed (74).

PHEOCHROMOCYTOMA

Over 100 years ago, pathologists recognized that certain tumors of the adrenal medulla developed a characteristic color reaction when exposed to chromium salts. The term "pheochromocytoma" has since been used to describe adrenal tumors that exhibit this reaction. It was soon realized that these tumors were associated with a constellation of symptoms and signs including headache, chest discomfort, palpitations, and hypertension. The first therapeutic surgical resection of such a tumor was performed by Dr.

Charles Mayo in 1927. After seeing the patient for the first time Dr. Mayo wrote, "Toxins are evidently intermittently discharged affecting the sympathetic." Since that time, physicians have become increasingly aware of this disorder with its striking and often dramatic clinical manifestations.

Pheochromocytoma is rare. The incidence is estimated at less than 0.1% of the hypertensive population. Nevertheless, the diagnosis is important since the hypertension is usually curable by surgical removal of the tumor. Furthermore, undetected pheochromocytoma is often fatal. This disease can masquerade as a variety of common disorders. For this reason, the astute clinician will at least consider this disorder in patients labeled with less esoteric diagnoses, such as essential or labile hypertension, anxiety neurosis, thyrotoxicosis, early diabetes mellitus, and functional bowel disease. **However, the characteristic hypertensive crisis is present in only approximately half of all patients with pheochromocytoma.** The majority of patients with pheochromocytoma will be hypertensive almost anytime the blood pressure is taken (76). Common symptoms during a paroxysm include headache, sweating, forceful palpitations, anxiety or fear of impending death, and tremor. Hypermetabolism, a history of weight loss, mild glucose intolerance, and orthostatic hypotension have also been observed in patients with pheochromocytoma.

Diagnosis

The diagnosis of pheochromocytoma is confirmed biochemically by measurement of catecholamines in urine or blood. For most patients, a 12-hour overnight urine collection for catecholamines is sufficient (77). Other studies have argued for the use of plasma catecholamines as the diagnostic test of choice (78, 79). In the study by Bravo et al. (79), the plasma catecholamine assay identified 23 of 24 patients with proved tumors versus 11 of 22 patients detected by the urinary assay. (However, the urinary assay was performed on a 24-hour collection and measured only vanillyl-mandelic acid (VMA) and metanephrines.) It is our practice to obtain a 12-hour overnight urinary collection for measurement of free catecholamines, metanephrines, and VMA. When the above method fails to establish the diagnosis in a patient strongly suspected to have a pheochromocytoma, the **clonidine suppression test** may be useful. This test is based on the ability of clonidine to suppress plasma norepinephrine levels in normals by stimulating central alpha-adrenergic receptors. However, in patients with pheochromocytoma, the release of catecholamines is presumed to be autonomous. Bravo et al. (80) studied 10 patients with surgically proven pheochromocytoma. All 10 patients failed to suppress their plasma norepinephrine after a single oral dose of 0.3 mg of clonidine. By contrast, in each of 15 essential hypertensive patients the plasma norepinephrine was suppressed.

Certain more subtle points in regard to the use and interpretation of these biochemical tests deserve emphasis. First, in those patients who are only hypertensive episodically, it is necessary to obtain urine collections during a period of hypertension, as samples obtained when normotensive might be normal. Secondly, one should know the capability and methodology employed by the laboratory. Some laboratories do not provide separate measurements of epinephrine and norepinephrine. Lastly, many laboratories are using newer, highly sensitive methods for determining catecholamines. The current state of the art appears to be the high pressure liquid chromatography system, which has eliminated many of the false-positive results due to certain drug interferences. With the newer methodologies, restrictions of diet and pharmacologic agents (with the exception of methyldopa) are unnecessary.

Preoperative Management

The preoperative and perioperative management of the patient with pheochromocytoma requires the coordinated expertise of the medical consultant, anesthesiolgist, and surgeon (Table 13.9). All patients undergoing exploratory surgery for a pheochromocytoma or needing urgent, unrelated surgery when a pheochromocytoma is present should be pretreated with adrenergic blocking agents. The alpha-blocking agents, phentolamine (Regitine), and phenoxybenzamine (Dibenzyline) are available for this purpose and each has a role in management. Phentolamine has a rapid onset and short duration of action. Although it is active orally, its major use is as an intravenous agent in the management of hypertensive crises. It is particularly useful intraoperatively for this purpose, since manipulation of the tumor by the surgeon can trigger catecholamine release and excessive rises in blood pressure. Phenoxybenzamine, on the other hand, has a long duration of action (perhaps 3–4 days) and is most useful as an oral agent in the management of surgically nonresectable met-

Table 13.9.   Pheochromocytoma

Clinical manifestations
   Hypertension, headache, chest pain, palpitations
Diagnosis
   12-hour overnight urinary catecholamines
   Occasionally, plasma catecholamines and clonidine suppression test may be helpful.
Management
   Preoperative
      Alpha-blocking agents—phenoxybenzamine
      Beta-blocking agents—propranolol (after alpha block)
      Tyrosine hydroxylase—alpha-methyl-p-tyrosine inhibitor
   Intraoperative emergencies
      Hypertensive crises—nitroprusside or phentolamine
      Arrhythmias—propranolol
   Postoperative
      Replace volume for hypotension.
      Repeat catecholamines for persistent hypertension.

astatic pheochromocytomas and in the preparation of patients for surgery. It is customary to pretreat the patient for several days with phenoxybenzamine up to the morning of surgery, reserving phentolamine for use intraoperatively. Phenoxybenzamine need only be give once daily. A dose of 40–60 mg per day is sufficient in most patients to achieve reasonable blood pressure control. The appearance of orthostatic hypotension and tachycardia suggest overdosage.

Propranolol, a beta-blocking agent, is particularly useful for the control of tachycardia, and intravenous propranolol is of great utility intraoperatively for the treatment of serious multiple tachyarrhythmias. The drug should not be administered until alpha-blockade is established in order to avoid a paradoxical rise in blood pressure mediated by unopposed alpha vasoconstricting effects. Low doses (1–2 mg intravenously) are oftentimes effective in abolishing these arrhythmias during surgery. Propranolol, as well as other beta-blocking agents, should be used with caution, however, since a significant proportion of these patients appear to have an occult (if not overt) catecholamine-induced cardiomyopathy, and beta-blockade could precipitate congestive heart failure.

Another approach, which is now available for the preoperative treatment of patients with pheochromocytoma, is the administration of **alpha-methyl-p-tyrosine** (Demser), which inhibits the enzyme, tyrosine hydroxylase, and results in a powerful inhibition of catecholamine synthesis. Oral doses of from 1–4 grams daily will produce a 50–80% inhibition of catecholamine synthesis as assessed by reduction in the urinary excretion of catecholamines and their metabolites. Usually 7–10 days of treatment are required for preoperative preparation. Side effects include sleepiness, diarrhea, and crystalluria. The overall effectiveness of the drug can be assessed by assaying urinary VMA frequently.

As mentioned above, preoperative pharmacologic preparation usually requires 5–10 days for the majority of patients with pheochromocytoma. However, prolonged medical therapy is often necessary for the post-myocardial infarct patient or women in their last trimester of pregnancy. The latter can be maintained on one of the above regimens until the infant is delivered, at which time surgical intervention can be undertaken.

In the past, surgery in patients with pheochromocytoma had been associated with a high mortality, but with thoughtful anticipation and prophylaxis, surgical morbidity and mortality has been significantly reduced. Hypertensive crises and the precipitation of arrhythmias are likely to occur during induction of anesthesia, intubation, and during surgical manipulation of the tumor. Phentolamine used to be the agent of choice for hypertensive crisis but nitroprusside has become more popular for the control of intraoperative hypertension (81). Prior to induction, intravenous and intra-arterial lines should be placed and electrocardiographic monitors connected. Intravenous phentolamine and propranolol should be readily available. In addition, the appropriate electrical equipment must be present for the treatment of cardiac arrhythmias resistant to pharmacologic intervention.

The choice of anesthetic agent is of extreme importance in patients undergoing surgery for pheochromocytoma. Previous experience has indicated that cyclopropane is contraindicated in these individuals, since it enhances the arrhythmic potential of catecholamines. More recently, the halogenated hydrocarbon anesthetics (halothane, ethrane, methoxyfluorane) have been used successfully. Although halothane can also enhance the arrhythmic activity of catecholamines, its well-recognized property of depressing sympathoadrenal activity, coupled with its ease of administration, relatively rapid induction, and recovery argue for its use in pheochromocytoma.

Following surgical extirpation of the tumor, the patient is likely to rapidly become hypotensive. **Volume replacement** is the preferred method of treatment. Because this problem occurs so predictably, some have recommended that the patient's intravascular volume be rendered euvolemic or even overexpanded with preoperative volume-expanding fluids, assuming that there are no contraindications such as congestive heart failure.

Although it is not uncommon for a patient to **continue to experience hypertensive episodes** during the first postoperative day, when the hypertension persists beyond this point, a number of etiologic possibilities should be considered. The possibility of residual or metastatic pheochromocytomas existing is suggested if the patient continues to exhibit a dramatic blood pressure lowering effect from intravenous phentolamine. To confirm this possibility, repeat urine collections for catecholamines must be obtained, but their collection should be delayed until at least the 4th or 5th postoperative day to avoid "false-positive" stress-related elevations. Overzealous preoperative volume expansion is another cause for postoperative hypertension in these patients. This possibility is suggested if the patient has a dramatic diuresis and blood pressure lowering effect from intravenous furosemide. Lastly, the inadvertent ligation of a renal artery (or branch) during surgery may cause the hypertension. This diagnostic possibility is best evaluated in the postoperative period by noninvasive nuclear renal scanning techniques or angiography. Diagnostic and management points are summarized in Table 13.9.

INAPPROPRIATE ANTIDIURETIC HORMONE SECRETION

Epidemiology and Pathophysiology

Hyponatremia is a common disorder of hospitalized patients. It occurs among 1–4% of hospitalized patients and is often associated with a poor prognosis. Nonosmotic secretion of vaopressin or "reset osmoreceptors" contribute to the hyponatremia of patients with heart failure, fatal postoperative fluid overload with unanticipated inappropriate ADH secretion, psychogenic water intoxication and other common causes of hyponatremia (85–88). SIADH is frequently associated with **six categories of clinical conditions** (Table 13.10): malignancies, central nervous system disorders, pulmonary diseases, metabolic and endocrine disorders, drugs and miscellaneous causes. The most common causes in surgical patients are drugs, mechanical ventilation, lung tumors and pneumonitis. Among neurosurgical patients, subarachnoid hemorrhages, skull fracture and brain tumors are common causes.

One of three physiologic mechanisms usually plays an important role in the development of this syndrome: *(a)* excess production of ADH or an ADH-like substance by non-hypothalamic tissues (oat cell carcinoma), *(b)* excess production and/or release of ADH by the central nervous system (skull fracture), and *(c)* potentia-

Table 13.10. Disorders Associated with SIADH

Malignancy: Adenocarcinoma and oat cell carcinoma of lung, pancreatic and duodenal carcinoma, thymoma
Central nervous system: Aneurysm, cerebrovascular disorders, herpes simplex encephalitis, Guillain-Barre, malformations, paroxysmal cerebral dysrhythmia, subarachnoid hemorrhage, trauma, tuberculosis, tumor
Pulmonary: Aspergillosis with cavitation, chronic lung infection, pneumonia, tuberculosis
Metabolic and endocrine: Myxedema, porphyria
Miscellaneous: Idiopathic, postcommissurotomy dilutional syndrome, postoperative states (pain, stress), prolonged mechanical ventilation
Drugs: Antineoplastics—vincristine, cyclophosphamide, others; diuretics—thiazides; Hypoglycemics—chlorpropamide, tolbutamide, phenformin; Tranquilizers—amitriptyline, barbiturates, carbamazepine, fluphenazine, thiothixene, thioridazine; Miscellaneous—acetaminophen, clofibrate, isoproterenol, morphine

tion of ADH effect on renal tubules (chlorpropamide).

Hyponatremia is usually the first manifestation but clinical symptoms correlate only roughly with serum sodium levels. Symptoms and signs are relatively unlikely to occur until the patient develops a serum sodium value of 120–125 meq/L. Hyponatremia produces progressive mental confusion, lethargy, headache, nausea, vomiting, and anorexia. Experimental evidence suggests that early cerebral edema has developed at these serum sodium levels. As the serum sodium falls to 110 meq/L or less, more severe symptoms and signs are likely: seizures, decreased or absent deep tendon reflexes, bilateral lower extremity clonus, Babinski signs, bulbar and pseudobulbar palsy, muscle weakness, hyperventilation, coma, and death. More severe symptoms develop at higher sodium levels when hyponatremia develops rapidly (89).

Diagnostic Tests

Confirm the diagnosis of SIADH by demonstrating that the patient's **urine is less than maximally dilute** (>200 mOsm) in the presence of **hypotonic serum** (<290 mOsm). The urinary sodium concentration is usually greater than 20 meq/L. Other conditions associated with hyponatremia, such as congestive heart failure, renal disease, cirrhosis, adrenal insufficiency, and hypothyroidism should be excluded before making a diagnosis of SIADH. Importantly, the water loading test does not distinguish adrenal insufficiency from SIADH.

The **water loading test** clarifies the occasional confusing clinical picture. Before testing, the patient's sodium must be maintained at 125 meq/L. Give the patient a water load of 20 ml/kg over 20 minutes. Collect hourly urine samples for the next 5 hours with the patient remaining recumbent. Measure the osmolality and volume of samples. Normal patients excrete 80% of this load by the 5th hour,

and the urinary osmolality will fall to less than 100 mOsm/kg (specific gravity, approximately 1.005). Patients with SIADH excrete less than 40% of the water load at 5 hours and fail to dilute the urine to hypotonic levels. Post-test fluid restrictions for 24 hours may be essential to avoid water intoxication of SIADH patients.

Treatment

Therapy consists of **fluid restriction** (500–1000 cc daily) for all patients. Fluid restriction effectively treats asymptomatic and mildly symptomatic patients with serum sodium levels of >120 meq/L. Some patients require hypertonic saline, diuretics, and demethylchlortetracycline. Symptomatic patients with serum sodium values lower than 120 meq/L require oral fluid restriction and 3–5% hypertonic saline infusions at 70–100 meq of sodium per hour. Large quantities of sodium are promptly excreted, as is potassium. Therefore, this measure is only transiently effective. The addition of intravenous furosemide to induce a diuresis and measurement of urinary sodium and potassium losses to guide electrolyte replacement can enhance the precision of therapy. Measure serum sodium and potassium levels hourly during acute, intensive therapy. Osmotic diuretics (mannitol, glycerol) have been effective in a few reported cases, but their use has not yet become widespread.

Demethylchlortetracycline (300 mg b.i.d. to q.i.d.) is the drug of choice for chronic therapy but it takes 5–14 days to be effective. The drug interferes with the action of ADH on renal tubules, and the effect lasts several days after drug withdrawal. A mixed syndrome of SIADH and mineralocorticoid deficiency has been reported among geriatric patients suffering severe head trauma. These patients respond to oral fludrocortisone acetate, 0.1–0.4 mg/d. The tendency to hyponatremia may persist several months after trauma.

DIABETES INSIPIDUS

Overview

Diabetes insipidus is encountered most commonly on surgical services among patients with brain tumors, following pituitary surgery, and after massive facial trauma. Occasionally, it occurs after major chest wounds with hypotension, hypoxic encephalopathy, drug overdose, brain death or profound coma. Hypernatremia and a 4–6 liter diuresis suggest possible diabetes insipidus.

Pathophysiology

Supraoptic and paraventricular nuclei control **vasopressin** release in response to osmoreceptor and other stimuli transmitted to the hypothalamus over the vagus nerves from volume receptors in the left atrium, carotids, and aorta. Pain, stress, emotions and drugs can enhance vasopressin release. Vasopressin (ADH) activates cyclic AMP of medullary nephron cells, which allow increased volumes of water to pass through the cells from renal tubules into the circulation, conserving body water and concentrating urine. In the presence of inadequate vasopressin or unresponsive kidneys (nephrogenic diabetes insipidus) polyuria, thirst, dehydration, and polydypsia follow. Stupor, coma, and associated surgical and medical problems often complicate the clinical picture.

Postoperative diabetes insipidus is a dynamic process that changes over hours to days. Twelve to 24 hours after trauma, cerebral edema develops and becomes most pronounced at 48–72 hours. Vasopressin deficiency and or excess frequently occurs during this period. The extent of CNS damage determines which of **four common patterns** dominate the clinical picture (95, 96). Most commonly, cerebral edema induces a transient polyuria that begins 1–3 days postoperatively and persists for about 1 week. When hypothalamic-pituitary structures are severely disrupted, polyuria begins about 1–2 days postoperatively, and over the ensuing week, normal urinary output returns for a day to several days. This is followed by persistent abnormally high urine outputs. Transient return of function probably represents utilization of existing vasopressin stores.

A third pattern is associated with a partial defect that is aggravated by cerebral edema. Polyuria develops 2–3 days after surgery, followed by a small decrease in urine volumes over several days. Finally, patients with profound damage exhibit immediate and permanent polyuria. Long-term prognosis is uncertain since a few patients regain function several months into recovery.

Diagnosis of Diabetes Insipidus

Use bedside observations and basic laboratory studies to distinguish the diuresis due to diabetes insipidus from a diuresis due to other causes. A postoperative diuresis is frequently due to one of three causes: (a) iatrogenic fluid overload, (b) solute excretion due to hyperglycemia, elevated urea levels or osmotic diuretics (e.g., mannitol) administered during neurosurgery, and (c) diabetes insipidus. Adrenal insufficiency, acute renal failure, postobstruction diuresis, hypercalcemia, hypokalemia and drugs (methoxyflurane, enflurane, narcotic antagonists) also induce a postoperative diuresis.

Clarify the nature of the diuresis by developing a comprehensive fluid and electrolyte flow sheet which records: perioperative weights, daily fluid and electrolyte input, fluid outputs, estimated insensible losses, daily fluid balance, serum electrolyte, glucose, calcium, BUN, and creatinine values, urine volumes, electrolytes, osmolity and specific gravity. Many of the causes of a diuresis listed above will be quickly identified.

The **diagnosis of diabetes insipidus** is confirmed by documenting a diuresis (output exceeds input by more than 2 liters) with a low specific gravity, and by measuring several simultaneous serum and urine osmolalities. In the absence of ADH, urine osmolality is inappropriately low in the presence of normal or increased serum osmolalities. Serum osmolality is conveniently estimated within 5% from the formula:

$$2 \times (Na + K \ meq/L) + \frac{blood \ glucose \ (mg/dl)}{18}$$
$$+ \frac{BUN \ (mg/dl)}{2.8}$$
$$= Serum \ Osmolality \ (mOsm)$$

Patients with **severe diabetes insipidus** exhibit a large volume diuresis (2–10 liters daily), characterized by a low urine specific gravity (1.001 to 1.005) and osmolality (50–200 mOsm/kg), normal or slightly increased serum sodium values (if the patient is drinking normally), and prominent complaints of thirst. Severe hypernatremia occurs among comatose or stuporous patients. The urine of patients diuresing from **iatrogenic fluid overload** is characterized by a low osmolality and high volume in the presence of a low plasma osmolality. A solute-induced diuresis is characterized by urine specific gravities between 1.009 and 1.035, urine osmolalities between 250 and 350 mOsm/kg of urine, and low or near normal serum sodium values. Occasionally, **mild diabetes insipidus** is associated with urine osmolality values of 290–600 mOsm/kg, since incomplete loss of ADH permits significant renal concentration. Patients with **unrecognized severe diabetes insipidus** who develop profound dehydration can concentrate their urine to a specific gravity of 1.010 or slightly greater and to 300 mOsm/kg of urine through compensatory renal mechanisms.

The **water deprivation test** with **pitressin administration** confirms the diagnosis (98). Begin by weighing the patient, recording blood pressure, pulse and urinary osmolality. For patients with a large volume diuresis (6–10 L/day), begin fluid restriction at 6 AM and hourly measurements of urinary osmolalities within 3 hours. For patients with a low volume diuresis, begin fluid restriction at midnight and hourly urine osmolality measurements should be underway by midmorning. Continue restriction and hourly measurements until three consecutive hourly urine samples reveal osmolalities that increase less than 30 mOsm/kg between hourly measurements. Once stable urine osmolalities are obtained, measure the serum osmolality to confirm adequate dehydration (serum osmolality of 288 mOsm/kg or more). Then give 5 units of aqueous pitressin subcutaneously and measure the patient's urine osmolality one-half hour after administration. Patients often lose 1–2 kilograms. Do not permit any patient to lose more than 5% of his baseline body weight. Stop the test if clinical evidence of volume depletion evolves.

Normal patients will reduce their urine flow to 0.5ml/min and increase their urine osmolality to 800 mOsm/kg (S.G. of approximately 1.020) if sufficiently water deprived. Normal patients do not increase their urine osmolality by more than 9% after pitressin. **Patients with diabetes insipidus** rarely achieve urine osmolalities of greater than 200 mOsm/kg (S.G. of 1.001–1.005) before stabilizing. With central diabetes insipidus, patients increase the urine osmolality at least 9% after subcutaneous pitressin. Chronically **fluid overloaded patients,** such as compulsive water drinkers, require prolonged periods of fluid restriction before a serum osmolality of 288 mOsm/kg or greater is achieved or a plateau in urine osmolality occurs. Moreover, these patients and those with severe debilitating diseases can suffer from a reduced renal medullary osmotic gradient. They often fail to increase their urine osmolality to 9% after vasopressin injection. **Nephrogenic diabetes insipidus patients,** those with **chronic hypokalemia** and **renal dis-**

ease alter their urinary and serum osmolalities little after dehydration and pitressin injection.

Treatment of Diabetes Insipidus

Monitor reliable parameters of fluid status. For a large volume diuresis measure urine output every 1–2 hours. Measure the output of other patients every 4–6 hours. Check the standing blood pressure and pulse of ambulatory patients every 6 hours and weigh daily to confirm the accuracy of input and output records.

Initial **fluid therapy** should consist of water or intravenous 5% D&W. Measured output should be equaled by input. Measure the serum sodium by hypernatremic patients every 6 hours until the patient's water deficit is corrected. If the serum sodium reaches 165 meq/dl the patient is at risk for permanent brain damage. Patients with this degree of water deficit need prompt intravenous therapy with 5% D&W. They will require some sodium replacement since obligatory sodium losses have occurred in this situation. (See Table 13.11 for a summary.)

Give **aqueous pitressin** (5–10 units) subcutaneously and monitor the patient's response. The short duration of action (4–6 hours) helps avoid water intoxication.

Table 13.11. Diabetes Insipidus

Symptoms and Signs
  Primarily brain trauma or surgery patients.
  Unexplained diuresis (output 2 liters > input).
  Serum sodium of 165 meq/L—urgent care required.
Diagnosis
  Low specific gravity diuresis (S.G. 1.001–1.005).
  Inappropriately low urine osmolality (50–200 mOsm/Kg) in the presence of a high serum osmolality.
  Positive water deprivation test with pitressin.
Treatment
  5% D&W (+ saline if severe dehydration is present).
  Aqueous pitressin 5 U sc, monitor response.
  Desmopressin 0.1–0.4 nasal insufflation b.i.d.

Give additional doses when two consecutive, high volume urine samples (>200 cc/hour) are obtained. The patient's dose requirements can change rapidly over several hours. Do not use longer acting agents until after several days of stable doses. An occasional patient will respond inadequately to subcutaneous therapy but will achieve a full response with a pitressin infusion (1 unit/hour).

Desmopressin (DDAVP), a synthetic vasopressin, is the long-term drug of choice. Twice daily intranasal insufflations (0.1 to 0.4 ml or 10 to 40 μg) are effective. Patients first learn to use the rhinyl catheter by insufflating saline and then test doses of 50, 100 and 200 μl are administered. A diuresis of 4 ml/min indicates a need for additional doses. Alternatively, control nocturia first with a 0.1 ml insufflation and then titrate higher doses according to the patient's needs. Headaches, slight increases in blood pressure and occasionally abdominal cramps complicate therapy.

Pitressin tannate in oil injections may be effective for 24–48 hours but can cause sterile abscesses and injection site discomfort. **Lysine vasopressin nasal spray** (Lypressin) must be insuflated 2–4 times daily and occasionally causes allergic and hypersensitivity reactions. Extended use may lead to a refractory state. A few patients with very mild insufficiency can be managed with oral **chlorpropamide** (Diabinese) 250–500 mg daily, which potentiates endogenous vasopressin effect on renal tubules.

PITUITARY INSUFFICIENCY

Epidemiology of Panhypopituitarism on Surgical Services

Acute panhypopituitarism on surgical services usually follows severe head trauma or pituitary apoplexy during anticoagulation or radiation therapy for pituitary tumors. Occasionally, surgical patients present with established pan-hypopituitarism or a patient will undergo pituitary ablation for diabetic retinopathy, breast carcinoma, or pituitary tumors. Spontaneous panhypopituitarism or pituitary apoplexy are uncommon.

Clinical Manifestations

Autopsies of as many as 40–50% of the patients who die of head trauma reveal hemorrhage and ischemic lesions of the pituitary. Yet, clinical panhypopituitarism is rare. The site and severity of hypothalamic-pituitary damage governs the clinical manifestations. Spontaneous panhypopituitarism and associated diabetes insipidus vary from obvious to extremely subtle. Some patients develop subtle clinical panhypopituitarism immediately after trauma, or limited dysfunction manifested as transient hypogonadism and hypothyroidism. Weeks or years can pass before the diagnosis is established. Others develop immediately obvious dysfunction within a short period after trauma and then gradually recover function over several years.

Pituitary dysfunction may be heralded by slowly progressive **stupor, easy fatigue, somnolence, cold intolerance, hypotension, hyponatremia, and coarse, dry skin** over several weeks. Any of the clinical manifestations of hypothyroidism or secondary adrenal insufficiency may be prominent while other signs and symptoms of panhypopituitarism are absent. The diagnosis is often suggested by a laboratory test, such as low T_4, or a decreased response to Cortrosyn stimulation. Primary insufficiency is confirmed by demonstrating a lack of growth hormone release following hypoglycemic stimulation, a failure of TSH release after TRF infusion, and abnormalities in prolactin, FSH, and LH secretion. The clinical manifestations of diabetes insipidus provide additional supportive evidence of pituitary dysfunction.

Pituitary Apoplexy

The acute onset of severe headache, meningismus, changes in vision, extraocular muscle dysfunction, syncope, and adrenal insufficiency heralds the onset of pituitary apoplexy among patients with functioning or nonfunctioning pituitary tumors. The syndrome is also encountered after head trauma, anticoagulation therapy, and radiation therapy for intracranial tumors. Rarely, symptoms evolve slowly, giving rise to more subtle and gradual clinical changes. The syndrome can cause acute deterioration of vision, which requires prompt surgical intervention to save the patient's sight. Cerebrospinal fluid analysis provides helpful information and usually reveals blood in the fluid.

Management of Hypopituitary Patients

Pituitary dysfunction includes a spectrum of hormonal deficiencies, ranging from isolated, single deficiencies to clinically dramatic panhypopituitarism. Management requires definition of the cause and extent of pituitary dysfunction.

ACTH deficiency may result in clinical symptoms within 36 hours of surgery. Some patients survive the acute stress of surgery and remain compensated for prolonged periods of time. When the status of adrenal function is unknown, provide substitution therapy prior to stressful diagnostic procedures. Anticipate postoperative loss of ACTH function after pituitary ablation and provide preoperative substitution therapy. Tumor surgery and other forms of surgery may involve brain dissection, which produces brain edema. Dexamethasone, which decreases CNS edema, can be given in 4-mg doses every 6 hours intravenously, and then tapered rapidly over 5–7 days. The discomfort related to pituitary surgery persists over 5–7 days, extending the period of perioperative stress and the need for stress level replacement therapy. Upon discharge, give the patient a preassembled syringe of dexamethasone (4 mg/ml) or hydrocortisone phosphate or hemisuccinate, 100 mg (Solu Cortef Mix-O-Vial) for use in the event of an acute crisis. Adequate daily adrenal replacement consists of oral cortisone acetate 25 mg in the AM and 12.5 mg in the PM or 7.5 mg of prednisone daily. Post-pituitary ablation or brain surgery-associated transient or permanent **diabetes insipidus** is managed as per recommendations in a previous section.

Thyroid insufficiency follows ablative surgery or severe head trauma but requires at least 8–10 days before early symptoms evolve. Adrenal replacement therapy must be given prior to thyroid replacement to avoid precipitating an adrenal crisis. Adequate replacement consists of Thyroxine (Synthroid, 0.1–0.2 mg/day orally), and therapy can be delayed a week or longer. Preoperative replacement is required only for patients who are hypothyroid prior to surgery.

The **insulin requirements of diabetic patients** decrease dramatically after ablative therapy. Monitor the blood glucose frequently and prepare for downward adjustments in dose of about 50%. Regular insulin is more effective than longer acting insulin during this period of changing needs.

Gonadotropin deficiencies may be covered in several ways. Testosterone deficiency may be treated after discharge from the hospital by injectable repository testosterone (testosterone enanthate or testosterone cypionate) in doses of 200 mg intramuscularly every 2–3 weeks, depending on the patient's response. Cyclic administration of female corticosteroids induces menstruation. Daily oral conjugated estrogens (0.625–1.25 mg of premarin or ethynil estradiol in 20 or 50 μg tablets) on days 1 through 25 of each cycle can be used in conjunction with 5–10 mg of medroxyprogesterone acetate on days 21 through 25.

HYPERPARATHYROIDISM AND HYPERCALCEMIA

Epidemiology

Primary hyperparathyroidism was once considered a rare disease characterized by bone disease and renal calculi. With the introduction of automated laboratory facilities, many more cases of previously unrecognized asymptomatic hyperparathyroidism have come to clinical attention. It is currently estimated that 2 patients per 1000 in a clinic or hospital population will have primary hyperparathyroidism (104, 105). Thus, primary hyperparathyroidism is now a relatively common problem seen routinely in both the inpatient and outpatient setting.

Diagnosis

The hallmark of hyperparathyroidism is hypercalcemia. The diagnosis most often comes to clinical attention by the detection of an asymptomatic elevation of serum calcium. Patients who are symptomatic generally present with renal colic; less often, patients may complain of fatigue, debility, weight loss, and anemia. About 40–50% of patients with primary hyperparathyroidism have a depressed serum phosphate concentration. The diagnosis is most often confirmed with an increase in the serum concentration of parathyroid hormone. However, the finding of an increased parathyroid hormone concentration must be interpreted in conjunction with the serum calcium level and renal function. The consultant must keep in mind the many other pathologic conditions associated with hypercalcemia including malignancy, multiple myeloma, hyperthyroidism, sarcoidosis, vitamin D intoxication, Paget's disease, and Addisonian crisis.

Management

Parathyroidectomy is the treatment of choice for the patient with hyperparathyroidism and established bone or renal disease. Medical management is usually reserved for patients who have coexisting medical problems that make neck operation a substantial risk or for those who have other diseases that portend a grim prognosis (106). The indications for surgical intervention are less clear in the asymptomatic patient with hyperparathyroidism. Proponents for surgery in the asymptomatic patient argue the high success rate and low morbidity rate of parathyroidectomy. On the other hand, because the natural course of uncomplicated hyperparathyroidism is probably benign (107), others advocate careful, regular observation combined with general and specific therapeutic measures such as estrogen in postmenopausal women (108). Definitive recommendations about the asymptomatic patient with hyperparathyroidism await a prospective comparison trial of surgical versus medical management.

For the patient undergoing parathyroidectomy, careful observation is essential. The serum concentrations of calcium and phosphorus should be obtained daily. The consultant must be aware of the transient hypocalcemia, which usually occurs on postoperative day three or four. As long as the serum calcium concentration does not drop below 7 mg/dl and the patient's symptoms are mild, supplemental calcium is probably not indicated. The serum calcium usually returns to normal within 1 week's time. If symptoms become severe (muscle cramping, numbness, twitching) or the hypocalcemia persists, intermittent intravenous calcium should be given (i.e., 10 ml of a calcium gluconate solution over 5–10 minutes). Occasionally, oral calcium and vitamin D are necessary for the patient with persistent hypocalcemia.

Hypercalcemia in the Surgical Patient

From time to time, the internist may be asked to see a patient scheduled for elective surgery who is found to have hypercalcemia on routine preoperative testing. The consultant must address the following questions: What is the etiology of the hypercalcemia? What are the implications for patient management? What risk does hypercalcemia impose on the surgical patient?

The differential diagnosis of hypercalcemia is discussed above. In most cases, the history and physical exam, routine laboratory testing, chest x-ray, and renal ultrasonography will reveal the cause of the hypercalcemia. Careful attention to the breast exam in women and prostrate exam in men is essential. If a malignancy is uncovered or strongly suspected, it may be prudent to postpone or cancel elective surgery until the patient's overall prognosis is better defined and the impact of this diagnosis on the surgical condition is considered.

Moderate hypercalcemia (i.e., calcium <12 mg/dl) poses no special perioperative management problems for the patient with normal renal and cardiovascular function. Because hypercalcemia can lead to hypovolemia, restoration of normal intravascular fluid and electrolyte status is a must. The EKG should be examined for signs of hypercalcemia (i.e., short PR and QT interval). For the patient with more **marked degrees of hypercalcemia (i.e., calcium >12–13 mg/dl) or with symptomatic hypercalcemia, surgery should be postponed** until the serum calcium is lowered by the methods outlined in Chapter 11.

READINGS

Diabetes Mellitus

1. Rossini AA: Why control blood glucose levels? *Arch Surg* 11:229–232, 1976.
2. Murry JF: Wound healing with diabetes mellitus. *Surg Clin North Am* 64:769–777, 1984.
3. Rifkin H (ed): The physician's guide to type II diabetes (NIDDM): Diagnosis and management. New York, American Diabetes Association, 1984.
4. Crapo PA: Simple versus complex carbohydrate use in the diabetic diet. *Ann Rev Nutr* 5:95–114, 1985.
5. Franz MJ: Diabetes and exercise: Guidelines

for safe and enjoyable activity. International Diabetes Center, Minneapolis, Mn. 1986.

6. Struthers AD: The choice of antihypertensive therapy in the diabetic patient. *Postgrad Med* 61; 563–569, 1985.

7. Delbridge L, Ctercteko G, Fowler C, et al.: The aetiology of diabetic neuropathic ulceration of the foot. *Br J Surg* 72:1–6, 1985.

8. Brand PW: The diabetic foot. In Ellenberg, M, Rifkin, H, *Diabetes Mellitus Theory and Practice,* New Hyde Park, NY. Medical Examiner Publications Co., Inc., 1983.

9. Page MM, Watkins PJ: Cardiorespiratory arrest and diabetic autonomic neuropathy. *Lancet* 1:14–16, 1978.

10. Larkin JG, Fier BM, Ireland JT: Diabetes mellitus and infection. *Postgrad Med J* 61:233–237, 1985.

11. Bergman M, Felig P: Self-monitoring of blood glucose levels in diabetes. *Arch Intern Med* 44:2029–2034, 1984.

12. Gerich JE: Sulfonylureas in the treatment of diabetes mellitus—1985. *Mayo Clin Proc* 60:439–443, 1985.

13. Podolsky S: Management of diabetes in the surgical patient. *Med Clin North Am* 66:1361–1372, 1982.

14. Meyer EJ, Lorenzi L, Bohannon NV, et al.: Diabetic management by insulin infusion during major surgery. *Am J Surg* 137:323–327, 1979.

15. Kitabchi AE, Ayyagari V, Guerra SMO: The efficacy of low-dose versus conventional therapy of insulin for the treatment of diabetic ketoacidosis. *Ann Intern Med* 84:633–638, 1976.

16. Knight AH, Williams DN, Ellis G, et al.: Significance of hyperamylasemia and abdominal pain in diabetic ketoacidosis. *Br Med J* 3:128–131, 1973.

17. Campbell IW, Duncan LJP, Innes JA, et al.: Abdominal pain in diabetic metabolic decompensation. Clinical significance. *JAMA* 233:166–168, 1975.

18. Levine RI, Glauser FL, Berk JE: Enhancement of the amylase-creatinine clearance ratio in disorders other than acute pancreatitis. *N Engl J Med* 292:329–332, 1975.

19. Munro JF, Campbell IW, McCuish AC, et al.: Euglycemic diabetic ketoacidosis. *Br Med J* 2:578–580, 1973.

20. Felig P: Insulin: Rates and routes of delivery. *N Engl J Med* 291:1031–1032, 1974.

21. Fisher JS, Kitabchi AE: A randomized study of phosphate therapy in the treatment of diabetic ketoacidosis. *J Clin Endocr and Metab* 57:177–180, 1982.

22. Morris LR, Murphy MB, Abbas EK: Bicarbonate therapy in severe diabetic ketoacidosis. *Ann Int Med* 105:836–840, 1986.

23. Young E, Bradley RF: Cerebral edema with irreversible coma in severe diabetic ketoacidosis. *N Engl J Med* 276:665–669, 1967.

24. Brenner WI, Lansky Z, Engelman RM, et al.: Hyperosmolar coma in surgical patients: An iatrogenic disease of increasing incidence. *Ann Surg* 178:651–654, 1973.

Hyperthyroidism

25. McArthur JW, Rawson RW, Means JH, et al.: Thyrotoxic crisis. *JAMA* 134:868–874, 1947.

26. Ronnov V, Kirkegaard C: Hyperthyroidism—A disease of old age? *Br Med J* 1:41, 1973.

27. Stiel JN, Hales IB, Reeve TS: Thyrotoxicosis in an elderly population. *Med J Aust* 2:986, 1972.

28. Davis PJ, Davis FB: Hyperthyroidism in patients over the age of 60 years. *Medicine* 53:161, 1974.

29. Cooper DS: Which anti-thyroid drug? *Am J Med* 80:1165, 1986.

30. Feed CM, Sawers JS, Irvine WJ, et al.: Combination of potassium iodide and propranolol in preparation of patients with Graves' disease for thyroid surgery. *N Engl J Med* 302:883–885, 1980.

31. Mackin JF, Canary JJ, Pittman CS: Thyroid storm and its management. *N Engl J Med* 291:1396–1398, 1974.

32. Thomas FB, Mazzaferri EL, Skillman TG: Apathetic thyrotoxicosis: A distinctive clinical and laboratory entity. *Ann Intern Med* 72:679–685, 1970.

33. Zonszein J, Santangelo RP, Macken JF, et al.: Propranolol therapy in thyrotoxicosis. *Am J Med* 66:411–416, 1979.

34. Nilsson OR, Karlberg BE, Kagedal B, et al.: Non-selective and selective beta-l-adrenoceptor blocking agents in the treatment of hyperthyroidism. *Acta Med Scand* 206:21–25, 1979.

35. Stehling LC: Anesthetic management of the patients with hyperthyroidism. *Anesthesiology* 41:585–595, 1974.

36. White VA, Kumogae LF: Preoperative endocrine and metabolic considerations. *Med Clin North Am* 63:1321–1334, 1979.

37. McArthur JW, et al.: Thyrotoxic crisis: Analysis of 36 cases seen at Massachusetts General Hospital during past 25 years. *JAMA* 134:868–874, 1947.

38. Waldstein SS, Slodki SU, Kaganiec I, et al.: A clinical study of thyroid storm. *Ann Intern Med* 52:626–642, 1960.

39. Mazzaferri EL, Skillman TG: Thyroid storm. A review of 22 episodes with special emphasis on the use of guanethidine. *Arch Intern Med* 124:684–690, 1969.

40. Nelson NC, Becker WF: Thyroid crisis, diagnosis, and treatment. *Ann Surg* 170:263–273, 1969.

41. Hoffenberg R: Thyroid emergencies. *Clin Endocrinol Metab* 9:503, 1980.

Hypothyroidism

42. Ladenson PW, Levin AA, Ridgway EC, et al.: Complications of surgery in hypothyroid patients. *Am J Med* 77:261, 1984.

43. Drucker DJ, Burrow GN: Cardiovascular surgery in the hypothyroid patient. *Arch Intern Med* 145:1585, 1985.

44. Wehmann RE et al.: Suppression of thyrotropin in the low-thyroxine state of severe non-thyroidal illness. *N Engl J Med* 312:546, 1985.

45. Bernecker C: Intermittent therapy with potassium iodide in chronic obstructive disease of the

airways: A review of 10 years' experience. *Acta Allergol* 24:216–225, 1969.

46. Evered D, Hall R (eds): Hypothyroidism and goiter. *Clin Endocrinol Metab* 8:1–180, 1979.

47. Kerber RE, Sherman B: Echocardiographic evaluation of pericardial effusion in myxedema: Incidence and biochemical and clinical correlations. *Circulation* 52:823–827, 1975.

48. Urbanix RC, Mazzaferri EL: Thyrotoxic crisis and myxedema coma. *Heart Lung* 7:435–447, 1978.

49. Ridgway EC, McCammon JA, Benotti J, et al.: Acute metabolic responses in myxedema to large doses of intravenous L-thyroxine. *Ann Intern Med* 77:549–555, 1972.

50. James ML: Endocrine disease and anaesthesia: A review of anaesthetic management in pituitary, adrenal, and thyroid diseases. *Anaesthesia* 25:232–252, 1970.

51. Hall R, Scanlon MF: Hypothyroidism: Clinical features and complications. *Clin Endocrinol Metab* 8:29, 1979.

52. Hoffenberg R: Thyroid emergencies. *Clin Endocrinol Metab* 9:503, 1980.

Adrenal Insufficiency

53. Steer M, Fromm D: Recognition of adrenal insufficiency in the postoperative patient. *Am J Surg* 139:443–446, 1980.

54. Axelrod L: Glucocorticoid therapy. *Medicine (Baltimore)* 55:39–65, 1976.

55. Graber AL, Ney RL, Nicholson WE, et al.: Natural history of pituitary-adrenal recovery following long-term suppression with corticosteroids. *J Clin Endocrinol Metab* 25:11–16, 1965.

56. Danowski TS, Bonessi JV, Sabeh G, et al.: Probabilities of pituitary-adrenal responsiveness after steroid therapy. *Arch Intern Med* 61:11–26, 1964.

57. Ackerman GL, Nolan CM: Adrenocortical responsiveness after alternate-day corticosteroid therapy. *N Engl J Med* 278:405–409, 1968.

58. May ME, Carey RM: Rapid adrenocorticotropic hormone test in practice: Retrospective review. *Am J Med* 79:679–683, 1985.

59. Plumpton FS, Besser GM, Cole PV: Corticosteroid treatment and surgery. An investigation of the indications for steroid cover. *Anaesthesia* 24:3–11, 1969.

60. Plumpton FS, Besser GM, Cole PV: Corticosteroid treatment and surgery. The management of steroid cover. *Anaesthesia* 24:12–18, 1969.

61. Bynny R: Preventing adrenal insufficiency during surgery. *Postgrad Med* 67:219–228, 1980.

62. Bynny R: Withdrawal of glucocorticoid therapy. *N Engl J Med* 295:30–32, 1976.

Selective Aldosterone Deficiency

63. DeFronzo RA: Hyperkalemia and hyporeninemic hypoaldosteronism. *Kidney Intern* 17:118–134, 1980.

64. Ashouri O: Hyperkalemic distal renal tubular acidosis and selective aldosterone deficiency. *Arch Intern Med* 145:1306–1307, 1985.

65. Schambelan M, Sebastian A, Biglieri EG: Prevalence, pathogenesis, and functional significance of aldosterone deficiency in hyperkalemic patients with chronic renal insufficiency. *Kidney Intern* 17:89–101, 1980.

66. Kokko JP: Primary acquired hypoaldosteronism. *Kid Intern* 27:690–702, 1985.

67. Batlle DC, Arruda JAL, Kurtzman NA: Hyperkalemic distal renal tubular acidosis associated with obstructive uropathy. *N Engl J Med* 304:373–380, 1981.

68. Perry GO, Lespier L, Jorge J, et al.: Hyporeninemia and hyperaldosteronism in diabetes mellitus. *Arch Intern Med* 137:852–855, 1977.

Primary Hyperaldosteronism

69. Conn JW: Primary aldosteronism: A new clinical syndrome. *J Lab Clin Med* 45:3–7, 1955.

70. Bravo EL, Taraz RC, Dustan HP, et al.: The changing clinical spectrum of primary aldosteronism. *Am J Med* 4:641–651, 1983.

71. Streeten DHP, Tomycz N, Anderson GH: Reliability of screening methods for the diagnosis of primary aldosteronism. *Am J Med* 67:403–413, 1979.

72. Weinberger MH, Grim CE, Hollifield JW, et al.: Primary aldosteronism: Diagnosis, localization, and treatment. *Ann Intern Med* 90:386–395, 1979.

73. Lyons DF, Kem DC, Brown RD, et al.: Single dose captopril as a diagnostic test for primary aldosteronism. *J Clin Endocrinol Metab* 57:892–896, 1983.

74. Kaplan NM: *Clinical Hypertension.* New York: Medcom Press, 1973, pp 252–253.

75. Ganguly A, Grim CE, Weinberger MH: Primary aldosteronism: The etiologic spectrum of disorders and their clinical differentiation. *Arch Intern Med* 142:813–815, 1982.

Pheochromocytoma

76. Hermann H, Mornex R: Clinical and physiopathological study of the pheochromocytomas. *Human Tumors Secreting Catecholamines.* Elmsford, New York, Pergamon Press, 1964.

77. Ganguly A, et al.: Diagnosis and localization of pheochromocytoma. *Am J Med* 67:21, 1979.

78. Hamberger B, et al.: Plasma catecholamine levels in the diagnosis and management of pheochromocytoma. *Surg Gynecol Obstet* 152:291–296, 1981.

79. Bravo EL, Taraz RC, Gifford RW, et al.: Circulating and urinary catecholamines in pheochromocytoma. *N Engl J Med* 301:682, 1979.

80. Bravo EL, Taraz RC, Fouad FM, et al.: Clonidine-suppression test: A useful aid in the diagnosis of pheochromocytoma. *N Engl J Med* 305:623, 1981.

81. Van Heerden JA, Sheps SH, Hamberger B, et al.: Pheochromocytoma: Current status and changing trends. *Surgery* 91:367, 1982.

82. Goldfrien A: Pheochromocytoma. *Clin Endocrinol Metab* 10:607, 1981.

83. Atuk NO: Pheochromocytoma: Diagnosis, localization, and treatment. *Hosp Prac* 187, 1983.

84. Desmonts JM, Le Houelleur J, Remond P, et

al.: Anesthetic management of patients with phaeochromocytoma: A review of 102 cases. *Br J Anaest* 49:991–997, 1977.

Inappropriate Antidiuretic Hormone Secretion

85. Anderson RJ, Hsiao-min C, Rudiger K, et al.: Hyponatremia: A prospective analysis of its epidemiology and the pathogenetic role of vasopressin. *Ann Int Med* 102:164–168, 1985.
86. Hariprasad MK, Eisinger RP, Nadler IM, et al.: Hyponatremia in psychogenic polydipsia. *Arch Intern Med* 140:1639–1642, 1980.
87. Arieff AI: Hyponatremia, convulsions, respiratory arrest, and permanent brain damage after elective surgery in healthy women. *N Engl J Med* 314:1529–1541, 1986.
88. Szatalowicz VL, Arnold PE, Chaimovitz C, et al.: Radioimmunoassay of plasma arginine vasopressin in hyponatremic patients with congestive heart failure. *N Engl J Med* 305:263–266, 1981.
89. Arieff AI, Llach F, Massry SG: Neurological manifestations and morbidity of hyponatremia: Correlation with brain water and electrolytes. *Medicine* 55:121–129, 1976.
90. Khokhar N: Inappropriate secretion of antidiuretic hormone: An overview of the syndrome. *Postgrad Med* 62:73–79, 1977.
91. Weinberg MS, Donohoe JF: Hyponatremia in the syndrome of inappropriate secretion of antidiuretic hormone: Rapid correction with osmotic agents. *Southern Med J* 78:348–350, 1985.
92. Miygawa CI: The pharmacologic management of the syndrome of inappropriate secretion of antidiuretic hormone. *Drug Intell Clin Phar* 20:527–531, 1986.
93. Ishikawa S, Toshikazu S, Kenzo K, et al.: Hyponatremia responsive to fluorocortisone acetate in elderly patients after head injury. *Ann Int Med* 106, 187–191, 1987.

Diabetes Insipidus

94. Moses AM, Miller M, Streeton DHP: Progress in endocrinology and metabolism: Pathophysiologic and pharmacologic alterations in the release and action of ADH. *Metabolism* 25:697–721, 1976.
95. Shucart WA, Jackson I: Management of diabetes insipidus in neurosurgical patients. *J Neurosurg* 44:65–71, 1976.
96. Hans P, Stevenaert A, Albert A: Study of hypotonic polyuria after trans-sphenoidal pitui-

tary adenomectomy. *Intensive Care Med* 12:95–99, 1986.
97. Miller M, Dalakos T, Moses AM, et al.: Recognition of partial defects in antidiuretic hormone secretion. *Ann Intern Med* 73:721–729, 1970.
98. Kreiger DT, Bardin WC (eds): Hypothalamic diabetes insipidus. In *Current Therapy in Endocrinology*. Philadelphia, BC Decker Inc., 1983.
99. Cobb WE, Spar S, Reichlin S: Neurogenic diabetes insipidus management with dDAVP (l-desamino-8-D arginine vasopressin). *Ann Intern Med* 88:183–188, 1978.

Pituitary Insufficiency

100. Winternitz WW, Dzur JA: Pituitary failure secondary to head trauma. *J Neurosurg* 44:504–505, 1976.
101. Kornblum RN, Fisher RS: Pituitary lesions in craniocerebral injuries. *Arch Pathol* 88:242–248, 1969.
102. Reid RL, Malachi EQ, Samuel SCY: Pituitary apoplexy. *Arch Neurol* 42:712–719, 1985.
103. Laws ER, Abboud CF, Kern EB: Perioperative management of patients with pituitary microadenoma. *Neurosurgery* 7:566–570, 1980.

Hyperparathyroidism and Hypercalcemia

104. Boonstra CE, Jackson CE: Serum calcium: Surgery for hyperparathyroidism: Results in 50,000 clinic patients. *Am J Clin Pathol* 55:523, 1971.
105. Mundy GR, Cove DH, Fisken R: Primary hyperparathyroidism: Changes in the pattern of clinical presentation. *Lancet* 1:1317–1320, 1980.
106. Bilezikian JP: The medical management of primary hyperparathyroidism. *Ann Int Med* 96:198, 1982.
107. Purnell DC, Scholz DA, Smith LH, et al.: Treatment of primary hyperparathyroidism. *Am J Med* 56:800, 1974.
108. Selby PL, Peacock M: Ethinyl estradiol and norethindrone in the treatment of primary hyperparathyroidism in postmenopausal women. *N Engl J Med* 314:1481, 1986.
109. Lafferty FW: Primary hyperparathyroidism. *Arch Int Med* 141:1761, 1981.
110. Wells SA, Leight GS, Ross AJ: Primary hyperparathyroidism. *Curr Probl Surg* 17:398, 1980.
111. Brennan MF: Primary hyperparathyroidism. *Adv Surg* 16:25, 1983.
112. Coe FL, Fauus MJ: Does mild asymptomatic hyperparathyroidism require surgery? *N Engl J Med* 302:224, 1980.

14

Hematology

Robert A. Gordon and James O. Ballard

The appropriate evaluation and management of hematologic disorders is essential for a successful outcome in patients undergoing surgery. Hematologic problems may be complex and require special expertise, but the non-hematologist can assess and care for many of the situations encountered during the pre- and postoperative periods. This chapter discusses general considerations and special problems of the hematologic system in the surgical patient.

THE PREOPERATIVE PATIENT WITH ANEMIA

The two major considerations in evaluating the anemic patient in the preoperative setting are, first, to determine as best as possible the cause for the anemia and, secondly, to assess the need for blood transfusion.

Diagnostic Activities

The patient should be questioned about prior history of anemia, bleeding, blood transfusion, current medications, dietary habits, history of renal, liver and thyroid diseases, and any family history of hematologic disorders. Women should be questioned in detail about menstrual periods and prior pregnancies. Ideally, the etiology of the anemia should be determined before elective surgery.

A review of the complete blood count, including indices by automated cell counter, reticulocyte count, peripheral smear and stool occult blood testing can be quickly accomplished. The anemia can then usually be classified as microcytic, macrocytic or normocytic, narrowing the diagnostic possibilities (Table 14.1). Even in emergency situations, a reticulocyte count should be obtained, since this test reflects the production rate of the erythroid bone marrow. The reticulocyte count more accurately indicates marrow red blood cell (RBC) production capacity when it is corrected for the degree of anemia and for the premature release of reticulocytes from the marrow during stress. The **reticulocyte production index (RPI)** corrects for both these factors:

$$RPI = \frac{\text{Observed retic} \times \dfrac{\text{Patient's hematocrit}}{45}}{\text{count (\%)}}{1 \text{ or } 2*}$$

[*Divide by 2 if bluish macrocytes (reticulocytes) seen on smear]

An RPI >3 is found with hemolysis, acute blood loss or erythroid response to replacement of a deficient hematinic, e.g., iron, B12, or folate. An RPI of 2 or less indicates inadequate erythroid production and suggests erythroid hypoplasia, marrow replacement or ineffective RBC maturation. In the absence of acute blood loss or recent repletion of iron, B12 or folate stores, an RPI >3 indicates hemolytic anemia. A direct and indirect Coombs' test should be performed to exclude immune hemolysis since finding compatible units of blood may be difficult and, therefore, transfusion could prove hazardous in this situation.

Clues to the underlying cause of the anemia are frequently found on the peripheral smear. In addition to assessing the hemoglobin content of RBCs, abnormalities such as spherocytes or frag-

Table 14.1. Causes of Anemia Classified by Indices and Peripheral Smear

Microcytic (MCV <80)
  Iron deficiency
  Thalassemia
  Polycythemia vera and iron deficiency
  Anemia of chronic disease
  Sideroblastic anemia
Macrocytic (MCV >100)
  Folate deficiency
  B12 deficiency
  Liver disease
  Alcoholism
  Drugs
  Hypothyroidism
  Refractory anemias
  Spurious (rouleaux formation)
  Reticulocytosis (marked)
Normocytic (MCV 80–100)
  Hypoproliferative (RPI <2)[a]
    Anemia of acute inflammation or chronic disease
    Early iron deficiency
    Endocrine insufficiency (thyroid, adrenal)
    Renal failure
    Bone marrow failure (infiltration, aplasia)
    Combined deficiency states (iron, B12, folate)
  Hemolysis (RPI >3)
    Autoimmune
    Hemolytic transfusion reactions
    Sepsis, DIC
    Microangiopathic hemolysis
    Hypersplenism
    Hemoglobinopathies and congenital hemolytic anemias
    Burns, trauma
    G-6-PD deficiency
  Hemorrhage (acute)

[a] RPI = Reticulocyte Production Index (see text).

mented RBCs may suggest specific forms of hemolytic anemia. Leukocyte and platelet abnormalities on the peripheral smear may lead to the diagnosis of an unsuspected leukemic disorder even when the total white blood cell (WBC) is within normal limits.

After classification of the anemia by indices, RPI and peripheral smear, serum should be obtained for ferritin, iron, total iron binding capacity, vitamin B12, and folate determinations before transfusion, since transfused blood will alter these values and confound diagnostic efforts. The red blood cell folate level provides a more reliable estimate of tissue folate reserves and is not affected by acute changes in dietary intake. When emergency surgery is required, there is little time to diagnose or treat specifically. A complete response to therapy with iron, vitamin B12 or folic acid takes several weeks; thus, replacement therapy is practical only in patients who require elective surgery.

Assessment for Blood Transfusion

Objective data correlating the hemoglobin level and the patient's risk from general anesthesia and surgery are lacking. Many surgeons and anesthesiologists use a predetermined hemoglobin level as adequate for surgery. A questionnaire study (1) found that a preoperative hemoglobin level of about 9 gm/dl was required by 88% of 1249 anesthesia departments surveyed. Experience with hemodialysis and renal transplant patients has shown some types of surgery can be done at hemoglobin levels as low as 6–7 gm/dl when a compensated intravascular volume exists. One study shows that patients who are at relatively increased risk for hypoxic complications can tolerate open heart surgery with preoperative hematocrits between 25–30% (3).

The decision to transfuse blood should be based on the patient's underlying clinical condition. Factors favoring transfusion are acute blood loss, underlying cardiopulmonary disease, and major procedures under general anesthesia with anticipated significant blood loss. Patients with ongoing bleeding should be transfused early since the hematocrit may not reflect the degree of blood loss because concomitant volume depletion and hemoconcentration are usually present. Cardiopulmonary compromise with dyspnea, angina, or congestive heart failure is also an indication for transfusion if these symptoms are attributable to the anemia (Table 14.2).

Transfusion for elective surgery

Table 14.2. Considerations for Preoperative Transfusion

Patient Factors
  Status of anemia (chronic vs. acute)
  Status of intravascular volume
  Ongoing blood loss
  Presence of pulmonary disease
  Presence of cardiovascular disease
  Symptoms due to anemia (cardiopulmonary, CNS)
Procedure
  Type of anesthesia (general vs. local)
  Type of surgery (major vs. minor)
  Anticipated blood loss

should be done at least 24 hours in advance for at least two reasons. Firstly, transfusion of packed red cells into a chronically anemic patient raises the total circulating blood volume, and heart failure may occur if transfusion is given too rapidly. Secondly, banked blood used for transfusion may have abnormal oxygen dissociation characteristics. Storage of blood depletes the level of 2,3-DPG, causing a significant displacement of the oxyhemoglobin dissociation curve to the left and prevents oxygen unloading to the tissues. The transfused red cells will regenerate 2,3-DPG, but with multiple unit transfusions an adequate level may not be restored for 24 hours or more.

Autologous Blood Transfusion

Blood transfusion is a therapy with significant potential complications. Although donor units may be tested for hepatitis B and human immunodeficiency virus (HIV), screening tests for the agent(s) causing non-A, non-B hepatitis, such as hepatitis C virus (HCV), are not yet clinically available. The use of serum ALT levels to detect occult liver disease in blood donors may reduce the incidence of non-A, non-B hepatitis. The patient's need for a blood transfusion should be clearly documented by the physician on the medical record.

Autologous transfusions have important benefits for the patient and the blood bank. There is no risk for the transmission of infectious diseases (hepatitis, syphilis, cytomegalovirus, or AIDS), and autologous transfusion avoids alloimmunization to erythrocyte, leukocyte, platelet, or protein antigens. Autologous transfusions are particularly valuable for patients who have rare blood types, a history of previous transfusion reactions and religious beliefs that prohibit homologous blood transfusions. Despite its advantages to patients and blood centers, autologous transfusion is not widely used (4).

Types of patients for whom autologous transfusion may be particularly appropriate include most patients anticipating elective surgery, especially plastic and orthopedic surgery. However, it can be used effectively for patients undergoing cardiopulmonary bypass and in women immediately after delivery.

Autologous blood can be stored for 21 days. Except in unusual circumstances, phlebotomy can be performed in most patients with a hemoglobin of 11 gm/dl or greater. Not more than 450 ± 45 ml or 12% of the estimated blood volume (whichever is less) should be withdrawn at a single donation. This amount of blood can ideally be withdrawn every 72 hours, and the last phlebotomy should be at least 72 hours before the operation. Iron supplementation should be started at least 1 week prior to the first donation and continued for 2–3 months after the last donation.

POSTOPERATIVE ANEMIAS

Diagnostic Activities

The approach to the patient with postoperative anemia requires attention to many factors. A careful history, physical examination, and record review should exclude anemias that existed postoperatively or those due to the patient's underlying disease. Stools should be obtained for occult blood, since gastrointestinal bleeding due to stress ulceration is common in the postoperative period. The operative report should be reviewed for estimated blood loss and all intake and output records, both intra- and postoperative, should be examined. If the postoperative drop in hematocrit is greater than one would expect from the blood loss at surgery, further causes should be considered. A useful clinical axiom is that **one unit of blood lost or given (250–350 cc) correlates with approximately three percentage points of the hematocrit.**

A review of the complete blood count, including indices, reticulocyte count, and peripheral smear, should classify the anemia into one of three major categories: microcytic, macrocytic, or normocytic (Table 14.3). A direct and indirect Coombs' test, LDH and bilirubin should be obtained to evaluate for hemolysis.

Most postoperative anemias are normocytic and normochromic and are generally multifactorial. The common causes are an underestimation of blood loss or continued bleeding, occult gastrointestinal stress bleeding, dilutional anemia due to excess fluid administration, repeated blood drawing for diagnostic tests ("nosocomial"), and acute

Table 14.3.   Causes of Anemia in the Postoperative Period

Most Common
  Normocytic (MCV 80–100)
    Bleeding (wound, occult, deep at operative site,
      GI, catheter sites)
    Dilutional
    Nosocomial (blood drawing)
    Acute inflammation/chronic disease
    Renal insufficiency
    Marrow suppression (drugs)
    Hemolysis (sepsis, drugs, transfusion reaction,
      underlying disease)
Uncommon
  Macrocytic (MCV >100)
    Folate deficiency
    Drugs
    Liver disease
  Microcytic (MCV <80)
    Anemia chronic disease
    Blood loss with iron deficiency

inflammation. In patients with borderline iron stores, a significant anemia can occur when complicated by blood loss at surgery.

Dilutional anemia is often overlooked. Overhydration during surgery and the postoperative period can cause significant dilution of the red blood cell mass. A comparison of fluid intake and output and preoperative and postoperative weights should be performed.

Blood drawing for diagnostic studies is a significant cause of anemia in ill hospitalized patients and has been termed **nosocomial anemia** (5). In one study of patients in coronary and pulmonary care units, a mean blood loss of approximately 55 ml per day was recorded. It was estimated that the hematocrit value may decrease by 6% during a hospitalization period averaging 21 days. This study concluded that for most seriously ill adults hospitalized for 3–4 weeks, an average of 500–1000 ml of blood will be withdrawn for diagnostic studies. In patients with nosocomial anemia, a reticulocytosis of 2–4% is common. However, most postoperative patients with preexisting medical illnesses will not be able to adequately increase their rate of red blood cell production to compensate for both surgical blood loss and frequent diagnostic blood studies.

The anemia associated with acute inflammation may be present with disorders such as infection, cancer, and collagen vascular disease. This type of anemia develops slowly and by itself should not produce a rapid fall in the hematocrit. However, postoperatively the decrease in marrow response caused by acute inflammation will contribute to a more rapid drop in hematocrit when combined with blood loss due to bleeding and blood drawing. Renal insufficiency postoperatively will also contribute to decreased red cell production.

Marrow suppression due to drugs must always be considered, especially if thrombocytopenia or leukopenia are also present. In unexplained anemias, all medications should be reviewed, including drugs used preoperatively.

Hemolysis is a less common cause of postoperative anemia, but should be strongly considered after blood loss and marrow underproduction have been excluded. Causes of postoperative hemolysis include:

(a) Hemolysis due to drugs: Penicillin, methyldopa, and quinidine are the more common causes. Also consider drug-induced hemolysis in a G-6-PD deficient patient. (b) Hemolysis due to sepsis: Some degree of hemolysis is often seen in sepsis or severe infection. Routine tests for hemolysis (e.g., Coombs' test) are usually negative. Disseminated intravascular coagulation may be present. (c) Hemolysis following transfusions: Acute severe transfusion reactions are easily recognized, but a delayed transfusion reaction with less severe hemolysis due to "minor" antibodies may be missed (See Delayed Transfusion Reaction). (d) Hemolysis due to the patient's underlying disease: Lymphoma, collagen vascular disease, and malignancies may be responsible. A mild preoperative hemolytic anemia may be missed if the reticulocyte response is adequate to maintain the hematocrit near normal. Helpful clues in diagnosing hemolysis are splenomegaly and an unexplained elevated preoperative reticulocyte count. If a preoperative reticulocyte count is unavailable, the peripheral smear can be examined for polychromatophilic erythrocytes.

Macrocytic anemias are uncommon postoperatively. An exception is the patient with prolonged hospitalization who may become folate deficient. Folate deficiency may manifest earlier if the patient was folate-depleted at the time of admission. Drugs implicated in producing macrocytosis, without necessarily causing anemia, include trimethoprim, triamaterene, hydantoin, and various chemotherapeutic agents. Liver disease or brisk reticulocytosis from blood loss or hemolysis should also be considered as a cause for postoperative macrocytosis.

Microcytic anemias rarely occur postoperatively since they require considerable time to develop. However, the patient with a prolonged pre- or postoperative course may develop an anemia of chronic disease.

THE TRANSFUSED PATIENT

Numerous clinical problems may accompany a blood transfusion. The physician should be aware that a blood transfusion reaction may produce a variety of clinical signs and symptoms, including anxiety, shortness of breath, chest pain, shaking chills, fever, hypotension, pulmonary edema, wheezing, and skin rashes. In approaching these clinical manifestations, a complete history and physical examination should be performed and the patient should always be **questioned about a previous blood transfusion.** Particular note should be made of the frequency and complications of previous pregnancies.

Transfusion reactions will be approached in the temporal sequence in which they usually arise rather than in the usual classification of immunologic and non-immunologic mediated transfusion reactions.

Immediate Reactions

HYPERSENSITIVITY SKIN REACTIONS

These reactions are characterized by urticaria, pruritis, or blotchy erythema. They usually begin within minutes of starting the transfusion and have been estimated to occur in approximately 3% of transfusions. It is generally agreed that these reactions arise from sensitization to foreign immunoglobulins. They occur with fresh-frozen plasma and cyroprecipitate, as well as with red blood cells. These reactions are treated with antihistamines and usually respond rapidly. They may be avoided or decreased by pretreatment with antihistamines, or less frequently, by the use of washed red blood cells.

ACUTE HEMOLYTIC TRANSFUSION REACTIONS

Although relatively rare, an acute hemolytic reaction is life-threatening. The most common form of acute hemolytic reaction results when incompatible red cells are transfused. The incompatibility is usually within the ABO system; Rh antibodies less commonly cause this type of reaction. The clinical symptoms include apprehension, facial flushing, chest or lumbar pain, chilliness or frank rigors, tachypnea, tachycardia, and nausea. These symptoms may be followed by signs of shock, acute oliguric renal failure, and diffuse bleeding. In a comatose or anesthetized patient, the first signs of this problem may be oozing from mucus membranes or the operative site, or hemoglobinuria.

The signs and symptoms in this type of reaction are due to two factors: *(a)* acute antigen-antibody reaction with subsequent activation of the complement, coagulation and the kallikrein systems; and *(b)* intravascular red blood cell destruction by isoantibodies.

When an acute hemolytic transfusion reaction is suspected, the transfusion should be stopped immediately. Careful attention should be directed to the blood pressure, urine output, and clinical evidence of bleeding. Laboratory studies of an acute hemolytic transfusion reaction include hemoglobinemia, hemoglobinuria, a depressed haptoglobin, and a transiently positive direct antiglobulin (Coombs') test. Since disseminated intravascular coagulation (DIC) may occur, coagulation studies including (PT), (PTT), platelet count, fibrinogen and fibrin split products should be performed. A citrated sample of blood should be centrifuged and the plasma examined, since a pink color to the plasma indicates free hemoglobin and rapidly confirms the diagnosis.

The **management of a patient with an acute hemolytic transfusion re-action** is the treatment of cardiovascular collapse, acute tubular necrosis and disseminated intravascular coagulation. Intravenous fluids should be infused as soon as the reaction is suspected. Pressors are indicated if hypotension supervenes. The urine output should be maintained at over 100 ml/hr. Mannitol (25 gm) or furosemide can be used for maintenance of urine output but only after appropriate fluid volume management. Shock is the most life-threatening complication of an acute hemolytic transfusion reaction, and diuretics can contribute to hypoperfusion if given indiscretely. The use of heparin for disseminated intravascular coagulation is controversial and depends on the clinical situation (See Management of DIC).

ANAPHYLACTIC REACTION

This reaction occurs very soon after beginning the transfusion and is characterized by shock-like symptoms with wheezing, abdominal, back or chest pain, and cyanosis. This reaction occurs in patients who are IgA-deficient. The incidence of IgA deficiency in a normal population has been estimated to vary between 1/600 to 1/800 individuals, but these reactions occur at a rate of less than 1 reaction per 20,000 units of blood products transfused. This reaction is due to the presence of anti-IgA antibodies. A prior history of transfusion or pregnancy is not required. Therapy is the same as for any anaphylactic reaction, with intravenous fluids, vasopressors, oxygen, steroids, and epinephrine. These reactions can be avoided by using completely washed red blood cells or blood components obtained from IgA-deficient donors.

ACUTE NONCARDIAC PULMONARY EDEMA

This complication is characterized by the abrupt onset of chills, fever, tachycardia, a nonproductive cough, and dyspnea. The chest x-ray reveals perihilar and lower lung field infiltrates without cardiac enlargement or pulmonary vascular engorgement. This reaction is due to antileukocyte antibodies that are obtained either from passively transfused antibodies reacting with the recipient's own leukocytes or due to alloimmunization to transfused granulocytes. Therapy consists of epinephrine and steroids, as well as additional measures for pulmonary edema.

Intermediate Reactions

THE FEBRILE TRANSFUSION REACTION

This is characterized by a flu-like syndrome consisting of malaise, fatigue, fever, myalgia, and headache. The onset varies and may begin within several minutes following the initiation of transfusion, but usually does not develop until 1–2 hours after transfusion. These reactions occur only in patients with a **history of prior transfusion or pregnancy.** The symptoms can persist for several hours. The frequency of these reactions is variable and dependent upon individual donors.

The febrile transfusion reaction is due to antileukocyte and antiplatelet antibodies. These reactions can be prevented or lessened in severity by transfusing leukocyte-depleted blood. This blood product can be obtained by various techniques. Leukocyte-poor red cells have about 80% of the leukocytes removed. Washed or frozen-thawed red cells have essentially zero leukocytes, but are two to three times as expensive to prepare. In the past several years, commercially available microaggregate filters have been shown to effectively reduce the leukocyte count in red blood cell units and to prevent most nonhemolytic febrile transfusion reactions. These filters have the advantages of saving time for the blood bank personnel and decreasing the cost of blood preparation.

Leukocyte-poor blood should be ordered when the multiply transfused patient begins to have symptomatic febrile transfusion reactions. Treatment is otherwise symptomatic using as-pirin or acetaminophen and diphenhydramine 25–50 mg orally or intravenously. In the unusual patient when reactions are frequent or severe, hydrocortisone 50–100 mg intravenously prior to the transfusion may be effective and meperidine 50 mg intravenously often reduces the severity of shaking chills. A hemolytic transfusion reaction and bacterial sepsis should be excluded with appropriate lab studies and blood cultures, depending on the severity of the patient's reaction.

VOLUME OVERLOAD

This is a common and often misdiagnosed complication in elderly patients with renal or cardiac insufficiency and chronic anemia. The patient may develop clinical manifestations varying from dyspnea to overt pulmonary edema. The onset may be delayed up to 24 hours after transfusion. This problem can be avoided by the awareness of this potential problem in elderly individuals, by slow transfusion of packed red blood cells (<2 ml/min), and by judicious use of diuretics. The use of small doses of intravenous furosemide between transfused units can prevent overload in patients at high risk.

Delayed Transfusion Reactions

Delayed hemolytic transfusion reactions are well recognized by blood bank personnel but often missed by the physician. A delayed transfusion reaction should be considered when there is an **unexplained decrease in the hematocrit 2–21 days after a transfusion.** The recipient has always been sensitized to blood group antigens by previous transfusion or pregnancy, but at the time of transfusion, antibody titers are below the level detectable by screening agglutination reactions. The transfusion initiates an anamnestic response and alloantibodies directed against the donor red blood cells are then produced causing hemolysis.

Most delayed transfusion reactions cause fever, a mild elevation of the indirect bilirubin, an elevated reticulocyte count, and a decrease in the hemoglobin and hematocrit concentrations. In one study (10), fever was the most common sign of an ongoing hemolytic process and occurred in 78% of those affected. Uncommonly, these reactions can be serious with patients developing oliguric renal failure and death. When these reactions are investigated early, the direct antiglobulin test is positive and one or more red blood cell antibodies are usually detected. However, it is important to remember that the direct Coombs' test becomes negative once donor red blood cells have been destroyed and cleared by the recipient's reticuloendothelial system. Therefore, a positive direct Coombs' test is very helpful, but a negative one does not preclude a diagnosis of a delayed transfusion reaction. The indirect Coombs' test remains positive for weeks following the reaction. Delayed hemolytic reactions may lead to the mistaken diagnosis of autoimmune hemolytic anemia. The **triad of anemia, fever,** and **recent blood transfusion** should alert the clinician to the possibility of a delayed hemolytic reaction. Because the serum alloantibody titer may become undetectable with time, it is advisable to provide these patients with a warning device (wristband or wallet card) listing the type of red blood cell antigen to which they are sensitized.

Massive Transfusion

A massive transfusion is defined as an amount of stored blood transfused exceeding the amount of the patient's normal blood volume. Among the potential problems of massive transfusion are electrolyte disorders and deficiency of platelets and clotting factors.

After 24 hours of storage, the platelet count of banked blood is essentially zero, and factors V and VIII are very low (approximately 10%). Blood is stored in an anticoagulant solution containing citrate, a compound that avidly binds ionized calcium. The potassium level in stored blood is approximately 30 meq per unit by the end of 3 weeks of storage, and ammonia levels become significantly elevated as well. Particles, consisting mainly of platelets, white blood cells, and fibrin, form in stored blood and are referred to as microaggregates. These features of stored blood may result in the complication of massive transfusion, which include thrombocytopenia, a dilutional coagulopathy, hypocalcemia, hyperkalemia, ammonia toxicity (especially in patients with hepatic insufficiency), and microembolization which may cause a respiratory distress syndrome (Table 14.4).

Many of these complications are avoidable. Calcium can be given as 10% calcium gluconate, administering 10 ml slowly intravenously for each 1000 ml of blood transfused. The calcium should be given in a vein remote from the transfusion site. The potassium level should be frequently checked. Six to eight units of platelets can be transfused for every 8–10 units of packed red cells depending on the platelet count. Two units of fresh frozen plasma are usually given for every 10 units of packed RBC transfused. If the factor VIII and/or fibrinogen levels are low, cryoprecipitate should be used. Six to eight pooled bags of cryoprecipitate should be adequate to restore the factor VIII and/or fibrinogen level (See Management of Coagulation Factor Disorders). The use of a filter finer than the standard 170-micron filter is effective in filtering the microaggregates and preventing microembolization.

Table 14.4. Problems Associated with Massive Transfusion

1. Thrombocytopenia
2. Dilutional coagulopathy (especially factors V and VIII)
3. Hypocalcemia
4. Hyperkalemia
5. Ammonia toxicity (pre-existing liver disease)
6. Respiratory distress syndrome (embolization of microaggregates)

SPECIAL OPERATIVE CONSIDERATIONS IN THE PATIENT WITH ERYTHROCYTE ABNORMALITIES

Sickle Cell Hemoglobinopathies

The common sickle hemoglobin disorders include homozygous sickle cell disease (Hgb SS), sickle cell trait (Hgb AS), sickle cell C disease (Hgb SC) and sickle cell-beta thalassemia. All these disorders except Hgb AS are characterized by recurrent microvascular occlusion under conditions predisposing to reduced tissue oxygenation. The sickle cell prep or the more rapid dithionite tube test are readily available screening tests for the detection of hemoglobins that sickle. A positive screening test should be followed by a hemoglobin electrophoresis on cellulose acetate to confirm hemoglobin S and to evaluate for combined hemoglobinopathies.

Patients with a sickle cell disorder other than Hgb AS present challenging diagnostic problems. For example, sickling in mesenteric and intestinal vessels can produce an abdominal crisis that mimics an acute surgical abdomen with abdominal pain, leukocytosis, fever and jaundice. Cholelithiasis and cholecystitis are common sequelae of the bilirubin stones formed as a result of chronic hemolytic anemia. Surgical intervention may be required in these circumstances; however, hepatic infarction, intrahepatic cholestasis and hepatitis must be considered in the differential diagnosis of abdominal pain and jaundice in these patients.

PREOPERATIVE MANAGEMENT

Hemoglobin AS does not increase the incidence of anesthetic or surgical complications. However, patients with the other forms of sickle hemoglobinopathies are at significant risk of developing acute episodes of sickling and tissue infarction if stressed by hypoxia, infection, dehydration, and acidosis. Hemoglobin values for patients with the more severe sickling disorders usually vary between 5.5–8.5 gm/dl. Elective surgery should be performed at a time when the hemoglobin is at its optimum value for the individual patient.

Preoperative blood studies should include a corrected reticulocyte count and serum bilirubin level to assess the status of bone marrow RBC production and the rate of hemolysis. Elective surgical procedures should be deferred until any infection, metabolic or fluid/electrolyte abnormalities are corrected. The general condition of the patient is equally as important as the absolute preoperative hemoglobin level.

Prophylactic packed RBC transfusions are frequently given prior to any major surgical procedure in an attempt to reduce the patient's hemoglobin S concentration and to suppress marrow production of hemoglobin S-containing RBCs. Although, theoretically, RBC transfusions could increase the viscosity of the blood and accentuate vascular occlusive crises, many clinicians favor preoperative transfusions to protect against inadvertent hypoxia during general anesthesia.

Hemoglobin S levels may be acutely lowered by manual or automated exchange transfusions with the general goal of lowering the hemoglobin S concentration to 40% or less. Exchange transfusion eliminates the potential problem of increasing blood viscosity with simple transfusion. The use of anti-sickling agents such as low-molecular-weight dextran or urea during surgery has proven to be of no clinical value. Alkalinization with sodium bicarbonate should be given if there is any degree of acidosis.

The choice of the anesthestic agent appears to be of less importance than the quality of the anesthetic management. The main objectives of **anesthetic management in the perioperative period** include 1) the provision of adequate oxygenation and ventilation; 2) the avoidance of hypothermia; and 3) the maintenance of adequate circulating volume and cardiac output.

POSTOPERATIVE MANAGEMENT

The patient with sickle cell hemoglobinopathy is subject to numerous potential postoperative problems. There is a well-recognized increased incidence of pulmonary complications related to these patients' inherent susceptibility to bacterial infection, especially due to encapsulated gram-positive species. Prevention of pulmonary atelectasis and prompt treatment of infection are essential. Since pre-existing heart disease and impaired renal function with hyposthenuria are common, meticulous attention to fluid intake (to prevent congestive heart failure) output (to avoid dehydration and sickling) and daily weights, are important features of the postoperative management of these patients. If there is evidence of worsening anemia or Coombs' negative hemolysis in the postoperative setting, the possibility of coexisting glucose-6-phosphate dehydrogenase deficiency with sickle cell hemoglobinopathy should be considered.

Immune Hemolytic Anemias

DIAGNOSTIC ACTIVITIES

Immune hemolytic anemias can be classified either on the basis of whether the antibody is warm or cold, or on the basis of the presence or absence of an underlying disorder. When an autoimmune hemolytic anemia is diagnosed, secondary causes should be identified. Lymphoproliferative disorders, various cancers, autoimmune disorders (especially systemic lupus erythematosus), infections (particularly viral infections, *Mycoplasma pneumoniae,* and subacute bacterial endocarditis), delayed transfusion reaction, and a variety of drugs should be considered. If an underlying disease cannot be determined, then the patient has idiopathic autoimmune hemolytic anemia (Table 14.5).

Immune hemolytic anemias in the postoperative period can be due to drugs or delayed transfusion reactions. Penicillin

Table 14.5.   Antibody-Induced Hemolytic Anemia

Warm antibody
 1. Drugs (common)
 2. Idiopathic
 3. Systemic lupus erythematosus
 4. Lymphoproliferative disorders: chronic lymphocytic leukemia, lymphomas
 5. Carcinomas (rare)
 6. Delayed transfusion reaction
Cold antibody
 1. Infection: mycoplasma, mononucleosis
 2. Lymphomas
 3. Idiopathic cold agglutinin disease

is an uncommon cause of immunohemolytic anemia. The usual clinical setting is a patient who has been given large doses of penicillin for 10 or more days. Renal insufficiency is often present. The penicillin becomes firmly bound to the red cell membrane and elicits an IgG antibody response. Other less common drugs causing hemolytic anemia are cephalosporins, quinidine, and methyldopa; rarely implicated drugs include antituberculosis, nonsteroidal anti-inflammatory, and anticonvulsant drugs. Cephalosporins may also cause a positive direct Coombs' test without hemolysis, and this is of no clinical importance except for its recognition. Sepsis is a common cause of postoperative Coombs' negative hemolytic anemia.

Laboratory data useful in establishing the diagnosis of an immune hemolytic anemia include a positive direct Coombs' test, elevated reticulocyte count, low to absent serum haptoglobin, an increase in serum LDH and indirect bilirubin, and an elevated cold-agglutinin titer.

MANAGEMENT OF WARM AUTOIMMUNE HEMOLYTIC ANEMIA

Patients with warm antibody-induced hemolytic anemia can present with severe anemia, and general cardiovascular support is of great importance. **Blood transfusions should be avoided whenever possible,** since they may result in accelerated hemolysis. However, blood transfusions are indicated for circulatory failure or hypoxemia due to severe anemia.

Although the transfused red blood cells will be eliminated rapidly, relatively small amounts of RBC may provide sufficient oxygen-carrying capacity to alleviate cardiopulmonary or CNS symptoms until corticosteroids become effective. The least amount of transfused RBC necessary to alleviate symptoms is the desirable endpoint. Transfusion to a predetermined hematocrit level should not be the goal in this setting. The history and physical examination are the most important factors in deciding the necessity for RBC transfusion. Exact cross-matching is often impossible. A blood bank experienced with these problems should be used to determine the most compatible units. Blood cells should be transfused slowly with close monitoring for symptoms of increased hemolysis, which require discontinuing the transfusion.

Corticosteroids are the initial treatment of warm antibody type autoimmune hemolytic disease. Prednisone or methylprednisolone should be given in a dosage of 1–2 mg/kg daily in divided doses; hydrocortisone in dosages of 100–200 mg every 6 hours can be given intravenously in the initial management. High-dose corticosteroids should be maintained until the hematocrit stabilizes at an acceptable value, after which the dosage of corticosteroids can be reduced gradually. Folic acid, 1 mg daily, should be given empirically. If autoimmune hemolytic anemia is associated with a known disease, therapy aimed at controlling that disease may ameliorate the hemolytic process.

Maintenance corticosteroid therapy should be given in the lowest dosage possible to maintain an asymptomatic patient with an acceptable stable hematocrit. **Splenectomy is indicated in patients not responding to high-dose steroids** or when steroids cannot be successfully tapered. Immunosuppressant agents should be reserved for patients with severe anemia, which is unresponsive to steroids and splenectomy.

Splenectomy, if necessary, can be performed with an acceptable complication rate and low mortality in patients who have been stabilized with steroids. The risk of splenectomy is significantly increased in patients with marked anemia unresponsive to medical management and in patients who are severely ill from their primary disease. Perioperative management includes the continuance of high-dose corticosteroids, maintenance of adequate oxygenation, and judicious transfusions of least incompatible packed red blood cells for unacceptably low hematocrits.

The incidence of thrombophlebitis and pulmonary embolism are increased in patients with autoimmune hemolytic disease, particularly in the idiopathic cases.

Hemolytic anemia caused by drugs usually resolves promptly after discontinuance of the drug. Corticosteroid therapy is usually of little value in treating drug-induced hemolytic states, but may be beneficial if hemolysis is prolonged. Blood transfusion can usually be employed safely and effectively if necessary to correct severe anemia.

EVALUATION AND MANAGEMENT OF COLD AUTOIMMUNE DISEASES

Cold autoimmune diseases are an uncommon group of immunologic disorders characterized by the abnormal production of autoantibodies, usually of the IgM class. These autoantibodies may cause agglutination and/or hemolysis.

Cold agglutinin autoantibodies may be found in idiopathic cold agglutinin disease, lymphoproliferative disorders, and in various infections, such as influenza, infectious mononucleosis, and acute **mycoplasma pneumonia** (see Table 14.5). The major perioperative problem in patients with cold autoantibodies is obstruction of the microcirculation. Gangrene of the peripheral parts, such as fingers, toes, and earlobes can occur. In patients undergoing systemic hypothermia, immune complex nephritis causing acute and chronic renal failure has been reported. The use of iced potassium cardioplegic solution during cardiac surgery may cause intracoronary hemagglutination with coronary thrombosis, subendocardial ischemia, and, possibly, myocardial infarction.

Cryoglobulinemia is more a syndrome complex than a primary immune disorder and can be idiopathic (essential) or associated with multiple myeloma or macroglobulinemia. These immunoglobulins do not cause hemolysis but will instead fix complement and precipitate in the serum on cold exposure. They may cause a leukocytoclastic vasculitis.

A directed management approach to patients with cold autoimmune disorders undergoing surgery is essential for a successful outcome. The most important concept in the preoperative evaluation of the cold autoimmune disorders is the **determination of the critical temperature of the cold antibodies** (the temperature above which activity as agglutinins and/or hemolysins ceases). This can be done in vitro by observing hemagglutination and noting the highest environmental or water bath temperature at which hemagglutination persists (14).

The preoperative recognition and treatment of the underlying condition associated with the cold agglutinins will prevent or decrease intraoperative risk. The efficacy of steroids and splenectomy have been poor in idiopathic cold agglutinin disease; long-term treatment with chlorambucil has been successful in some patients. Chemotherapy for plasma cell dyscrasias and lymphomas will frequently control the disease process and reduce the titer of the cold autoantibodies. When cold agglutinins are caused by an infectious process, elective surgery should be postponed until this process resolves naturally or with specific therapy. In addition, preoperative plasmapheresis can be used to rapidly reduce high antibody titers for patients with clinically important cold agglutinins in whom surgical hypothermia will be induced.

Perioperative management is directed at **warming the patient** above the critical temperature of the cold autoantibodies. Intraoperative temperature monitoring and maintenance of critical temperature is essential. Intravenous fluids should be given at normal body temperature. If transfusions are necessary, red cells should be washed to eliminate plasma complement and then given through a blood warmer.

Following surgery, and for several postoperative days, laboratory studies should include peripheral blood smear, hemoglobin, hematocrit, serum and urine hemoglobin to evaluate for persistent agglutination and hemolysis.

Erythrocytosis

Erythrocytosis is defined as an increase in the number of red blood cells in the circulation. The increase in red blood cells usually reflects an increase in the quantity of hemoglobin and in the volume of packed red cells. **The hematocrit should be considered elevated when it is greater than 54% in men and 48% in women.** In approaching the problem of an elevated hematocrit, the consultant should have two strategies in mind. The first should be to determine the cause of the erythrocytosis. Secondly, it is important to determine whether the patient is symptomatic from hyperviscosity and to appreciate the complications of hemorrhage and thrombosis in patients with significant erythrocytosis.

An elevated hemoglobin and hematocrit represents either a true increase or a relative increase in the red blood cell mass. Relative erythrocytosis occurs when there is a loss or contraction of plasma. This decrease in plasma volume may occur because of loss of plasma into the interstitial fluid or a third space; extracellular losses due to persistent vomiting, diarrhea, or severe sweating; inadequate fluid intake; or diuretic therapy. The term *stress polycythemia* is used when the red cell mass is normal and there is no obvious cause for the erythrocytosis.

The first step in the evaluation of erythrocytosis is to document an absolute increase in the erythrocytes by **measurement of the red blood cell mass.** If the red blood cell mass is elevated (in men ≥ 36 ml/kg and in women ≥ 32 ml/kg), then two categories of disease need to be considered. The first includes causes of erythrocytosis resulting from either an appropriate increase in erythropoietin secondary to hypoxemia or abnormal hemoglobin function, or as a result of an inappropriate increase in erythropoietin, usually from tumor or renal disease. The second major consideration is polycythemia vera, an autonomous myeloproliferative disorder.

Clinical and laboratory information are necessary to differentiate the types of erythrocytosis due to a true increase in RBC mass. If the patient has an increased red blood cell mass along with an arterial oxygen saturation of $>92\%$ and splenomegaly, the diagnosis of polycythemia vera can be made. However, in the absence of splenomegaly, which occurs in about 25% of patients with polycythemia vera on presentation, the patient requires two of the following four abnormalities: thrombocytosis, with a platelet count of greater than 400,000/mm^3; leukocytosis, with a white count of greater than 12,000/mm^3 in the absence of fever or infection; an elevated leukocyte alkaline phosphatase score; or an increased serum B12 level or unbound B12 binding capacity. Other findings that support a diagnosis of polycythemia vera include an elevated basophil and eosinophil count, abnormal platelet morphology, and an elevated uric acid.

If absolute erythrocytosis is present and criteria cannot be met for polycythemia vera, then one must determine whether the patient has an appropriate or inappropriate erythrocytosis. Hypoxemia is a common cause for an appropriate increase in red blood cell mass. This occurs from pulmonary disease, cardiac disease with right to left shunts, alveolar hypoventilation, and high altitude residence.

These patients have an arterial oxygen saturation of less than 92%. If the arterial oxygen saturation is normal, then abnormal hemoglobin function or an ectopic production of erythropoietin should be sought. The most common cause of abnormal hemoglobin function is the presence of carboxyhemoglobin in cigarette smokers. Patients with **smoker's polycythemia** have an elevated carboxyhemoglobin level and the oxyhemoglobin dissociation curve is shifted to the left with a lower P_{50} (18). (P_{50} is the partial pressure of oxygen at which hemoglobin is 50% saturated.) Rare congenital hemoglobins may also be responsible for a shift of the P_{50} to the left. If an appropriate cause for erythrocytosis cannot be found, the patient is not a smoker, and the P_{50} is normal, then one needs to consider an autonomous increase in erythropoietin. Renal lesions, particularly hypernephroma and polycystic kidney disease, are the most likely causes of inappropriate secondary erythrocytosis. Hepatomas, uterine tumors, and pheochromocytoma are other rarer causes.

The pathophysiologic consequences of true erythrocytosis include hyperviscosity, hypervolemia, and decreased systemic oxygen transport. At hematocrit levels about 50%, the viscosity of blood increases exponentially (Fig. 14.1). This increase in viscosity is responsible for many of the signs and symptoms of polycythemia. Complaints of altered circulation such as dizziness, headache, vertigo, tinnitus, and visual alterations, including scotomata and double or blurred vision, should be sought. Cerebral blood flow has been found to be significantly lower in patients with hematocrits between 47–53% when compared to patients with hematocrits between 36–46% (16). Reduction to the lower hematocrit range by phlebotomy increases cerebral blood flow by a mean of 50%.

Thromboses are particularly common in polycythemia vera but also occur from any cause of true erythrocytosis. Paradoxically, hemorrhage is also a common prob-

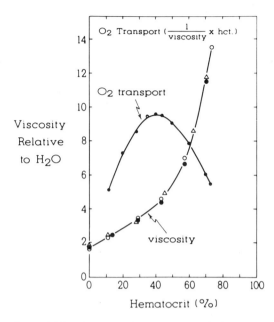

O_2 Transport $(\frac{1}{viscosity} \times hct.)$

O_2 transport

Viscosity Relative to H_2O

viscosity

Hematocrit (%)

Figure 14.1. Oxygen Transport as Calculated from Blood Oxygen-carrying Capacity (hematocrit) and Blood Flow (reciprocal of viscosity). (From Ersley AJ, Gabuzda TG: *Pathophysiology of Blood,* 2nd ed. Philadelphia, WB Saunders, 1979, p 35.)

lem, especially in polycythemia vera. Hemorrhages from mucous membranes can be attributed to blood vessel distention, circulatory stagnation, which causes ischemia and necrosis, and poor clot retractability. Gastrointestinal tract bleeding is particularly common. In polycythemia vera, intrinsic platelet dysfunction contributes to bleeding.

Hyperviscosity results in sluggish blood flow and a decrease in the transport of oxygen to tissues. The optimal hematocrit for oxygen transport is between 40–45% (Fig. 14.1). An increased blood viscosity also elevates pulmonary arterial pressure. If erythrocytosis occurs from hypoxemia, the combined elevation of pulmonary vascular resistance together with the elevated pulmonary arterial pressure contributes to the development or worsening of cor pulmonale.

The treatment of erythrocytosis is dependent upon its cause. **Patients with polycythemia vera and a hematocrit** **above 45% should undergo phlebotomy.** Phlebotomy is especially important in patients with polycythemia vera who must undergo surgery. The intra- and postoperative morbidity and mortality are 4–5 times greater in patients with polycythemia vera who have not been phlebotomized as compared to phlebotomized patients (15). Much of the increased risk is due to thrombosis and hemorrhage. In addition, patients with effective and prolonged control of their polycythemia vera are at less risk of complications from surgery than polycythemic patients who require acute control.

In an emergency situation, the red blood cell mass can be reduced acutely by phlebotomy with a suitable plasma replacement to prevent vascular instability associated with too rapid a reduction in total blood volume. **If thrombocytosis is present in a patient with polycythemia vera, elective surgery is contraindicated.** If surgery is emergent, the platelet count should be acutely reduced. (Refer to the section entitled, "Treatment of Thrombocytosis.") If surgery is not emergent, the platelet count can be reduced by a cytotoxic agent such as hydroxyurea. Surgery can then be performed after normalization of the platelet count and red cell mass.

WHITE BLOOD CELL DISORDERS

Neutrophilia

An absolute neutrophil count greater than 10,000/mm^3 is considered elevated. The consultant's main objective in approaching the preoperative patient with neutrophilia is to differentiate a myeloproliferative disorder, particularly, **chronic granulocytic leukemia versus a leukemoid reaction.** The physical examination may demonstrate splenomegaly, and a careful review of the peripheral smear, looking for basophilia, eosinophilia, and immature myeloid cells is often helpful in supporting the diagnosis of chronic granulocytic leukemia.

Characteristically in a leukemoid reaction, the elevated white count is due to an increase in polymorphonuclear cells, with a mild increase in bands and metamyelocytes. Myelocytes in the peripheral blood are unusual, and the presence of promyelocytes is usually indicative of chronic myelogenous leukemia. Toxic granulations and cytoplasmic vacuolization of the neutrophils may be seen in a leukemoid reaction due to infection. The leukocyte alkaline phosphatase is a very helpful laboratory study and is low to zero in chronic granulocytic leukemia and usually elevated in a leukemoid reaction. A bone marrow examination may be helpful in differentiating chronic granulocytic leukemia (CGL) from a leukemoid reaction, especially when marrow cytogenetic analysis demonstrates the Philadelphia chromosome (t9; 22) which is present in 90% of patients with CGL.

Operating on patients with chronic granulocytic leukemia with white counts of less than 50,000/mm^3 presents no real difficulty as long as the red blood cell count and platelet count are normal. However, white blood counts of greater than 100,000/mm^3 if associated with blast crisis may predispose to capillary sludging, particularly in the brain and lungs, resulting in cerebral hemorrhage and hypoxemia.

Because patients with myeloproliferative disorders frequently have an elevated serum uric acid, adequate hydration, urine alkalinization, and allopurinol therapy may prevent postoperative gout and uric acid nephropathy.

The postoperative approach to neutrophilia is usually straightforward: infection must be ruled out. A transient elevation in the neutrophil count may occur postoperatively due to the stress of surgery and usually does not exceed 15,000–30,000 white cells/mm^3.

Neutropenia

The term neutropenia is used when the absolute neutrophil count is less than

Table 14.6. Common Causes for Neutropenia

Benign (chronic idiopathic, familial)
Bone marrow disorders (myelodysplastic syndrome, leukemia, aplasia)
Infection (bacterial sepsis, viral)
Nutritional deficiency (B12/folate)
Immune disorders (autoimmune, SLE)
Felty's Syndrome (complex mechanisms)
Hypersplenism
Drug induced (most common drugs)
  Idiosyncratic
    Antibiotics (penicillins, chloramphenicol, vancomycin, sulfonamides)
    Anticonvulsants (hydantoin, carbamazepine)
    Anti-inflammatory (phenylbutazone, indomethacin, gold salts, penicillamine)
    Anti-thyroid (propylthiouracil, methimazole)
    Cardiovascular (procainamide, quinidine, captopril)
    Phenothiazines (chlorpromazine)
    Antidepressants (tricyclics)
    Miscellaneous (cimetidine, allopurinol, ethanol)
  Predictable (antineoplastic and immunosuppressant therapy)

3,000/mm^3. Commonly encountered causes for neutropenia are listed in Table 14.6.

A neutrophil count of less than 2,000/mm^3 is uncommon, and its cause should be elucidated before surgery is undertaken. When the absolute neutrophil count is below 1,500/mm^3, the risk of infection begins to increase, but a serious risk of infection is usually not encountered until the absolute neutrophil count is less than 500/mm^3. In addition to the neutrophil count, the risk of infection is related to the primary disease process. Patients with chronic idiopathic neutropenia with neutrophil counts less than 500/mm^3 develop infection infrequently; however, patients with hypoproliferative neutropenia or bone marrow infiltrative disorders are almost certain to become infected with similarly low white counts. A history of previous bacterial infections will allow the consultant to decide the clinical significance of the neutropenia. (Associated anemia and thrombocytopenia require additional evaluation.) A bone marrow examination is necessary to determine if the neutropenia is caused by decreased production, ineffective production, or increased destruction.

Surgery should be postponed in patients with an absolute neutrophil count less than 1,500/mm³ if the process causing the neutropenia is reversible. If the neutropenia is unresolvable, a clinical decision regarding the urgency of the surgery must be made. If surgery is necessary, broad-spectrum prophylactic antibiotics should be given immediately pre- and postoperatively. Granulocyte transfusions may rarely be indicated in patients who are severely neutropenic (absolute neutrophils <500/mm³) and in those who have culture proven bacterial infections which are unresponsive to appropriate antibiotics after 24–48 hours. The granulocytes are usually given for a minimum of 5 days but should be continued until a clinical response occurs. Other indications for granulocyte transfusions in neutropenic patients are not well defined, and there is increasing evidence that these transfusions are less effective than originally believed because of the inability to procure adequate numbers of donor granulocytes. There is no role for prophylactic granulocyte transfusion regardless of the cause of neutropenia. Granulocyte transfusions may have significant side effects, particularly when HLA-matched granulocytes are not used. Pulmonary infiltrates caused by a leukoagglutinin reaction, high fevers and severe shaking chills are not uncommon.

The neutropenic patient should be placed in reverse isolation postoperatively until wound healing is satisfactory. Any postoperative fever should be assumed to represent infection. Broad-spectrum antibiotics should be instituted immediately after cultures are obtained.

Lymphocytosis

Lymphocytosis is defined as an absolute lymphocyte count above 4,000/mm³. The causes for lymphocytosis in the adult surgical patient are limited. The differential diagnosis is between a viral infection (infectious mononucleosis, viral hepatitis, cytomegalovirus) and chronic lymphocytic leukemia (CLL). A study of the peripheral blood smear will usually distinguish between a viral infection with reactive atypical lymphs and CLL in which small lymphocytes predominate.

There is no contradication to surgery in patients with CLL and a marked lymphocytosis. A lymphocyte count of 100 to 200,000/mm³ does not cause vascular stasis since lymphocytes are deformable through the microcirculation. An associated anemia and/or thrombocytopenia should be evaluated with a reticulocyte count and bone marrow examination, since these cytopenias can result from bone marrow replacement or autoimmune disorders. Quantitative immunoglobulin levels should be measured since patients with CLL may be hypogammaglobulinemic, which may predispose them to serious bacterial infections. If such an infection occurs, intravenous gammaglobulin should be given together with broad-spectrum antibiotics.

Lymphocytopenia

Lymphocytopenia occurs when the absolute lymphocyte count is below 1,500/mm³. Lymphocytopenia is often associated with altered host immune response. The importance of chronic lymphocytopenia is in the identification of an underlying disorder which may predispose to or be associated with infection. Common causes for lymphocytopenia include malignancies, malnourishment, acquired immunodeficiency syndrome, corticosteroid therapy and systemic lupus erythematosus.

EVALUATION AND MANAGEMENT OF HEMOSTASIS IN THE SURGICAL PATIENT

Evaluation of the Hemostatic System

A thorough history that is targeted to certain key questions (Table 14.7) is the single most valuable screening technique

Table 14.7. Key Questions for Evaluation of the Hemostatic System[a]

1. Do you develop large bruises without a good reason? Have you bled a long time after minor cuts or trauma to your tongue, cheek or lip? If so, how old were you when this began?
2. Have you had teeth extracted? If so, which ones? How long did you bleed after extraction? Did bleeding start up again a day or so later?
3. What operations have you had? Was bleeding after surgery or childbirth hard to stop? Were transfusions necessary? Did your wounds heal well?
4. Have you had general medical problems? What are these and how are they being treated? Have you had kidney, liver or arthritic diseases?
5. What medicines do you take? Do you use over-the-counter drugs for colds, allergy, headaches, arthritis, menstrual cramps, back aches or other pains? Have you taken any medicines, including antibiotics within the last 7–10 days?
6. Do you have any blood relatives who have experienced prolonged or excessive bleeding?

[a] Modified from Rappaport, SI: Preoperative hemostatic evaluation: Which tests, if any? *Blood* 61:229–231, 1983.

in evaluating patients for bleeding disorders and for ensuring adequate hemostasis during surgery (20). Although preoperative laboratory tests to exclude platelet and coagulation factor abnormalities are readily available and reasonably sensitive, the result of these **tests must be interpreted in light of the history.** On the other hand, if the patient is a poor historian or minimizes symptoms, laboratory testing assumes more importance in estimating operative risk. In addition, an abnormal coagulation test result may be the first evidence of a mild congenital coagulation factor deficiency or platelet disorder in the patient who has never had a prior surgical challenge or significant trauma.

Careful screening by history and laboratory testing is especially indicated when patients are scheduled for major surgical procedures known to be associated with a higher risk of operative bleeding. These include prostatic surgery and cardiac surgery in which the pump-oxygenator is used.

The same degree of caution is warranted in the evaluation of patients undergoing ophthalmologic and neurological surgery, since even small amounts of bleeding could be detrimental.

When the screening history is positive for excessive and/or prolonged bleeding in the past, determining the age of onset will help define whether the bleeding disorder is congenital or acquired. Next, the pattern of bleeding episodes should be established. For example, a history of bleeding predominantly from skin and mucosal surfaces (oral, nasal, GI and/or GU tracts), which is spontaneous or occurs immediately after minimal trauma, is suggestive of a quantitative or qualitative platelet deficiency. By contrast, coagulation factor deficiency is more likely to manifest as bleeding into muscles and joints, and may be delayed in onset for several hours following trauma. Gastrointestinal and genitourinary tract bleeding are common in thrombocytopenia or platelet dysfunction but are also seen with coagulopathies and vasculitis.

Questions regarding general medical problems (especially renal, liver and autoimmune diseases), as well as a detailed listing of medications are of obvious importance. The patient may not realize that medications purchased over the counter contain aspirin or nonsteroidal anti-inflammatory agents. Finally, the family history obtained from the patient or relatives is an essential part of the preoperative evaluation.

The physical examination may provide clues that are helpful in differentiating the etiology of abnormal bleeding. Petechiae, small pinpoint capillary hemorrhages, seen most frequently on the feet and legs, are commonly present with thrombocytopenia or platelet dysfunction. Ecchymoses greater than 4 cm in diameter, hematomas, hemarthroses, and flexion contractures of joints suggest coagulation factor deficiency. Purpura, irregularly shaped purple macular lesions with clearly defined margins, may have

Table 14.8.   Screening Lab Tests for a Patient with Suspected Bleeding Diathesis or Undergoing High-Risk Surgery

1. Platelet count
2. Template bleeding time: measures adequacy of platelet number and function
3. Prothrombin time: measures extrinsic coagulation system (factor VII) and common pathway
4. Partial thromboplastin time: measures intrinsic coagulation system and common pathway
5. Thrombin time: measures the rate of fibrinogen to fibrin conversion when thrombin is added to plasma
6. Fibrinogen
7. Factor XIII (fibrin-stabilizing factor) screen: factor XIII is not detected by any other standard coagulation test

the same significance as petechiae. However, purpura is quite common on the dorsal surfaces of the arms and hands of otherwise healthy elderly individuals (senile purpura). It is also commonly seen on the extremities of patients receiving chronic corticosteroid therapy, and in these patients is not indicative of a coagulation abnormality. Palpable purpuric lesions in patients with a generalized illness should suggest the diagnosis of vasculitis. Generalized oozing from mucosal surfaces and venipuncture sites occurs with hemostatic disorders affecting both platelets and coagulation factors, such as disseminated intravascular coagulation (DIC).

In situations where the screening history and/or physical exam are abnormal, an accurate history is unobtainable, or the patient is to undergo a high-risk surgical procedure, a platelet count, template bleeding time, prothrombin time (PT), activated partial thromboplastin time (aPTT), thrombin time, fibrinogen level, and screen for factor XIII deficiency should be obtained (Table 14.8). These tests permit the identification of the area of the hemostatic mechanism that may be affected and indicate the need for other, more specific tests to determine the precise nature of the defect. Figure 14.2 depicts an approach to the initial laboratory screen for a defect in hemostasis.

The platelet count and bleeding time are usually considered in conjunction with each other. If the platelet count is low, this may result from underproduction by the marrow, increased sequestration by the spleen, or increased consumption of platelets (e.g., immunologic thrombocytopenia or DIC). If the platelet count is normal but the template bleeding time is longer than 10 minutes, platelet dysfunction should be suspected. This is commonly caused by drugs such as aspirin but may be due to von Willebrand's disease, renal insufficiency, liver disease or congenital thrombocytopathy. In the absence of a history of drugs, further testing including platelet aggregation studies may be indicated. Platelet related problems can be excluded when both bleeding time and platelet count are normal.

The prothrombin time, which measures the extrinsic coagulation system and those clotting factors common to both the intrinsic and extrinsic systems, is the next test in the screening sequence. If the prothrombin time is prolonged and the partial thromboplastin time normal, a defect of the extrinsic system is present. This may be caused by a deficiency in Factor VII, which is rare, or by commonly acquired problems, including a mild combined defect in the vitamin K dependent clotting factors (II, VII, IX and X) as a result of vitamin K deficiency, liver disease, or the early effect of coumarin anticoagulants. Factor VII has the shortest half-life of all coagulation factors (approximately 5 hrs), which explains an isolated prolonged PT early in the course of these disorders.

If both the prothrombin time and the activated partial thromboplastin time are prolonged, single or multiple common pathway factor deficiencies are present. Common causes for these results are severe vitamin K deficiency, liver diseases, coumarin anticoagulation, congenital factor X or V deficiency and, rarely, prothrombin (II) deficiency.

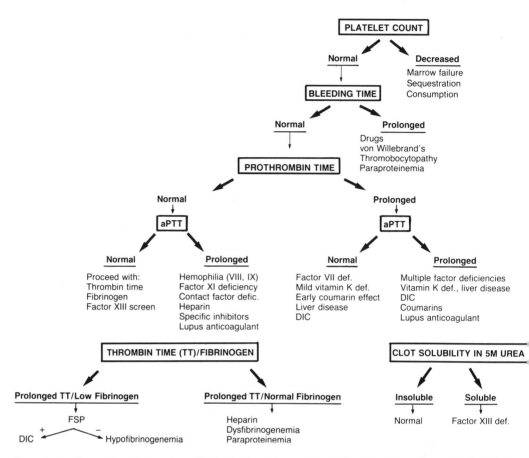

Figure 14.2. Screening Laboratory Tests in the Diagnosis of Bleeding Disorders. (Modified from Edwards RL and Rickles FR: The Evaluation of the Patient with a Bleeding Disorder. MA Lichtman (ed): *Hematology and Oncology,* New York, Grune & Stratton, 1980, p. 208.)

When the activated partial thromboplastin time is prolonged while the prothrombin time is normal, a defect in the intrinsic system is the problem. The physician should confirm that an isolated prolongation of the aPTT is not a laboratory error by **repeating the test on a carefully collected specimen.** The finding of an isolated prolongation of the aPTT in a patient without an abnormal bleeding history, and with previous uncomplicated surgery or trauma, suggests a deficiency of factor XII or one of the contact factors (prekallikrein [Fletcher factor] or high-molecular-weight kininogen [Fitzgerald factor]. Once identified, these patients can be operated on safely. In the patient with abnormal bleeding, an isolated prolonged

aPTT will usually be due to a form of hemophilia (factor VIII or IX deficiency) or due to factor XI deficiency. When both the activated partial thromboplastin time and template bleeding time are prolonged, von Willebrand's disease is the likely diagnosis (Fig. 14.3).

The thrombin time and fibrinogen level should be evaluated in conjunction with each other. These tests monitor the final stage of clot formation in which fibrinogen is converted to fibrin. The thrombin time and fibrinogen level should be normal in all of the specific disorders mentioned thus far. If the fibrinogen is low and the thrombin time prolonged, a test for fibrin split products should also be obtained. The combination of elevated fibrin split prod-

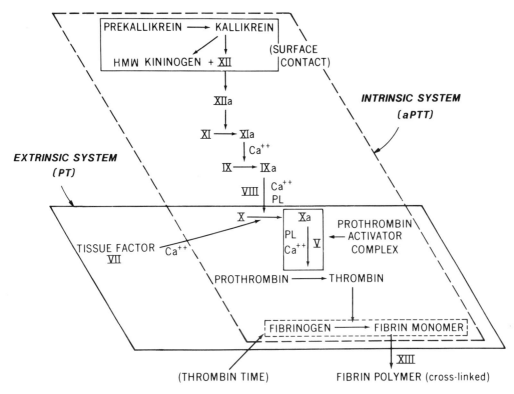

Figure 14.3. Coagulation Scheme. *PL,* Phospholipid (platelet membrane); *a,* activated; *HMW,* High Molecular Weight.

ucts (FSP), decreased fibrinogen, and a low platelet count is a good indicator of ongoing disseminated intravascular coagulation. In the absence of FSP, hypofibrinogenemia from decreased synthesis should be suspected. If the fibrinogen is normal or high and the thrombin time prolonged, the presence of heparin or an abnormal fibrinogen (dysfibrinogenemia) should be considered (Table 14.9).

If all the above tests are normal in a patient with a history of bleeding, wound dehiscence or keloid formation, factor XIII deficiency should be sought by determining if the fibrin clot is soluble in 5 molar urea. Factor XIII deficiency results in a

Table 14.9. Diagnosis of Common Clotting Disorders[a]

Disorder	PT	aPTT	Fibrinogen	Fibrin-Split Products	Thrombin Time	Platelet Count	Template Bleeding Time
Hemophilia A (VIII)	N	A	N	−	N	N	N
von Willebrand's disease	N	A or N	N	−	N	N	A
Hemophilia B (IX)	N	A	N	−	N	N	N
Vitamin K deficiency	A	N or A	N	−	N	N	N
Coumarin excess	A	A	N	−	N	N	N
Liver disease	A	A	N or A	+ or −	N or A	N orA	N or A
DIC	N or A	N or A	N or A	+	A	N or A	N or A

[a]The abbreviations used are: N, normal; A, abnormal; −, absent; +, present.

non-cross-linked clot, which readily dissolves in this solution. This test represents the only screening test for this disorder. Factor XIII deficiency is usually congenital. Inhibitors to factor XIII may be acquired after long-term exposure to certain drugs such as isoniazid or phenytoin.

A major consideration in evaluating the cause of an abnormal screening test is the need to **establish whether the abnormality reflects a decreased level of clotting factor(s) or the presence of circulating coagulation inhibitors.** The latter are substances, frequently antibodies, which circulate in plasma and interfere with the normal function of one or more clotting factors. They may produce bleeding that is as severe as that which occurs with congenital coagulation factor deficiencies, or they may interfere only with the in vitro clotting test without causing actual clinical bleeding (e.g., lupus anticoagulant). The presence of an inhibitor can usually be demonstrated by repeating the abnormal clotting test (PT, PTT, or TT) on a mixture of equal parts of the patient's plasma and normal plasma. A clinically significant coagulation inhibitor in the patient's plasma will prolong the PTT of the normal plasma, and the PTT on the mixture will remain prolonged. By contrast, if the initial test is abnormal because of deficiency in one or more of the coagulation factors, the addition of normal plasma will provide approximately 50% of the missing factor(s) and correct the test. As mentioned, heparin, even in small quantities, prolongs the thrombin time because of its antithrombin properties. Addition of normal plasma will not correct the thrombin time in a patient receiving heparin since the drug remains in the mixture.

Management of Coagulation Factor Disorders in the Surgical Patient

PREOPERATIVE CHECKLIST

Before the patient with a coagulation factor disorder is taken to surgery, all of the following questions must be addressed: *(a)* Has the diagnosis been firmly established? Does the patient have more than one hemostatic defect? *(b)* Is there an associated platelet deficiency or qualitative platelet defect? *(c)* Is there evidence of a coagulation factor inhibitor? *(d)* Can the blood bank provide adequate clotting factor replacement for the entire pre- and postoperative periods? *(e)* What mode of therapy would pose the least risk of transmission of hepatitis and the acquired immunodeficiency syndrome? *(f)* Is a hematology consultant available? Is a specialized coagulation laboratory available? Where can the patient best be cared for?

A care plan that details the frequency and amounts of clotting factor support and the timing of coagulation testing should be developed prior to surgery and circulated to all individuals involved in the care of the patient. **Intramuscular injections, anti-platelet medications and anticoagulants must be avoided** in patients with coagulation factor disorders. Invasive procedures and vigorous physical therapy should be preceded by clotting factor replacement.

Management of Congenital Clotting Factor Disorders

The most common congenital clotting disorders are hemophilia A (factor VIII deficiency), hemophilia B (factor IX deficiency), and von Willebrand's disease. Rare deficiency states that would also require replacement therapy for surgery include deficiency of factor XI, VII, X, V, XIII and prothrombin and fibrinogen.

The patient with **hemophilia** due either to factor VIII or IX deficiency demonstrates an isolated prolongation of the aPTT unless the deficiency is very mild (plasma factor level >30%), in which case the aPTT is frequently normal. The diagnosis of hemophilia is occasionally first established in the postoperative period in mild hemophiliacs who have escaped prior surgery and trauma.

Circulating inhibitors to factor VIII develop in approximately 15% of patients with severe factor VIII deficiency and are somewhat less common in factor IX deficiency. A **test for inhibitors** should be performed prior to any surgical procedure and at intervals during the postoperative period of factor replacement, since an inhibitor may first appear during intensive factor replacement for surgery. Elective surgery is contraindicated in the hemophiliac with an inhibitor or a history of an inhibitor, especially if the antibody has been shown to be of the high-titer, easily stimulated type. In the event emergency surgery is required, the procedure should be carried out at a center that provides specialized resources for the management of such patients.

In the absence of an inhibitor, either cryoprecipitate or factor VIII concentrate (heat-treated to inactivate the human immunodeficiency virus) is used for factor VIII replacement. Fresh frozen plasma or prothrombin complex concentrates are sources of factor IX for the treatment of factor IX deficiency (Table 14.10). Both factor VIII and factor IX concentrates are prepared from the pooled plasmas of many thousand donors, and these forms of therapy carry a high risk for transmission of hepatitis B and non-A, non-B hepatitis.

The plasma half-life of transfused clotting factor is 8–12 hours for factor VIII

Table 14.10. Blood Component Therapy of Common Clotting Disorders

Disorder	Deficient Factor(s)	Blood Component	Initial[b] (dose per kg)	Maintenance (dose per kg/hrs)
			Dosage[a]	
Congenital				
Hemophilia A	VIII: C[c]	Cryoprecipitate	0.2–0.5 bags	0.1–0.3 bags/12
		AHF concentrate	20–40 units	10–20 units/12
		Plasma	20–40 ml	10–20 ml/12
von Willebrand's	VIII: C/VIII:VWF[c] {	Cryoprecipitate	0.1 bag	0.1 bag/24[d]
		Plasma	10–15 ml	10–15 ml/24
Hemophilia B	IX	Plasma	20–60 ml	5–10 ml/12
		Prothrombin complex concentrate	40–60 units	5–10 units/12
Acquired				
Vitamin K deficiency	II (prothrombin) VII, IX, X	Plasma	10–20 ml	10 ml/6–12
Coumarin excess		Prothrombin complex concentrate	20–40 units	10–20 units/24
Liver disease	II (prothrombin), VII, IX, X, V, I (fibrinogen) if severe	Plasma	10–20 ml	10 ml/6–12

[a] Extremes of dosage and duration are dependent on severity of bleeding disorder.
[b] Treatment of congenital clotting disorders can be managed by the internist in an emergency situation. However, the pre- and postoperative management of these patients should be left to the physician experienced in their care. Lower dosage is indicated for minor hemarthroses. Higher dosage should be given for head or neck injury or CNS bleeding. Intermediate dosage is adequate therapy for severe joint or muscle hemorrhage and gastrointestinal bleeding.
[c] VIII:C = Factor VIII procoagulant activity; VIII:VWF = Factor VIII von Willebrand's factor.
[d] Cryoprecipitate is the preferred component for von Willebrand's disease. In the treatment of mucosal hemorrhage, more frequent dosing intervals may be necessary to maintain a normal template bleeding time.

and 18–24 hours for factor IX. The calculation of dosage and planning of treatment schedules should be carried out in collaboration with the hematology consultant and should take into account the patient's plasma volume (~40 ml/kg), the percent of normal clotting factor desired to control or prevent bleeding, the half-life of the transfused factor, and the concentration of clotting factor in the replacement product. The in vivo recovery and survival of a test dose of clotting factor should be determined prior to surgery, and these studies should be repeated at regular intervals during prolonged periods of postoperative replacement.

Hemophiliacs with moderate or mild factor VIII deficiency may show as much as a 2-to 3-fold rise in baseline factor VIII levels following the intravenous infusion of desmopressin acetate (DDAVP). The maximum increase occurs immediately at the end of the infusion and is transient. Tachyphylaxis may occur when more than two doses are given within a 24-hour period. This form of therapy is feasible only for minor surgical procedures and dental extractions; however, it spares the patient with moderate or mild hemophilia the exposure to plasma components with their potential for transmission of viral infections. A test infusion of DDAVP with measurement of preinfusion and postinfusion factor VIII levels should be completed at least 7 days prior to the minor procedure to confirm a rise in factor VIII level.

Von Willebrand's disease (VWD) produces a combined deficiency of factor VIII clotting activity and the factor VIII von Willebrand factor (VWF), which is necessary for normal platelet adhesion to vascular subendothelium. Thus, both a mildly prolonged aPTT and a prolonged template bleeding time are characteristic of most cases of this disorder. Several variants of the disease have been described, including cases in which the factor VIII von Willebrand protein is dysfunctional rather than deficient.

Experience has shown that the control of surgical bleeding in patients with VWD is, in general, more dependent on achieving normal levels of factor VIII clotting factor activity than on correcting the prolonged bleeding time. On the other hand, arrest of bleeding from mucosal surfaces appears to require at least temporary elevation of the factor VIII VWF concentration and the accompanying correction of the bleeding time. **Cryoprecipitate,** but not factor VIII concentrate, is enriched in the higher-molecular-weight forms of factor VIII VWF and is, therefore, the **therapy of choice** for patients with VWD who are undergoing major surgical procedures.

Patients with this disorder may also respond to intravenous infusion of DDAVP with an increase in factor VIII clotting factor activity with or without a rise in factor VIII VWF. If a test infusion confirms an adequate rise in factor VIII levels with DDAVP, this drug can be used for transient augmentation of factor VIII in preparation for minor surgery. Patients with variant VWD may show no response (Type III, severe homozygous form) or may develop severe thrombocytopenia (Type IIB) after DDAVP infusion; therefore, this form of therapy should be reserved for the management of Types I and IIA VWD.

Management of Acquired Clotting Factor Disorders

An acquired coagulopathy may be discovered during preoperative evaluation (history, exam and/or lab screening), in which case the goal should be to make the correct diagnosis and, if possible, to reverse the abnormality prior to surgery. More commonly, acquired clotting factor deficiency may develop in the postoperative period, especially if surgery or recovery are complicated by hypotension, infection, poor nutrition, or massive blood transfusion. Acquired coagulopathies usually involve deficiencies of more than one clotting factor, and the correct diagnosis is suggested by the clinical setting combined with the pattern of screening laboratory tests (Table 14.9).

Vitamin K deficiency is a very common problem, particularly in the ill postoperative patient. Body stores of vitamin K are limited, and a deficiency state may develop as quickly as 1–3 weeks in the following situations: *(a)* prolonged inadequate oral intake of food in combination with antibiotic therapy, especially when the gut flora responsible for vitamin K_2 synthesis are eliminated; *(b)* intestinal malabsorption; and *(c)* oral anticoagulant therapy.

Vitamin K absorption depends on fat absorption, and conditions such as celiac disease, biliary tract obstruction, pancreatitis, regional enteritis and cholestyramine therapy can result in the deficiency state. Broad-spectrum antibiotics, especially neomycin and certain cephalosporins, such as cefamandole, cefoperazone and moxalactam, can promptly interfere with the normal synthesis of the vitamin K dependent clotting factors (II, VII, IX and X). Early in the course of vitamin K deficiency, only the prothrombin time is prolonged, but with time, the aPTT also becomes abnormal.

Correction of this coagulopathy is dependent upon the urgency of the clinical situation. If bleeding is absent or surgery is elective, Vitamin K_1 (Aquamephyton) can be given subcutaneously, intramuscularly, or intravenously in doses of 10–20 mg. Intravenous administration should be avoided if possible since it has been occasionally associated with anaphylactic reactions. If vitamin K_1 must be given intravenously, it should be diluted with saline or dextrose and given at a rate not to exceed 1 mg/min. Vitamin K_1 requires 10–12 hours for correction of the abnormal clotting tests. Response to therapy should always be confirmed by repeating the prothrombin time. If the prothrombin time is not satisfactorily shortened within 24 hours, the dose may be repeated, but failure to correct the prothrombin time within this time period usually signifies the presence of hepatocellular disease or concomitant non-vitamin K dependent coagulation factor deficiencies.

In patients who have serious bleeding or in those who require urgent surgery, fresh frozen plasma at 10–20 ml/kg will immediately replace vitamin K dependent clotting factors (Table 14.10). Vitamin K_1 at a dose of 20 mg should be given concurrently with the administration of fresh frozen plasma. Fresh frozen plasma will also rapidly reverse the anticoagulant effect of coumarin drugs and is the treatment of choice when emergency surgery is required in a patient on chronic warfarin therapy.

If parenteral hyperalimentation is being administered, vitamin K_1 should be given prophylactically at a dose of 10 mg once weekly. It is also recommended that vitamin K_1 be given prophylactically prior to initiation of antibiotic therapy with third generation cephalosporins and at least once weekly during therapy.

Liver disease is one of the commonest causes of an acquired coagulation disorder. These patients pose complex problems since multiple factors contribute to their hemostatic defects. There is defective synthesis of factors II (prothrombin), VII, IX, and X, which are the vitamin K-dependent clotting factors, and also factor V, when liver disease is more severe. In very severe liver disease, there is deficient, and rarely, defective synthesis of fibrinogen. These patients also may be thrombocytopenic, particularly when portal hypertension leads to splenomegaly and splenic pooling of platelets. In addition, there is an increase in the fibrinolytic activity because the liver is the site of synthesis of antiplasmin and the site of clearance of plasminogen activators. The contribution of each of these factors differs depending on the associated clinical circumstances. However, defective coagulation factor synthesis is usually the most important and the most common. In patients with liver disease, it is common to have both a prolonged aPTT and prothrombin time. In severe liver disease, the plasma fibrinogen level may be low and the thrombin time prolonged.

In managing these patients preoperatively or before a lesser procedure such as a liver biopsy, infusion of fresh frozen plasma should be given until the coagulation studies return to normal. Vitamin K_1 therapy is ineffective since the liver is incapable of producing the vitamin K-dependent factors, but should be administered because vitamin K deficiency due to malabsorption or inadequate intake may accompany liver disease. Infusion of prothrombin complex concentrates should be avoided since it may precipitate intravascular clotting (Table 14.10). A template bleeding time should also be performed prior to any surgical procedure, since a qualitative platelet abnormality may coexist. Unfortunately, complete correction of the coagulation and platelet abnormalities associated with liver disease is not always possible.

Disseminated intravascular coagulation (DIC) represents the consumption of coagulation factors following the intravascular activation of coagulation during the course of a serious underlying condition. This disorder should be thought of as a syndrome and as a complication of a number of clinical disorders. Common triggers for DIC are listed in Table 14.11.

The clinical manifestations of disseminated intravascular coagulation are variable and may range from an acute onset with shock, generalized bleeding from multiple sites and organ damage from ischemia, to being asymptomatic and running a chronic or subacute course. The diagnosis of disseminated intravascular coagulation is confirmed by demonstrating the consumption of prothrombin, factor V, factor VIII, fibrinogen, and platelets. The abnormalities of coagulation factors and platelets are reflected by a prolonged prothrombin time, partial thromboplastin time, and thrombin time,

Table 14.11. Conditions Triggering DIC

Acute DIC
  Bacterial or fungal sepsis
  Shock
  Obstetrical emergencies
      Abruptio placenta
      Amniotic fluid embolism
  Burns
  Severe trauma
  Heat stroke
  Aortic aneurysm (localized consumption)
  Acute pulmonary embolism (localized consumption)
  Adult respiratory distress syndrome
  Promyelocytic leukemia
  Acute hemolytic transfusion reaction
  Viremia
  Rocky Mountain Spotted Fever
  Snakebite
Chronic DIC
  Visceral malignancies (especially mucin positive carcinomas)
  Large arteriovenous malformations; hemangiomas
  Obstetrical problems
      Toxemia
      Retained dead fetus
  Malignant hypertension
  Hepatic cirrhosis

and by the presence of thrombocytopenia and fibrin degradation products.

It is important to understand that not all of the coagulation factors that are consumed during the coagulation process are necessarily depressed below normal limits in individual patients with disseminated intravascular coagulation. This occurs because the initial concentration and the rates of regeneration of these clotting factors vary from individual to individual. Since fibrinogen is an acute phase reactant, it may be elevated before the onset of intravascular coagulation. Although it will be consumed, the fibrinogen level may be normal and therefore there is only a relative decrease in the fibrinogen level. This is also true for platelets, factor V, and factor VIII. Therefore, the routine screening tests of the prothrombin time, partial thromboplastin time, and the platelet count may be normal early in the course of DIC and especially if thrombosis is the only clinical manifestation of the syndrome. However, the fibrin split products should be present, and the thrombin time will usually be prolonged (Table 14.9).

The first approach to the management of the patient with intravascular coagulation is to identify and reverse, if possible, the underlying disorder. Intravascular coagulation associated with placental separation or with fetal death should be treated by removal of the uterine contents. In a patient with septicemia, appropriate antibiotic therapy is the initial requirement. Every effort should be made to reverse shock with replacement of fluids and maintenance of adequate blood pressure to prevent vasoconstriction, venous stasis, acidosis, and hypoxemia.

Even with meticulous attention to the appropriate medical problems, there is a population of patients in whom the underlying disorder causing the intravascular coagulation cannot be reversed. The **initial management of patients with DIC** is based primarily on whether the patient with intravascular coagulation has bleeding, organ dysfunction due to thrombi, or both.

If bleeding is the only problem, then the appropriate clotting factors need to be replaced. If thromboembolic phenomena are present, heparin therapy is indicated. Fortunately, the need to use heparin is rare. If simultaneous bleeding and clotting are present, then the use of heparin requires careful strategy.

Heparin will inhibit intravascular clotting and permit improvement of the clotting factor levels. However, bleeding is frequently enhanced by heparin alone, and it is imperative to initially administer platelets if the platelet count is significantly low (usually between 20,000–50,000/mm^3, and to replace the consumable clotting factors specifically factor VIII and fibrinogen, if the fibrinogen level is less than 100 mg/dl.

A reasonable initial dosage of platelets in adults is 8–10 units. Consumable factors can be replaced with fresh frozen plasma (prothrombin and factor V) and cryoprecipitate (fibrinogen and factor VIII). Fresh frozen plasma can be given at a dosage of 10 ml/kg. The dosage of cryoprecipitate to restore the fibrinogen and factor VIII to adequate levels is empiric; an initial trial of 0.1 bags/kg should be given to the adult. Fresh frozen plasma and cryoprecipitate can be repeated every 12–24 hours if necessary, as indicated by serial aPTT and fibrinogen levels.

After the fibrinogen level and platelet count have been restored to safe levels, heparin therapy can be initiated if thrombosis is documented. Heparin at 100 units/kg of body weight should be given initially as a bolus, followed by 10 units/kg/hr by constant intravenous infusion. The loading dose of heparin should be eliminated if bleeding is apparent. Significantly smaller doses of heparin should be used in the presence of thrombocytopenia since heparinization under this circumstance puts the patient at a very high risk for dangerous hemorrhage.

The best index of hemostatic effectiveness is cessation or reduction of bleeding. **The most sensitive laboratory indicator of response to heparinization is a rise in the level of fibrinogen.** In the responsive patient, the level of fibrinogen returns toward normal within 24–48 hours, and the platelet count rises more slowly. A reduction in the fibrin degradation products may be delayed but provides evidence that intravascular fibrinolysis has been interrupted. The other coagulation abnormalities revert to normal more slowly. These tests are less sensitive indicators in following the intravascular clotting process.

The use of the fibrinolytic inhibitor, epsilon-aminocaproic acid (ϵ-ACA), is rarely indicated in the treatment of intravascular coagulation. The only clinical condition in which the use of this drug should be considered occurs when excessive fibrinolytic activity exists following prostatectomy or in patients with a prostatic carcinoma. In this situation, adequate heparinization must be accomplished before the use of ϵ-ACA, since its use alone could produce a disastrous thrombotic tendency.

Massive Transfusion Syndrome (refer to section on The Transfused Patient, page 317).

Circulating anticoagulants develop in a variety of clinical situations, including hemophiliacs receiving clotting factor replacement, some postpartum women, patients with autoimmune disorders and drug reactions, and occasionally in otherwise healthy, elderly patients with no apparent underlying disease. The clue to the presence of a circulating anticoagulant is the failure to correct the abnormal clotting test when repeated, using a mixture of the patient's plasma and normal plasma. Inhibitors to all of the clotting factors have been described; however, those directed against factor VIII and the lupus anticoagulant are most common. The patient with a factor VIII inhibitor usually has a severe hemorrhagic tendency. The control of bleeding in these patients is very difficult. Elective surgery is contraindicated in patients with coagulation factor inhibitors, and specialized laboratory investigations and therapeutic maneuvers are required in the management of these patients.

On the other hand, a bleeding tendency does not usually accompany patients with the lupus anticoagulant unless thrombocytopenia or low prothrombin levels are also present. Surgery can be performed without the fear of excessive bleeding in the absence of these deficiencies. The lupus anticoagulant is a spontaneously acquired antibody that may appear during the course of SLE or other autoimmune diseases, malignancies, therapy with drugs, such as chlorpromazine, hydralazine and procainamide, and also in patients with no apparent underlying disease. This "anticoagulant" interferes with in vitro clotting tests and prolongs the partial thromboplastin time, and occasionally the prothrombin time, but, paradoxically, has been shown to be associated with an increased risk of thrombosis (see "Hypercoagulable States").

HYPERCOAGULABLE STATES

The term "hypercoagulable state" refers to a number of conditions which may predispose an individual to inappropriate and excessive thrombosis (27). This enhanced tendency to form blood clots may be acquired during the course of an illness that causes alterations in coagulation factors, platelet function, blood vessels, or blood flow properties (Table 14.12). Alternatively, it may be the result of a congenital deficiency of one of the naturally occurring plasma anticoagulants or fibrinolytic proteins, which under normal circumstances limit the extent of thrombus formation following vascular injury.

Table 14.12. Risk Factors for Thromboembolism

Secondary Risk Factors
  Advancing age
  Obesity
  Immobilization
  Prior thromboembolism
  Stasis (CHF, myocardial infarction, cardiomyopathy, constrictive pericarditis, anasarca, venous insufficiency)
  Estrogen therapy
  Malignancy
  Nephrotic syndrome
  Hyperviscosity (erythrocytosis, paraproteinemia)
  Paroxysmal nocturnal hemoglobinuria
  Myeloproliferative disorders
  Inflammatory bowel disease
  Diabetes Mellitus
  Artificial surfaces (cardiac valves, vascular grafts)
  Postoperative state
Primary Risk Factors
  Antithrombin III Deficiency
  Protein C Deficiency
  Protein S Deficiency
  Dysfibrinogenemia
  Disorders of Fibrinolysis
  Lupus Anticoagulant

(Modified from Schafer AI: The Hypercoagulable States. *Ann Int Med* 102:814–828, 1985.)

Diagnostic Approach

The **preoperative assessment of thromboembolic risk begins with the history,** which should identify factors known to be associated with an increased thrombotic tendency in the postoperative period. These include advanced age, obesity, past history of repeated thromboembolism, venous insufficiency, estrogen therapy, malignancy and medical illnesses, such as congestive heart failure. Even in the absence of clearly defined predisposing factors, patients undergoing surgical procedures such as orthopedic, abdominal, urologic, gynecologic, and neurosurgical operations are at substantially increased risk of developing deep venous thrombosis and pulmonary embolism.

Certain historical findings suggest the possibility of a primary hypercoagulable state due to a congenital deficiency or abnormality of one of the naturally occurring anticoagulants or fibrinolytic enzymes. These include: (a) family history of repeated thrombosis, especially occurring at a young age; (b) history of recurrent thrombosis without precipitating factors; (c) history of thrombosis occurring in adolescence or early adulthood; (d) history of clot formation in unusual anatomic locations (mesenteric or hepatic veins); and (e) history of resistance to heparin anticoagulation. Evaluation for these primary conditions requires access to a laboratory that can provide assays for antithrombin III, proteins C and S, and the lupus anticoagulant. Rarely, studies to exclude abnormalities in the fibrinolytic system or abnormal fibrinogens may also be necessary.

The clinical expression and mode of inheritance of deficiency of antithrombin III, the major physiologic antagonist of thrombin and other activated clotting factors, is the prototype of the primary hypercoagulable states. Typically, a quantitative or qualitative abnormality in the antithrombin III molecule is inherited in an autosomal dominant fashion. Patients frequently develop venous thrombosis and/or pulmonary embolism first in adolescence or young adulthood, but they may also present with thrombosis in unusual anatomic locations. Most symptomatic heterozygotes have antithrombin III levels of 30–50% of normal and the severity of disease expression may vary considerably within affected families. Patients with a deficiency of protein C (inactivator of activated coagulation factors VIII and V) or protein S (a cofactor for protein C) appear to have a similar clinical presentation and mode of inheritance as antithrombin III deficiency. Both proteins C and S are vitamin K-dependent proteins.

Risk Reduction and Treatment

Prior to elective surgery, an attempt should be made to eliminate any reversible causes of hypercoagulability. For example, oral contraceptives should be discontinued several weeks before the elective procedure. The treatment of congestive heart failure and other edematous states should be maximized. Hyperviscosity from increased red blood cell mass (erythrocytosis) or increased serum paraprotein concentrations (macroglobulinemia and other plasma cell dyscrasias) should be corrected with phlebotomy and plasmapheresis, respectively.

Available data support the use of **prophylactic subcutaneous heparin** (5,000 units subcutaneously every 8 or 12 hours) in patients at high risk for thrombosis who are to undergo general surgical, urologic, or gynecologic procedures. This therapy is begun 2 hours before surgery and continued at least until the patient is ambulatory. The aPTT usually remains normal during low-dose subcutaneous heparin therapy. Intravenous dextran is an alternative agent, which may also provide antithrombotic prophylaxis in these settings.

Both prophylactic heparin and dextran increase the risk of bleeding and hematoma formation at the operative site, but the risk of life-threatening bleeding complications from these agents is minimal. Low-dose heparin has not been shown to provide effective prophylaxis in orthopedic patients and is considered contraindicated in patients undergoing neurosurgical operations for intracranial or spinal lesions. For orthopedic patients, dextran, low-dose warfarin or adjusted-dose heparin may provide adequate prophylaxis. Such physical measures as gradient compression stockings, early ambulation, and physical therapy are important antithrombotic adjuncts for surgical patients in general and should not be overlooked.

The perioperative management of patients with one of the primary hypercoagulable states, such an antithrombin III deficiency, protein C or S deficiency, and the lupus anticoagulant, should be carried out in conjunction with a specialist who is familiar with the treatment of these fairly uncommon disorders. As with all surgical patients, risk factors such as obesity, pregnancy, immobilization, and estrogen-containing medication will further increase the potential for thrombosis in these individuals. Prophylactic replacement of antithrombin III with fresh frozen plasma or commercially prepared antithrombin III concentrate, with or without low-dose heparin therapy, is recommended for surgical patients with congenital deficiency of this important protein. Fresh frozen plasma and commercially available prothrombin complex concentrates are sources of proteins C and S, which can be used for replacement therapy. Prothrombin complex concentrate therapy, however, carries a substantial risk of transmitting viral hepatitis and has, by itself, been occasionally associated with thrombotic manifestations. Patients with congenital deficiency of antithrombin III and proteins C and S will usually require chronic, long-term anticoagulation with warfarin.

The lupus anticoagulant may disappear during treatment of the underlying condition or with corticosteroid therapy. If emergency surgery is required in such a patient, low-dose heparin prophylaxis should be considered, and measures such as early ambulation and gradient compression stockings emphasized.

MANAGEMENT OF PLATELET DISORDERS IN THE SURGICAL PATIENT

Preoperative Diagnostic Studies

Platelets arrest bleeding from small vessels by forming a plug at the site of vascular damage within 2–10 minutes of injury. To succeed in this process, platelets must circulate at a minimum concentration of $100,000/ml^3$ and must function normally. **The template bleeding time reflects the adequacy of platelet number and function.**

Some authors have proposed that a bleeding time should be done on all surgical candidates as part of the preoperative screen for hemostatic defects. In a retrospective study of preoperative bleeding time done at a single institution, Barber et al. found that 110 of 1,941 routine preoperative bleeding times were prolonged. However, in approximately 75% of these patients, the abnormality could have been predicted since there was a recorded history of recent ingestion of aspirin or nonsteroidal anti-inflammatory drugs, azotemia, or thrombocytopenia. Furthermore, an isolated, prolonged bleeding time did not always correlate with the degree of surgical bleeding (31).

It seems most reasonable to perform **preoperative bleeding times on selected patients at high risk** for surgical bleeding as identified by a careful history (Table 14.5), together with information regarding the type of surgery planned. Neurosurgical procedures and cardiopulmonary bypass are examples of operations that require careful preoperative screening for bleeding disorders.

Thrombocytopenia

As the platelet count decreases below 100,000/mm³, there is a proportional increase in the template bleeding time and an increase in the risk of surgical bleeding. It is unusual for bleeding to occur after surgery or injury when the platelet count is above 75,000/mm³ if platelet function is normal. Spontaneous bleeding may occur when the platelet count is between 10,000–20,000/mm³. However, it is not only the absolute number of platelets but the underlying process causing the thrombocytopenia, the presence or absence of other hemostatic defects, the duration of thrombocytopenia, and any coexisting qualitative platelet abnormalities, that must also be considered. For example, patients with autoimmune thrombocytopenia have platelets that appear to be hemostatically more active, and life-threatening bleeding is unusual in this disorder, even with platelet counts below 10,000/mm³ (Fig. 14.4).

Minor procedures involving surgical sites that are easily visualized can usually be safely performed when the platelet count is only moderately reduced (platelet counts above 50,000/mm³). Below this count, hemorrhage is more likely, and major elective procedures should be deferred until a higher platelet count is achieved. Prior to emergency surgery, every attempt should be made to obtain a platelet count of 50–80,000/mm³ or higher.

Thrombocytopenia in the adult patient is usually acquired by one of four mechanisms: (a) decreased or ineffective platelet production; (b) increased platelet destruction; (c) abnormal platelet distribution; and (d) platelet dilution. Specific causes for each mechanism are shown in Table 14.13.

Decreased platelet production occurs with systemic infection (especially

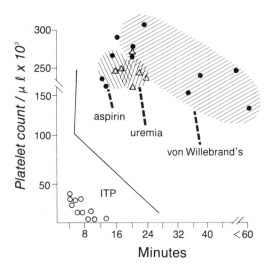

Figure 14.4. Relationship of Template Bleeding Time to Platelet Count. (Modified from Harker LA: *Hemostasis Manual*, 2nd ed. Philadelphia, F.A. Davis Company, 1974, page 9.)

viral), B12 and folate deficiencies, various drugs, chemotherapy and bone marrow involvement by fibrosis, infection, or malignancy. It may be part of bone marrow

Table 14.13. Causes of Thrombocytopenia

Decreased or ineffective production
 Drugs (e.g., ethanol, thiazides, anticonvulsants)
 Viral infection
 B12 and folic acid deficiency
 Aplastic anemia, hematologic malignancy
 Myelophthisis (fibrosis, granulomas, cancer)
 Chemotherapy
 Radiation
Increased platelet destruction
 Drug-induced immune thrombocytopenia
  heparin, quinidine and quinine, thiazides, gold, imipramine, phenothiazines, sulfonamides, penicillins, cephalosporins, digitoxin, chlorpromamide
 Autoimmune thrombocytopenia (ITP, SLE and other autoimmune disorders, carcinoma)
 Immune complex mediated thrombocytopenia
  sepsis, bacterial endocarditis, intravenous drug abuse, post-transfusion purpura, AIDS
 DIC and TTP
 Mechanical (e.g., prosthetic heart valves, grafts)
Abnormal platelet distribution or dilution
 Hypersplenism
 Massive transfusion syndrome

aplasia affecting all cell lines or, less commonly, can be seen as an isolated deficiency of platelet production. Drugs that inhibit platelet production include agents such as ethanol, thiazides, and anticonvulsants. A bone marrow aspirate showing severely reduced or absent megakaryocytes confirms this diagnosis.

Treatment or prevention of serious hemorrhage is with platelet concentrates. Usually 6–8 units of platelet concentrates are infused, and platelet counts are obtained 1 and 12 hours post-infusion to estimate platelet recovery and survival. When patients have been alloimmunized by prior transfusions or pregnancies, random donor platelets may be ineffective. Platelets obtained from relatives or from HLA-matched donors may be required for these patients.

Increased platelet destruction is the most common mechanism responsible for acquired thrombocytopenia in general clinical practice. Severe thrombocytopenia with a bone marrow aspirate showing abundant megakaryocytes and no other abnormality is consistent with platelet destruction in the circulation. Drug-associated immune thrombocytopenia occurs with some of the most commonly prescribed medications (Table 14.13).

There has been a recent awareness of the syndrome of immune-mediated **thrombocytopenia associated with heparin,** which can occur in as many as 10% of patients receiving heparin by any route or dosage schedule. In patients who have previously received heparin, thrombocytopenia may develop as early as 2 days after initiating therapy. These patients are not only at increased risk for bleeding, but paradoxically, may develop fatal arterial, or rarely, venous thrombosis. The heparinized patient should be monitored for the development of thrombocytopenia, and if a falling platelet count cannot be explained by other causes, heparin must be discontinued in favor of other methods of anticoagulation. Dextran, warfarin, or fibrinolytic therapy may be substituted for heparin depending on the clinical situation.

Autoimmune thrombocytopenic purpura is a form of destructive thrombocytopenia caused by the spontaneous development of an IgG antibody directed against the host's platelets. It is frequently idiopathic in nature (ITP) but may be secondary to other diseases, such as lymphoid malignancies and systemic autoimmune disorders. The initial approach to treatment is with several weeks of oral corticosteroids in high dosage (equivalent of prednisone, 1–2 mg/kg). However, the majority of adult patients with autoimmune thrombocytopenia will fail to achieve a lasting remission when steroid doses are tapered, and **splenectomy is frequently necessary.** A significant improvement in platelet count during corticosteroid treatment seems to be predictive of the ability to achieve a complete remission with splenectomy if this procedure is subsequently required. Because of the potential of adrenal suppression from chronic steroid use and in order to maintain the highest possible platelet count, corticosteroids should be continued throughout the pre- and postoperative periods.

Patients with autoimmune thrombocytopenia who fail to respond to corticosteroids require splenectomy at a time when they are severely thrombocytopenic and generally unresponsive to platelet transfusion. Intraoperative and postoperative bleeding is usually surprisingly mild in these patients. Once the splenic pedicle is clamped, the platelet count frequently rises spontaneously. If thrombocytopenia persists and bleeding occurs, platelet transfusion and steroid therapy may be somewhat more effective after splenectomy.

Three patterns of response to splenectomy are recognized. Approximately 70–75% of patients achieve a complete remission, and platelet counts rise sharply in the first 1–2 weeks after surgery. Another 20% have improvement in platelet counts to a hemostatically safe, although not normal, level. The remaining 5–10% remain severely thrombocytopenic and require other treatment modalities for refractory ITP including treatment with danazol, high-dose intravenous gamma-globulin (IgG) or immunosuppressive agents (33).

Other forms of destructive thrombocytopenia include immune-complex mediated thrombocytopenia associated with sepsis, bacterial endocarditis, intravenous drug abuse, post-transfusion purpura, and the acquired immunodeficiency syndrome. Thrombin-induced platelet consumption occurs in DIC (see section "Management of Coagulation Factor Disorders in the Surgical Patient"). The constellation of intravascular platelet consumption, hemolytic anemia, fever, renal dysfunction, and CNS abnormalities constitute the pentad of findings diagnostic of thrombotic thrombocytopenic purpura. Recognition of this syndrome is important since treatment with plasma infusions and/or plasma exchange may be lifesaving.

Abnormal platelet distribution and platelet dilution occur commonly with hypersplenism and the massive transfusion syndrome, respectively. (Refer to discussion of splenomegaly and the massive transfusion syndrome.)

Qualitative Platelet Dysfunction

A prolonged bleeding time with a normal or near normal platelet count indicates abnormal platelet function. The hemostatic history will often detect these functional platelet disorders preoperatively and help determine whether the abnormality is congenital or acquired.

Patients with **congenital platelet dysfunction** give a longstanding history of bruising and mucosal bleeding that may be exacerbated by the use of antiplatelet drugs. These drugs are also an important cause of acquired platelet dysfunction, and a history of their use within 1–2 weeks of preoperative evaluation should be sought.

Von Willebrand's disease is a hereditary disorder in which the platelets fail to adhere to the vascular subendothelium. This abnormality is not intrinsic to the platelet but is caused by a deficiency of plasma factor VIII von Willebrand factor, which is corrected by cryoprecipitate (see p. 332). Hereditary defects of platelet function are relatively common causes of mild bleeding disorders, especially in women. A family history is often positive for mucosal or skin bleeding and menorrhagia. These patients should be evaluated preoperatively with platelet aggregation studies and studies to exclude von Willebrand's disease. These qualitative platelet disorders are often poorly characterized, but the platelet release type defect is the most common of these disorders. If a platelet release type defect is confirmed by platelet aggregation testing, preoperative therapy with prednisone will frequently decrease the bleeding time to normal or near normal. If prednisone is ineffective, DDAVP may be beneficial (42). Platelet transfusions are indicated if excessive bleeding occurs during surgery. As in the management of all hemostatic disorders, close communication between the internist and surgeon are important to ensure patient safety.

Acquired platelet dysfunction (Table 14.14) occurs most commonly with aspirin and other nonsteroidal anti-inflammatory drugs, which inhibit platelet cyclooxygenase, a key enzyme required for normal platelet aggregation. The duration of antiplatelet effect varies among these agents. Aspirin irreversibly acetylates cyclooxygenase resulting in an antiplatelet effect lasting for up to 1 week. Other nonsteroidal drugs have antiplatelet effects lasting less than 24 hours. Penicillins, especially carbenicillin, and the third generation cephalosporin, moxalactam, causes a dose-related prolongation of the bleeding time and may produce a bleeding diathesis, especially in patients with renal insufficiency. The antiplatelet effect persists as long as 4–5 days after

Table 14.14. Causes of Acquired Platelet Dysfunction

Drugs
  (aspirin and other nonsteroidal anti-inflammatory drugs, dipyridamole, carbenicillin and other penicillins, moxalactam, clofibrate, dextran, hydroxychloroquine)
Uremia
Cirrhosis
Ethanol
Platelet dyspoiesis
  (leukemia, myeloproliferative syndrome, myelodysplastic syndrome)
Paraproteinemias
  (multiple myeloma, Waldenstrom's macroglobulinemia)
Cardiopulmonary bypass
Fibrin degradation products
  (DIC, fibronolytic therapy)

these drugs are stopped. In addition to discontinuation of the drug, serious bleeding due to drug-induced platelet dysfunction should be treated with platelet transfusion.

Acquired defects in platelet function can accompany several types of systemic illnesses. The hemorrhagic tendency associated with uremia seems to parallel the progressive loss of renal function and may relate to the kidney's failure to clear metabolic products. Partial or complete correction of the bleeding tendency in uremia has been reported following both peritoneal and hemodialysis, cryoprecipitate infusion, intravenous DDAVP and estrogen therapy. The shortening of the bleeding time is transient after DDAVP infusion, lasting only approximately 6 hours (41). Cryoprecipitate (10 bags infused over 30 min) may shorten the bleeding time. The maximum shortening of the bleeding time occurs between 1 and 12 hours after the cryoprecipitate infusion and usually returns to pretreatment levels by 24 hours. It is clear that responses to these treatments are variable from patient to patient, and frequently all modalities must be utilized to prepare a patient for an invasive procedure or to treat established bleeding. A repeat bleeding time should

be performed prior to the procedure to document the efficacy of the therapy.

Platelet dysfunction is also seen in paraproteinemic states such as multiple myeloma, in myeloproliferative diseases, DIC, and hepatic cirrhosis. Response to platelet transfusion may be less than optimum in these conditions, and treatment of the primary disease process is an important aspect of management. Alkylating agents may correct the qualitative platelet abnormality in myeloproliferative syndromes. DDAVP can occasionally shorten the bleeding time in patients with cirrhosis (43). Plasmapheresis will remove paraproteins and correct the bleeding time prolongation due to these abnormal globulins.

Several studies have implicated acquired platelet defects as the major hemostatic abnormality that occurs during cardiopulmonary bypass (see "Hemostatic Problems in Cardiac Surgery").

Thrombocytosis

A platelet count in excess of 400,000/mm^3 is encountered in a variety of clinical circumstances. The problem arises as to whether the thrombocytosis reflects a primary marrow disorder, that is, a myeloproliferative disorder, or is secondary to an underlying disease, i.e., secondary or reactive thrombocytosis. A clear-cut distinction may be difficult, but because of the prognostic implications, a differentiation is essential.

Secondary thrombocytosis occurs in various clinical conditions, including malignancy, infections, rheumatoid arthritis, other collagen vascular disorders, iron deficiency anemia, inflammatory bowel disease, and the postsplenectomy state. The platelets in these disorders function normally. These patients are usually not at increased risk for thromboembolic phenomenon, even with platelet counts in excess of 1,000,000/mm^3.

The platelets in patients with myeloproliferative disorders (polycythemia vera, essential thrombocythemia, and myelofibrosis) can be hyperaggregable, hypoactive, or normal. These patients are at substantial risk for thromboembolic phenomena and/or bleeding. Surgery poses an increased risk in these individuals until normal platelet function can be established, and the platelet number is reduced.

A template bleeding time should be performed on all preoperative patients with thrombocytosis due to a myeloproliferative disorder. The template bleeding time may be prolonged or normal in these patients. If the template bleeding time is prolonged, then platelet dysfunction is present and abnormal bleeding can be expected.

The preoperative approach to the patient with thrombocytosis due to a myeloproliferative disorder is dependent upon the platelet count and the urgency of surgery. A platelet count in excess of 1,000,000/mm^3 should be reduced. Busulfan or hydroxyurea will reduce the platelet count over several weeks to months. Nitrogen mustard and plateletpheresis will reduce the platelet count within 7–10 days. If surgery is emergent, then plateletpheresis should be instituted immediately, and nitrogen mustard can be given concomitantly to reduce the megakaryocytic mass. It is crucial to reduce the platelet count to normal or near normal levels in these patients since life-threatening thromboembolic phenomena or hemorrhage can occur.

SPECIAL HEMATOLOGIC MANAGEMENT PROBLEMS IN THE SURGICAL PATIENT

Hemostatic Problems in Cardiac Surgery

The use of cardiopulmonary bypass (CPB) for cardiac surgery is a common procedure today. The patient who has undergone CPB surgery presents some unique management problems. The internist is often called on to evaluate these patients postoperatively because of bleeding. Prophylactic therapy to reduce bleeding is becoming an important aspect of care.

DIAGNOSTIC ACTIVITIES

Postoperative bleeding most commonly occurs from an open vessel, which may require reoperation. Occasionally, however, systemic bleeding occurs, which requires an accurate diagnosis for appropriate therapy.

The consulting internist needs to understand the complex hemostatic changes that occur during CPB surgery. The CPB procedure produces changes in the coagulation system, the fibrinolytic system, and in the quantity and quality of platelets. These changes are considered "physiologic" in patients undergoing CPB.

After initiation of cardiopulmonary bypass, there is a decrease in all clotting factors, antithrombin-III, platelets, and plasminogen due to hemodilution effect of priming the pump with 2 liters of crystalloid solution. By the end of CPB, most of these factor levels remain low, approximating 50% of baseline normal. For unknown reasons, factor V levels decrease markedly to less than 20% of baseline. Since a 30% level of most coagulation protein is adequate for hemostasis, it is difficult to attribute the bleeding that occurs to inadequate coagulation proteins; however, the low factor V level is an exception and may contribute to bleeding in an occasional patient. Measurement of the PT and aPTT will help determine the extent of the deficiencies. The low factor V level makes the use of fresh frozen plasma rational if the aPTT is prolonged. All coagulation factors return to baseline normal by 48 hours (49).

Heparin anticoagulation is necessary during cardiopulmonary bypass. Although its use is indispensable, it has given rise to abnormal bleeding during and after the surgical procedure. The etiology of such hemorrhage has been traced to administration of excessive heparin during surgery, failure of neutralization of the heparin by protamine sulfate at the end of surgery, and heparin rebound. Heparin rebound refers to the reappearance of hypocoagulability after adequate neutralization has been accomplished. A prolonged activated clotting time suggests excessive heparinization.

There is a significant decrease in the platelet count when patients are placed on the bypass machine, and this decrease persists for 48–96 hours postoperatively. It is unusual for the platelet count to decrease much below 80,000/mm^3, and therefore bleeding from thrombocytopenia as the sole mechanism is uncommon.

However, the bleeding time is often prolonged with a near normal platelet count, which substantiates a qualitative platelet defect. Thus, **loss of platelet function is the most significant hematologic consequence of CPB and is the main contributor to postoperative bleeding.** Several hypotheses have been proposed to explain this loss of platelet function: *(a)* the alteration of platelet membrane receptors during surface contact with oxygenator systems renders the platelets refractory to physical and chemical stimuli; and *(b)* the release and depletion of alpha granules causes a reduction in the platelet's ability to aggregate.

PROPHYLAXIS AND TREATMENT

Prophylactic treatment to prevent bleeding in patients undergoing cardiopulmonary bypass cardiac surgery has gained increased importance. In a randomized prospective double-blind study, the administration of DDAVP (0.3 μg/kg) after CPB significantly reduced blood loss during the operation and in the first 24 hours after CPB in **complicated cardiac operations** (valve replacement and repeat CABG). Patients undergoing uncomplicated coronary artery bypass graft surgery were not included in this study (49). This treatment appears to be highly effective in reducing bleeding after CPB in this setting and has not been associated with any significant complications.

The prophylactic use of platelet transfusions has been studied and shown to be ineffective.

Every attempt to identify the specific hemostatic defect(s) should be pursued if bleeding occurs after CPB, and specific therapy should be tailored to the defect(s). The **therapeutic modalities** available include the use of platelet concentrates, DDAVP, cryoprecipitate, and fresh frozen plasma. The preceding discussion regarding causes of bleeding makes the use of these products understandable.

The use of platelet concentrates is usually the first step in attempting to control bleeding if the PT, aPTT, and platelet count are normal, and the template bleeding time is prolonged. DDAVP has not been used as extensively once bleeding has occurred in this situation, but the use of this agent remains an important consideration. In the less common situation in which bleeding cannot be attributed to platelet dysfunction, fresh frozen plasma to replace factor V and cryoprecipitate to supplement factor VIII and fibrinogen can be given empirically. If bleeding fails to be controlled after a reasonable attempt with multiple products, **reoperation to explore for an open vessel** must occur.

Splenomegaly: Pre- and Postoperative Management

The preoperative management of a patient with marked splenomegaly requires an understanding of the hemodynamic and hematologic changes that occur with progressive splenic enlargement (50). With marked splenic enlargement from whatever cause, blood flow through the organ increases from a normal value of 5% to as much as 50% of the cardiac output. With massive splenomegaly, the splenic blood volume may increase, such that the spleen contains as much as 25% of the total blood volume. Blood flow through the portal system increases dramatically, and at the same time, blood is shunted away from other intravascular spaces including the renal circulation. This stimulates the renin-angiotensin-aldosterone system, causing retention of sodium and water. The patient with a massively enlarged spleen characteristically shows evidence of high cardiac output and wide pulse pressure on physical exam. Care must be exercised to avoid further volume expansion with vigorous hydration or rapid transfusion. Following surgical removal of the spleen, the expanded intravascular volume slowly returns to normal over several months.

Hypersplenism is a term used to describe the increased sequestration of the formed elements in the blood that occurs as the splenic blood pool enlarges. Anemia, neutropenia or thrombocytopenia may exist in any combination. The bone marrow compensates for the peripheral cytopenias by increasing its basal rate of blood cell production. The anemia seen with splenomegaly is a result of both hemodilution from the expanded blood volume and increased red blood cell trapping in the spleen.

The thrombocytopenia seen with hypersplenism is usually moderate in severity with platelet counts in the 30–50,000/mm^3 range. The markedly enlarged spleen may sequester as much as 90% of the total body pool of platelets. Transfused platelets are rapidly removed from the circulation in hypersplenic states. However, if bleeding is present, platelet transfusions should be given, since bleeding may respond even though a platelet increment cannot be achieved. When significant thrombocytopenia is present prior to splenectomy, the blood bank should be requested to have 10–20 units of platelet concentrates available for emergency use if excessive operative bleeding develops. Platelet transfusion will be more effective in raising the platelet count once the surgeon has clamped the splenic pedicle.

Following splenectomy for any cause, the platelet count commonly rises above 600,000/mm^3 and often exceeds 1 million/mm^3. **Post-splenectomy thrombocy-tosis** usually resolves within weeks to a few months after surgery; however, marked platelet count elevations may persist indefinitely in patients with underlying myeloproliferative disorders (e.g., chronic myelogenous leukemia, polycythemia vera, agnogenic myeloid metaplasia and essential thrombocythemia) and in individuals with acquired idiopathic sideroblastic anemia.

Thrombocytosis after splenectomy may be of such magnitude that the physician considers antithrombotic therapy as prophylaxis against thromboembolism. One study suggests that the incidence of thrombotic complications among patients with platelet counts above 1 million is not significantly different from those with normal platelet counts as long as patients with myeloproliferative disorders are excluded (51). Therefore, the routine use of aspirin or anticoagulants for prevention of post-splenectomy thrombosis in patients **without** myeloproliferative disorders cannot be substantiated. Furthermore, the use of antiplatelet drugs may enhance bleeding in patients with myeloproliferative disorders.

When splenectomy is performed on patients with myeloproliferative diseases, there is special danger because of excess production of platelets, which may also be qualitatively abnormal. Myelosuppressive therapy should be given preoperatively to normalize both the platelet count and the platelet function (see "Management of Thrombocytosis"). Even when this is done, however, an unexpected thrombocytosis may occur in these patients.

Asplenic adult patients are at increased risk of developing fulminant sepsis due primarily to encapsulated bacteria such as *Strep pneumoniae, Hemophilus influenzae,* and meningococcus. The risk appears to be greater for infants and young children, and the underlying cause for which the spleen is removed is also an important determinant of this complication. The incidence appears greatest in splenectomized patients with thalassemia or malignant hematologic disorders. The risk is greatest within 2–3 years of splenectomy but is present at a lower probability for several years thereafter. Mortality rates from postsplenectomy sepsis are as high as 50%; therefore, prophylactic immunization which pneumococcal vaccine, preferably several weeks before splenectomy, is of importance in preventing this complication. Also, patients must be counseled that fever and infection may indicate a life-threatening situation, and these symptoms should be reported to their physician immediately.

Hematologic Problems in Pregnancy

Discussed in Chapter 22.

READINGS

Preoperative Evaluation and Anesthesia

1. Kowalshyn TJ, Praeger D, Young J: A review of the present status of preoperative hemoglobin requirements. *Anesth Analg* 51:75–77, 1972 (with comments by Jacoby JA, pp 77–78, Jenkins MT, pp 78–79).
2. Gillies I: Anemia and anesthesia. *Br J Anaesth* 46:589–602, 1974.
3. Bayer WL, Coenen WM, Jenkins DC, et al.: The use of blood and blood components in 1,769 patients undergoing open-heart surgery. *Ann Thor Surg* 29:117–122, 1980.
4. Toy P, Strauss RG, Stehling LC, et al.: Predeposited autologous blood for elective surgery. *N Engl J Med* 316:517–520, 1987.
5. Eyster E, Bernene J: Nosocomial anemia. *JAMA* 223:73–74, 1973.
6. Searle J: Anaesthesia in sickle cell states. *Anaesthesia* 28:48–58, 1973.
7. Sears D: The morbidity of sickle cell trait. A review of the literature. *Am J Med* 64:1021–1036, 1978.
8. Alavi JB: Sickle cell anemia: Pathophysiology and treatment. *Med Clin North Am* 68:545–556, 1984.

The Transfused Patient

9. Goldfinger D: Acute hemolytic transfusion reactions: A fresh look at pathogenesis and considerations regarding therapy. *Transfusion* 17:85–98, 1977.
10. Pineda A, Taswell H, Brzica S: Delayed hemolytic transfusion reaction. An immunologic hazard of blood transfusion. *Transfusion* 18:1–7, 1978.
11. Collins J: Massive blood transfusion. *Clin Haematol* 5:201–222, 1976.

Immune Hemolytic Anemia

12. Pirofsky B: Immune hemolytic disease: The autoimmune hemolytic anemias. *Clin Haematol* 4:167–180, 1975.
13. Petz LD: Autoimmune hemolytic anemia: Transfusion in special situations. *Human Pathol* 14:251–255, 1983.
14. Diaz JH, Cooper ES, Ochsner JL: Cold hemagglutination pathophysiology: Evaluation and management of patients undergoing cardiac surgery with induced hypothermia. *Arch Intern Med* 144:1639–1641, 1984.

Polycythemia

15. Wasserman L, Gilbert H: Surgery in polycythemia vera. *N Engl J Med* 269:1226–1230, 1963.
16. Thomas D, Marshall J, Du Boulay GH, et al.: Cerebral blood-flow in polycythemia. *Lancet* 2:161–163, 1977.
17. York EL, Jones RL, Sproule BJ, et al.: Management of secondary polycythemia with hypoxic lung disease. *Am Heart J* 100:267–269, 1980.
18. Smith JR, Landaw SA: Smoker's polycythemia. *N Engl J Med* 298:6–10, 1978.

White Blood Cells

19. Strauss RG: Granulocyte transfusion therapy. *Clin Oncol* 2(3):635–655, 1983.

Hemostasis/Coagulopathy

20. Rapaport, SI: Preoperative hemostatic evaluation: Which tests, if any? *Blood* 61:229–231, 1983.
21. Ansell JE, Kumar R, Deykin D: The spectrum of vitamin K deficiency. *JAMA* 238:40–42, 1977.
22. Lechner K, Niessney H, Thaler E: Coagulation abnormalities in liver disease. *Semin Thromb Hemostasis* 4:40–56, 1977.
23. Cederbaum A, Blatt P, Roberts H: Intravascular coagulation with use of human prothrombin complex concentrates. *Ann Intern Med* 84:683–687, 1976.
24. Egan E, et al.: Effect of surgical operations on certain tests used to diagnose intravascular coagulation and fibrinolysis. *Mayo Clin Proc* 49:658–664, 1974.
25. Colman R, Robboy S: Postoperative disseminated intravascular coagulation and fibrinolysis. *Urol Clin North Am* 3:379–392, 1976.
26. Bussel JB: Circulating anticoagulants: Physiologic and pathophysiologic. *Hosp Prac* 18(2):169–186, 1983.

Hypercoagulability/Thrombosis

27. Schafer AI: The hypercoagulable states. *Ann Intern Med* 102:814–828, 1985.
28. Rodgers GM, Shuman MA: Congenital thrombotic disorders. *Am J Hematol* 21:419–430, 1986.
29. NIH Consensus Conference: Prevention of venous thrombosis and pulmonary embolism. *JAMA* 256:744–749, 1986.
30. Mueh J, Herbst K, Rapaport S: Thrombosis in

patients with the lupus anticoagulant. *Ann Intern Med* 92:156–159, 1980.

Evaluation/Management of Platelet Disorders

31. Barber A, Green D, Galluzzo T, et al.: The bleeding time as a preoperative screening test. *Am J Med* 78:761–764, 1985.
32. Lind SE: Prolonged bleeding time. *Am J Med* 77:305–312, 1984.
33. Karpatkin S: Autoimmune thrombocytopenic purpura. *Blood* 56:329–343, 1980.
34. Carr JM, Kruskall MS, Kaye JA, et al.: Efficacy of platelet transfusions in immune thrombocytopenia. *Am J Med* 80:1051–1054, 1986.
35. Kelton JG, Levine MN: Heparin-induced thrombocytopenia. *Sem Thromb Hemost* 12:59–62, 1986.
36. Poskitt TR, Poskitt PK: Thrombocytopenia of sepsis. The role of circulating IgG-containing immune complexes. *Arch Intern Med* 145:891–894, 1985.
37. Malpass TW, Harker LA: Acquired disorders of platelet function. *Sem Hematol* 17(4):242–258, 1980.
38. Sattler FR, Weitekamp MR, Ballard JO: Potential for bleeding with the new beta-lactam antibiotics. *Ann Intern Med* 105:924–931, 1986.
39. Davies D, Steward D: Unexpected excessive bleeding during operation: Role of acetylsalicyclic acid. *Can Anaesth Soc J* 24:452–458, 1977.
40. Mannucci PM, Remuzzi G, Pusineri F, et al.: Deamino-8-arginine vasopressin shortens the bleeding time in uremia. *N Engl J Med* 308:8–12, 1983.
41. Janson P, Jubelirer S, Weinstein M, et al.: Treatment of the bleeding tendency in uremia with cryoprecipitate. *N Engl J Med* 303:1318–1322, 1980.
42. Kobrinsky NL, Israels ED, Gerrard JM, et al.: Shortening of bleeding time by 1-deamino-8-D-arginine vasopressin in various bleeding disorders. *Lancet* 1:1145–1148, May, 1984.
43. Mannucci PM, Vicante V, Vianello L, et al.: Controlled trial of desmopressin in liver cirrhosis and other conditions associated with a prolonged bleeding time. *Blood* 67:1148–1153, 1986.
44. Kelton JG, Ali AM: Platelet Transfusions: A critical appraisal. *Clin Oncol* 2(3):549–585, 1983.
45. Schafer AI: Bleeding and thrombosis in the myeloproliferative disorders. *Blood* 64:1–12, 1984.
46. Hoagland H, Perry M: Thrombocythemia (thrombocytosis). *JAMA* 235:2330–2331, 1976.
47. Taft E, Babcock R, Scharfman W, et al.: Platelpheresis in the management of thrombocytosis. *Blood* 50:927–933, 1977.

Hemostasis in Cardiopulmonary Bypass Surgery

48. Mammen EF, Koets MH, Washington BC, et al.: Hemostasis changes during cardiopulmonary bypass surgery. *Sem Thromb Hemost* 11(3):281–292, 1985.
49. Salzman EW, Weinstein MJ, Weintraub RM, et al.: Treatment with desmopressin acetate to reduce blood loss after cardiac surgery: A double-blind randomized trial. *N Engl J Med* 314:1402–1406, 1986.

Spleen

50. Hess C, Ayers C, Sandusky W, et al.: Mechanism of dilutional anemia in massive splenomegaly. *Blood* 47:629–644, 1976.
51. Boxer M, Braun J, Ellman L: Thromboembolic risk of postsplenectomy thrombocytosis. *Arch Surg* 113:808–809, 1978.
52. Krivit W: Overwhelming postsplenectomy infection. *Am J Hematol* 2:193–201, 1977.

15

Oncology

Robert A. Gordon

Numerous medical and surgical complications occur in cancer patients. Many of the hematologic, metabolic, and infectious problems are dealt with in other chapters. This section will emphasize principles the internist should know when performing perioperative consultations on patients with cancer. Management of specific complications caused by metastatic cancer will also be presented.

The surgical cancer patient can be classified into two general groups:

1. The cancer patient who is presently undergoing treatment or has been previously treated and requires surgery that is unrelated to his cancer.

2. The cancer patient who is recently diagnosed and requires therapeutic cancer surgery.

INCIDENTAL SURGERY IN CANCER PATIENTS

Cancer patients undergoing chemotherapy and/or radiation therapy may present with acute problems unrelated to their cancer that require surgery. These patients may have concurrent infections, poor nutritional status, bleeding, and metabolic abnormalities. A knowledgeable estimate of the patient's prognosis as it relates to his cancer is clearly important. If these patients are potentially curable, aggressive medical and surgical management is indicated. Correction of the underlying acute problem is most critical.

Acute **abdominal pain in patients with neutropenia** following chemotherapy for malignancy is a common reason for combined medical and surgical collab-

oration. Localized abdominal pain is more likely to be caused by a surgically correctable condition than is generalized abdominal pain. Surgery should be avoided unless pain is accompanied by specific signs or x-ray findings. Neutropenic patients undergoing operations tolerate these procedures well if aggressive supportive care is administered and granulocyte recovery is rapid. Prolonged neutropenia following surgery portends a poor outcome.

Perirectal infections are relatively common in neutropenic patients and are associated with a high mortality rate. The usual physical findings of fluctuance and erythema are uncommon because of the neutropenia, but fever, pain, and induration are present. A study of perirectal infections in acute leukemics who were severely neutropenic showed that early surgical incision and debridement was associated with rapid relief of pain, excellent healing, and improved survival (1).

Remote Organ Toxicity Caused by Cancer Therapy

When surgery is indicated in patients who have been previously treated with chemotherapy and/or radiation therapy, there are several potential complications due to the remote effects of such treatment on organ systems. These potential complications are usually preventable and require special consideration.

LUNGS

Bleomycin has major toxicity on the lung and can cause chronic pneumonitis progressing to pulmonary fibrosis. It is important to identify the associated risk factors that increase the incidence of pulmonary toxicity in patients undergoing general anesthesia. These risk factors include the following:

1. Cumulative dose of bleomycin; the incidence of pulmonary fibrosis increases significantly after a total dose of 400 units;
2. Age >70 years old;
3. Prior or concomitant thoracic radiation therapy;
4. The concurrent use of cyclophosphamide or Adriamycin;
5. Administration by intravenous bolus technique causes more toxicity than the constant infusion technique;
6. Exposure to high-dose oxygen;
7. Pre-existing lung disease, especially emphysema.

The importance of the use of **high oxygen concentration** in a patient previously treated with bleomycin deserves special emphasis. There appears to be a synergistic effect between prior bleomycin and high-oxygen concentration used during anesthesia. This synergistic effect is toxic to lung tissue and can cause progressive pulmonary fibrosis. Since many patients who receive bleomycin are young, have been cured of their malignancy (testicular cancer, Hodgkin's disease, and lymphomas), and may require incidental surgery in the future, this point should not be overlooked. It is recommended that inspiratory **oxygen concentration not exceed 40%** at any time during or after surgery. The internist should assure that the surgeon and anesthesiologist are aware of the patient's chemotherapy history prior to surgery.

Since bleomycin will frequently decrease the lung volumes and cause a diffusion abnormality, a careful pulmonary evaluation including spirometry, DLco, and arterial blood gas prior to major surgery is indicated.

Mitomycin is an additional chemotherapeutic drug that will increase the risk of pulmonary toxicity when a patient is exposed to high-oxygen concentration. The same guidelines recommended for bleomycin apply to patients who have received mitomycin.

HEART

Doxorubicin (Adriamycin) is one of the most commonly used anti-cancer drugs and is an active agent against many malignancies. An important toxicity is a cumulative, **dose-dependent cardiomyopathy** that can result in congestive heart failure. The frequency of this cardiomyopathy ranges from a few percent to over 50% depending on the population treated and the techniques used to study cardiac function.

Risk factors for Adriamycin-induced cardiomyopathy include:

1. Cumulative dose (significant increase when dose is $\geq$ 550 mg/m^2);
2. Dose schedule (lower incidence when weekly or infusion schedule used compared to "standard" every 3 week schedule);
3. Age older than 40 years;
4. Mediastinal radiation therapy;
5. Previous underlying cardiac disease;
6. The concurrent use of cyclophosphamide (possible).

At least one-third of patients with Adriamycin-induced cardiomyopathy are asymptomatic, and left ventricular dysfunction is only abnormal when evaluated by radionuclide angiography associated with exercise. This group of patients should be identified prior to the stresses of major surgery so that appropriate cardiac monitoring can be employed. The left ventricular dysfunction lasts for years but tends to be stable and nonprogressive, and is not a contraindication to necessary surgery.

KIDNEYS

Cisplatin (Platinol) commonly causes a subclinical reduction in kidney function, which appears to be **irreversible.** Even when the BUN and creatinine are normal or only minimally elevated, a marked decrease in the creatinine clearance can be documented.

Hypomagnesemia occurs in a substantial number of patients who have received cisplatin. This is due to renal wasting of magnesium caused by a toxic effect on the renal tubules by the cisplatin. Hypocalcemia and hypokalemia may be associated abnormalities.

Several recommendations can be made regarding surgery in patients who have received cisplatin. Adequate hydration and a urinary output of 100 ml/hr during and after surgery may prevent additional renal injury. Mannitol (25–50 gm) should be used to ensure diuresis during surgery. Avoidance of nephrotoxic drugs, especially aminoglycoside antibiotics and combination aminoglycoside-cephalosporin agents, is recommended.

Magnesium, calcium, and potassium measurements should be a part of the preoperative evaluation and appropriate replacement is indicated for low levels.

INTESTINES

Radiation injury to the small intestine and colon is a significant complication of radiation therapy for pelvic and abdominal malignancies. The incidence has been estimated to approach 10%. This complication usually occurs several years after radiation therapy. The most common presenting signs and symptoms are related to bowel obstruction, although fistula formation, ulceration, or perforation also occur.

Several important **principles regarding management** of radiation enteropathy include the following:

1. Early diagnosis and surgical intervention is critical.

2. Total parenteral nutrition should be instituted before and after definitive surgery.

3. Broad-spectrum antibiotic coverage is necessary. Non-absorbable antibiotics should be given either orally or through a long intestinal tube preoperatively and parenteral antibiotics, which cover bowel flora, should be given preoperatively and for at least 3–5 days postoperatively.

Preoperative consideration of the effects of previous cancer therapy on organ systems may prevent significant postoperative complications.

THERAPEUTIC SURGERY IN CANCER PATIENTS

Cancer patients undergo therapeutic surgery for many reasons at different times during the natural course of their cancer.

Early in therapy, surgery is often indicated to remove a localized cancer for potential care. Regionally advanced cancers may be treated initially with chemotherapy and/or radiation therapy to make surgery possible in the future. "Second-look" surgery may be recommended to evaluate a therapeutic effect or to debulk tumor. On occasion, surgery may be performed on selected cancer patients with a single or few metastases (see Table 15.1).

Table 15.1. Evaluation of the Surgical Cancer Patient

I. *Incidental Surgery*
 1. Carefully evaluate metabolic, infectious, and hematologic abnormalities associated with cancer and treatment.
 2. Anticipate or prevent problems related to previous or current cancer therapy. Consider remote effects of chemotherapy and radiation therapy on organ systems.

II. *Therapeutic Surgery*
 1. Evaluate the extent of the cancer preoperatively. (Stage and anticipate intraoperative therapy.)
 2. Understand the changing role for initial chemotherapy and/or radiation therapy prior to or in place of surgery (neoadjuvant therapy).
 3. Recognize the benefit and limitations of postoperative adjuvant therapy for specific cancers.
 4. Appreciate the indications for "second look" surgery.
 5. Consider resectability of a single or few metastases.

Preoperative Evaluation of the Newly Diagnosed Cancer Patient

Each specific cancer should be thought of as a unique disease with its own natural history and patterns of spread. When evaluating the more common malignancies, the literature recommends certain studies depending on the initial clinical stage of the cancer. As a general rule, there is little evidence that the initial surgical procedure will be altered in **early** stage cancer patients who are **asymptomatic** and have **normal** routine laboratory studies. Therefore, preoperative scans should be ordered thoughtfully.

When evaluating an asymptomatic woman with a clinical stage I or II **breast cancer** (see Appendix for stage), there is no benefit in obtaining a brain or liver scan since metastases to these organs are extremely uncommon on initial presentation.

Although bone scanning is often considered a routine procedure prior to mastectomy for breast cancer, objective data do not support its use in early breast cancer (Stage I or II) (8). The risk of metastases at presentation and for recurrent disease is best determined by the size of the primary tumor, presence or absence of metastases in the axillary lymph nodes (LN), and the number of lymph nodes involved. It is unusual (approximately 1%) for women with a primary tumor <2 cm and negative axillary LN to have a "truly" positive bone scan. When the primary tumor is between 2–5 cm and axillary LN are positive, the incidence of positive bone scans is approximately 5%, and less than half of these patients with positive scans will have proven bony metastases. The extra cost, time, and anxiety of additional tests, such as skeletal roentgenograms, bone biopsies, and computed tomography required to clarify spurious findings on bone scans is significant. Bone scans need not be part of the routine workup of patients free of musculoskeletal complaints and normal chemistry profiles before their initial treatment of truly early breast cancer.

On the other hand, in a woman with stage III (local-regional advanced) breast cancer, there is a greater likelihood of metastases, which would alter the treatment, and a bone scan is indicated. A liver scan is not necessary if liver function tests and physical exam are normal.

Colorectal cancer is a malignancy that usually requires surgery regardless of the stage. A preoperative liver scan is not indicated unless liver function tests are abnormal. This cancer rarely metastasizes to bone on presentation, so a routine bone scan is not indicated.

In the patient with colorectal cancer and abnormal liver function tests, an evaluation for liver metastases is important prior to surgery. A CAT scan or sonogram of the liver will show better delineation of liver metastases than a radionuclide scan. If limited liver metastases are documented, surgical resection of these lesions should be considered. A patient with unresectable liver metastases could be a candidate for the placement of an implantable *Infusaid* pump for continuous infusion of chemotherapy through the hepatic artery. It is important to identify these patients preoperatively since a preoperative arteriogram is necessary to evaluate the vascular supply to the liver. Although there is controversy regarding whether treatment of liver metastases by means of the *Infusaid* pump prolongs life, there is good evidence that response rates in the liver are very high, and such treatment does change the natural history of colorectal carcinoma with metastases to the liver. If these patients are carefully selected, prolonged life and good paliation can occur.

A patient with newly diagnosed **non-small cell lung carcinoma** requires thorough evaluation to determine operability. If the tumor is unresectable because of the presence of mediastinal lymph node metastases or poor pulmonary function, then multiple scans are not indicated if the patient is asymptomatic from brain, bone, or intra-abdominal metastases. Radiation therapy is the treatment of choice in such a patient. Systemic chemotherapy is of limited value. If the patient is a surgical candidate for cure, then an evaluation for common sites of potential metastases is indicated since asymptomatic adrenal, liver, or bone metastases would clearly preclude curative surgery. In this case a CAT scan of the upper abdomen including the adrenals and a bone scan is warranted.

Prostate carcinoma is a common malignancy in elderly men. Since surgical therapy can range between a palliative TURP to a potentially curative radical prostatectomy and pelvic lymphadenectomy, a careful preoperative staging evaluation may be necessary. Bone metastases are common on initial presentation and are occasionally asymptomatic or confused with symptoms of arthritis; for this reason, a preoperative bone scan should be performed.

As a general rule, the more extensive the surgical procedure, the greater the chance that surgery will be curative, but the higher the risk of patient morbidity, and the more important it is to accurately determine the extent of the malignancy preoperatively.

Neoadjuvant Therapy

It is important for the internist to understand the changing priorities of chemotherapy, radiation therapy, and surgery available to the newly diagnosed cancer patient. There are several important malignancies that are best treated and even cured with initial chemotherapy and/or radiation therapy (neoadjuvant therapy), with or without surgery, which were previously approached only by surgery (Table 15.2).

Anal carcinoma is an uncommon malignancy that was previously treated surgically, often requiring an anterior-posterior (A-P) resection and colostomy. Systemic recurrences and death were still common. Presently, initial chemotherapy with mitomycin and 5-fluorouracil, given by a continuous 4-day infusion, and simultaneous radiation therapy have essentially eliminated the need for surgery. Cure rates are high (13).

Table 15.2.   Cancers Which Should Be Treated with Initial Chemotherapy and/or Radiation Therapy

1. Anal carcinoma
2. Advanced squamous cell head and neck cancer
3. Local-regional advanced and inflammatory breast cancer
4. Squamous cell carcinoma of the esophagus (investigational)
5. Small cell lung carcinoma
6. High-grade, high-stage transitional cell carcinoma of the bladder (investigational)

Advanced head and neck malignancies have a poor prognosis, and these patients are often not surgical candidates. Chemotherapy with Platinol and a 5-day infusion of 5-fluorouracil have given dramatic responses when used as initial therapy. Radiation therapy is usually given after initial chemotherapy. Surgery may be recommended for selected patients with minimal residual disease. This combined modality approach improves local control, but its benefit to overall survival is unknown.

Squamous cell esophageal carcinoma has a poor prognosis with a 5-year survival of only approximately 5%. Complete responses have been obtained in patients with local-regional disease using multimodality therapy, consisting of initial chemotherapy with Platinol and infusional 5-fluorouracil and simultaneous radiation therapy followed by surgical resection. Unfortunately, treatment toxicity is significant and surgical mortality is high. Such therapy remains investigational, and standard treatment for local-regional esophageal carcinoma continues to be surgery or radiation.

Local-regional advanced breast cancer (Stage IIIB) and **inflammatory breast carcinoma** are not surgically approachable and are best treated with initial chemotherapy, followed by radiation therapy and/or mastectomy. This combined approach offers the best chance for local-regional control. Improvement in long-term survival is less easily measured.

Small cell carcinoma of the lung has been known for many years to contraindicate surgery. This is a systemic disease and initial chemotherapy is indicated. Initial response rates are high, but long-term survival beyond 2 years is very uncommon.

Standard therapy for high-grade, high-stage **transitional cell carcinoma of the urinary bladder** (muscle invasion) is radical cystectomy and urinary diversion, with or without pre- or postoperative irradiation. Such treatment has provided unacceptable long-term 5-year survival rates ranging from 30–50%. The development of the combination chemotherapy regimen M-VAC (Methotrexate, Vinblastine, Adriamycin and Cisplatin) has been shown to downstage and convert unresectable bladder cancer to resectable disease in a significant percentage of patients. The neoadjuvant use of M-VAC is very promising but requires additional clinical trials.

Postoperative Adjuvant Therapy in Common Cancers

The risk factors for recurrence for most of the common malignancies involve the stage and the histologic grading of the cancer (see Appendix). The estrogen and progesterone receptor status are additional prognostic factors for breast cancer. Patients who are at increased risk for recurrence after the initial surgical procedure should be considered for adjuvant therapy. The goal of such adjuvant therapies is to eradicate micrometastatic cancer cells, which would potentially result in eventual death.

Despite the theoretical advantage of the use of adjuvant chemotherapy to eliminate these occult micrometastatic cancer cells, there have been few studies in the common solid malignancies that substantiate an unequivocal improvement in survival when systemic chemotherapy is compared to surgery alone. Nevertheless, there are several instances in which adjuvant therapy has been proven beneficial.

Postoperative adjuvant combination chemotherapy in **premenopausal women with lymph node involvement** does prolong the disease-free interval and cures approximately 20–25% of women whose cancers would otherwise recur. The use of combination chemotherapy in postmenopausal women with lymph node involvement remains controversial, but is recommended in those postmenopausal women who are younger and/or have estrogen receptor negative tumors. Tamoxifen is recommended as adjuvant systemic therapy in postmenopausal women who have lymph node involvement and have estrogen receptor rich tumors (21).

Two studies have shown the efficacy of treating **lymph node negative, estrogen receptor negative** breast cancer patients with adjuvant chemotherapy. Chemotherapy significantly prolonged the disease-free survival after a 4-year follow-up in both pre- and postmenopausal women. A survival advantage has not been observed during this short follow-up period (22, 23).

A randomized, double-blind, placebo-controlled trial of postoperative therapy with tamoxifen in 2644 patients with **lymph node negative, estrogen receptor positive** breast cancer revealed a significant prolongation of the disease-free survival among pre- and postmenopausal women treated with tamoxifen. Tamoxifen reduced the rate of recurrences at both local and distant sites and decreased the incidence of tumor recurrence after lumpectomy and breast irradiation. No survival advantage was observed during a 4-year follow-up period (24).

Despite encouraging improvement in the disease-free survival and survival of women with the various subsets of breast cancer treated with either adjuvant chemotherapy or hormonal therapy, ideal therapy for any of these groups is yet to be achieved. Newly diagnosed breast cancer patients should be encouraged to participate in ongoing clinical trials.

Patients with **rectal carcinoma stage B-2 and C** (penetration through the bowel wall or LN involvement) are at increased risk of local as well as systemic recurrence. Radiation therapy in these patients has been shown to decrease local recurrences. Radiation therapy along with 5-fluorouracil and methyl CCNU has been found to prolong the disease-free interval and possibly overall survival (21). Unfortunately, this treatment cannot be routinely employed at this time because methyl CCNU is not available and is also associated with an increased incidence of hematologic problems, including leukemia and preleukemic conditions.

The use of adjuvant chemotherapy after curative resection of **colon cancer in patients who are at high risk for recurrence** (stage B_2 and C) has been a controversial subject. Recently, a well performed randomized 3 arm study compared a control population to levamisole and to 5-fluorouracil (5-FU) and levamisole. This study revealed a statistically significant improvement in the recurrence rate, as well as a delay in those recurrences. There was a significant survival improvement in the subset stage C patients (lymph node involvement) who were treated with 5-FU and levamisole (26). Although physicians should encourage their patients to enter clinical trials, adjuvant therapy with 5-FU and levamisole in patients with stage C colon cancer appears effective and offers these patients an improvement in survival with acceptable patient tolerance.

"Second Look" Surgery

Second look operations to evaluate the effectiveness of chemotherapy and to remove local recurrent cancer for potential cure is valuable in selected patients.

Chemotherapy responses to advanced **ovarian carcinoma** are impressive. Unfortunately, cure is uncommon and these patients often have residual carcinoma at "second look" surgery. Preoperative evaluation by CAT scan is of limited value since the CAT scan usually does not visualize small residual ovarian carcinoma. The tumor marker CA-125 is useful in determining the efficacy of therapy and the development of progressive disease; however, its sensitivity is low in patients with small volume tumors. Extensive surgical debulking of residual carcinoma with bowel resection, if necessary, can prolong life and palliate symptoms. It is debatable whether overall survival is influenced, however.

"Second look" surgery in **colorectal carcinoma** can be palliative and curative in selected individuals. An **increasing CEA** level on follow-up care is an indication for evaluation of recurrence. "Second look" surgery in this situation, even when residual carcinoma is not found by non-invasive studies, is indicated in good-risk patients. Resection of a local recurrence or resection of liver metastases can prolong life and may be potentially curative (28).

RESECTION OF A SINGLE OR FEW METASTASES

The presence of an isolated metastasis or several metastases in an important organ should be considered for surgical resection. Depending on the solid tumor histology, the number of metastases and the disease-free interval, prolonged survival and even cure can be anticipated. Metastases from certain solid tumors make surgical resection most considerable. The different tumor types are discussed below in the organ of metastases.

Pulmonary Metastases

The lung is a common site of metastases for many cancers, including osteogenic and soft tissue sarcomas, melanoma, non-seminomatous germ-cell tumors of the testes, head and neck, colorectal, renal, endometrial, cervical, and breast carcinomas. Although lung metastases usually represent only one site of extensive spread, important exceptions should be considered.

Osteogenic and soft tissue sarcomas frequently metastasize to the lungs, and the pulmonary metastases are often exclusive from other sites. Surgical resection has been shown to prolong survival and may even be curative.

Patient selection is important and patients should meet the following criteria:

1. The primary site must be controlled;
2. The patient must be a good surgical candidate;
3. No extrapulmonary metastases may be present;
4. The tumor doubling time should be calculated as greater than 20 days;
5. The disease-free interval should be greater than 12 months;
6. Less than 5 nodules should be present on preoperative lung tomograms or chest CAT scan;
7. Adequate functioning lung should be preserved after potential resection.

A median sternotomy approach is recommended so that both lungs can be explored.

Pulmonary nodules occurring in patients with a previous diagnosis of head and neck cancer represent an important subject since these patients have a second primary lung cancer at least as often as metastases from their primary head and neck cancer. Since preoperative radiologic estimates of metastases versus a primary lung cancer are inaccurate, surgery should be considered. Patients who are good surgical candidates, show no evidence of distant metastases or mediastinal involvement, and have a disease-free interval of at least one year, should undergo thoracotomy.

Pulmonary metastases from all other primary cancer sites are less well studied and individual judgment is necessary.

Liver Metastases

It is unknown whether resection of solitary or a few liver metastases is of any palliative or curative benefit to patients. If liver resection is contemplated, it should be considered a curative, not a palliative procedure.

Only two groups of adult cancer patients should be considered for resection of their liver metastases. The first group should include highly selected patients with primary colon and rectal cancers who have localized liver metastases as their only manifestation of recurrent or persistent disease. The second and even more unusual group of patients are those with endocrine tumors, such as carcinoid or islet-cell tumors, that have disabling symptoms from liver metastases. These malignancies are usually slow growing, and surgical resection may benefit these patients if widespread metastases are not evident.

Liver resection for patients with carcinoma metastatic from other common sites, such as the pancreas, stomach, lung, breast, and melanoma is not justified.

Brain Metastases

The use of combination chemotherapy to control systemic cancer has led to an increased incidence of brain metastases, since most chemotherapeutic agents are unable to cross the blood-brain barrier. Brain metastases may be the only symptomatic site of recurring cancer. Lung and breast are the most common primary malignancies to metastasize to brain, but melanoma, renal cell, and unknown histologies occur with important frequency.

Most brain metastases are treated with radiation therapy. However, there is a subset of patients who benefit from resection of metastases followed by radiotherapy. These patients have the following characteristics:

1. They are ambulatory;
2. The brain metastasis is solitary and localized to the cerebrum, especially in an area of the brain where resection will not cause significant neurologic deficit;
3. The primary cancer site is controlled;
4. There is no evidence of metastatic disease outside the brain.

SPECIAL CONSIDERATIONS IN THE CANCER PATIENT

There are special considerations in cancer patients that require the internist and surgeon to work closely together.

Superior Vena Cava Syndrome

The superior vena cava (SVC) syndrome may be acute, but is more often a subacute syndrome that is usually caused by a malignant tumor. The most common causes for the syndrome include lymphomas, Hodgkin's disease and bronchogenic carcinomas, both small cell and non-small cell types. Thymic, testicular, and other metastatic tumors are less common causes.

The treatment approach and prognosis is very different among these malignancies, and a **definitive histologic diagnosis should be established before therapy** is instituted.

Previous teaching that the SVC syndrome was an acute emergency and that invasive diagnostic procedures were dangerous have been proven wrong. To the contrary, the SVC syndrome usually presents with subacute symptoms and invasive diagnostic procedures, i.e., mediastinoscopy, bronchoscopy or even thoracotomy, can be performed safely. It is the unusual patient who presents with life-threatening symptoms for whom a tissue diagnosis should be deferred prior to therapy.

Chemotherapy is the initial treatment for SVC syndrome caused by small cell lung carcinoma and histiocytic lymphoma and is highly effective in alleviating symptoms rapidly. Radiation therapy should be the initial therapy for non-small cell lung cancers. Chemotherapy and/or radiation therapy may be the initial therapy for Hodgkin's disease depending on the clinical circumstances.

Malignant Pleural Effusion

A malignant pleural effusion requires treatment when the patient has respiratory symptoms. Since many different types of malignancies can cause a pleural effusion, the treatment is directed against the specific cancer. Pleural effusion from lymphomas, germ cell cancer, small cell lung cancer, and breast cancer usually respond to systemic chemotherapy or hormonal therapy in the case of breast cancer. However, many solid malignancies, such as colon and lung cancers, that cause pleural effusions are unresponsive to systemic therapy. Following thoracentesis, there is usually a rapid reaccumulation of the effusion.

The best approach to control a malignant pleural effusion is to place a large bore chest tube into the pleural cavity with closed tube suction drainage followed by installation of a sclerosing agent into the pleural cavity. Successful management is more likely if thoracostomy drainage is continued for 48–72 hours or until complete drainage is achieved. Complete drainage may not be possible and drainage limited to 50–100 cc/day may have to be acceptable. Many sclerosing agents have been used, but it is the obliteration of the pleural space and not the agent that determines the effectiveness of therapy. **Tetracycline** instillation (1 gram mixed with 70 cc of normal saline) appears to be as effective as any agent and has less toxicity than most other drugs. Routine use of 20 ml of lidocaine 1% mixed with the tetracycline and normal saline will often eliminate associated pleuritic pain. To ensure patient comfort, parenteral administration of a narcotic 1 hour before installation of sclerosing therapy is recommended. After installation of this mixture, the chest tube is clamped for 4–6 hours, with the patient instructed to change positions frequently to distribute the sclerosing agent throughout the pleural cavity. The tube can then be unclamped, and if there is no significant drainage during the subsequent 12 hours, the tube can be removed.

Neoplastic Pericardial Effusion

Pericardial involvement in cancer patients can occur either from contiguous extension by an adjacent cancer in the lung or mediastinum or from metastases from a distant primary cancer. Lung cancer, breast cancer, leukemia, Hodgkin's and non-Hodgkin's lymphoma account for more than three-fourths of the cases involving the pericardium. Radiation-induced pericardial injury may manifest itself as an acute pericarditis either during the course of the treatment, or weeks or months after its completion, or as a chronic form occurring several months to many years after the treatment. The importance of differentiating and managing radiation-induced pericarditis in a patient who may be cured of his cancer from progressive malignant disease with pericardial metastases is obvious.

The echocardiogram is the easiest and most sensitive method to detect a pericardial effusion and may detect impending cardiac tamponade. Total electrical alternans on ECG, involving both atrial and ventricular complexes, is virtually pathognomonic of cardiac tamponade. Approximately three-fourths of documented malignant pericardial effusions will have

a positive cytology. Therefore, negative cytologic results may not differentiate cancer from radiation as the cause for the pericardial effusion. There are no other characteristics of the effusion that will help in the differentiation.

The management of pericardial effusion is dependent on the clinical setting. Cardiac tamponade is an emergency situation and pericardiocentesis should be performed immediately, preferably under electrocardiographic monitoring. The pericardial effusion usually recurs within 1–2 days after the initial pericardiocentesis. Therefore, additional therapy will be required and should be planned depending on the cause of the effusion, the type of the effusion (effusive or constrictive), and the patient's medical condition and long-term prognosis.

If therapy is aimed at short-term palliation because of extensive metastatic disease, then a transcutaneous catheter can be placed into the pericardial space to drain the pericardial effusion. Tetracycline (500 mg in 20 cc NSS) can subsequently be instilled through the catheter to sclerose the pericardial surfaces and obliterate the pericardial space. This method is efficacious in preventing recurrent pericardial tamponade. Additional radiation therapy or chemotherapy can be given, depending on the chemo-radiosensitivity of the cancer.

In a patient with a malignant pericardial effusion and a good prognosis, prolonged palliation can be obtained by the surgical placement of a pleuropericardial window. This procedure is well tolerated, but there is a risk that the window will eventually close due to the development of adhesions. In addition, this surgical procedure may be technically difficult if the tumor encases the heart and pericardium.

Pericardectomy is the treatment of choice for radiation-induced pericardial effusion causing cardiac tamponade. This surgical procedure is more extensive, requiring a thoracotomy, and has significant morbidity associated with it. This surgery is rarely justifiable in a patient with a malignant pericardial effusion and a limited life span.

Malignant Ascites

Malignant ascites refractory to systemic anticancer therapy is a common and difficult management problem. The use of spironolactone, a low salt diet, and repeated paracentesis are the mainstays of treatment, but are often ineffective. Intraperitoneal administration of radioactive elements is not available to most patients. Many chemotherapeutic agents have been instilled intra-abdominally with limited success and frequent morbidity.

The use of **peritoneovenous shunting** in the palliative management of intractable malignant ascites should be considered in carefully selected cancer patients. The main problem is clotting of the shunt, which renders it nonfunctional. Cancer patients with a positive cytology, high ascitic fluid protein content, and bloody ascites have frequent clotting of these shunts. Peritoneovenous shunting is best avoided in these patients, although these contraindications are relative. Absolute contraindications to the placement of these shunts include recent or concurrent infection, liver failure, loculated intraperitoneal fluid, and preoperative coagulopathy.

Complications of peritoneovenous shunting include disseminated intravascular coagulation, which is usually subclinical and does not require treatment; pulmonary edema, which can occur in the immediate postoperative period from large volumes of peritoneal fluid shunted into the systemic circulation, and infection.

Biliary Obstruction

Obstructive jaundice in cancer patients may be caused by tumors that are intra- or extrahepatic. Extrahepatic biliary tract obstruction is far more common. Proper radiologic evaluation is important. Percutaneous transhepatic cholangiography gives the most accurate and specific information regarding the site of obstruction and possible role of surgery. The prognosis in most of these patients is so poor that it is the unusual patient who is a surgical candidate for definitive extirpative surgery. The role of surgery is usually limited to biliary tract decompression. These patients usually tolerate surgery poorly and recuperate slowly.

Drainage of an obstructed biliary tree can also be achieved by percutaneous catheter placement. Although this technique may be considered as an alternative to surgery, it is associated with a high rate of sepsis, bleeding, and catheter malfunction. Temporary palliation of a terminally ill patient may be achieved by this technique, but outpatient management is difficult.

External beam irradiation to radiosensitive tumors or metastatic porta hepatis lymph nodes may occasionally be palliative.

Ureteral Obstruction

Bilateral complete obstruction of the ureters is a life-threatening condition. The most common primary tumors causing ureteral obstruction are cervix, ovary, bladder, prostate, and rectum. The diagnosis of upper tract obstruction is best made by renal ultrasonography. The intravenous administration of contrast medium should be avoided in the azotemic patient since it may result in further renal damage.

Percutaneous nephrostomy with antegrade pyelogram will determine the site and nature of obstruction and provide drainage of the obstructed kidney. A percutaneous nephrostomy will provide temporary relief of obstruction, but should not be considered a permanent form of drainage because of the difficulty in maintaining the tubes and patient discomfort.

Permanent indwelling ureteral stents can be positioned by retrograde ureteral catheterization over a guidewire and are well tolerated by the patient. Permanent surgical urinary diversion techniques may be indicated, depending on the clinical circumstances.

Management of Pathologic and Impending Pathologic Fractures of Long Bone

The occurrence of bone metastases is common in cancer patients. More than three-fourths of adults who develop bone metastases have common malignancies, including breast, lung, and prostate carcinomas. Involvement of the proximal femur accounts for more than half of all pathologic long bone fractures and causes significant morbidity because of immobilization. Metastases distal to the elbow or knees are uncommon except in preterminal patients and accounted for only 10% of pathologic fractures in one series.

A pathologic fracture of a long bone should not be interpreted as a terminal event in most cancer patients. In fact, directed management of such a fracture can result in marked improvement in the quality of life for many cancer patients, especially patients with breast and prostate cancers. Prosthetic replacement or internal fixation of proximal femoral pathologic fractures is the best approach to ensure early ambulation and alleviation of pain. Selection of patients for such surgery is an important decision. Harrington has recommended that the **following criteria be met before this surgery** is performed: (a) life expectancy of at least 2 months and the general condition of the patient such that major surgery can be tolerated; (b) the procedure must be expected to expedite mobilization of the patient or facilitate general care; and (c) the quality of bone proximal and distal to the fracture site must be adequate to support metallic fixation or to secure prosthetic seating (38).

Harrington developed a technique in which the diseased bone and tumor tissue is replaced by methylmethacrylate supplemented by metal internal fixation devices or prostheses, resulting in a structural capacity to withstand the stresses of early weight bearing. In his experience, 94% of 400 patients who were ambulatory prior to pathologic fractures regained the ability to walk postoperatively, and pain relief was rated as excellent or good in 85% and as poor in only 2% (38).

Some metastatic bone lesions, particularly renal, pancreas, and colon, tend to be highly vascular, and blood loss at the time of attempted fixation or even biopsy may become prohibitive. If such situations can be anticipated preoperatively, the technique of arterial embolization of the bone tumor site may be attempted.

The **prophylactic fixation of an impending fracture of the femur** should be performed when there is a high risk of fracture. Criteria that should be used to assess this high risk include the following: (a) primarily lytic lesion; (b) size of 2.5 cm or more; (c) cortical involvement; (d) lytic lesion, involving more than 50% of the diameter of the femur; and (e) persistent pain despite irradiation.

Complications specifically related to the operative fixation or prosthetic replacement of malignant pathologic fractures include infection, thromboemboli, local tumor seeding and delayed wound healing. The complication rate is acceptable particularly considering the physiologic fragility of these patients.

Radiation therapy should be given to the involved area after internal fixation or prosthetic replacement. The radiation therapy can usually be initiated safely 10–14 days after surgery. The prognosis for union of a pathologic fracture is dependent upon rigid fixation and the tumor cell type. Fractures secondary to metastatic breast or prostate carcinomas, myeloma or lymphoma unite far more frequently than malignant tumors of the lung, kidney, or gastrointestinal tract. Fortunately, metastatic breast cancer is the most common cause for pathologic fracture of long bones, and internal fixation followed by irradiation results in good local tumor control and fracture union in most patients.

Spinal Cord Compression

Spinal cord compression is a common complication of metastatic cancer and often causes severe disability. An early diagnosis requires a high index of suspicion for this problem. Therapy must be instituted rapidly to prevent morbidity.

Spinal cord compression by epidural tumor is **almost always preceded by back pain.** Typically, the pain has been present for weeks to months and is located over the spinal column with or without radicular radiation. Motor weakness, autonomic dysfunction, sensory loss, and ataxia are late signs and often indicate irreversible neurologic impairment.

Plain films of the spine usually show vertebral involvement. Despite the increased sensitivity of bone scans in detecting bone metastases, their predictive value in detecting spinal cord compression is inferior to the plain film. The role of the CAT and MRI scan in evaluating the patient for suspect early spinal cord compression is less well studied but can give important information regarding vertebral destruction and tumor involvement near the spinal cord and spinal nerves.

A cancer patient with back pain and a plain film showing vertebral involvement should have a myelogram, even though the neurologic exam is normal. Using this approach, a high incidence of epidural spinal metastases will be found on myelography, and institution of appropriate therapy will usually prevent neurologic morbidity.

The appropriate treatment for epidural spinal cord compression is controversial and is dependent upon the primary cancer, the level of the block, the rapidity of onset, and the patient's overall clinical condition and prognosis. Treatment options include surgery or radiation therapy alone or in combination. No single therapy has been proven superior to another. Early diagnosis and patient selection are the critical factors in predicting a successful outcome.

Lymphoma and myeloma patients who develop spinal cord compression are usually treated with radiation therapy alone, since these tumors are rapidly radiosensitive.

Indications for an aggressive surgical approach may include relapse after radiation therapy, neurologic deterioration during radiotherapy, or the absence of a histologic diagnosis of the tumor.

Dexamethasone should be used when the diagnosis of spinal cord compression is established. The optimal dosage is not established but ranges from 16–100 mg of dexamethasone daily. Dexamethasone at 100 mg daily has been shown to be oncolytic in some patients. Patient tolerance is initially acceptable at this dosage, but the dose should be rapidly tapered after 3 days.

MISCELLANEOUS SURGICAL ONCOLOGY TOPICS

Conservative Breast Surgery

Conservative surgery for early stage breast cancer (Stage I and II) is an acceptable alternative to mastectomy for selected women. Although breast cancer appears clinically localized, hematogenous micrometastases frequently occur, resulting in ultimate relapse, and prove the concept that breast cancer is a systemic disease.

A randomized study of over 1800 women with Stage I and II breast tumors ≤4 cm in size compared total mastectomy to segmental mastectomy with and without breast irradiation. The results indicated similar distant disease-free and overall survival at 8 years (40). The incidence of local recurrence was significantly greater in the women who underwent segmental mastectomy without irradiation.

More and more women will elect conservative surgery as their primary therapy for breast cancer. An **axillary lymph node dissection is necessary** for staging of the disease. **Adjuvant radiation therapy to the breast only** is an integral part of the therapy since local recurrence rates are unacceptably high if irradiation is not given (41).

It is important that the internist understand the indications and contraindications for conservative breast surgery since such surgery is not indicated in all women. Before any treatment options are discussed with the patient, mammograms of both breasts must be obtained. The mammograms are critical in evaluating the size and location of the primary tumor, the presence and extent of microcalcifications, the presence of multicentric disease, and the status of the contralateral breast. Consultation between the internist, surgeon and radiation therapist is often necessary (Table 15.3).

There are several conservative surgical techniques that can be performed, including wide local excision (lumpectomy) or quadrantectomy. Whichever technique is used, it is crucial that all tumor be removed and that the resected margins are free of tumor. Lumpectomy generally gives a better cosmetic result, although this technique is not always feasible. The optimal axillary staging procedure is controversial.

Table 15.3. Breast Cancer Patient Selection for Conservative Surgery and Radiation

Indications	Relative Contraindications
Small to moderately large breast	Large pendulous breast
Primary tumor ≤ 4–5 cm	Large tumor in a small breast
Single discrete tumor	Several tumors in one breast
Circumscribed micro-calcifications	Widespread microcalcifications
Clinically negative or clinically positive non-fixed axillary nodes	Subareolar primary

Reproduced, with permission, from Danoff BF, Haller DG, Glich JH, Goodman RL: Conservative Surgery and Irradiation in the Treatment of Early Breast Cancer. *Ann Int Med* 102:634–642, 1985.

Adjuvant chemotherapy will be indicated in some women after conservative surgery. The optimal integration of adjuvant chemotherapy and irradiation after surgery has not yet been established.

Pelvic Exenteration

Refer to chapter 21.

Radical Neck Surgery

Refer to chapter 21.

APPENDIX

Staging of Common Cancers

Breast Cancer TNM Classification
(abridged)

T - Primary Tumor

T1: tumor 2 cm or less in greatest dimension

T2: Tumor 2–5 cm in greatest dimension

T3: Tumor more than 5 cm in greatest dimension

T4: Tumor of any size with direct extension to chest wall or skin (Inflammatory carcinoma included)

N - Regional Lymph Nodes

N0: No regional lymph node metastasis

N1: Metastasis to movable ipsilateral axillary lymph node(s)

N2: Metastasis to ipsilateral axillary lymph node(s) fixed to one another or to other structures

N3: Metastasis to ipsilateral internal mammary lymph node(s)

M – Distant Metastases

M0: No evidence of distant metastases

M1: Distant metastases [includes metastasis to ipsilateral supraclavicular lymph node(s)]

Stage Grouping

Stage I:	T1 N0 M0
Stage IIA:	T1 N1 M0
	T2 N0 M0
Stage IIB:	T2 N1 M0
	T3 N0 M0
Stage IIIA:	T0-3 N2 M0
	T3 N1 M0
Stage IIIB:	Any T, N3, M0
	T4, Any N, M0
Stage IV:	Any T, Any N, M1

Colorectal Cancer Astler-Collier (modified Duke's) Staging

A: Limited to mucosa; nodes negative

B1: Extension through mucosa but still within bowel wall; nodes negative

B2: Extension through entire bowel wall; nodes negative

C1: Limited to bowel wall; nodes positive

C2: Extension through entire bowel wall; nodes positive

Prostate Cancer American Urologic Staging System

A1: No tumor palpable; focal involvement; well-differentiated

A2: No tumor palpable; diffuse involvement; poorly differentiated

B1: Tumor less than 2 cm, involving 1 lobe

B2: Tumor greater than 2 cm or diffuse involvement

C: Tumor extension beyond the prostate capsule without evidence of metastases

D1: Any tumor size involving pelvic lymph nodes below the aortic bifurcation

D2: Any tumor size involving lymph nodes above the aortic bifurcation and/or distant metastases to other sites

Readings

1. Barnes SG, Sattler FR, Ballard JO: Perirectal infections in acute leukemia. *Ann Int Med* 101:515–518, 1984.
2. Ginsburg SJ, Comis RL: The pulmonary toxicity of antineoplastic agents. *Sem Onc* 9:34–51, 1982.
3. Von Hoff DD, et al.: Risk factors for doxorubicin-induced congestive heart failure. *Ann Int Med* 91:710–717, 1979.
4. Gottdiener JS, Mathisen DJ, Borer JS, et al.: Doxorubicin cardiotoxicity: Assessment of late left ventricular dysfunction by radionuclide cineangiography. *Ann Int Med* 94:430–435, 1981.
5. Dentino M, Luft FC, Yum MN, et al.: Long term effect of Cis-Diamminedichloride Platinum (CDDP) on renal function and structure in man. *Cancer* 41:1274–1281, 1978.
6. Lyman NW, Hemalatha C, Viscuso RL, et al.: Cisplatin-induced hypocalcemia and hypomagnesemia. *Arch Int Med* 140:1513–1514, 1980.
7. Marks G, Mohiudden M: The surgical management of radiation-injured intestine. *Surg Clin North Am* 63(1):81–96, 1983.
8. Lee YN: Bone scanning in patients with early breast carcinoma: Should it be a routine staging procedure? *Cancer* 47:486–495, 1981.
9. Ciatto S, et al.: Preoperative staging of primary breast cancer. A multicentric study. *Cancer* 61:1038–1040, 1988.
10. Lahr CJ, Soong SJ, Cloud G, et al.: A multifactorial analysis of prognostic factors in patients with liver metastases from colorectal carcinoma. *J Clin Oncol* 1:720–726, 1983.
11. Stagg RJ, Lewis BJ, Friedman MA, et al.: Hepatic arterial chemotherapy for colorectal cancer metastatic to the liver. *Ann Int Med* 100:736–743, 1984.
12. Armstrong JD, Bragg DG: Thoracic neoplasm: Imaging requirements for diagnosis and staging. *Int J Rad Onc Biol Phys* 10:109–135, 1984.

13. Leichman L, Nigro N, Vaitkevicius VK, et al.: Cancer of the anal canal: Model for preoperative adjuvant combined modality therapy. *Am J Med* 78:211–215, 1985.

14. Mead GM, Jacobs C: Changing role of chemotherapy in treatment of head and neck cancer. *Am J Med* 73:582–595, 1982.

15. Poplin E, Fleming T, Leichman L, et al: Combined therapies for squamous-cell carcinoma of the esophagus, a Southwest Oncology Group study. *J Clin Oncol* 5:622–628, 1987.

16. Rouesse J, Friedman S, Sarrazin D, et al.: Primary chemotherapy in the treatment of inflammatory breast carcinoma: A study of 230 cases from the Institut Gustave-Roussy. *J Clin Oncol* 4:1765–1771, 1986.

17. Hortobagyi GN, Blumenschein GR, Sapnos W, et al.: Multimodality treatment of locoregionally advanced breast cancer. *Cancer* 51:763–768, 1983.

18. Zincke H, Sen SE, Hahn RG, et al.: Neoadjuvant chemotherapy for locally advanced transitional cell carcinoma of the bladder: Do local findings suggest a potential for salvage of the bladder? *Mayo Clin Proc* 63:16–22, 1988.

19. Parl FF, Schmidt BP, Dupont WD, et al.: Prognostic significance of estrogen receptor status in breast cancer in relation to tumor stage, axillary node metastasis, and histopathologic grading. *Cancer* 54:2237–2242, 1984.

20. NIH Consensus Conference. Adjuvant chemotherapy for breast cancer. *JAMA* 254:3461–3463, 1985.

21. Cummings FJ, Gray R, Davis TE, et al.: Adjuvant tamoxifen treatment of elderly women with stage II breast cancer, *Ann Int Med* 103:324–329, 1985.

22. Fisher B, et al.: A randomized clinical trial evaluating sequential methotrexate and fluorouracil in the treatment of patients with node-negative breast cancer who have estrogen-receptor-negative tumors. *N Engl J Med* 320:473–478, 1989.

23. Mansour EG, et al.: Efficacy of adjuvant chemotherapy in high-risk node-negative breast cancer. An Intergroup Study. *N Engl J Med* 320:485–490, 1989.

24. Fisher B, et al.: A randomized clinical trial evaluating tamoxifen in the treatment of patients with node-negative breast cancer who have estrogen-receptor-positive tumors. *N Engl J Med* 320:479–484, 1989.

25. Gastrointestinal Tumor Study Group. Prolongation of the disease-free interval in surgically treated rectal carcinoma. *N Engl J Med* 312:1465–1472, 1985.

26. Laurie JA, et al.: Surgical adjuvant therapy of large-bowel carcinoma: an evaluation of Levamisole and combination Levamisole and Fluorouracil. *J Clin Oncol* 7:1447–1456, 1989.

27. Clarke-Pearson DL, Bandy LC, Dudzinski M, et al.: Computed tomography in evaluation of patients with ovarian carcinoma in complete clinical remission. *JAMA* 255:627–630, 1986.

28. Minton JP, Hoehn JL, et al. Results of a 400-patient carcinoembryonic antigen second-look colorectal cancer study. *Cancer* 55:1284–1290, 1985.

29. Putnam JB, Roth JA, Wesley MN, et al.: Analysis of prognostic factors in patients undergoing resection of pulmonary metastases from soft tissue sarcomas. *J Thorac Cardiovasc Surg* 87:260–268, 1984.

30. Ahmann FR: A reassessment of the clinical implications of the superior vena caval syndrome. *J Clin Oncol* 2:961–969, 1984.

31. Hausheer FH, Yarbro JW: Diagnosis and treatment of malignant pleural effusion. *Sem Onc* 12:54–75, 1985.

32. Posner MR, Cohen GI, Skavin AT: Pericardial disease in patients with cancer. The differentiation of malignant from idiopathic and radiation-induced pericarditis. *Am J Med* 71:407–414, 1981.

33. Davis S, Rambotti P, Grignani F: Intrapericardial tetracycline sclerosis in the treatment of malignant pericardial effusion: An analysis of thirty-three cases. *J Clin Oncol* 2:631–636, 1984.

34. Lacy JH, Wieman TJ: Management of malignant ascites. *Surg Gyn Onc* 159:397–412, 1984.

35. Cheung DK, Raaf JH: Selection of patients with malignant ascites for a peritoneovenous shunt. *Cancer* 50:1204–1209, 1982.

36. Joseph PK, Bizer LS, Sprayregen SS, et al.: Percutaneous transhepatic biliary drainage. *JAMA* 255:2763–2767, 1986.

37. Sise JG, Grichlow RW: Obstruction due to malignant tumors. *Sem Onc* 5:213–224, 1978.

38. Harrington KD: The role of surgery in the management of pathologic fractures. *Ortho Clin North Am* 8(4):841–859, 1977.

39. Rodichok LD, Harper GR, Ruckdeschel JC, et al.: Early diagnosis of spinal epidural metastases. *Am J Med* 70:1181–1187, 1981.

40. Fisher B, et al.: Eight-year results of a randomized clinical trial comparing total mastectomy and lumpectomy with or without irradiation in the treatment of breast cancer. *N Engl J Med* 320:822–828, 1989.

41. Danoff BF, Haller DG, Glick JH, et al.: Conservative surgery and irradiation in the treatment of early breast cancer. *Ann Int Med* 102:634–642, 1985.

16

Infectious Disease

John Stuckey and Richard J. Gross

Surgical procedures are frequently complicated by infections at the operative or distant sites (1, 1A, 4, 8–12, 15–17, 25). Nosocomial infections occur in 4–7% of surgical patients, and nosocomial bacteremia occurs in about 0.9% of surgical cases.

The reported incidence of localized infections varies widely. About 85% of post-surgical infections involve the wound (32%), urinary tract (40%), and respiratory tract (15%). The urinary tract is the most common cause of fever and bacteremia, mainly due to catheterization. Although the third most common cause of infection, respiratory infections are the leading cause of death from nosocomial infection in the postoperative patient (8–10, 241) (Table 16.1). Wound infection rates ranged widely from 3–11% in different hospitals and from 0–25% for different operations (Table 16.2) (15).

The most common organisms involved have been *Staphylococcus aureus* and gram-negative organisms. Over the past decade, gram-negative organisms other than *Escherichia coli* have increased in frequency, especially *Pseudomonas, Klebsiella,* and *Serratia.* An increase in fungal infections has occurred, especially candida albicans.

The most important factors contributing to infection are the type of surgery and instrumentation perioperatively. Other important predisposing causes are preceding antibiotic usage, use of steroids and immunosuppressives, and instrumentation (especially Foley catheters, endotracheal tubes, and intravenous lines).

This chapter will first consider the prevention of surgical infection by prophylactic antibiotics. It must not be forgotten that proper surgical technique, postoperative care, and appropriate use of invasive catheters are of primary importance in prevention of postoperative infection (18).

Secondly, management will be discussed for the occasional patient having an infection unrelated to the reason for surgery in whom surgery cannot be postponed.

Table 16.1. Nosocomial and Surgical Infection Rates[a]

	Wound	Urine	Respiratory	Bacteremia	Skin	Other	Total
			rate/100 admissions				
University of Virginia	4.33	2.57	1.95	1.53		0.74	11.12
(surgical service)	(38.9%)	(23.1%)	(17.5%)	(13.8%)		(6.7%)	(100%)
University of Virginia	1.54	2.41	1.01	0.88		1.35	7.19
(all infections)	(21.6%)	(33.8%)	(14.1%)	(12.4%)		(18.9%)	(100%)
NNIS 1971–1974	0.76	1.38	0.57	0.26	0.18	0.38	3.46
(all infections)	(22%)	(39.9%)	(16.5%)	(7.7%)	(5.2%)	(8.7%)	(100%)

[a]From Wenzel RP: Nosocomial infections, in Mandel GL, Douglas RG, Bennett JE (eds): *Principles and Practice of Infectious Disease.* New York, John Wiley & Sons, 1979, with permission.

Table 16.2.   Incidence of Wound Infections in Selected Procedures (14–16)

	Multicenter Study (15)	Cruse (15a, 16–17)
All operations	7.5%[a]	5.1%
Non-body cavity		
Mastectomy (modified radical)		4.2%
Fractured hip		4.2%
Menisectomy		0.5%
Abdominal		
"Negative" laparotomy	1.9%	0.5%
Partial gastrectomy	10.1%	14.4%
Partial colectomy	10.0%[b]	17.6%
Cholecystectomy	6.9%	2.0%
Inguinal hernia	1.9%	.5%
Appendectomy	11.4%	6.4%
Pelvic		
Abdominal hysterectomy	6.1%	4.2%
Thoracic		
Pulmonary resection (lobectomy)	6.9%	5.5%
Vascular		
Femoral-popliteal bypass		8%

[a] Range 3–11% in different hospitals.
[b] Range 5–20% in different hospitals.

The last topic considered will be the diagnosis and management of major infections in the postoperative period.

PROPHYLACTIC ANTIBIOTICS

Antibiotics are widely used to prevent postoperative infections. Postoperative infections contribute significantly to postoperative mortality, patient discomfort, late or permanent complications (such as enlarged scars or adhesions), prolonged hospitalization (an average of 7–9 days for wound infections), and hospital cost. *Against the risk of postoperative infection must be balanced the staggering extent of antibiotic use for prophylaxis of surgical infections.* Prophylactic antibiotics are used in about 20% of surgical patients, and account for 30% of all antimicrobial drugs used in hospitals (21–22). Major criticisms of prophylactic antibiotics have included widespread use for pro-

cedures where no benefit was apparent (such as hernia repair) and administration of irrational drug regimens.

Internists are increasingly involved in the pros and cons of surgical antibiotic prophylaxis because of questions from antibiotic utilization committees, and the need to know the limitations of prophylaxis in giving postoperative consultation. The introduction below will outline basic principles of surgical prophylaxis and general clinical guidelines for administering prophylactic antibiotics. Major clinical trials will be reviewed by type of surgical procedure in the following sections.

The *definition* of prophylactic antibiotics is the use of antibiotics *prior to establishment* of organisms at a given site to prevent development of clinical infection.

Recent contamination is included within the definition of prophylaxis by many authors. Some contaminated and most dirty procedures fall in this category (e.g., perforated viscus, abdominal trauma). There are important theoretical and empirical differences when antibiotics are administered after, rather than prior to, contamination, including risk of infection, timing, and duration of "prophylaxis." The effectiveness of antibiotics decreases linearly with the time since the introduction of bacteria. Antibiotics were ineffective when administered 3 hours after contamination in an animal model (23–24) (Fig. 16.1). Antibiotic treatment may be required for a longer period when gross spillage from a viscus occurs.

The type(s) of infection prevented by prophylactic antibiotics needs to be clearly understood. Most prophylactic antibiotics in surgery are given to prevent a single infectious complication, i.e., wound infection. Prevention of deeper infection (e.g., at the site of intestinal anastomosis) is a less common reason. Other common reasons for administering antibiotics are prevention of infection at the site of a foreign body (or graft insertion) and sepsis. Attempts to prevent "all infections" have failed because of the many types of bac-

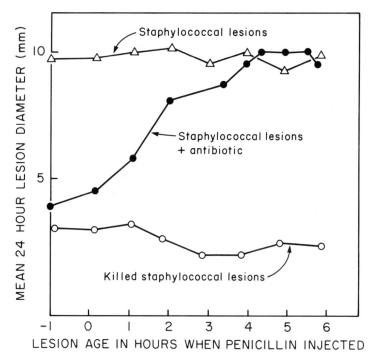

Figure 16.1. Prevention of wound infection by antibiotics in a guinea pig model. The size of the lesion was related to the timing of antibiotics and infection. The antibiotic (penicillin) was most effective when given before introduction of staphylococci. No difference in treated and untreated animals was seen when antibiotics were given 4 hours or longer after infection. (From Burke JF: The effective period of preventive antibiotic action on experimental infections and dermal lesions. *Surgery* 50:162, 1961, with permission.)

teria and varying times of introduction. With few exceptions, antibiotics are not effective in preventing infections that are remote from the operative site and not directly related to surgery, such as pneumonia or urinary tract infection.

Wound infections have a low mortality unless other factors (e.g., malnutrition) are present; morbidity is frequent, including discomfort and scarring. Thus, the prevention of morbidity is quantitatively more important than mortality. This issue is important in evaluating antibiotic trials because sample sizes often are not large enough to demonstrate a difference in mortality.

Multiple reasons (Table 16.3) have been cited for and against use of prophylactic antibiotics. However, no convincing deci-sion can be made strictly from theoretical arguments.

The discussion below will focus on wound infection, where a substantial amount of data has been accumulated (other types of infections will be discussed under individual headings).

Pathophysiology of Wound Infection

The development of a wound infection depends upon three factors: (a) bacterial contamination, (b) systemic resistance, and (c) local factors (24–25, 332).

A surgical wound may be contaminated by bacteria originating from incompletely prepped skin, breaks in the sterility of operative technique, surgery on infected or contaminated tissue, perforation of vis-

Table 16.3. Reasons for and against Use of Prophylactic Antibiotics

For	Against

1. Prevent frequent morbidity and mortality	1. a. Many human trials equivocal or negative
	   b. Increased risk of superinfection and/or resistant organisms
	   c. Toxicity of antibiotics

2. Decrease hospitalization and cost (by preventing complications)	2. High cost of antibiotics; use in large numbers of patients
3. Animal data support efficacy	3. Only good animal model is for wound infections; some experiments negative
4. a. Do no harm b. Avert use of toxic antibiotics for prolonged periods to treat infection	4. Toxicity of antibiotics; use in large numbers of patients
5. Theoretically should work	5. Do not work in practice in many situations
6. Certain patients at high risk of infection (impaired defenses; certain operations)	6. Risk factors and natural history of infections often not well understood (exception: wound infections)

cus, and contamination of operating room environment. Less common sources of bacterial contamination are bacteremic seeding from distant sites and contaminated prosthetic devices or instruments (24).

The quantity of bacteria is a determinant of wound infection. The type of bacteria is also important since certain species such as *Staphylococcus* are more likely to produce actual infection. Contamination by more than one bacterial species may also influence development of infection.

The major systemic factor influencing infection rates is nutrition. Other important systemic factors are age of the patient and diseases decreasing host response to infection (23, 26).

Local defenses at the wound site are important in determining whether infection occurs after contamination. Important local factors are presence of nonviable tissue, presence of a foreign body or drainage, ability to mount a local inflammatory response, and duration of surgery. Surgical skill is a real but poorly defined factor, as shown by the widely varying wound infection rate between hospitals and surgeons (15–16).

The importance of timing of antibiotic administration was shown by Burke (23–24) in a classic series of experiments. Antibiotics were effective in preventing experimental staphylococcal wound infections when given from 1 hour before to 3 hours after the introduction of bacteria. Animals given antibiotics more than 3 hours after bacterial contamination had similar wound infection rates as controls. Infection rates were lowest when antibiotics were given 1 hour prior to introduction of bacteria, and rose linearly until 3 hours after colonization when infection rates were similar to controls (Fig. 16.1). A few human trials have shown that a single preoperative dose alone is as effective as when antibiotic prophylaxis is continued postoperatively. The data from these experiments have been used to justify the need to start prophylactic antibiotics before the operative procedure and the ineffectiveness of prophylaxis past 0–48 hours postoperatively.

In clinical (human) studies, contamination of the wound at surgery is the major determinant of wound infection. A standard classification of wounds is based on the degree of contamination at the time of surgery. The degree of contami-

Table 16.4.   Classification of Surgical Wounds (14–16, 23)

Clean: Operation not involving infected areas, traumatic wounds, or entrance into the gastrointestinal, genitourinary, or respiratory tracts. No break in aseptic technique occurred. (If acute inflammation is not present, cholecystectomy, appendectomy, hysterectomy, and urinary tract operations are included in this category.)

Clean-Contaminated: The gastrointestinal or respiratory (bronchi or oropharynx) tracts are entered but no significant spillage or contamination occurs.

Contaminated: Operations involving acute inflammation without pus, major breaks in sterile technique, or fresh traumatic wounds. (Some authors include spillage from a hollow viscus during surgery.)

Dirty: Operations on perforated viscera, abscesses, old (>4 hr) traumatic wounds, or where pus is encountered.

Table 16.4a.   Wound Infection Risk Index (330)

Factor	Points
1. Abdominal operation	1
2. Operation lasting > 2 hours	1
3. Contaminated or dirty infected operation (by traditional wound classification system)	1
4. Having ≥ 3 diagnoses	1
Total possible points	0–4

Total Points	Wound Infection Risk (%)
0	1%
1	4%
2	9%
3	17%
4	27%

*See text for explanation of terms.

nation has closely paralleled the incidence of wound infection in several studies (Tables 16.4 and 16.5) (15–17).*

Prophylactic antibiotics are not indicated for most clean surgery because of the low rates of infection. Since by its nature prophylaxis will only prevent a proportion of infections, substantial ben-

Table 16.5.   Infection Rates by Wound Classification

	Multicenter Study (15)	Cruse (15a, 16–17)
1. Clean	5.1%	1.5%
2. Clean-Contaminated	10.8%	7.7%
3. Contaminated	16.3%	15.2%
4. Dirty	28.6%	40.0%
Total	7.5%	4.7%

*Dirty wounds occupy the gray area between prophylaxis and treatment. By definition, bacteria are present in most dirty wounds prior to surgery, but often will present to the physician within the 3-hour period when antibiotics are effective. Since antibiotic effectiveness declines even within the 3-hour period after bacterial contamination, we prefer to consider antibiotic therapy of dirty wounds as early treatment.

efit will be difficult to achieve if the baseline infection rates are very low.

Surgical wounds should be classified (Table 16.4) both to decide on the need for prophylaxis in the individual patient and to assess the need for prophylactic antibiotics for a given procedure.

Recent studies (330) have shown better prediction of wound infection when additional operative and patient susceptibility factors (Table 16.4a) are considered in addition to the traditional wound classification (Table 16.4). In addition to the wound classification, this index incorporates location (abdominal) of operation, duration of surgery, and over 3 diagnoses at discharge (a proxy factor incorporating how "ill" the patient was generally and how susceptible to infection). The index was about twice as proficient at predicting wound infection as the traditional wound classification. A few patients undergoing "clean" surgery were at higher risk (because of multiple other risk factors) than patients undergoing contaminated surgery (330, 339).

Other risk factors were less important than the type of wound in determining the wound infection rate in human studies. Significant determinants include increasing age, steroid therapy, obesity, duration of preoperative hospitalization, proper skin preparation, duration of surgery, and number of patients on the ward. Certain factors have not been correlated with wound infection, including air colonization (except possibly for very clean wounds) and diabetes (15–17).

Principles for Use of Prophylactic Antibiotics

Several factors are frequently cited as common elements of an effective prophylactic antibiotic regimen (Table 16.6). These principles have been developed on the basis of clinical experience and by comparing successful and unsuccessful prophylactic regimens.

Ideally, prophylaxis is given for infections that are caused by a single or few organisms, and introduced during a relatively short period of time. The infection should occur with sufficient frequency and/or severity that the benefits outweigh the risks of prophylaxis. Wound infections are

Table 16.6. Principles of Successful Prophylactic Antibiotic Regimens

Procedure
1. Infection to be prevented clearly specified (e.g., wound)
2. Period when bacteria can be introduced brief
3. One or few organisms cause most infections
4. High enough risk of infection that prophylaxis beneficial

Antibiotics
5. Antibiotics cover important organisms; narrow spectrum (all organisms need not be covered)
6. Least toxic drugs
7. Avoid "first line" antibiotics that may be needed for infection, if other agents effective (because of resistance). Use least expensive drugs.
8. Administer prior to contamination
9. Therapeutic serum-tissue levels through entire period of operation when contamination occurs
10. Administer for as short duration as possible and only during period prophylaxis effective. Avoid administration >1 hr pre-op and prolonged administration (usually >48 hr) post-op

generally preventable because they are caused by a few species of bacteria introduced at the time of surgery. Conversely, postoperative urinary tract infections and pneumonia are poor targets for prophylaxis because they can be caused by a large variety of bacteria at any time during hospitalization.

The antibiotic used should cover most or all important organisms, but all possible infecting agents need not (and often cannot) be covered. Antibiotics used should be of the narrowest spectrum possible, least toxic, and the lowest cost. Where multiple antibiotic regimens are equivalent, "first line" antibiotics should be avoided to decrease the acquisition of resistance by organisms within the hospital. The antibiotics should be administered for as briefly as possible (usually less than 1 hour preoperatively and less than 24 hours postoperatively; often 1–2 doses total are sufficient), administered prior to contamination, and in adequate doses to achieve therapeutic serum-tissue levels throughout the entire operative period. Additional doses of antibiotics may need to be given during surgery for prolonged operations or where the half-life of the antibiotic is short.

Infections will still occur despite prophylactic antibiotics due to local factors and resistant organisms. Infections remote from the site targeted for prophylaxis will not be decreased, and may be increased, especially if prophylaxis is prolonged.

Human Trials

A large number of clinical trials have been conducted in the past 15 years to determine appropriate indications and use of prophylactic antibiotics. Most of the studies have had faulty study designs (26–28, 328). In reviewing the studies under individual procedures below, the selected major points of study design listed in Table 16.7 should be considered. The most important points of study design are rep-

Table 16.7. Criteria for Adequate Study Design for Clinical Trials of Antibiotic Prophylaxis[a]

1. Prospective, randomized design (includes concurrent controls)
2. Sample stratified by risk or extent of disease before randomization
3. Adequate sample size from a defined, representative population undergoing a single procedure
4. Double-blinded design
5. Antibiotic present before bacteria introduced (prophylaxis vs. treatment)
6. Diagnostic criteria for infection objective and specific. Relevant outcomes measured (mortality, number of infections). All possible infections cultured.
7. Antibiotic active against relevant organisms; first dose administered preoperatively; adequate dose and limited duration of administration. Proof target organisms are susceptible.
8. Count antibiotic complications including drug toxicity, superinfection and change in resistance patterns
9. All patients randomized included in analysis
10. Statistical testing performed

[a]Variables that are not adequate end points are fever, change in colonization, and sterile cultures in absence of clinical infection.

resentative patient samples, randomization, clear definition of the type of infection to be prevented, and adequate, blinded evaluation of the patient.

Because of the large number of studies comparing new cephalosporin drugs and space limitations, only major or representative studies of these drugs are summarized in the tables. Prophylactic antibiotics are covered in other chapters for burns (see p. 568), urinary tract infections (see p. 177) and ENT procedures (see p. 575).

Recommended prophylactic antibiotic regimens are summarized in Table 16.8.

Pneumonia

RATIONALE

Postoperative pneumonia accounts for 16% of postoperative infections, and is the leading cause of death from nosocomial infection. The mortality of nosocomial pneumonia ranges from 30–70% (9–10, 12, 19, 49) (see also p. 415). The gram-

Table 16.8. Recommended Antimicrobial Prophylaxis for Surgery[a,b]

Type of Surgery	Recommended Regimens		Specific Regimens	Postoperative Frequency and Duration[a]	Notes
	First Choice	Alternative			
Gastro-intestinal					
Upper gastro-intestinal	Cephalosporin	Uncertain	Cefazolin (1 gm)	Every 6–8 hours for 1 dose to 24 hours	Not indicated for uncomplicated peptic ulcer surgery
Colon and rectum	1. Neomycin-erythromycin ± 2. Cephalosporin high-risk patients only	1. Cephalosporin or 2. Metronidazole ± aminoglycoside	Neomycin (1 gm) and erythromycin base (1 gm) at 1 PM, 2 PM, 11 PM day before surgery	None given post-op	Neomycin and erythromycin preferable for high-risk patients
			Cephalothin (2 gm) 6 PM day before and 12 AM, 6 AM day of surgery Cefoxitin (2 gm)	Every 6 hours for 2–6 doses	
Cholecystectomy	Cephalosporin	Uncertain	Cefazolin (1 gm)	Every 6–8 hours for 12–48 hours	High-risk patients only

Table continues next page

Table 16.8. *Continued*

Type of Surgery	Recommended Regimens		Specific Regimens	Postoperative Frequency and Duration[a]	Notes
	First Choice	Alternative			
Orthopaedics					
Hip fractures	Cephalosporin	Semisynthetic penicillin	Nafcillin (500 mg–1 gm)	Every 6 hours for 24 hours	
Total hip replacement	Cephalosporin	Semisynthetic penicillin	Cefazolin (1 gm)	Every 6 hours for 24 hours	
Lower extremity amputation for ischemia	Cefoxitin	Uncertain	Cefixitin (2 gm)	Every 6 hours for 24 hours	
Otolaryngology	Cephalosporin	Uncertain	Cefazolin (1 gm)	Every 6 hours for 4 doses	Indicated only for extensive cancer surgery or entry into oropharynx
Pulmonary					See text
Gynecology					
Vaginal hysterectomy	Cephalosporin	? Ampicillin	Cephalothin (1–2 gm); cefazolin (1 gm)	Every 6 hours for 12–18 hours	? Premenopausal only
Abdominal hysterectomy					See text
Urology					
Transurethral prostate resection					Treat preoperative infection by sensitivities; no routine prophylaxis if urine sterile
Neurosurgery					See text
Vascular surgery	Cephalosporin	Uncertain	Cefazolin (1 gm)	Every 6 hours for 4 doses	Not indicated for upper extremity procedures

[a] Timing of administration. **Initial dose:** all regimens require one dose preoperatively within 1 hour of surgery; a second dose in the operating room may be necessary for surgery lasting more than 4 hours or the expected duration of action of the antibiotic. **Duration:** most regimens should be stopped within 24 hours postoperatively. Data for most procedures suggest 1–3 total doses (including preoperative dose) are sufficient (see text) (43); colorectal procedures may be an exception.

[b] See references 35–38; text.

[c] For most indications, 2nd and 3rd generation cephalosporins have not been shown to be superior to 1st generation (40, 47).

negative pneumonias carry the highest mortality ranging from 40–70%.

High-risk groups include patients who are in coma, in intensive care units, on respirators, intubated, using respiratory care equipment, or debilitated (50). Postoperative pneumonia does not fit the criteria for prophylaxis (Table 16.6) because of the wide variety of possible organisms, the rapid acquisition of new organisms, and the prolonged period the patient is at risk.

CLINICAL STUDIES

Antibiotics alone do not decrease postoperative production of purulent sputum (51). Antibiotic prophylaxis increased the incidence of pneumonia in a comparative trial of unconscious patients (52). Broad-spectrum antibiotic use has been implicated in the development of gram-negative pneumonias in surgical patients (49). Aerosolized polymyxin decreased the occurrence of *Pseudomonas* pneumonia in a controlled trial, but an increased incidence of pneumonia caused by unusual polymyxin-resistant organisms occurred after prolonged use (49–50). Several studies of antibiotic prophylaxis for wound infection have not found a decreased incidence of respiratory infections in antibiotic-treated patients (63, 72, 74, 82).

RECOMMENDATIONS

Antibiotics should not be used for prophylaxis of pneumonia in surgical patients.

Appendectomy

RATIONALE

Wound infection is the only common complication of appendectomy to be considered for antibiotic prophylaxis. Appendectomy is classified as clean, contaminated surgery because the colonized lower bowel is transected. The incidence of wound infection after appendectomies is proportionally high at about 10% (Table 16.2). When the appendix is perforated, the incidence of wound infection is much higher; in addition, peritonitis or abscess may occur. Antibiotics used for perforated appendices should be considered treatment, rather than prophylaxis, because bacteria are present before the antibiotic is administered.

CLINICAL STUDIES

Uncontrolled and comparative studies have found conflicting results in using antibiotics for appendectomies (42–43, 53–54). A randomized trial of ampicillin or tetracycline compared to control found no effect on wound infection (15–20%) or duration of postoperative fever in uncomplicated acute appendicitis (normal appendix or acute, unperforated appendix). A higher incidence of intraperitoneal

abscess occurred in the patients not receiving antibiotics, but most were in patients with perforated appendices (53).

RECOMMENDATIONS

Prophylactic antibiotics are controversial for uncomplicated appendectomy. The weight of evidence is beginning to favor prophylaxis with a second generation cephalosporin. Antibiotic treatment should be given for complications of appendicitis, including peritonitis and abscess. Antibiotic treatment depends on the sensitivities of the organism(s) found and is of a longer duration than prophylaxis.

Cholecystectomy

RATIONALE

Antibiotics are given to patients undergoing cholecystectomy to prevent wound infection and cholangitis with resulting septicemia. Cholangitis and septicemia presumably result from instrumentation and manipulation of a previously colonized biliary tract during surgery.

CLINICAL STUDIES

The incidence of wound infection after cholecystectomy ranges from 1–21% (Tables 16.2 and 16.9). The risk of wound infection is substantially higher in the presence of infected bile and/or complications of cholelithiasis. A high-risk group with a wound infection rate of 20–27% can be identified by five factors: (a) age over 70, (b) obstructive jaundice, (c) common duct stones, (d) emergent acute cholecystitis, and (e) cholangitis (58). Diabetes may also be a risk factor.

Patients with none of these factors have an incidence of infected bile of about 17%. The risk of wound infection with sterile bile or none of the above complications ranges from 1–2% (15a, 44, 54).

The organisms causing wound infection after cholecystectomy are usually the same gram-negative organisms found in the biliary tree.

Statistically significant reduction in

Table 16.9.   Biliary Surgery: Antibiotic Prophylaxis[e]

Study (Year)	Patient Group	Antibiotic Regimen	Number (Antibiotic/ Control)	Wound Infection		Sepsis	
				Antibiotic	Control	Antibiotic	Control
Keighley (1975)	All patients	Gentamicin × 5 days	100 (49/48)	3 (6%)	10 (21%)[a]	1 (1%)	5 (10%) NS[b]
Moran (1978)	All patients	Cotrimoxazide × 1 dose	95 (48/47)	28 (4%)	10 (21%)[a]	1 (2%)	5 (11%)[c]
Stone (1976)	All patients	Cefazolin × 2 days (start pre-op)	131 (60/38)	1 (2%)	4 (11%)[a]		
		Cefazolin × ½ days (start post-op)	(33/38)	3 (9%)	4 (11%)		
Strachan (1977)	All patients	Cefazolin × 1 dose	201 (63/65)	2 (3%)	11 (17%)[a]		
		Cefazolin × 5 days	(73/65)	4 (6%)	11 (17%)[a]		
Evans (1973)	All patients	Cephaloridine × 3 doses	59 (31/28)	2 (6%)	6 (21%)[c]		
Elliott (1977)	High risk	Cephaloridine × 4 doses	140 (78/62)	6 (8%)	3 (5%)[c]	1 (1%)	7 (11%)[c]
Kauffman (1984)	All patients	Gentamicin × 4 doses	105 (56/49)	2 (4%)	12 (25%)[a]		
Lewis (1987)	High risk	Cefazolin × 1 dose	92 (52/40)	1 (5%)	10 (25%)		

[a] $p < 0.05$.
[b] NS, not significant.
[c] Statistical testing not done.
[d] $p < 0.05$.
[e] See also reference 43.

wound infection from 11–21% to 2–6% was found in five randomized studies (54–57, 61). Two additional studies showed a similar trend favoring antibiotics, but did not have separate statistical analysis (43–44, 58). A single preoperative dose or three doses immediately perioperatively were as effective as a 5-day course of antibiotics (43, 56, 63).

The incidence of sepsis following cholecystectomy in patients not treated with antibiotics is up to 10% (Table 16.9). A decreased rate of sepsis has been shown in three controlled studies of prophylactic antibiotics, but no statistical analysis was performed or the sample sizes were too small to demonstrate statistical significance. Risk factors for sepsis are similar to those for wound infection above.

Many patients with acute cholecystitis have high fever and leukocytosis. Preoperatively, it may be impossible to tell whether cholangitis, sepsis, or biliary infection is present. In this setting, antibiotic usage represents treatment of a suspected infection, rather than prophylaxis.

RECOMMENDATIONS

Antibiotics are not recommended for uncomplicated cholecystectomy in the absence of clinical cholecystitis or other risk factors (age > 70, jaundice, common duct stone, cholecystitis, diabetes mellitus). In the presence of these risk factors, prophylaxis is usually administered, but is not required in all cases. A cephalosporin antibiotic is recommended, since most studies have used this group of antibiotics. Single studies have indicted that both cotrimoxazole and gentamycin are effective; ampicillin should also be effective, although studies are lacking.

Most studies have administered one dose preoperatively and continue prophylaxis for 1–2 days postoperatively, although 1–3 perioperative doses are as effective (43, 56–58, 62–63).

Upper Gastrointestinal Surgery

RATIONALE

A moderately high incidence of wound infection has been reported following gastroduodenal surgery. Other types of infection and sepsis are unusual in the absence of preexisting infection or perforation.

CLINICAL STUDIES

The incidence of wound infection following surgery on the stomach or duodenum ranges from 10–30% (Tables 16.2 and 16.10) (55, 62, 64–65). The risk is much higher for gastric ulcer or cancer (22–23%) than uncomplicated duodenal ulcer (4–5%). The difference has been related to the higher incidence and colony count of bacterial colonization in stomachs with low acidity (65, 65a). Some au-

thors have found an increased incidence of wound infection following emergency surgery for actively bleeding ulcers (65).

Patients with gastroduodenal resections were included in four randomized studies, although only one studied solely upper gastrointestinal surgery. A statistically significant reduction in wound infections from 20–35% to 0–5% was found (Table 16.10) (42–43, 47, 55–62, 64–65a). A cephalosporin was given for a duration of three doses to 5 days (65).

RECOMMENDATIONS

Antibiotics are not indicated for surgery for uncomplicated duodenal ulcer. Prophylaxis should be given when surgery is performed for gastric carcinoma, for gastric bypass for obesity, or in the presence of achlorhydria due to other reasons (atrophic gastritis, prior gastric resection). Inadequate data are available to make a recommendation for gastric ulcer or emergency surgery for gastrointestinal bleeding.

The recommended regimen is a single dose of a cephalosporin given 1 hour preoperatively, followed postoperatively for a postoperative duration from 2 doses to 1 day.

Table 16.10. Upper Gastrointestinal Surgery: Prophylactic Antibiotics

				Wound Infections		
Study (Year)	Patient Group	Antibiotic Regimen	Number	Antibiotic Group	Control Group	P
Stone (1976)	Stomach only	Cefazolin × 3 days	96	2 (4%)	5 (22%)	<0.01
Evans (1973)	Vagotomy-pyloroplasty; gastrectomy	Cephaloridine × 3 doses	66	1 (3%)	6 (20%)	Not done
Polk (1969)	Gastroduodenal	Cephaloridine × 3 doses	68	0 (0%)	11 (30%)	<0.001
Nichols (1982)	Gastroduodenal	Cefamandole × 3 doses	39	1 (5%)	7 (35%)	<.01
Feltis (1967)	Gastroduodenal		104	2 (5%)	14 (22%)	<.02
Lewis (1979)	Gastroduodenal	Cephaloridine × 2 doses	83	0 (0%)	11 (26%)	<.02

[a] See reference 42.

Lower Gastrointestinal (Colorectal) Surgery

RATIONALE

The clearest rationale for prophylactic antibiotics is present for surgery on the colon and rectum. The most common postoperative infection after colon surgery is wound infection; less common but more serious complications are intraperitoneal abscess, anastomotic breakdown, and sepsis. Infectious complications are a significant contributor to mortality after colectomy (66–68). Although significant colony counts of multiple aerobic gram-negative organisms may be cultured from the colon, a much larger number of anaerobes are present.

CLINICAL STUDIES

Wound infection occurs in 10–60% of patients undergoing elective colectomy without antibiotics (Table 16.11). Wound infection rates have varied from 5–20% (Table 16.2) among hospitals using a variety of prophylactic regimens. An increased risk of anastomotic breakdown accompanies local infections of any type, but uncertainty exists whether infection of the suture line is the cause, or the result of the breakdown of the colonic anastomosis. The risk of bacteremia or septicemia after colectomy ranges from 2–10%. A significant proportion of the postoperative mortality is related to postoperative infections of the wound, peritoneum, distant organs, and sepsis (Table 16.11) (66–72).

Wound infection has been significantly reduced in randomized studies using neomycin-erythromycin (42–43, 66–67, 69, 74); neomycin-other antibiotic (42–43, 72–73), and cephalosporins (42–43, 47, 62, 64, 67, 74) (Tables 16.11 and 16.12). Limited evidence suggests that anastomotic dehiscence and deep intra-abdominal abscesses are also reduced by prophylactic oral antibiotics (329).

The carefully done, randomized Veterans Administration trial demonstrated that a neomycin-erythromycin combina-

tion was superior to a cephalosporin with a 6 vs. 30% wound infection rate (67). A statistically significant reduction was obtained for all infectious complications combined (39 vs. 6%), and bacteremia-septicemia (7 vs. 1%). There was a slight reduction in mortality from 4/67 (6%) in the cephalosporin to 2/126 (2%) in the neomycin-erythromycin group, which was not statistically significant.

Several trials have demonstrated that a cephalosporin will reduce the incidence of wound infection compared to groups receiving placebo (Table 16.11) (62, 66, 74). The degree of reduction in wound infections differs in various trials, in part because of markedly different rates of infection in the control group. A combination of neomycin-erythromycin and a cephalosporin further reduced the wound infection rate in one study (74); a repeat trial is underway (67).

Most studies have administered three doses of neomycin-erythromycin within less than 24 hours preoperatively. Cephalosporins have been administered as one dose preoperatively and continued postoperatively for a total of three doses to five days.

Several older trials have tested the efficacy of multiple parenteral antibiotics, including an aminoglycoside or combinations of an aminoglycoside with non-absorbable antibiotics (Tables 16.11 and 16.12) (69, 72, 76–78). Most of these studies were inconclusive in demonstrating a therapeutic effect. An increased incidence of staphylococcal enterocolitis was found when parenteral and oral non-absorbable antibiotics were combined (77–79).

Metronidazole has been shown to decrease wound infections both alone and in combination with aminoglycosides (68, 70, 76, 80, 92). Metronidazole has not been used widely for prophylaxis in the United States because of fears of carcinogenesis.

Mechanical preparation of the bowel by laxatives and enemas decreases the quantity of feces, and the chance of fecal spil-

Table 16.11. Colon Surgery: Prophylactic Antibiotics

Study (Year)	Antibiotic Regimen[a]	Number	Wound Infections		Other Infectious Complications (Antibiotic vs. Control %)	
			Antibiotic Group	Control Group	Bacteremia Sepsis	Mortality
Clarke (1977)	Neo + Ery × 3 doses	116	5 (9%)[b]	21 (35%)	2% vs. 10%	2% vs. 12%
Evans (1973)	Cephal × 3 doses	69	10 (29%)	15 (43%)		
Eykyn (1979)	Metron	83	6 (14%)	20 (51%)		
Goldring (1975)	Metron + Kan × 3 days	50	2 (5%)[b]	11 (44%)		4% vs. 8%
Hughes (1979)	Pen × 1 dose	108	5 (9%)	11 (23%)		6% vs. 6%
Nichols (1973)	Neo + Ery × 3 doses	20	0 (0%)	3 (30%)		
Polk (1969)	Cephal × 3 doses	104	4 (7%)[b]	15 (30%)		
Rosenberg (1971)	PTS × 5 days or PTS + Neo × 2 days	128	(47%)[b]	(73%)		
Stone (1976)	Cz × 2 days + Neo + Ery × 2 days	190	6 (6%)[b]	7 (16%)		
Washington (1974)	Neo Neo & Tobra	196	28 (41%) 3 (5%)[b]	27 (43%)	6; 3% vs. 6%	3; 3% vs. 8%
Willis (1977)	Metron	46	0 (0%)[b]	11 (58%)		
Burdon (1977)	Cephal × 2 doses	42	5 (28%)	11 (46%)		
Burdon (1977)	Cephal × 2 doses	51	13 (46%)	13 (56%)		
Kjellgren (1977)	Ceph. × 4 days		10 (17%)	26 (53%)[b]		

[a] Neo, neomycin; Ery, erythromycin; Ceph, cephalothin; Cephal, cephalordine; Metron, metronidazole; Kan, kanamycin; Lin, lincomycin; Tobra, tobramycin, PTS, phthalysalphathiazole; Bac, bacitracin; Cz, cephazolin.
[b] Statistically significant ($p \leq 0.05$) difference between antibiotics and control groups.
[c] See reference 42.

lage, but not the concentration of bacteria in the colon. Thus, mechanical preparation is important in preventing fecal spillage but is not equivalent to antibiotic prophylaxis in reducing bacterial concentration (67, 79).

Antibiotic prophylaxis for local infection does not reduce the incidence of distant pulmonary and urinary tract infections (63, 72, 74, 82). Cephalosporins have been administered from one dose to 5 days. Stone (63) found similar wound infection rates for three perioperative doses of cephalosporin compared to 5 days of administration in various types of abdominal surgery. Among patients undergoing

Table 16.12. Colon Surgery: Comparisons of Different Prophylactic Antibiotic Regimens

Study (Year)	Antibiotic Regimen	Number	Wound Infections (%)	Other Infectious Complications		
				Total	Bacteremia/septicemia	Mortality
Altemeier (1966)	Neomycin & sulfathaladine & penicillin & tetracycline × 4 days	19	1 (5%)			
	Paromomycin & penicillin & tetracycline × 4 days	18	2 (11%)			
	Sulfathaladine & penicillin & tetracycline × 7 days	16	0 (0%)			
	Neomycin & sulfathaladine pre-op only × 1 day	23	3 (13%)			
	Penicillin & tetracycline post-op only × 3 days	17	0 (0%)			
Condon (1979)	Cephalothin × 4 days	67	20 (30%)	26 (39%)[a]	5 (7%)[a]	4 (6%)
	Neomycin-erythromycin × 3 doses (+ cephalothin × 4 days)	126	7 (6%)[a]	7 (6%)	1 (1%)	2 (2%)
Sellwood (1969)	PTS[b] × 96 hr	35		10 (62%)		
	Neomycin & bacitracin & Nystatin × 48 hr	16 19		4 (21%)		
Washington (1974)	Neomycin	68	28 (41%)	4 (6%)	2 (3%)	
	Neomycin & tetracycline	65	3 (5%)[a]	2 (3%)	2 (3%)	
Brass (1976)	Metron[b]	39	2 (5%)			
	Erythromycin	40	10 (25%)			
Keighley (1979)	Metron & kanamycin (oral)	47	17 (36%)			
	Metron & kanamycin (IV)	46	3 (6%)[a]			

[a] Statistically significant ($p \leq 0.05$) from other regimen in study.
[b] PTS, phthalysulphathiazole; Metron, metronidazole.

colon resection, 5/54 (9%) of three-dose and 5/47 (11%) of 5-day regimen patients had wound infections; 2/54 (4%) of three-dose and 1/47 (2%) of 5-day regimen patients had intraabdominal infections (63). Subsequent studies show about 24 hours postoperative antibiotics is as effective as longer courses. Single dose prophylaxis preoperatively alone is less effective than when combined with 2–4 postoperative doses.

RECOMMENDATIONS

Antibiotic prophylaxis is clearly indicated for colon surgery because of the high rate of wound infections, peritoneal infections, and sepsis. Multiple trials have indicated that antibiotic prophylaxis at least reduces the incidence of wound infections. Neomycin-erythromycin (Table 16.8) is an effective regimen. A cephalosporin administered for one dose preoperatively and for less than 48 hours postoperatively does reduce the rate of wound infections. A cephalosporin is probably less effective than neomycin-erythromycin, at least in the setting where a high rate of infection is suspected.

Neomycin-erythromycin orally is the first choice prophylactic regimen. In high-risk patients, addition of a parenteral cephalosporin for more than one dose but no more than 24 hours seems to give added benefit. Cephalothin has been shown to be effective; at least theoretically, a cephalosporin with anaerobic activity should be more effective, but this has not been convincingly demonstrated in clinical trials. Mechanical preparation with laxatives and enemas should be used in all patients. Regimens that should NOT be used are parenteral, non-absorbable antibiotic combinations (with the possible exception of cephalosporin with neomycin-erythromycin), parenteral aminoglycosides (as first choice), administration of antibiotics only after surgery, and prolonged antibiotic administration beyond 48 hours postoperatively.

Abdominal Trauma

Antibiotics are administered for abdominal trauma because of the possibility of perforation of the gastrointestinal tract. This use of antibiotics represents treatment because bacterial contamination occurs at the time of trauma prior to institution of antibiotics. Thus, antibiotics for abdominal trauma are discussed in detail in the section on peritoneal infections (see p. 426).

Vascular Surgery

RATIONALE

The results of infection of synthetic vascular grafts are devastating in terms of mortality and loss of tissue (i.e., amputation) due to loss of vascular supply. Antibiotic prophylaxis is used to avoid this devastating consequence, although the incidence of infection is felt to be low. A secondary consideration is wound infection. The most common organisms are skin and bowel organisms (99).

CLINICAL STUDIES

The incidence of graft infections is about 2% after vascular surgery. The incidence of wound infection ranges from 5–15% (Table 16.13) (62, 96, 98–99).

Two of three randomized trials showed that a cephalosporin given as one dose immediately preoperatively and for 24 hours postoperatively reduced the rate of wound and possibly graft infections (Table 16.11). Vascular surgery on the upper extremity (brachiocephalic) has a low risk of infection and may not require prophy-

Table 16.13.   Vascular Surgery: Antibiotic Prophylaxis

Study (year)	Antibiotic	Number (Antibiotic/ Placebo)	Infection Studied	Infections (%) Antibiotic Group	Control Group
Kaiser (1978)	Cefazolin (1 gm × 5 doses)	462 (225/237)	All	2 (0.9%)	16 (6.8%)
			Graft	0 (0%)	4 (1.7%)
			Wound	2 (0.9%)	12 (5.1%)
Evans and Pollack (1973)	Cephaloridine (1 gm × 3 doses)	73 (27/46)	Wound	6 (22%)	7 (15%)
Hasselgren (1984)	Cefuroxime	211 (121/66)	Wound	5 (4%)	11 (17%)
			Graft	0 (0%)	1 (2%)

laxis (96). Wound infection in amputation of an ischemic lower extremity was reduced by antibiotics (100).

RECOMMENDATIONS

Prophylactic antibiotics are recommended for vascular surgery, with the possible exception of upper extremity procedures, based upon the devastating effects of graft infection despite the low (2%) incidence. Administration of a first generation cephalosporin immediately preoperatively and for 24 hours postoperatively is the recommended regimen. Prophylaxis with cefoxitin for 24 hours is recommended for ischemic lower extremity amputations.

Gynecologic Surgery

VAGINAL HYSTERECTOMY

Rationale

A high incidence of wound infections in the vaginal cuff accompanies vaginal hysterectomy. More serious but less common infections are pelvic cellulitis and adenexal abscesses. Prophylactic antibiotics are mainly given to prevent vaginal cuff infections.

Clinical Studies

Studies have used two criteria for postoperative infections after vaginal hysterectomy because of the difficulty of being certain of infections at the end of the vaginal cuff (wound infection). "Febrile morbidity" has been defined as a temperature greater than 100.4°–100.6°F on two separate occasions separated by 6–24 hours. "Wound infections" have been defined clinically by the appearance of the vaginal cuff and culture of pathogenic bacteria from swabs of the vaginal apex. The incidence of febrile morbidity has ranged from 28–74% and of clinical vaginal cuff infections from 17–64% (Table 16.14). The risk is higher in premenopausal patients.

Multiple studies have shown a reduction in wound infection with antibiotics

(42, 101–111). The most commonly used antibiotics have been cephalosporins. Efficacy in preventing vaginal cuff infections has also been demonstrated for ampicillin-streptomycin (101–107). A single dose preoperatively or one dose preoperatively plus two doses postoperatively are as effective as a longer duration of therapy (101–107).

Prophylactic antibiotics have reduced febrile morbidity from 32–74% to 0–24% (Table 16.14) (101–111). Clinical wound infections were reduced from 13–64% to 0–20%.

Unlike most other surgical procedures, prophylaxis for vaginal hysterectomy also reduces the incidence of urinary tract infection in most studies (31, 101–105, 108, 110).

Recommendations

Antibiotic prophylaxis should be administered to women undergoing vaginal hysterectomy. Some authorities would restrict use to premenopausal women or to institutions where infection rates are high (7, 31). Cephalosporins have been the most widely evaluated, but ampicillin may be adequate. Aminoglycosides are not recommended because less toxic antibiotics are effective. Duration of prophylaxis should be 12–18 hours postoperatively.

ABDOMINAL HYSTERECTOMY

Rationale

Wound infections are less common with abdominal hysterectomy compared to vaginal technique. The major use of prophylactic antibiotics has been in prevention of wound infections.

Clinical Studies

Substantially less information is available on the usefulness of antibiotics after abdominal hysterectomy compared to vaginal hysterectomy. Similar to vaginal hysterectomy, infectious complications have been defined as febrile morbidity (temperature greater than 100.4°–100.6°F on two occasions) and clinical wound in-

Table 16.14. Vaginal Hysterectomy: Prophylactic Antibiotics

Study (Year)	Antibiotic Regimen	Febrile Morbidity (t > 100.4)			Wound, Pelvic Infections	
		Number	Antibiotic Group	Control Group	Antibiotic Group	Control Group
Bivens (1975)	Cephalothin Cephalexin × 48 hr	60	4 (13%)	13 (43%)[a]	4 (20%)	6 (13%) NS[b]
Breeden (1974)	Cephaloridine × 12 hr	120	6 (9%)	29 (52%)[a]	2 (3%)	11 (19%)[a]
Allen (1972)	Cephalothin × 5 days	98	2 (4%)	25 (50%)[a]	2 (4%)	20 (40%)[c]
Grossman (1979)	Penicillin × 48 hr	78	5 (19%)	17 (71%)[c]	2 (8%)	6 (25%)[c]
	Cefazolin × 48 hr		5 (18%)		1 (4%)	
Harrolson (1974)	Penicillin + strepto-mycin × 48 hr	200	8 (8%)	37 (37%)[c]	1 (10%)	19 (19%)[c]
Jennings (1978)	Cefazolin-cephaloxin > 24 hr	101	10 (21%)	32 (74%)[a]	1 (2%)	14 (33%)[a]
Ledger (1973)	Cephaloridine × 24 hr	100	12 (24%)	23 (46%)[a]	4 (8%)	17 (34%)[a]
Mendelson (1979)	Cephradine × 1 dose	66	2 (9%)	16 (73%)[a]	1 (4%)	14 (64%)[a]
	Cephradine × 24 hr	0		0 (0%)		
Ohm (1975)	Cephalordine × 5 days	48	0 (0%)	11 (48%)[a]	0 (0%)	5 (22%)[c]
Bolling (1973)	Ampicillin or te-traycline × 7 days	296	9 (7%)	57 (32%)[c]	(27%)	(4%)[c]
Forney (1976)	Cephaloridine × 4 days	32	0 (0%)	6 (44%)	0 (0%)	4 (29%)[c]
Swantz (1976)	Cephalozin × 3 doses	96	10 (24%)	28 (52%)[a]		
Lett (1977)[d]	Cafazolin × 1 dose or Cephaloridine × 3 doses	153			6 (14%)	29 (61%)[a]
Holman (1976)[d]	Cefazolin × 3 dose	84	2 (5%)	13 (30%)[a]	?0 (%)	10 (23%)[a]
Roberts (1976)[d]	Carbenicillin × 5 doses	52	2 (8%)	9 (35%)[a]	0 (0%)	3 (12%)[c]
Mathews (1979)[d]	TMP-SMT × dose	50			(8%)	(16%)
Polk (1980)[d]	Cefazolin × 3 doses	86	(14%)	(31%)[a]	(2%)	(21%)[a]
Hemsell (1980)[d]	Cefoxitin × 3 doses	99			(8%)	(57%)[a]
Michell (1980)[d]	Cefoxitin × 3 doses	125			7 (10%)	17 (30%)[a]

[a] p < 0.05.
[b] NS, not significant.
[c] Statistical testing not done.
[d] See reference 42.

Table 16.15. Abdominal Hysterectomy: Prophylactic Antibiotics

Study (Year)	Antibiotic Regimen	Febrile Morbidity (t>100.6)			Wound, Pelvic Infections	
		Number	Antibiotic Group	Control Group	Antibiotic Group	Control Group
Allen (1972)	Cephalothin × 5 days	168	12 (14%)	34 (41%)[a]	7 (8%)	18 (22%)[b]
Grossman (1979)	Penicillin × 48 hr	239	24 (32%)	22 (26%)[c]	4 (5%)	9 (11%)[c]
	Cefazolin × 48 hr		28 (35%)[c]		9 (11%)[c]	
Jennings (1978)	Cefazolin cephalexin (>24 hr) Cephalexin (>24 hr)	102	40 (8%)	17 (33%)[a]	0 (0%)	6 (12%)[a]
Ohm (1976)	Cephaloridine × 5 days	93	17 (15%)	18 (39%)[b]	3 (6%)	8 (15%)[b]
Swantz (1976)	Cefalozin × 3 doses	135	9 (16%)	18 (23%)[a]		
Holman[d]	Cefazolin × 3 doses	80	6 (14%)	17 (45%)	(5%)	(34%)[a]
Roberts[d]	Carbenicillin × 5 doses	47	1 (4%)	12 (54%)[a]	1 (4%)	3 (14%)[c]
Polk[d]	Cefazolin × 3 doses	429	(14%)	(20%)[a]	(14%)	(21%)[a]
Mathews[d]	TMP-SMX	59			(27%)	(38%)
Schapens[d]	Cefoxitin	103			(6%)	(16%)
Duff[d]	Cefoxitin × 2 doses	91			8 (18%)	12 (24%)[c]

[a] p < .05.
[b] Statistical testing not done.
[c] Not significant.
[d] See ref. 42.

fection. The incidence of febrile morbidity after abdominal hysterectomy has ranged from 26–41%, and clinical wound infection from 11–22% (Table 16.15) (113–116).

Prophylactic antibiotics have reduced the incidence of febrile morbidity from 23–39% to 8–32% (Table 16.15), and of wound infections from 11–22% to 0–11% (Table 16.15).

Authorities are less convinced of the need for prophylactic antibiotics after abdominal hysterectomy because of the lower incidences of infection and the fewer, less well-designed studies (7, 31, 42, 112).

Recommendations

Inadequate data exist to make a recommendation on prophylactic antibiotic use for abdominal hysterectomies. An exception would be institutions or settings where a high incidence of wound infection is expected. When antibiotics are used, the recommended regimen is a cephalosporin given one dose preoperatively through 12–18 hours postoperatively.

Transurethral Prostate Resection (TURP)

RATIONALE

Traditionally, prostatectomy has been associated with a high incidence of morbidity and mortality due to sepsis. The high incidence of septic complications was seen with open prostatectomy and transurethral prostatectomy by older techniques. Newer techniques of transure-

Table 16.16. **Transurethral Prostate Surgery: Risk of Bacteriuria, Bacteremia, and Sepsis in Patients Not Receiving Antibiotics**[a]

Study (Year)	Number without Antibiotics	Bacteriuria	Bacteremia	Sepsis
Sterile pre-op				
Plorde (1965)	15	6 (40%)	1 (7%)	0 (0%)
Morris (1976)	53	14 (26%)	6 (11%)	3 (6%)
Gibbon (1978)	50	6 (12%)		
Matthew (1978)	40	10 (25%)	0 (0%)	0 (0%)
Creevy (1954)	94		43 (46%)	
McGuire (1974)	44		4 (9%)	
Lacy (1971)	24	(54%)		
Genster (1970)	43	(70%)		
Landes (1976)	156	(14%)		
Gonzalez (1976)	49	20 (41%)		
Bacteriuria pre-op				
Plorde (1965)	22	19 (86%)	2 (9%)	0 (0%)
Appleton (1956)	50	50 (100%)		4 (8%)
McGuire (1974)	13		0 (0%)	
Genster (1970)	40	(100%)		
Landes (1976)	81	(28%)		

[a] See also reference 134.

thral resection have a low but significant incidence of asymptomatic bacteremia and a smaller incidence of clinical sepsis. The major focus of antibiotic prophylaxis is postoperative bacteriuria and symptomatic urinary tract infection.

CLINICAL STUDIES

Infectious morbidity after transurethral prostate resection has been measured as postoperative fever, bacteriuria (positive urine cultures regardless of symptomology), bacteremia (positive blood cultures), and clinical sepsis (positive blood cultures and clinical picture). The incidence of bacteriuria after TURP has ranged widely from 10–100% in different studies (Table 16.16). A major influence is the presence or absence of infection in the preoperative urine. When the preoperative urine is sterile, the incidence of postoperative bacteriuria ranges from 12–54% (Table 16.16). Infected preoperative urine is followed by a 28–100% incidence of postoperative bacteriuria (Table 16.16) (7, 123, 134). If routine postoperative blood cultures are taken in patients with sterile

preoperative urine, the incidence of bacteremia ranges from 0–11% and clinical sepsis occurs in 0–6% of patients (7, 123). An increased incidence of bacteremia would seem to occur in patients with infected urine preoperatively, although data is conflicting (Table 16.16) (42, 134).

Postoperative bacteriuria is not restricted to those with preoperative infections, since infections may be introduced at the time of surgery or during postoperative catheter drainage. A large number of studies have been done on the effectiveness of antibiotics in preventing postoperative bacteriuria and bacteremia (Table 16.17) (123–131). Most studies cannot be evaluated because of lack of randomization, inadequate control groups, lack of statistical analysis, and inappropriate antibiotic regimens. The evaluable studies (Table 16.17) indicate a decrease in the incidence of postoperative bacteriuria, although the differences are not convincing. Plorde (120) found a decreased incidence of postoperative bacteriuria only in patients without preoperative infection. Inadequate data exist to tell whether

Table 16.17. Transurethral Prostate Resection (TURP): Prophylactic Antibiotics[c]

Study (Year)	Antibiotic	Number	Preop Urine	Bacteriuria (%) Antibiotic Group	Control Group	Bacteremia Antibiotic	Control	Sepsis Antibiotic	Control
Plorde (1975)[a]	Nitrofurantoin 100 mg q.i.d.			17 (50%)	25 (68%)	1 (3%)		0 (0%)	0 (0%)
	Kanamycin 0.5 gm q 8 hr	112	Sterile + infected	4 (13%)		0 (0%)	3 (8%)		
Morris (1976)	Kanamycin 1 gm, then cotramoxazole 2 tablets b.i.d.	101	Sterile	2 (5%)	14 (26%)	4 (10%)	6 (1%)	1 (2%)	3 (6%)
Gibbons (1978)	Kanamycin 500 mg preop, then q 8 hr	100	Sterile	3 (6%)	6 (12%)				
Matthew (1978)	Nitrofurantoin 100 mg preop, then t.i.d. × 10 days	87	Sterile	0 (0%)	10 (25%)	0 (0%)	0 (0%)	0 (0%)	0 (0%)
Lacy (1971)	Cephaloridine 1 gm q 6 h	108	Sterile + infected	(25%)	(54%)				
Hills (1976)	Cotriamoxazole	34	Sterile + infected	0 (0%)	6 (35%)				
Gonzalez (1976)	Cephalothin	90	Sterile	0 (0%)	20 (41%)				
Goldwasser (1983)	SMZ-TMP	81	Sterile	2 (4%)	8 (32%)				

[a] Includes patients with other types of prostate resection.
[b] Not studied.
[c] See also reference 134.

antibiotics prevent symptomatic urinary tract infection, bacteremia, or clinical sepsis (Table 16.17) (7, 124).

RECOMMENDATIONS

A firm recommendation cannot be made because of the lack of data. Patients undergoing TURP should have a preoperative urine culture. If the urine is infected, a therapeutic course of an appropriate antibacterial should be given in an attempt to cure the infection. The chances of sterilizing the urine temporarily are fair, although the relapse rate will be high. Patients infected immediately preoperatively should have a short course of antibiotics until after the catheter is removed, unless catheter drainage is prolonged. Patients with sterile preoperative urine should not receive prophylactic antibiotics because there is little evidence of short- or long-term benefit. Following TURP, all patients should be followed closely for sepsis and treated appropriately. Prophylaxis for bacterial endocarditis is *also* indicated in susceptible patients.

Orthopaedics

HIP FRACTURE

Rationale

Antibiotics are often used prophylactically in repair of hip fractures because of the moderate incidence of wound infections, and the risk of infection in an implanted foreign body. Hip fractures represent a heterogenous group, since a variety of procedures are done involving nails, more complex plate-like devices, and total hip replacements.

Table 16.18. Orthopaedic Surgery: Prophylactic Antibiotics

Study (Year)	Procedure	Antibiotic Regimen	Number (Antibiotic/ Control)	Wound Infections Antibiotic Group	Control Group	p
Boyd (1973)	Hip fracture	Nafcillin × 48 hr	348 (135/145)	1 (0.8%)	7 (5%)	<0.04
Ericson (1973)[b]	Hip operations	Cloxicillin × 14 days	171 (83/88)	0 (0%)	12 (14%)	<0.004
Hill (1981)[b]	Hip replacement	Cefazolin × 5 days	2137 (1070/1067)	10 (3%)	35 (.9%)	
Patzakis (1974)	Open fractures	Cephalothin × 10 days	310 (84/79)	2 (2%)	11 (14%)	<0.05
		Penicillin + streptomycin × 10 days	171 (92/79)	9 (10%)		
Pavell (1974)	All orthopaedic procedures (except open fractures)	Cephaloridine × 2 days	1591 (887/704)	25 (3%)	35 (5%)	—[a]
Gatell (1984)	Procedures with metal devices	Cefamandol × 24 hrs	284 (134/150)	0 (0%)	7 (5%)	<0.05

[a] Statistical testing not done.
[b] Also found a decrease in late deep hip infections (42, 147).

Clinical Studies

The incidence of wound infection following hip fracture repair is about 5% (Tables 16.1 and 16.18). The incidence of deep wound and prosthesis infection is not stated separately in most studies. Boyd (135) found 10 of 13 patients with wound infection had major problems but the exact incidence of infection of prostheses was uncertain.

The incidence of wound infection was reduced from 5% to 0.8% in a well-done randomized study, using nafcillin one dose preoperatively and eight doses postoperatively. A smaller study with oral cloxicillin found similar results (138) (Table 16.18).

Total hip replacements may become infected due to sepsis from distant sources, especially the urinary tract (136, 139).

Recommendations

Reviews of antimicrobial prophylaxis for repair of hip fracture (6, 7, 31) have reached conflicting results because of the low incidence of infection and the uncertain incidence of more serious deep infection. Pending further studies, an antistaphylococcal semisynthetic penicillin or a cephalosporin should be administered for one dose preoperatively and for 1 dose to 24 hours postoperatively. Duration of prophylaxis will also depend on whether a total artificial hip replacement is inserted (see below). In cases where prolonged surgery exceeds the duration of action of the antibiotic, a second dose may be needed intraoperatively. Distant infections, especially of the urinary tract, should be treated preoperatively because of the chance of hematogenous seeding of prosthetic devices.

TOTAL HIP REPLACEMENT

Rationale

The infection of a prosthetic joint has serious consequence, including requirement for removal of the prosthesis, and prolonged antibiotic therapy to eradicate the infection.

Clinical Studies

Two randomized trials demonstrated decreased wound infections and late deep hip infections with antibiotic prophylaxis for hip replacement (42, 138, 147, 148). Retrospective studies indicate a decreased incidence of infected prosthesis when antibiotic prophylaxis is used (7, 145), but control groups are not adequate. A decreased incidence of wound infections was found in a small randomized study (135).

Total hip prosthesis may be infected by bacteremia from distant infections, especially the urinary tract and skin (136, 139, 139a). Infections from seeding from dental and surgical procedures are rare (137, 139c, 148).

Recommendations

A cephalosporin (cefazolin) or a penicillinase-resistant penicillin (second choice) should be administered preoperatively and for 24–48 hours postoperatively. A second dose of the antibiotic should be given intraoperatively if the procedure exceeds 4 hours or the expected duration of action of the antibiotic. Patients with distant infections (especially skin and urinary tract infections), should be treated with antibiotics and should have their operations delayed until the infection is cleared.

FRACTURES AND CLEAN ORTHOPAEDIC SURGERY

Rationale

Antibiotics are administered after fractures and clean orthopaedic surgery to decrease the incidence of wound infection. Antibiotics are also administered to prevent postoperative osteomyelitis, especially after open fractures. Antibiotic administration to open fractures should be considered treatment because bacteria are introduced at the time of fracture and prior to antibiotic administration (open fractures will not be discussed below).

Clinical Studies

The incidence of wound infections following clean orthopaedic surgery and repair of closed fractures ranges from 1–5% (Table 16.18) (7). A significant reduction in wound infections from 5–3% was found in a randomized trial using two doses of cephalosporin (142). This small difference was significant because of the large size of the trial. Antibiotics reduced wound but not deep infections when metal devices were inserted to repair fractures (146).

Recommendations

Prophylactic antibiotics should not be used in clean orthopaedic surgery or repair of closed fractures. The single randomized study is insufficient to recommend prophylaxis because of the low baseline rate of infection and small reduction in infection rates. A cephalosporin *may* be used when metal devices are inserted.

Otolaryngology

See page 575, "Radical Neck Surgery."

Noncardiac Thoracic Surgery

RATIONALE

Antibiotics are used to prevent wound infections after thoracic and pulmonary surgery. Some surgeons use antibiotics to prevent other complications, including pneumonia, empyema, or purulent bronchitis.

CLINICAL STUDIES

The incidence of wound infections in general hospitals for pulmonary resection is 5–6% (Table 16.2). The incidence of other types of infections following pulmonary surgery has been 17–40% in placebo groups in various trials (Table 16.19).

Studies using cephalosporins for 2 or more days perioperatively have yielded conflicting results in part due to varying underlying infection rates. Most studies have shown at least a trend toward lower wound infection rates in the group receiving prophylactic antibiotics. Consistent

Table 16.19. Noncardiac Thoracic Surgery: Prophylactic Antibiotics

Study (Year)	Antibiotic Regimen	Number	All Infections		
			Antibiotic Group	Control Group	p
Truesdale (1979)	Cefazolin-cephalothin × 48 hours	57	5 (8%)	5 (17%)	NS[a]
Kvale (1977)	Cephalosporin × 5 days	90	9 (19%)	17 (40%)	<.03
Ilves (1981)[b]	Cephalothin × 2 doses	211	6 (6%)	22 (24%)	<.05
Frimodt-Moller (1982)[b]	Pen G × 6 doses	92	2 (4%)	9 (19%)	= .03
Cameron (1981)[b]	Cephalothin × 3 doses	171	16 (18%)	23 (28%)	NS[a]

[a] NS, not significant.
[b] See reference 42.

lowering of infection rates has not been shown for more serious infections, such as empyema or pneumonia.

Empyema occurs in 1–20% of patients with penetrating chest wounds; the effects of antibiotics have not been established (42, 100).

RECOMMENDATIONS

The available data are not sufficient to make a recommendation regarding the use of prophylactic antibiotics for chest surgery (7, 42). If prophylaxis is given, cefazolin for a total of 2–3 doses is recommended. Some authorities (6, 42) recommend antibiotic prophylaxis for lung resection or penetrating wounds.

Neurosurgery

SKULL FRACTURES

Rationale

Prophylactic antibiotics are used after skull fracture to prevent meningitis, especially in the presence of a cerebrospinal fluid leak.

Clinical Studies

The incidence of meningitis after skull fracture has ranged from 0–5%. The risk is higher if there is a clinical or subclinical cerebrospinal fluid leak. (Table 16.20). No large randomized trial has been done

with separation of patients based on the presence of CSF leak. Available studies are conflicting on whether antibiotic prophylaxis reduces the incidence of meningitis. No study indicated benefit in skull fractures without CSF leak; the data are inadequate to evaluate effectiveness in the presence of CSF leak (153–158).

Recommendations

Antibiotics should not be administered to patients with uncomplicated skull fractures without CSF leak (6, 7). Although antibiotics are commonly used, data are inadequate to show benefit in patients with CSF leak, and no specific antibiotic regimen can be recommended.

Table 16.20. Incidence of Meningitis after Skull Fractures

Study	Group	Number (without Antibiotics)	Number with Meningitis (%)
Ignelizi (1975)	Skull fracture	50	0 (0%)
Hoff (1976)	Skull fracture	80	0 (0%)
MacGee (1971) (series and literature review)	CSF leak	77	4 (5%)
Klastersky (1976)	CSF Leak	26	1 (4%)

Rationale

The major concern in using prophylactic antibiotics for neurosurgery is the prevention of meningitis and infection in prosthetic shunts. Wound infections are a secondary consideration.

Clinical Studies

No adequate, randomized study has been done of prophylactic antibiotics in clean neurosurgery, using postoperative meningitis, abscess, or shunt infections (158a) as the end result. A small study using clindamycin found a decreased incidence of wound infections, but the results were uninterpretable because of an epidemic of infections occurring during the study (158). Wound infections were confined to patients undergoing surgery for more than 6 hours.

Recommendations

Prophylactic antibiotics are not indicated for clean neurosurgery (6, 7). Some authorities recommend a short course of prophylactic therapy when CSF shunts are inserted. No recommendations can be given for the type or duration of antibiotics because of the lack of data and the multiple possible organisms. If prophylactic antibiotics are used for CSF shunts, the type of antibiotic should be based on local experience with the type of infecting organisms and ability of the antibiotic to cross uninflamed meninges.

Subacute Bacterial Endocarditis

RATIONALE

Antibiotic prophylaxis is recommended for patients at risk of developing bacterial endocarditis because of the devastating consequences of endocarditis.

CLINICAL STUDIES

Despite *uniform agreement that prophylaxis is required for patients at risk of bacterial endocarditis,* there has never been a retrospective or prospective study demonstrating its effectiveness. The problem of prophylaxis of endocarditis is made more difficult by the lack of data on the risk of endocarditis in various patient groups.

The pathogenesis of endocarditis depends on three factors: (*a*) a preexisting valvular lesion; (*b*) bacteremia; (*c*) immunological response (165).

A *bacteremia* is the initiating event in bacterial endocarditis. The most common portals of entry associated with clinical endocarditis are the mouth (dental work), gastrointestinal, and genitourinary tracts. However, an entry site for bacteria can be discovered by history in only 24–60% of cases of endocarditis (163, 175). Only in the minority of the cases having a clear precipitating event would prophylaxis be practical.

Multiple events can cause transient bacteremias (6, 159, 162–165, 175) (Table 16.21). A high frequency of bacteremia is associated with the classical precipitating causes of endocarditis. Frequent bacteremias are seen with procedures not usually associated with endocarditis, such as barium enema and sigmoidoscopy. Transient bacteremia has been reported in 1% of normal persons without mucus membrane trauma; however, its significance is controversial because the rate approaches the contamination rate of blood cultures and most of the organisms isolated could be considered skin contaminants. Transient bacteremia have been demonstrated to occur after such routine daily activities as having a bowel movement, chewing candy or gum, or teeth cleaning with irrigation devices (164).

Little data are available relating the risk of endocarditis to transient bacteremia (164). One study of 350 children with rheumatic heart disease undergoing tooth extraction found a 52% incidence of streptococcal bacteremia and a 1% incidence of endocarditis. The risk of endocarditis may be lower in children than adults. In addition to the risk of bacter-

Table 16.21.   Incidence of Bacteremia following Procedures[a]

High Risk	Intermediate Risk	Low Risk

Prostatectomy (infected urine)
  Transurethral 58%
  Retropubic 82%
	Prostatectomy (sterile urine)
	  Transurethral 11%
	  Retropubic 13%
		Sigmodoscopy 2–10%
		Colonoscopy 3–6%
		Esophageal dilatation, sterile dilator 0%

Esophageal dilatation, unsterile dilator 100% Tonsillectomy 28–38% Dental extraction 18–85% Periodontal surgery 21–88%	Barium enema 11% Liver biopsy 3–13% Rigid bronchoscopy 15% Nasotracheal intubation 10% Nasotracheal suctioning, intensive care patients 16%	Fiberoptic bronchoscopy 0% Orotracheal intubation 0% Parturition 0–5% IUD insertion 0%
Burn surgery 46% Surgery of infected areas 54%		

[a] From Flynn NM, Lawrence RM: Antimicrobial prophylaxis. *Med Clin North Am* 63:1230, 1979. Used by permission. See also reference 164.

emia, the risk of endocarditis has been felt to depend upon the number of organisms present and the duration of bacteremia (163–165). Data are lacking to confirm the importance of duration and intensity of bacteremia. The nature of the bacteremia probably also depends on the mucosal surface, since more frequent bacteremia are seen in patients with gingival disease.

Only a few gram-positive organisms commonly cause bacterial endocarditis, including viridans *Streptococci, Enterococcus,* other group D *Streptococci* and *Staphylococcus.* Multiple organisms not commonly causing endocarditis can be recovered during bacteremia, including aerobic gram-negative rods and anaerobes. An important factor may be the immunological nature of certain gram-positive cocci. These cocci produce an antibody response which assists adherence to valves or sterile platelet-fibrin vegetations (165).

Recommendations for endocarditis prophylaxis are made based on the specific organisms from a given site or procedure presenting a major risk of endocarditis. The most common organism causing endocarditis from dental procedures is viridans streptococci. From gastrointestinal or genitourinary procedures, the most common organism is group D streptococci (which includes the enterococcus). Subacute endocarditis is usually believed to occur in patients with *underlying heart disease* (acute endocarditis more frequently occurs on normal valves). In older classic studies, the most frequent underlying cardiac disease in patients with endocarditis is rheumatic valvular disease, which is present in 40–60% of cases. Second most frequent is congenital heart disease, which is present in 7–16% of patients (163). The presence of mitral valve prolapse is being increasingly found in patients with endocarditis, although the exact proportion is unknown.

An increasing proportion of patients with endocarditis are elderly (over the age of 60) with degenerative heart disease. A large number of these patients have no *clinically* recognizable cardiac disease, although it is difficult to exclude hemodynamically insignificant lesions such as aortic sclerosis. Other degenerative problems in which endocarditis has been reported include bicuspid aortic valves, calcific aortic stenosis, and calcification of the mitral annulus. Endocarditis has been reported but is rare in certain lesions, including uncomplicated ostium secundum atrial septal defect and idiopathic hypertrophic subaortic stenosis. Infective endocarditis very rarely occurs in patients with cardiac pacemakers.

The distribution of types of valvular disease currently among patients with endocarditis is probably different from classic studies. Mitral valve prolapse and diseases found in elderly patients are much more common and rheumatic valvular disease less common, but a recent study has not been done.

Approximately 20–40% of patients with endocarditis have no clinically recognizable cardiac disease (163). Some of these cases can be explained by inaccurate diagnosis or subclinical heart disease; others are due to acute endocarditis with virulent organisms. However, a proportion of cases of subacute endocarditis remain with no underlying disease.

Finally, the risk of recurrent endocarditis in patients with one attack is 9% and a third episode will occur in 25% of patients having a second attack (163).

When all the available data are summarized, 25–60% of patients with endocarditis have a known initiating event and 60–80% have underlying heart disease. Since only patients with both underlying heart disease and an initiating event would be practical candidates for prophylaxis, *less than one-half of patients with endocarditis are potentially preventable by prophylaxis.*

No controlled study has been done on the effectiveness of prophylactic antibiotics in preventing endocarditis because of the severe nature of the disease. The small number of patients at risk of actually developing endocarditis would make such a trial impractical, even if it were ethically allowable.

Prophylactic antibiotics have been shown to reduce the incidence of bacteremia and, possibly, the number of bacteria after certain procedures (162–163, 175). The reduction is in part an artifact, since bacteria will less frequently grow in blood cultures where antibiotic is present. The incidence of bacteremia after prophylactic antibiotics rises when penicillinase is added to the blood culture flask.

Prophylactic antibiotics have been tested by evaluating their efficiency in preventing endocarditis in a rabbit model. Older, lower dose regimens did not prevent endocarditis, while higher dose regimens were effective (163, 166–167). The animal model has been criticized because the concentration of organisms used is much higher than in human bacteremia and because of the use of foreign catheters to initiate a valvular nidus.

The only direct human evidence for efficacy of antibiotic prophylaxis comes from reported cases of prophylactic failures (160, 163, 177). Only a few cases of endocarditis have been *reported* in patients receiving older low-dose regimens (160, 163, 175, 177). Many of these patients received doses lower than those the American Heart Association (AHA) recommends. Failures of prophylaxis have been reported in patients receiving the newer higher doses recommended by the American Heart Association (160, 177). Most of the failures were in patients receiving antibiotic regimens other than the AHA recommendations (160). Only limited conclusions can be drawn from reports of antibiotic failure because of: (a) incomplete reporting of cases; (b) the fact that only a minority of patients at risk receive prophylaxis; and (c) incomplete data in many reports.

Prophylactic antibiotics are not given to many patients who would be considered candidates for prophylaxis. Several studies of dental patients with valvular disease showed the majority of patients were unaware of the need for prophylaxis, their dentist was uninformed of their heart disease, and many dentists were not using recommended antibiotic regimens (161). The fact that many or most patients with underlying heart disease do not receive prophylactic antibiotics indicates a failure of "accepted" care and complicates the interpretation of case reports of antibiotic failure.

Despite the gaps in data, authorities

Table 16.22. Prophylaxis of Bacterial Endocarditis: Underlying Cardiac Disease [a]

Heart Disease

Accepted

Congenital heart disease (except secundum atrial septal defect) [b]

Rheumatic valvular disease

Acquired valvular disease

Idiopathic hypertrophic subaortic stenosis (IHSS)

Mitral prolapse

Prosthetic heart valves (including porcine heterografts)

Surgically constructed systemic–pulmonary shunts.

Previous bacterial endocarditis [c]

Uncertain

Dialysis A-V shunts

Ventriculoatrial shunts for hydrocephalus

Not indicated

Closed secundum ASD by suture (at least 6 months earlier) (without patch) [b]

Ligated patent ductus arteriosus (at least 6 months earlier)

Coronary artery bypass grafts

Transvenous pacemakers [b]

---

[a] From Committee on Prevention of Rheumatic Fever and Bacterial Endocarditis: Prevention of bacterial endocarditis. *Circulation* 70:1123A–1127A, 1984, with permission of the American Heart Assn.

[b] Some authorities recommend prophylaxis for secundum ASD or pacemakers.

[c] Even in the absence of clinical valvular disease.

strongly recommend prophylactic antibiotics for patients at risk of bacterial endocarditis, because of the severe consequences of the disease. Current regimens adopted by American Heart Association expert panels are controversial because of the lack of data. Animal models (167) have served as a major impetus for the American Heart Association to switch from low-dose regimens to current high-dose regimens (159, 166).

RECOMMENDATIONS

Most authorities recommend antibiotic prophylaxis be given to patients who: (*a*) have underlying heart disease on which endocarditis can develop (Table 16.22), and (*b*) are undergoing procedures (Table 16.23) recognized as having a risk of bacteremia related to development of endocarditis. The prophylactic antibiotic regimens recommended by the Committee on Prevention of Rheumatic Fever and Bacterial Endocarditis of the American Heart Association are given in Table 16.24.

Several qualifications to the recommendations should be noted:

1. Patients with prosthetic heart valves

Table 16.23. Prophylaxis of Bacterial Endocarditis: Procedures [a]

Procedures

Accepted

Dental procedures (except shedding of deciduous teeth, simple adjustment of orthodontic appliances)

Upper respiratory tract: surgery, procedures, instrumentation [b]

Gastrointestinal tract: surgery, instrumentation (including gallbladder)

Genitourinary tract: instrumentation, surgery (including urethral catheterization with uninfected urine, prostate manipulation, obstetrical infections)

Surgery/procedures in infected tissues (including abscess drainage)

Uncertain [c]

Vaginal delivery (uncomplicated)

Sigmoidoscopy (without biopsy)

Barium enema

Dilation and curettage (uncomplicated)

IUD insertion, removal (uncomplicated)

UGI endoscopy (without biopsy)

Liver biopsy

---

[a] From Committee on Prevention of Rheumatic Fever and Bacterial Endocarditis: Prevention of bacterial endocarditis. *Circulation* 70:1123A–1127A, 1984, with permission of the American Heart Assn.

[b] Including bronchoscopy, tonsillectomy, adenoidectomy, and procedures disrupting respiratory mucosa.

[c] Uncertain status applies only to uncomplicated procedures. Procedures involving infected tissue, prolonged manipulation, or biopsy require prophylaxis.

Table 16.24. Prophylaxis for Bacterial Endocarditis: Dental-Upper Respiratory and Gastrointestinal-Genitourinary Procedures[a]

	Penicillin (or Equivalent)	PLUS	Aminoglycoside
A. Dental-upper respiratory			
1. Oral	Penicillin V 2.0 gm orally } 1.0 hr before procedure **then** Penicillin V 1 gm orally 6 hours after initial dose		None
2. Parenteral	Aqueous penicillin G 2,000,000 units } IM or IV 0.5–1.0 hr before procedure **then** Aqueous penicillin G 1,000,000 units 6 hours after initial dose		None
3. Penicillin-allergic patients	Vancomycin 1 gm IV[c] } 1.0 hr before procedure or Erythromycin 1 gm orally } 1 hr before procedure **then** Erythromycin 500 mg orally 6 hours after initial dose[d]		None
4. High risk (include prosthetic heart valve)	Ampicillin 1.0–2.0 gm IM or IV } 0.5 hr before procedure	PLUS	Gentamicin 1.5 mg/kg IM or IV
	then Penicillin V 1.0 gm orally 6 hours after initial dose		None
a. Penicillin-allergic high-risk patient	Vancomycin 1 gm IV[c] } 0.5–1.0 hr before procedure **then** No repeat dose is necessary		None
B. GI/GU procedures			
1. Parenteral	Ampicillin 2 gm IV or IM **Initial dose:** 0.5–1.0 hr before procedures **Then:** Repeat[b] 8 hours after initial dose	PLUS	Gentamycin 1.5 mg/kg IV or IM
2. Penicillin-allergic patients	Vanomycin 1 gm IV[c] **Initial dose:** 0–1.0 hr before procedure **Then:** Single dose probably sufficient, except for complicated situations; may repeat × 1 dose in 12 hr	PLUS	Gentamicin 1.5 mg IM or IV

[a] From Committee on Prevention of Rheumatic Fever and Bacterial Endocarditis: Prevention of bacterial endocarditis. *Circulation* 70:1123A–1127A, 1984, with permission of the American Heart Association.
[b] Both penicillin and aminoglycoside should be given at the same time.
[c] Vancomycin should be infused over 1 hour. Infusion should begin 30 min–1 hour prior to the procedure.
[d] Single dose; no repeat dose is necessary if vancomycin is used.

should receive the more intensive regimen for upper respiratory tract procedures (i.e., penicillin plus an aminoglycoside).

2. Patients with prosthetic heart valves may be at higher risk for staphylococcal endocarditis when the skin is incised or surgery involves other sites of staphylococcal colonization. Some authorities suggest that these patients receive a parenteral semisynthetic penicillin such as nafcillin or cephalosporin such as cefazolin in addition to the other recommendations.

3. Although not in the AHA list of recommendations, antibiotic prophylaxis should obviously be given for surgery on infected or contaminated tissue such as abscesses or intraabdominal emergencies. In these cases antibiotic selection will need to be individualized according to the expected bacteriology, but antibiotics effective against *Staphylococcus aureus* should be included in most instances.

4. Surgery involving infected areas (e.g., abscesses) should include prophylaxis for suspected or commonly encountered organisms in addition to the listed recommendations.

5. Most authorities do not recommend prophylaxis for procedures with low risk of bacteremia or unassociated with clinical endocarditis, such as sigmoidoscopy without biopsy. An exception is in patients with prosthetic valves.

6. Uncomplicated vaginal delivery has a low incidence of bacteremia and infrequent occurrence of endocarditis in a large study (182a). The risk of endocarditis from dilation and curettage and manipulation of intrauterine devices is rare. The use of prophylaxis for these procedures is controversial. However, patients with prosthetic valves probably should receive prophylaxis.

7. Prophylaxis should be given for several "non-surgical" procedures, including routine professional cleaning of teeth and Foley catheterization of the urinary tract.

8. Antibiotics should be given for a longer period of time than recommended in patients undergoing prolonged procedures or at a prolonged risk of bacteremia because of delayed healing or infection.

9. The indications and benefits for prophylaxis are not clear in patients with noncardiac vascular devices such as renal dialysis arteriovenous shunts and fistulae, vascular prostheses, prosthetic joints, and cerebrospinal fluid shunts. Many authorities recommend prophylaxis for these groups. These patients incur the risk of infection of the foreign material as well as, in some, the risk of endocarditis (due to arteriovenous shunts). Although data are lacking, we recommend prophylaxis in patients with CSF shunts (because of the consequences of infections) and dialysis shunts. Prophylaxis is provided to recent prosthetic vascular devices less than 6 months old.

10. Prophylactic antibiotics are probably not required for cardiac catheterization, angiography, and angioplasty. Subacute bacterial endocarditis prophylaxis is not required for most transvenous pacemakers in most situations, but may be given (159). Since the most common infections associated with pacemakers are due to staphylococci, consideration of coverage for this organism should be given when antibiotics are used.

11. It should be stressed that prophylaxis against acute rheumatic fever is INADEQUATE for bacterial endocarditis because of the substantially lower doses. Patients receiving chronic prophylaxis for rheumatic fever have developed endocarditis with penicillin-resistant organisms. Consideration should be given the use of other antibiotics in patients receiving chronic penicillin for rheumatic fever prophylaxis, such as erythromycin, vancomycin, or the addition of an aminoglycoside.

PREOPERATIVE RESPIRATORY INFECTION

Epidemiology

Most anesthesia textbooks suggest waiting 2 weeks after an acute upper respiratory infection before undergoing general anesthesia. The recommendation to postpone surgery after upper respiratory infections is based on very old series and case reports of sudden deaths in children. A 1933 series found postoperative respiratory complications doubled from 6 to 11% in the presence of pharyngitis, and to 11% when "oral sepsis" was present (185). Statistical testing was not done; these findings may not be applicable to modern anesthetic techniques or other types of respiratory infections.

Secondly, a small number of cases have been reported of acute upper airway obstruction (laryngospasm) and sudden death in previously healthy children who underwent elective surgery soon after a respiratory infection. Most of the children were less than 6 months of age. Similar complications have not been frequently reported in adults.

No empirical data are available on the duration of time that should lapse between an upper respiratory infection and elective surgery. Most anesthesia textbooks recommend a 2-week wait between an upper respiratory infection and elective surgery.

The risk of surgery after pneumonia has not been documented in either a prospective or a retrospective series.

Diagnostic Activities and Approaches

Patients undergoing surgery should be asked whether they have had symptoms of an acute upper respiratory infection in the past 2 weeks. Examination of the ears, nose, and oropharynx may confirm current infection. The temperature, white blood cell count, and differential are useful in ascertaining the activity of respiratory infections.

A chest x-ray should be obtained in patients with recent respiratory symptoms to exclude a mild, resolving pneumonia. Gram stain and culture of sputum should be performed in patients producing purulent sputum.

Some patients undergoing surgery with respiratory infections should have an arterial blood gas to detect unsuspected hypoxemia and to serve as a baseline.

Preoperative Management

Most authorities recommend waiting 2 weeks after an uncomplicated upper respiratory infection before undergoing nonemergency surgery. Although empirical documentation is lacking for postponement of surgery, the medicolegal consequences must be considered should complications occur.

Guidelines for delaying elective surgery in patients with pneumonia are not stated in most anesthesia texts. Surgery should be delayed until all signs and symptoms of pneumonia have cleared, including infiltrates by chest x-rays, sputum production, and temperature. Six to eight weeks may be required for chest x-ray clearing.

A few patients will require operation soon after an upper respiratory infection or pneumonia. Patients with postoperative pneumonia may require reoperation for intraabdominal sepsis or surgical complications. Although documentation is lacking, the risk of postoperative respiratory failure, superinfection, and hypoxia are probably increased. Patients undergoing urgent surgery during a respiratory infection should have a baseline preoperative blood gas and, if possible, spirometry. These patients need to be followed closely postoperatively for respiratory complications and should be observed in an ICU for at least 24 hours postoperatively. Therapy for pneumonia should be continued postoperatively with strong emphasis on pulmonary toilet.

Preoperative Urinary Tract Infection

For information see page 177.

POSTOPERATIVE PROBLEMS

Evaluation of the febrile postoperative patient is a frequent reason for consultation. The surgeon will usually diagnose the routine infection of the wound, lungs, and urinary tract. Common reasons for consultation include prolonged fever of undetermined origin, a severely ill or septic patient, interpretation of unusual microbiology results, or usage of antibiotics.

The internist contributing to the case requires a background knowledge of the common causes of postoperative fever (see Table 16.28) and the common reasons for misdiagnosis and failure to respond to antibiotic therapy (see Table 16.31).

The internist's most valuable contribution may be in sorting out those causes unrelated to the specific surgical procedure (e.g., drug fever), in recognizing a non-infectious cause of fever (e.g., phlebitis, pleural effusion) or in recognizing a second complicating infection (e.g., distant seeding from a urinary tract infection, infection in a preexisting vascular graft after prostatic surgery). Another particular contribution is the evaluation of the deteriorating postoperative patient, usually already on antibiotics, frequently days or weeks after surgery.

The evaluation of the febrile postoperative patient is often an urgent one. Therefore, direct verbal communication between the referring physician and the consultant is mandatory as historical information can be shared and diagnostic and therapeutic maneuvers coordinated. If reexploration is a possibility, joint planning between internist and surgeon is required.

The internist should be aware of local hospital infection rates, common nosocomial organisms, local antibiotic susceptibility patterns, and any recent pattern of nosocomial infections. The infection control nurse and microbiology laboratory staff are invaluable resources for additional information. The internist should be aware of methods of disease transmission and infection control in the hospital (1, 18, 25, 194).

The Febrile Postoperative Patient

EPIDEMIOLOGY AND PATHOPHYSIOLOGY

Although fever is an undisputed indicator of disease, its clinical usefulness in determining the etiology of temperature elevation is very limited. Some understanding of the nature of the febrile response is important to interpret changes.

Most clinical fevers result from resetting the hypothalamic regulatory center by endogenous pyrogens (4, 187, 189). The synthesis and release of the pyrogen by fixed and circulating phagocytes and some tumor cells is influenced by phagocytosis, endotoxin, antigen-antibody complexes, and pyrogenic steroids, though the exact mechanism of resetting is unclear. There is a normal circadian rhythm influencing the thermoregulatory center, and many febrile conditions merely accentuate this normal diurnal temperature variation.

"Normal" oral temperatures range from 96.6°–99.6°F with a low in the morning to a high between 4 PM and midnight. In general, the elderly have lower temperature ranges between 96.6°F to perhaps a 97.6°F maximum late in the day, while a 99.6°–100°F maximum is not unusual for a young individual in the late afternoon. Diurnal variations range from 0.9°F–2.7°F.

In evaluating fever, one should be aware that small variations in thermometers may cause large variations in temperature readings. Roe (193) showed that the range of temperatures of 40 thermometers in a constant temperature bath at 98.6°F varied from 97°–100°F. Additionally, significant temperature elevations occurring between charting intervals have been noted in nursing progress notes and not recorded on the temperature graph.

Temperature elevation in the postoperative period is very common and by itself lacks sensitivity and specificity as an indicator of disease. Data are sparse but a few general comments can be made. Dykes (190) found that of 162 non-obstetric general anesthesia patients, 133 (82%) developed a postoperative rise in oral temperature. In 72 (55%), rises of temperature could not be explained by a complication or continuation of a preoperative fever. Most of the temperature elevations for four common procedures followed a typi-

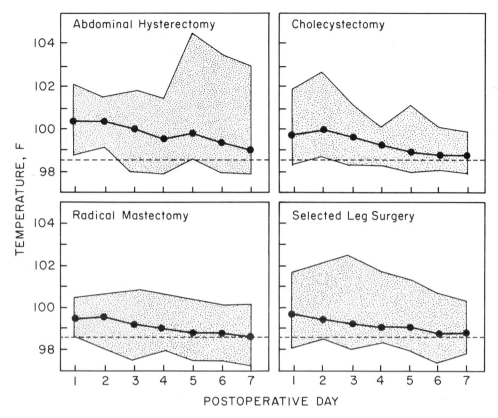

Figure 16.2.   Unexplained fever following four common surgical procedures. The mean, minimum, and maximum temperatures are given for patients with no "apparent" cause for fever. (From Dykes MH: Unexplained postoperative fever: Its value as a sign of halothane sensitization. *JAMA* 216:641, 1971. Copyright 1971, American Medical Assn. Used by permission.)

cal declining pattern (Fig. 16.2). A few patients had high (≥102°F) unexplained febrile episodes.

The location of the operation also influences the incidence of unexplained fever. Livelli et al. (191) noted temperatures greater than 100°F in 99% of 219 cardiac surgery patients during the first week, with a similar declining fever curve. After day 6, 73% of the patients remained febrile and 54% of these were unexplained. Bell (192) reported on 189 patients postcardiac valve surgery. The maximum temperature of 154 patients without documented infection was 101.2°F on day 1 and fell to an average of 100°F by day 8. These temperature elevations are often thought to be due to tissue trauma, blood in closed spaces, drain tubes, etc., but the

exact cause is unknown. Roe (193) studied a group of patients in whom an intraoperative drop in temperature was followed by a postoperative rebound to 101°F by 24 hours with a return to normal by 32 hours. If the intraoperative temperature was controlled and not allowed to decline, there was no postoperative elevation, suggesting to the investigators an anesthetic "paralysis" of the hypothalamic regulatory mechanism followed by a rebound phenomenon.

Whatever the cause, mild low-grade fever is expected in the first 24–48 hours followed by a gradual decline over 2–5 days, but may occasionally persist into the second week. An arbitrary temperature of 101°F is widely used as an indicator for more in-depth evaluation. Lower temperatures of 99.6°–100°F may have the same significance in elderly compromised host or debilitated patients. Temperatures to 102°–104°F are more commonly due to an infectious cause, but should not be ignored. The duration of fever, the clinical status of the patient, possible sources of infection, and the time since surgery must be considered, in addition to the height of the temperature.

Fever patterns only rarely assist in diagnosis of the cause of elevated temperature. Fever patterns may be classified as: (*a*) **Continuous:** temperature elevated throughout 24-hour period with fluctuation less than 1°C. (*b*) **Remittent:** temperature elevated throughout 24-hour period, but varying by more than 1°C. (*c*) **Intermittent:** temperature is normal for part of the day and elevated for part of the day with large daily oscillations more than 2–5°F (most common pattern); a *hectic fever* is a remittent fever with large daily oscillations of more than 2.5°F. (*d*) **Relapsing fever:** febrile periods separated by days of normal temperature.

Musher et al. (188) reviewed the fever patterns of 200 consecutive cases referred to an infectious disease service (Table 16.25) and concluded that no pattern had diagnostic value. Eighty-three per cent of patients had intermittent or remittent fevers and, of these, 90% had diurnal variations. The lack of *diurnal variation* was thought to give slight support to a non-infectious cause since this pattern was seen in about 50% of non-infectious febrile entities. *Sustained fever* was seen with gram-negative pneumonia and CNS damage with enough frequency to suggest one of these diagnoses. Beyond these loose associations, the clinician should not look to fever patterns as a clue to the diagnosis. The height of the fever also has variable diagnostic significance.

The concurrence of fever in a well-looking patient classically suggests abscess; however, any non-infectious cause of fever may give a well-appearing febrile patient, including drug fever, atelectasis, thromboembolic disease, and tumor.

DIAGNOSTIC APPROACH TO THE FEBRILE POSTOPERATIVE PATIENT

Eliciting the cause of a postoperative fever can be a complex clinical challenge for both surgeon and internist (Table 16.26). *A systematic but individualized approach is suggested.* It is helpful to think in terms of (*a*) the most common febrile complications, (*b*) infectious complications of the primary surgical disease, (*c*) the temporal relation of the fever to the operation, and, (*d*) the type and location of surgery performed (Table 16.27). Beyond this, a systematic regional approach and well-planned diagnostic work-up appropriate to the condition of the patient is essential.

The work-up and management of most individual conditions causing fever will be described in subsequent sections; this section gives a general approach to the febrile patient.

The most common sites of postoperative fever are the surgical wound and the urinary and pulmonary tracts (Table 16.28) (see also Table 16.1). Less common are deep infections such as intraperitoneal abscesses and infections of prostheses. Non-infected surgical hematomas may also cause postoperative fevers. Although usually not listed, common causes of postoperative fever include sites of instrumentation (e.g., intravenous line, Foley catheters), drug or anesthetic allergy, thromboembolic disease, diarrhea (*C. difficile*) and dehydration. Rare causes of postoperative fever include myocardial infarction and transfusion reactions. A low-grade, self-limited, unexplained fever is common after any major surgical procedure; the cause of these fevers is unknown. The temperature is usually less than 101°F but may reach 102°–103°F for brief periods, declining gradually (a temperature elevation over 101°F should prompt an historical review of the case and a physical examination).

Table 16.25.   The Lack of Relationship of Fever Patterns and the Cause of Fever[a]

| | Pneumonia | | Lung Abscess | Empyema of the Thorax | Intra-abdominal Abscess | Urinary Tract Infection | Osteo-myelitis | Bacterial Endo-carditis | Drug Fever | Solid Tumors | Leu-kemia | Miscel-laneous Non-infectious Febrile Conditions | Fever Associated with CNS Damage |
	Gram Positive	Gram Negative											
Remittent	3	3	13	12	14	15	18	4	8	6	3	14	1
Intermittent	1	1	5	5	4	9	5	1	4	4	2	10	1
Sustained	0	5	0	0	0	0	0	0	0	0	0	0	6
Hectic	1	1	2	3	2	1	2	3	2	0	2	6	2
Total	5	10	20	20	20	25	25	8	14	10	7	30	10
Patients with diurnal variation	5	3	16	16	18	22	24	6	13	10	5	16	1

[a]From Musher DM, Fainstein V, et al.: Fever patterns: Their lack of clinical significance. *Arch Intern Med* 139:1226, 1979. Copyright, American Medical Assn. Used with permission.

Table 16.26. Postoperative Fever

Diagnostic Possibility	Approximate Peak Incidence	Clinical Clue
Benign post-op fever	48–72 hr	Normal exam, temp < 101°F
Urinary infection	48 hr	Catheter, instrumentation
Wound infection	4–10 days	Purulent drainage
IV catheter infection	72 hr	"Phlebitis," unexplained fever
Atelectasis	24 hr	Rales, diminished breath sounds
Aspiration	Anytime	Debilitation, putrid sputum
Pneumonia	24–48 hr	Consolidation, purulent sputum
Venous thrombosis	7–10 days	± Leg pain, swelling
Pulmonary embolus	7–10 days	Unexplained tachypnea
Transfusion reaction	24 hr	Abrupt onset posttransfusion
Drug fever	Anytime	Suspect with any drug
Monitoring devices	72 hr	Unexplained fever/bacteremia
Parotitis	2 weeks	Dehydration, parotid swelling
Otitis media	Anytime	Ear pain, nasogastric tube
Acute cholecystitis	48 hr	RUQ symptoms/signs
Pancreatitis	Anytime	Epigastric tenderness, N&V
Malignant hyperthermia	During anesthesia; recovery room	
Endocrine-related	24 hr	
Intraabdominal abscess	4 days–weeks	Mass, persistent fever, bacteremia
Prostatitis	Anytime	Prostatic tenderness
Endocarditis		Murmur, anemia, peripheral emboli
Trauma-related	48–72 hr	Significant tissue damage
Hepatitis		
Viral	8–12 weeks	RUQ tenderness, jaundice, SGOT
Cytomegalovirus		Splenomegally, atypical lymphocytosis
Halothane		Previous exposure
Intramuscular injection	48 hr	Fluctuance
Decubitus ulcer	Anytime	Necrotic/devitalized tissue
Vertebral osteo	Anytime	Low back pain, previous UTI
Perinephric abscess		"Pyelonephritis" with fever 5 days
Osteitis pubis	Anytime	Pubic tenderness, thigh pain
Pudendal/psoas abscess	48 hr	Paracervical block, hip pain
Prosthetic graft	Anytime	GI bleeding, bacteremia
Skeletal prosthesis	Anytime	Pain, loosening of prosthesis
Endometritis/salpingitis		
Pelvic thrombophlebitis		Hectic fever despite appropriate antibiotic
Hematoma		Mass
Starch peritonitis	2–3 weeks	Diffuse abdominal symptoms
Factitious fever	Anytime	Normal exam, lab
CNS infection		Mental status change
Epidural abscess		Spinal anesthesia; back pain
Alcohol/drug withdrawal	2–5 days	History of use

Special attention should be directed toward atypical presentation of the six most common causes of fever: pulmonary (atelectasis or aspiration), wound infection, urinary tract infection, thrombophlebitis, intravenous catheter infections, and drug allergy. Infection specific to the type of surgical procedure should be considered, such as infected prosthesis or disc space infection.

Before initiating an extended laboratory work-up, special attention is placed on specific *historical information* and pertinent physical examination. The time of

Table 16.27. Approach to the Febrile Postoperative Patient

1. Most common febrile complications of surgery (in general)[a]
2. Common infectious complications and sequelae of primary surgical disease
3. Type and location of the surgery
4. The temporal relationship of the fever to the operation
5. Obvious clinical clues

[a] See Table 16.28.

onset of the fever after surgery is relevant, but of limited diagnostic value. For example, atelectasis often occurs in the first 24–48 hours, intravenous catheter infections at 48–72 hours, and wound infections in 4–10 days. Unlike more common wound infections, group A streptococcal and *Clostridium perfringens* wound infections may occur within 24 hours of surgery. Nursing notes should be reviewed for any temperature elevations not on the temperature chart. Historical information should be obtained with reference to preexisting bacterial or viral infection, allergies, pertinent drugs (alcohol, barbiturates, steroids), prior sensitivities (halothane), or special conditions such as prosthetic devices or vascular grafts. Alcohol or other drug withdrawal, as well

Table 16.28. Most Common Etiologies of Postoperative Fever

Surgical site
  Wound
  Deep (e.g., abscess, peritonitis)
  Specific to the procedure (e.g., infected prosthesis)
Remote
  Pulmonary (atelectasis, pneumonia)
  Urinary tract infection
  Diarrhea (C. difficile)
  Instrumentation (e.g., IV,[a] CVP lines)
Usually non-bacterial
  Drug or anesthetic allergy
  Dehydration
  Intravenous catheter phlebitis[a]
  Thrombophlebitis and pulmonary emboli
Unexplained

[a] Can also be infected (septic phlebitis).

as alcoholic hepatitis, may present in the postoperative period. Hepatitis of several types may present as a fever of uncertain origin postoperatively. Fever alone is a common presentation of anesthesia or drug-induced hepatitis. "Short incubation" post-transfusion hepatitis (non-A, non-B hepatitis) may present as early as 10–14 days post-transfusion.

Anesthesiology and recovery room notes should be reviewed for temperature elevations, drugs or transfusions administered, or notation of aspiration. Clues from the notes and the early postoperative course should point to an endocrine cause such as thyroid storm or adrenal crises. The medication list should be reviewed, and the patient questioned about nonprescription drugs he/she may have at the bedside.

The *physical examination* should be systematic and thorough. A depressed level of consciousness may suggest aspiration. The eardrums should be checked for otitis media caused by obstruction from a nasogastric tube or nasotracheal tube. An ophthalmologic exam may be helpful in selected instances such as candida endopthalmitis, or endocarditis. The sinuses should be palpated for tenderness; the nose checked for purulent discharge. Parotid or submaxillary tenderness should be noted and, if present, attempts made to express pus from the ducts.

A careful pulmonary exam may reveal atelectasis or consolidation. Atelectasis may be present without causing fever and thus a secondary cause should always be considered. Persistent atelectasis may be a sign of subphrenic or pancreatic abscess or pulmonary embolism.

New heart murmurs from endocarditis may appear in the postoperative period and, if present, a diligent search should be begun for additional subtle signs of endocarditis. Intravenous cannula sites should be examined closely for erythema, tenderness, or pus. Intravenous catheters in the febrile patient should be removed and cultured. Hyperalimentation lines, central venous pressure lines, and arterial pressure transducers are potential sources of infection. Abdominal findings of right upper quadrant tenderness may suggest postoperative cholecystitis, hepatitis, cholangitis, hepatic, or perihepatic abscess. Although rare, postoperative pancreatitis should not be overlooked. Signs of intraabdominal abscess may not be present at this point, although a tender mass would be suggestive.

All wounds should be carefully observed for signs of infection. If major trauma and tissue necrosis has occurred, a temperature of 102°F is not unusual. A rectal exam is mandatory to rule out rectal or prostatic abscess or prostatitis. Suprapubic tenderness or inner thigh pain after genitourinary surgery suggests osteoitis pubis. The gynecologist will perform postoperative pelvic exams for cuff abscess, endometritis, pelvic abscess, and septic pelvic thrombophlebitis, but it is well to remember subgluteal or retroposal abscess after paracervical or pudendal block, especially with hip pain. After spinal anesthesia or back surgery, carefully palpate for tenderness, which would suggest epidural abscess or vertebral osteomyelitis.

Soft tissue sites should be examined for intramuscular infection, hematoma, or abscess. Pressure points are observed for decubitus ulcers. Tender, swollen joints should be obvious. Joint symptoms may suggest crystal induced arthropathy or infection. Septic joint should prompt a search for a distant infection. The lower extremities may provide a clue to thrombophlebitis. In specific neurosurgical, or-

Table 16.29. Initial Laboratory Evaluation of Postoperative Fever

Complete blood count, differential
Chest x-ray
Induced sputum culture/gram stain
Blood cultures
Urinalysis/culture/gram stain
Culture intravenous catheter
Wound culture/gram stain

thopaedic, and urologic procedures, the referring surgeon will be familiar with causes of fever unique to that procedure.

Initial *laboratory investigation* should include complete blood count, chest x-ray, sputum for gram stain and culture, urinalysis, urine culture and gram stain, removal and culture of intravenous catheters, gram stain and culture of any wound drainage, and blood cultures (Table 16.29).

The absence of leukocytosis does not rule out an infectious cause of postoperative fever. The presence of a leukocytosis helps support an infectious cause, especially after the first 24–72 hours, but there are many other non-infectious causes of postoperative leukocytosis. Leukocytosis is common in uninfected patients immediately postoperatively (<24 to ? hours), especially with major or intraabdominal surgery in our experience; a finding of leukocytosis during this time period is less specific for infection.

If a presumptive diagnosis of infection can be made and the patient is ill, antibiotics can be initiated based on the site of presumed infection and most likely organisms (Table 16.30). If definite infection cannot be identified and the patient

Table 16.30. Infections in Surgical Patients: Initial Empirical Antibiotic Choices [a-f]

Infection	Clinical Situation	Antibiotic Choice	Alternate(s)
Urinary tract	Cystitis or pyelonephritis; no sepsis, catheter, or instrumentation; patient not acutely ill	Cephalosporin, ampicillin, trimethoprim/ sulfamethoxazole	Aminoglycoside
	Pyelonephritis ± sepsis with catheter, instrumentation or prior antibiotics	Ampicillin + Aminoglycoside	Vancomycin + Aminoglycoside

Table 16.30. *Continued*

Infection	Clinical Situation	Antibiotic Choice	Alternate(s)
Urinary tract	Perinephric abscess With staphylococcal sepsis	PRSP	Cephalosporin (first generation)
	With pyelonephritis	Aminoglycoside + PRSP	
Lung	Acute aspiration of gastric contents	By gram stain	
	"Aspiration pneumonia"	Clindamycin ± aminoglycoside	Penicillin G ± aminoglycoside
	Lobar pneumonia Postoperative ± Tracheostomy	By gram stain	
	Compromised host	Ticarcillin + aminoglycoside + cephalosporin or PRSP	Vancomycin + aminoglycoside
Sepsis	Unknown source Noncompromised host	PRSP + aminoglycoside	Clindamycin or cephalosporin + aminoglycoside
	Compromised host	Ticarcillin + PRSP + aminoglycoside	
	Suspected intraabdominal source	Clindamycin + aminoglycoside	Cefoxitin or cefotetan or ampicillin-sulbactam + aminoglycoside
Intraabdominal abscess or Peritonitis	Bowel perforation Traumatic injury Abdominal surgery	Penicillin + clindamycin + aminoglycoside	Cefoxitin + aminoglycoside
Cholecystitis	Complicated	Ampicillin + aminoglycoside	Clindamycin or cefoxitin[e] + aminoglycoside
Cholangitis	Stones/stricture	Ampicillin + aminoglycoside	Clindamycin or cefoxitin + aminoglycoside
Hepatic abscess		Same as for intraabdominal abscess; add metronidazole if amebiasis suspected	
Septic thrombophlebitis	Intravenous catheter	PRSP + aminoglycoside	Vancomycin + aminoglycoside
Joint	Septic arthritis postoperative	PRSP + aminoglycoside	Cephalosporin (first generation) or vancomycin + aminoglycoside
Skin	Postoperative wound *with* sepsis	PRSP + aminoglycoside	Clindamycin + aminoglycoside
	Decubitus ulcer with sepsis	PRSP + aminoglycoside	Clindamycin + aminoglycoside
	Necrotizing fasciitis	Penicillin G + clindamycin + aminoglycoside	Cefoxitin[e] + aminoglycoside
Muscle	Gas gangrene (clostridial myonecrosis)	Penicillin G	

[a] Sources: Stanford JP: *Guide to Antimicrobial Therapy,* 1988. *Handbook of Antimicrobial Therapy.* New Rochelle: Medical Letter, 1986. Dupont HL: *Practical Antimicrobial Therapy.* New York, Appleton-Century Crofts, 1978.

[b] PRSP = penicillinase-resistant synthetic penicillin (methicillin, oxacillin, nafcillin).

[c] Aminoglycoside: gentamicin, tobramycin, amikacin; choice depends on local sensitivity patterns.

[d] Cephalosporins—*first generation:* cephalothin, cefazolin, cephapirin, cephradine
second generation: cefamandole, cefoxitin, cefuroxime, cefonicid, cefotetan, cefordanide
third generation: cefotaxime, moxalactam, cefoperazone, ceftizoxime, ceftriaxone, ceftazidime

[e] or Cefotetan

[f] Metronidazole and ampicillin-sulbactam are alternatives for anaerobic infections.

does not appear seriously ill, antibiotics can usually be withheld to prevent masking of an abscess or drug allergy. An **exception** is the patient with an intravascular prosthesis (heart valve, vascular graft) or other prosthesis, where bacterial seeding of the prosthesis can have devastating consequences; these patients should be treated empirically if clinical circumstances suggest that a risk of seeding exists. Prophylactic antibiotics given beyond 48 hours should be discontinued.

An *extended work-up for fever* should be focused on likely causes suggested by findings and the type of surgery. Repeated physical examination will often yield diagnostic clues. Liver function tests and repeated cultures should be obtained. X-ray examinations should be directed at likely causes, especially deep abscesses at the operative site. For abdominal surgery, ultrasound, gallium or indium scans, and computerized tomography are better primary studies for occult abscesses than standard contrast x-rays (see p. 408).

The diagnosis of occult deep abscesses can be particularly difficult; conversely, extended searches for abscesses are frequently done in patients with other causes of fever (see p. 404). The most important, common circumstances that should initiate a work-up for a deep abscess are *a*) a procedure in which abscesses are a common complication (abdominal trauma, colon resection, pelvic surgery, perforated viscus), and *b*) a prolonged course. Localized symptoms and signs are valuable if present but are frequently absent, especially early in the course. The classic timing of fever several days or weeks postoperatively is not specific, and many patients with abscesses will have early postoperative fevers for other reasons. The appearance of a fever in a well patient suggests either abscess or a nonbacterial cause, especially drug fever and pulmonary causes.

The presence of concomittent unexplained multiple organ failure (pulmonary, renal, liver, less commonly cardiac) and fever suggests abscess and the need for urgent drainage (196–197, 200, 211–213).

Particularly difficult diagnoses, because of the paucity of signs, include suppurative cholangitis, perinephric abscess, retroperitoneal hematoma or abscess, prostatic abscess, pulmonary emboli, and intravenous device infections without obvious suppuration. *Clostridium difficile* colitis may present as a fever of uncertain origin postoperatively. The fever may overshadow minor or atypical (e.g., ileus without diarrhea) gastrointestinal presentations. A marked leukocytosis may be present.

Failure to determine the cause of fever is usually due to an inadequate history, failure to order an important test, or improper evaluation of a previously ordered test (Table 16.31).

A complete review should be made of the history, hospital course, medication, and laboratory data, including personal review of x-rays and gram stains. Three possibilities should be considered: *a*) Was an infection common to the operative procedure not considered? *b*) Was an infection consistent with the clinical picture not considered? and *c*) Is this an atypical presentation of a common disease? Complications should be considered that are remote from the operative site (e.g., liver abscess), are non-bacterial (e.g., parapneumonic effusion), or result from inadequate drainage.

In a prolonged postoperative fever evaluation, entities unrelated to surgery or nosocomial infection must be considered, including drug allergy, collagen vascular disease, drug withdrawal, viral infection, alcoholic hepatitis, and reactivation of tuberculosis. If not already done, all intravenous catheters should be removed and cultured, and unnecessary drugs discontinued.

Factitious fever has been reemphasized as a cause of obscure fever. Medical personnel are frequently involved, with additional clues being a well-appearing pa-

Table 16.31.   Common Reasons for Failure to Diagnose Cause of Fever (or of Fever to Respond to Therapy)

Common
1. Incorrect initial diagnosis of prolonged fever
2. Incorrect interpretation of laboratory data
    Gram stain: not done or misinterpreted
    Culture, sensitivity results
    X-rays not reviewed by clinician
3. Failure to suspect/treat appropriate organism(s) for clinical situation
4. Normal variation in clinical course
5. Antibiotic
    Incorrect administration (transcription of order)
    Antibiotic used to which organism sensitive, but incorrect for clinical situation
6. Drainage of infection not considered, not done or inadequate
    a) Abscess
    b) Obstruction (biliary, renal, respiratory)
    c) Necrotic tissue
    d) Foreign body
    e) Intraabdominal surgical disease (e.g., perforated viscus)
7. Remote complication (e.g. meningitis, liver abscess, infected distant prosthesis)
8. Non-bacterial complication (e.g. atelectasis, parapneumonic effusion)
9. Development of unrelated non-bacterial source
    Drug or anesthetic allergy
    IV Phlebitis
    Thromboembolism
    Dehydration
    Aspiration
10. Superinfection; Colonization after antibiotics misinterpreted as infection
11. Reinfection (e.g. repeated aspiration; undiscovered perforation)
12. Second, unrelated infection
13. Preceding major disease, but unrelated to surgery causing fever (e.g. lymphoma, collagen disease) or
    slowing response (e.g. myeloma)
Not common (But important!)
1. Organism: acquired resistance
2. Antibiotic
    Incorrect dose, or route
    Combination of multiple antibiotics required
3. Immune deficiency not discovered
4. Drug interaction or incompatibility
5. Drug penetration
6. Development of L-forms
7. Tuberculosis, fungal or viral infection
8. Liver disease (hepatitis)
9. Fever unrelated to surgery (e.g. viral, respiratory infection)

tient with a normal physical examination and laboratory studies (including sedimentation rate and blood count), failure of the fever to follow a diurnal variation, rapid defervescence without diaphoresis, temperature greater than 42°C, and absence of tachycardia. Methods of detection include observed rectal temperatures, checking thermometer serial numbers, and measurement of urine temperatures.

Reexploration is often considered when evaluating a deteriorating patient on antibiotics, with persistent bacteremia (see p. 411), or with prolonged unexplained fever. The decision to reexplore the patient should be based on the total clinical circumstance and total laboratory information, not isolated pieces of data.

The number of blind explorations should be reduced by a careful clinical evaluation and use of modern diagnostic modalities, including computerized axial tomography. However, a clinically ill patient with a clear indication of unexplained infection should not be denied drainage until the site is localized by radiographic studies (196–197, 211–213) (see below).

Intraabdominal Abscesses

EPIDEMIOLOGY

Intraabdominal abscesses continue to cause significant morbidity and mortality in the postoperative patient. The most common abdominal operations followed by abscess formation are appendectomy, colon resection, pelvic and gynecologic surgery, and surgery for abdominal trauma (Table 16.32) (203). Biliary, pancreatic, and genitourinary sources are less common. Abscesses are also frequent in surgery for perforated viscus and abdominal trauma.

Abscesses can be either intraperitoneal, retroperitoneal, or visceral (Fig. 16.3) (203).

Table 16.32.   Sources of Infection in Intraabdominal Abscess[a]

Primary Disease	No. of Cases	Percentage
Appendicitis	97	19
Pancreatitis or pancreatic tumor	60	12
Lesions of genitourinary tract	91	18
Lesions of biliary tract	41	8
Diverticulitis	37	7
Actinomycosis	19	4
Septicemia	20	4
Osteomyelitis of spine or 12th rib	18	4
Perforating tumors	17	3
Trauma	17	3
Peptic ulcer	8	2
Leaking anastomotic suture line	7	2
Amebiasis	5	1
Regional enteritis	3	0.6
Miscellaneous	19	4
Unknown	42	9
Total	501	100

[a] From Altemeier WA, Culbertson WR, Fullen WD, Shook CD: Intraabdominal abscesses. *Am J Surg* 125:74, 1973, with permission.

The most common postsurgical site is intraabdominal. The location of the abscess will bear some relation to the site of the primary disease (4, 25, 203–204). The most common sites of abscess location in order of frequency are: right lower quadrant, perihepatic, left lower quadrant, pelvic, and left subphrenic (4, 203). Colonic surgery and trauma are the most frequent causes of subphrenic abscess (205). A recent review by Wang (205) indicated that abscesses in more than one location occur in 20%. Visceral abscesses are uncommon postoperatively, but may occur in the liver, pancreas, and kidney.

BACTERIOLOGY

The bacteriology of intraabdominal abscesses is polymicrobial. Finegold (207) reported an average of 4.5 organisms per infection (Table 16.33). Wang's series of subphrenic abscesses revealed *E. coli* 96%, *Klebsiella* 21%, *Proteus* 38%, *Bacteroides* 83%, *Clostridia* 50%, and anaerobic cocci 50%. Intraabdominal infection of the female genital tract consists usually of *E. coli*, non-enterococcal streptococci, and several anaerobes. Anaerobic organisms are more commonly predominant in chronic abscesses presenting weeks or months after surgery, especially after initial brief antibiotic therapy.

DIAGNOSTIC ACTIVITIES

In Wang's series of patients, the main interval from surgery to drainage of the subphrenic abscess was 5½ weeks. This statistic indicates the indolent nature of many abscesses and the difficulty in making the diagnosis. The usual situation involves the patient who undergoes a major abdominal operation, begins to improve or is placed on antibiotics for suspected postoperative infection, and then plateaus or deteriorates into a period of morbidity with malaise, weight loss, weakness, anorexia, distention, nausea, and vomiting. The other common presentation is fever beginning early in the postoperative course unresponsive to antibiotics.

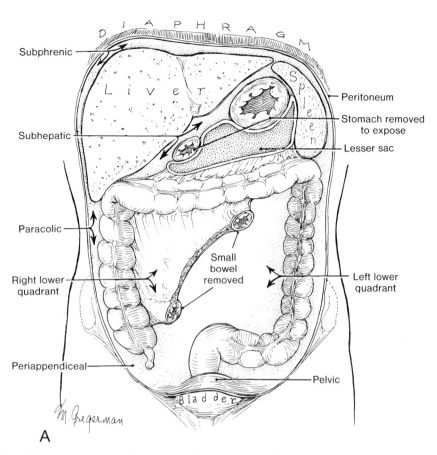

Subphrenic

D I A P H R A G M

L i v e r

S p l e e n

Peritoneum

Stomach removed to expose

Subhepatic

Lesser sac

Paracolic

Small bowel removed

Right lower quadrant

Left lower quadrant

Periappendiceal

Pelvic

Bladder

M. Gregerman

A

Figure 16.3. The most common locations of abscesses and their anatomical relationships. Abscesses may be (A) intraperitoneal (subphrenic, subhepatic, lesser sac, paracolic, periappendiceal, pelvic); (B) visceral (e.g., hepatic, splenic, pancreatic, renal, tuboovarian); or (C) retroperitoneal (anterior/posterior retrosperitoneal; perinephric). The retroperitoneal space is bounded by the peritoneum anteriorly and the transversalis fascia posteriorly. The anterior lamina of the perirenal fascia subdivides the anterior and posterior compartments of the retroperitoneal space. (Adapted from Altemeier WA, Alexander JW: Retroperitoneal abscess. *Arch Surg* 83:512–524, 1961. Copyright 1961, American Medical Assn.; and Altemeier WA, et al.: Intraabdominal abscesses. *Am J Surg* 125:70–77, 1973, with permission.)

The dangers of an unrecognized abscess are sepsis, progressive debilitation, multiple organ failure, fistula formation, rupture (into the abdomen, a blood vessel, or through the diaphragm, producing empyema or pneumonia) and death.

The diagnosis of occult deep abscesses can be particularly difficult; conversely, extended searches for abscesses are frequently done in patients with other causes of fever. The most important, common circumstances that should initiate a workup for a deep abscess are a procedure in which abscesses are a common complication (abdominal trauma, colon resection, pelvic surgery, perforated viscus), and a prolonged course. Localized symptoms and signs are valuable if present but are frequently absent, especially early in the course. The classic timing of fever several days or weeks postoperatively is not specific, and many patients with abscesses will have early postoperative fevers for other reasons. The appearance of a fever in a well patient suggests either abscess or a non-bacterial cause, especially **drug**

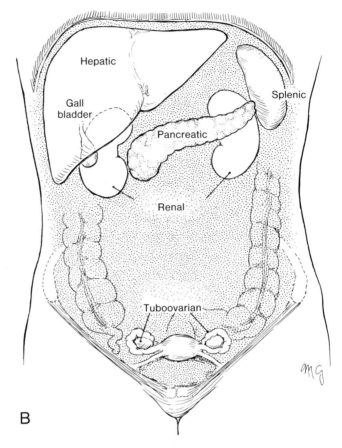

Figure 16.3. *(B)*

fever and pulmonary causes. Suggestive clues are continued fever despite the use of antibiotics and persistent gram-negative bacteremia. The presence of concomitant, unexplained multiple or remote organ failure (pulmonary, renal, liver; less often cardiac) and fever suggests occult infection, often from an intraabdominal site or abscess (and the need for urgent drainage) (196–197, 200, 211–213). Unexplained and unresponsive pulmonary, renal, or liver failure may result from occult intraabdominal abscesses and will improve with drainage.

Symptoms of unlocalized abdominal pain and tenderness, leukocytosis, and chills are common but not specific. When local pain, tenderness, and a mass are present there is usually no problem in making the diagnosis, but most patients lack clear-cut localizing signs.

Subphrenic abscesses characteristically produce few local signs but may be suggested by intercostal tenderness, shoulder pain, elevation of a hemidiaphragm, atelectasis, or pleural effusion. Unless localized pain or a mass is found in a continuously febrile patient, the nonspecific symptoms merely serve as a stimulus to search for the source of continued illness.

Liver abscesses are related to biliary tract disease in 25–40% of cases, but have been reported following a wide variety of surgical procedures from both continuous and hematogenous spread (208). Multiple hepatic abscesses are more likely to be acute (average duration of symptoms 5 days), associated with more dramatic signs

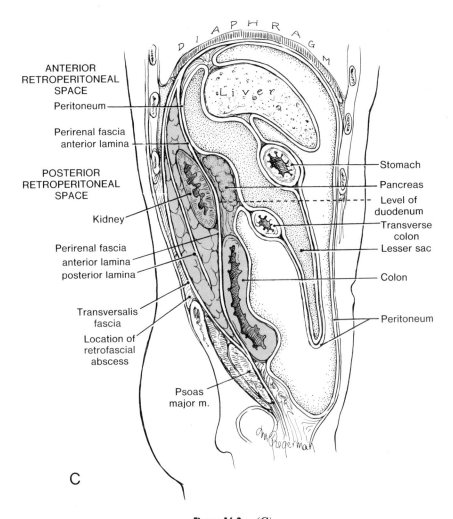

ANTERIOR
RETROPERITONEAL
SPACE
Peritoneum

Perirenal fascia
anterior lamina

POSTERIOR
RETROPERITONEAL
SPACE

Kidney

Perirenal fascia
anterior lamina
posterior lamina

Transversalis
fascia

Location of
retrofascial
abscess

Psoas
major m.

Stomach

Pancreas

Level of
duodenum

Transverse
colon

Lesser sac

Colon

Peritoneum

C

Figure 16.3. *(C)*

and symptoms of cholangitis secondary to biliary obstruction, and carry a higher mortality. Solitary abscesses are more indolent (average duration of symptoms 5 weeks) and jaundice, pain, mass, or tenderness may be absent. Malaise, anorexia, and weight loss may predominate. Patients are often thought to have fever of unknown origin, pulmonary embolus, cholecystitis, pancreatitis, or other infection before an enlarged liver or abnormal liver enzymes call attention to the diagnosis.

Pancreatic abscesses following surgery are rare but have not been eliminated with the use of prophylactic antibiotics. Manipulation of the biliary tract, pancreas, or stomach usually precedes this complication (209) (Table 16.34). Pancreatic abscess usually occurs in the setting of postoperative pancreatitis. Fever, leukocytosis, abdominal distention, and tenderness are the most frequent findings, but are non-specific. Serum amylase is not helpful.

Splenic abscesses only rarely follow intraabdominal surgery (231). Most cases are related to infective endocarditis, urinary infection, and non-penetrating trauma. Symptoms are non-specific and

Table 16.33. Bacteriology of Intraabdominal Abscesses [a]

	No. of Isolates (67 Patients)[b]
ANAEROBES	
Bacteroides	71
Fusobacterium	14
Peptococcus and *Peptostreptococcus*	29
Eubacterium	24
Clostridia	43
AEROBES	
GRAM-NEGATIVE	
E. coli	44
Proteus	15
Klebsiella	13
Enterobacter	9
Pseudomonas	10
GRAM-POSITIVE	
Staphylococcus aureus	3
Enterococcus	10
Streptococcus (other)	7

[a] Modified from Finegold SM, et al.: Management of anaerobic infections. *Ann Intern Med* 83:375–389, 1975.
[b] Number of isolates exceeds the number of patients because of the isolation of more than one species per patient.

Table 16.34. Previous Operations in Patients with Postoperative Pancreatitis and Pancreatic Abscess [a]

Operation	No. of Patients
Cholecystectomy	6
Choledochotomy	12
Choledochotomy and transduodenal sphincterotomy	6
Excision of cystic duct stump	1
Cholecystojejunostomy	1
Choledochoduodenostomy	3
Subtotal gastrectomy (Billroth II)	8
Distal pancreatectomy	2
Pancreatoduodenectomy	3
Splenectomy	2
Adrenalectomy	1
Parathyroidectomy	2
Total	47

[a] From Camer SJ, Tan EGC, Warren KW, Braasch JW: Pancreatic abscess: A critical analysis of 113 cases. *Am J Surg* 129:427, 1975.

only a high degree of suspicion will suggest the diagnosis.

The radiographic approach to a suspected abscess should proceed in a well-planned fashion to avoid delays. Routine studies include chest x-ray, which may reveal abnormalities suggestive of a subdiaphragmatic process including pleural effusion, elevation of the diaphragm, atelectasis, extraluminal air fluid level, and a subdiaphragmatic gas pattern. For other abscesses, flat, upright, or lateral decubitus abdominal films detect abnormal gas patterns, soft tissue masses, abnormalities of the psoas shadow, loss of the renal outline, and bony destruction in the spine or 12th rib. Combined liver-lung scan is useful to detect subdiaphragmatic abscesses.

The use of ultrasound, gallium citrate scanning, and computerized axial tomography (CAT) has revolutionized the workup of abscesses (215–217). Insufficient comparative information is available for indium-leukocyte scans. Each technique has its own advantages and disadvantages. Biello et al. (215) reviewed a number of mostly retrospective series with the three techniques (Table 16.35).

Retrospective studies have found that any one of the three radiologic modalities (ultrasound, gallium, CAT scans) has about a 90% sensitivity and 95% specificity in identifying abscesses (Table 16.35) (215, 217, 334). However, a careful, blinded prospective study including a wider spectrum of patients (216) (Table 16.36) found

Table 16.35. Radiology in the Diagnosis of Intraabdominal Abscesses [a]

	Total Patients	Sensitivity	Specificity	Accuracy
Gallium	613	91%	93%	
Ultrasound	433	90%	97%	95%
Computerized tomography	70			90%

[a] From Biello PR, Levitt RG, Nelson GD: The role of gallium G7 sclentography, ultrasonography, and computerized tomography in the detection of abdominal abscesses. *Semin Nucleic Med* 9:58, 1979, adapted with permission.

Table 16.36. Yield of Three Radiologic Modalities (Ultrasound, Gallium Scans, CAT Scans) in Identifying Focal Causes of Fever[a,b]

	Sensitivity	False Positive Rate
One study +	60%	15%
One of any two studies +	90%	25%

[a] Data from McNeil BJ, et al.: A prospective study of computed tomography, ultrasound, and gallium imaging in patients with fever. *Radiology* 139:647–653, 1981.
[b] Focal causes of fever included abscess, lesions of the biliary system, kidney, intestines (such as hematoma, or tumor).

the sensitivity was 60%, and false positive rate 15% for identification of *any* focal cause of fever. If any two of the three modalities were positive, the sensitivity rose from 60–90%, but the false positive rate also rose from 15–25%. We believe the lower, prospective figures more closely approximate actual clinical practice, because of a more representative patient population and more objective ascertainment of accuracy.

Since the three studies have similar yield, Biello (215) has noted the following clinical considerations. Gallium citrate may accumulate in a recent wound and show as a localized mass, necessitating lateral and oblique views. Gallium may not always distinguish between inflammation and tumor, nor can it determine a fluctuant from a nonfluctuant mass. The time required for scanning is 24–72 hours, and a bowel preparation is usually necessary to avoid false-positives due to excretion of gallium into the gastrointestinal tract. Its main advantage is a full body view with the ability to locate other sites of inflammation. Indium leukocyte scanning is a new nuclear medicine technique with too little comparative data for a definitive statement. It does not accumulate in tumors or the surgical wound as does gallium and *may* be more specific in this setting. With ultrasound, fluid-filled bowel loops and edematous anasta-

moses will give false-positives or prevent optimal visualization of an area. Hematomas, pseudocysts, and ascites sometimes resemble abscesses. Both ultrasound and CAT scan can differentiate a nonfluctuant mass from a fluid-filled abscess, and both can direct diagnostic and therapeutic aspirations.

When physical and routine x-ray findings suggest the location of an abscess, its presence should be confirmed by ultrasound, computerized tomography, or contrast x-ray, depending on the location and the facilities available. Ultrasound or computerized tomography will usually be done first. Barium or hypaque studies of the gastrointestinal tract are useful when perforation with an adjoining viscus is likely, as with diverticulitis, perforated colon carcinoma, or ulcer. The intravenous pyelogram is useful for perinephric abscesses and, occasionally, in detecting retroperitoneal abscesses.

A modified scheme may be used for the diagnosis of abscesses where the location is not apparent (Fig. 16.4). After plain chest and abdominal films, a liver-lung scan is done, if hepatic or subphrenic abscesses are being considered. If masses are found, then either ultrasound or CAT scanning is recommended.

If the patient is acutely ill or has localizing signs, then ultrasound or CAT scanning are performed directly. Ultrasound is favored if there is a suspected diaphragmatic location or the patient is unable to suspend respiration. CAT is done if there are open wounds, dressings over the suspected area, or an ileus is present. The experience of the institution must be considered in selecting between ultrasound and CAT scanning. If either is negative, the other study is performed if the patient is acutely ill; gallium scanning follows if the patient is stable enough for a 24–72 hour study. If positive, then ultrasound or CAT scanning is repeated in the area in question.

If there are no localizing signs and the patient is stable gallium or indium scan-

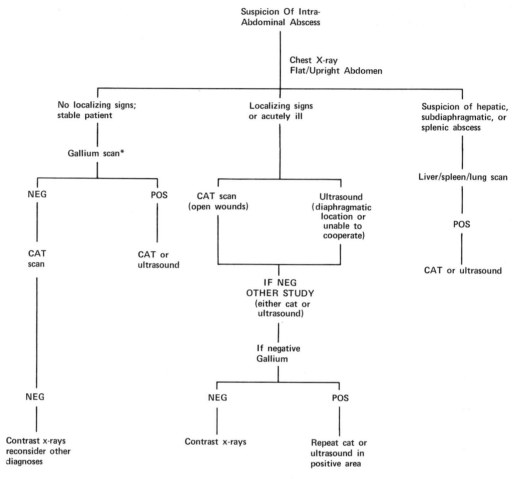

Figure 16.4. Radiographic approach to suspected abscess with no localizing signs. *CAT scanning is recommended as a first step by many authorities. (Adapted from Bielle DR, et al.: The role of gallium G7 sclentography, ultrasonography, and computerized tomography in the detection of abdominal abscesses. *Semin Nucl Med* 9:58, 1979, adapted with permission.)

ning may be done first, recognizing that full scanning will take 48 hours. If abnormal, then CAT or ultrasound is done in the area of abnormality.

Previously, barium contrast x-rays and intravenous pyelograms were performed first to locate abscesses. These techniques are less sensitive, interfere with subsequent scanning, and require more time (if there are no clues to the location of the abscess), compared to CAT scanning and ultrasound. Contrast x-rays are useful when localized findings are present or if a leaking viscus (e.g., colon) or stomach is the suspected source.

If x-rays, gallium, and CAT scans are normal, then another etiology for fever should be seriously considered. A decision will have to be made about reexploration if abscess is considered likely.

The decision to reexplore a patient to diagnose a suspected, unidentified abscess must be based on the total clinical and laboratory situation (196–197, 333). The best clinical indications of abscess are preceding surgical procedures at high risk of abscess formation (perforated viscus, abdominal trauma, colon, pelvic, or gynecologic surgery), prolonged fever and leukocytosis without identified cause, peritoneal irritation, or mass formation. Drainage should not be unduly delayed in an obvious clinical situation because of the lack of absolute radiographic confirmation, nor rushed into in a stable patient without adequate study. The appropriate time for reexploration in an individual patient remains a clinical decision.

MANAGEMENT

Once the diagnosis is suspected, every effort should be made to confirm and locate the abscess. If the patient is not acutely ill or septic, antibiotics may cautiously be discontinued to facilitate the diagnosis, obtain cultures, and exclude drug fever. Once a diagnosis has been made and blood cultures drawn, antibiotics should be given pending results of surgical drainage. Prompt drainage is imperative. The type of drainage will depend on the individual situation and the surgeon. Ultrasound or CAT-guided aspiration for culture, limited drainage, or definitive drainage can be attempted in selected cases.

Empirical antibiotics are directed against anaerobes and gram-negative rods. Clindamycin and an aminoglycoside provide adequate initial coverage. Penicillin or ampicillin may be added to cover enterococcus. Alternate regimens would include cefoxitin alone or with an aminoglycoside. Another alternative is ampicillin-sulbactam with an aminoglycoside. Repeat cultures of blood and purulent drainage should be used to guide changes in antibiotics.

Continued fever on a previous antibiotic regimen does not necessarily indicate antibiotic resistance; the presence of an inadequately drained abscess should be strongly considered. The duration of antibiotic treatment depends on the site of infection, continued searching, and drainage. The surgical literature generally recommends continuing antibiotics for 1–3 weeks after the patient is afebrile.

The outcome of intraabdominal infections is not good. The poor outcome is due to delayed diagnosis and drainage, malnutrition, and the underlying surgical problem. The poor prognosis of abscesses may be improved with earlier diagnosis by CAT, ultrasound, and gallium scanning, and by improved support with hyperalimentation.

Prompt, adequate drainage, combined with antibiotics and nutritional support (by hyperalimentation if necessary), are the three major therapeutic modalities.

Bacteremia

EPIDEMIOLOGY

Gram-negative bacteremia continues to increase in frequency. Risk factors include manipulative procedures, antibiotics, steroids, antimetabolites, elderly, and severely ill patients (218–219).

The most frequent source of gram-negative bacteremia is the urinary tract (30%). Fifty-two per cent of those with a urinary source have indwelling catheters, cystoscopy, surgery, or biopsy of the urinary tract. Seventy per cent of those with respiratory origin for the bacteremia have endotrachial intubation, tracheostomy, respiratory assistance devices, surgery, or biopsy of the respiratory tract. These statistics emphasize the importance of respiratory and urinary tract instrumentation. The gastrointestinal tract operative site may be the source of bacteremia (218, 221). In many postoperative situations, the gastrointestinal tract is the obvious reservoir of bacteria, but it must be realized that indwelling catheters, drainage tubes, monitoring devices, intravenous fluids, diagnostic instruments, inhalation therapy equipment, and hospital food and equipment are also sources of colonization and infection.

The bacteriology of gram-negative bacteremia in several series indicates that *E. coli* is most common, followed by *Klebsiella, Enterobacter, Serratia, Pseudo-*

monas, Proteus, Providencia, and *Bacteroides. S. aureus* represents about 10–15% of bacteremias. Approximately 10% of bacteremias are polymicrobial, usually indicating a source from an abscess, the gastrointestinal tract, a neutropenic patient, or a contaminant.

Gram-positive bacteremia usually originates from the skin, wound, intravenous or intra-arterial lines in surgical patients. The urinary and respiratory tracts are less common sources. Anaerobic bacteremia is usually from a gastrointestinal source; female pelvic infections are next most common.

Persistent "breakthrough" bacteremia while on antibiotics is most frequently seen in patients with steroids, diabetes mellitus, moderate renal failure and leukopenia. Continuing bacteremia suggests the existence of an abscess, other focal, undrained sources of infection (e.g., gallbladder, obstructed urinary tract), other intra-abdominal foci of infection (biliary or bowel source), or an intravascular infection (e.g., intravenous lines) especially if gram-negative rods are present or multiple episodes of breakthrough bacteremia occur (194). Subtherapeutic antibiotic levels may be another reason for persistent bacteremia; antibiotic levels should be measured in this situation (194).

DIAGNOSTIC ACTIVITIES

A frequent problem in postoperative consultation is determining the cause of persistent bacteremia. The most common sources are intravascular foci (intravenous lines, prosthesis, endocarditis), abdominal abscesses, and gastrointestinal or genitourinary foci (194, 223–224). Recent surgical instrumentation or manipulation should be considered as a source of transient bacteremia. When the patient repeatedly has positive blood cultures with an organism sensitive to the antibiotic being administered, several possibilities should be considered. Intravascular foci should be searched for, including intra-

venous devices, prostheses, septic nonsuppurative thrombophlebitis, and bacterial endocarditis. Focal undrained sources of infection should be considered including abscesses, undrained infection (gallbladder or obstructed urinary tract, and intra-abdominal foci (biliary, bowel) sources. Occult infection in the abdomen should be sought with special attention to the liver, gallbladder, kidneys, appendix, colon, and intraabdominal abscesses. Susceptibility testing should be reviewed with the microbiology laboratory, and drug incompatibilities and the dose-route of antibiotic administration should be checked. A second source of error is an inadequate dose of aminoglycoside.

If no source can be found after extensive and prolonged search, then a decision on abdominal exploration will need to be made.

The deteriorating patient already on appropriate antibiotics for bacterial sepsis must always be considered to have a surgical lesion requiring drainage until proven otherwise.

Management. Of particular importance is determination of the source of bacteremia, since elimination of the focus of infection is necessary for cure. Table 16.37 lists common sources of bacteremia for several organisms. Initial treatment of bacteremia in the surgical patient depends on the most likely site (see Table 16.30).

Initial therapy for suspected bacteremia of unknown origin should include a penicillinase-resistant penicillin and aminoglycoside. Vancomycin should be considered in institutions or settings where a high rate of methicillin-resistant *staphylococci* are present. When intraabdominal infection is suspected, clindamycin, metronidazole, or ampicillin-sulbactam should be added. Combinations of first generation cephalosporins and an aminoglycoside should be avoided because of increased risk of renal failure. Focal sources of infection should be drained or removed.

Table 16.37.   Common Sources of Bacteremia

Staphylococcus aureus	Lung
	Wound
	Intravenous catheter
	Skin
Staphylococcus epidermidis	Prosthetic heart valves
	Ventriculo-atrial shunts
	Intravenous catheter
	Urinary procedures
	Valvular heart diseases
	Contaminant
Escherichia coli	Urinary procedures
	GI tract
	Abdominal abscesses
	Peritonitis
Klebsiella	Abdominal wounds
	GI tract
	Intravenous catheter
	Lung
Enterobacter	Contaminated blood products
	Contaminated intravenous fluids
	Intravenous catheter
	Urinary procedures
Serratia	Intravenous catheter
	Urinary procedures
	Pneumonia following respirator use
Pseudomonas	Respiratory tract
	Urinary tract
	Wound infection
	Intravenous catheter
Proteus	Wound infection
	Urinary tract
Bacteroides	Female genital tract
	GI tract
	Postoperative abdominal abscesses
	Liver abscess
Citrobacter	Urinary tract
Acinetobacter	Intravenous catheter
Erwinia	Intravenous infusion set
Providencia	Urinary tract

Fungemia

EPIDEMIOLOGY

Hospital-acquired fungemia is assuming new importance in infectious complications of hospitalized patients. The Boston Collaborative Drug Surveillance Program reported antibiotic-related superinfection in 0.9% of 14,000 medical patients. Seventy-one per cent of the episodes were caused by yeast or fungi, principally *Candida* (227). The incidence on surgical units may be higher due to the more frequent use of hyperalimentation. Overall mortality with established fungemia is high at 50–80% (229).

The typical patient at risk is the severely ill postoperative patient with a serious bacterial infection who is receiving antibiotics and hyperalimentation, has multiple intravenous lines, and a Foley catheter (336). Additional risk factors are hyperglycemia, immunosuppression, and steroids. In two series (226, 229), 100% had intravenous catheters, 99% were on antibiotics, 89% had a Foley catheter, 88% had concomitant bacterial infection, 47% had recent abdominal surgery, 21% other recent surgery, 21% had diabetes, 54% were on corticosteroids and 60% were receiving hyperalimentation.

Diagnostic Activities. Clinical clues of significant fungemia are any change in the fever pattern, new unexplained change in mental status, or new hypotension. The clinical picture can be indistinguishable from gram-negative septicemia. Many patients are treated for gram-negative septicemia and continue to deteriorate. It is important to recognize that there may be a 2–3 week period of latent infection; only after bloodstream invasion does the infection become fulminant.

Physical examination is consistent with sepsis. However, especially important features include a cheesy white exudate expressed from the catheter site, erythematous macronodular skin lesions, and pathognomonic white retinal exudates. A funduscopic exam by an ophthalmologist is strongly recommended if a diagnosis of fungemia is suspected. Other organ systems involvement may aid diagnosis, especially arthritis, pulmonary disease, osteomyelitis, and myocarditis.

Scrapings from skin lesions should be examined microscopically and cultured. Burn wounds would be biopsied for histology and quantitative culture.

Candida may be cultured from wounds, peritoneum (335), urine, sputum, or feces. Since colonization of these areas is common, cultures are not diagnostic of invasive disease. In the presence of a Foley catheter, fungal colony counts cannot distinguish between invasive disease and colonization of the bladder. Since renal involvement is present in 80% of systemic candidiasis, it is an important but difficult distinction. Evaluation of precipitin tests and counterimmunoelectrophoresis to detect candida antigenemia have yielded conflicting results. While positive serologic tests support the diagnosis of disseminated candidiasis in a high-risk setting, they are not diagnostic. A negative serologic test is not useful in excluding disseminated disease because of the high rate of false-negative results. The finding by culture of *Candida* colonizing multiple body sites in a high-risk patient should raise a high suspicion of invasive candidiasis, since a substantial percentage of these patients have invasive infection. However, the documentation of multiple colonized sites is not sufficient to prove invasive infection.

A definitive diagnosis must be based on positive tissue biopsy, blood cultures, fundoscopic findings and skin lesions. While other findings are strongly suggestive, they are not diagnostic.

MANAGEMENT

Management of fungal infection is beyond the scope of this text (See references 4, 25).

Drug Fever

EPIDEMIOLOGY AND PATHOPHYSIOLOGY

Febrile reactions to drugs, especially antibiotics, complicate the evaluation of the postoperative patient. Diagnosis of a drug fever is difficult in the seriously ill patient in whom withholding of possible offending agents may make management difficult or may not be possible.

Drug fevers occur in about 0.5% of hospitalized patients, nearly all of whom receive at least one medication (230). About 30–60% of surgical patients receive anti-

biotics of which 10–20% receive antibiotics for prophylaxis. Drug fever is a particular problem with antibiotics because they are commonly administered and are a common cause of febrile reactions.

Although no comprehensive study is available, the drugs most commonly implicated in drug fever include penicillin, cephalosporins, sulfonamides, allopurinol, procainamide, quinidine, methyldopa, phenytoin, barbiturates, iodine, propylthiouracil, methimazole, and antihistamines. Other drugs causing fever include salicylates, cimetidine, nitrofurantoin, isoniazid, rifampin, and hydralazine. Digitalis and insulin rarely, if ever, cause fever (230).

Hypersensitivity reaction is the best established mechanism for drug fever, but does not account for all episodes. Other postulated mechanisms are direct pyrogenic effect of the injected material (e.g., amphotericin), alteration of thermoregulatory mechanisms, pharmacologic action, side effects (e.g., hemolytic anemia, vasculitis), local phlebitis at the site of injection, and idiosyncratic responses (230).

DIAGNOSTIC ACTIVITIES

The onset of a new fever should prompt a review of the medication record. A thorough history should be obtained of prior allergy to medication, medication before hospitalization, and bedside drugs from home. All drugs should be suspected, with priority to common agents listed above.

The onset of drug fever occurs 7–10 days after initial administration of the agent in hypersensitivity reactions. The fever may begin earlier if there was prior exposure to the agent or if caused by another mechanism. The presentation may be an increased or recrudescent fever when the primary illness is improving (e.g., pneumonia). Other signs of hypersensitivity reaction are rash, eosinophilia, and recurrence with repeat challenge. Patients with drug fever often appear well, without leukocytosis, and have a relative bradycardia. Other organs may be affected, such as hepatitis or interstitial nephritis, but usually are not affected initially.

The clinical spectrum of drug fevers varies widely from the classic hypersensitivity reaction. Drug fevers may occur at any time from the first day to after months of therapy; accompanying signs such as rash or hepatitis may be absent. The patient may appear acutely ill mimicking sepsis with high fever to 104°F, rigors, hypotension, and hypoxia.

No particular fever pattern is characteristic of drug fever, as sustained, intermittent, remittent, and hectic patterns have been described. Almost any drug may be responsible, although a few drugs are common offenders.

Most drug fevers will improve within 48–72 hours of stopping the offending agent. Occasionally a week or more is necessary for deferverscence, especially if the course is complicated by drug-induced serum sickness, or hepatitis.

In the febrile patient, the initial assessment should establish if an infection or other non-drug cause is responsible for fever. The administration of drugs commonly causing fever, temporal relationship of drug administration to fever, and other signs of drug reaction (fever, eosinophilia) should be established. If a drug fever is suspected, the suspected offending drug should be discontinued or changed.

The clinical situation, availability of alternative drugs, and need for medication will determine if all remaining drugs should be stopped or changed together, or if this should be done sequentially. Sequential discontinuation is helpful diagnostically, but exposes the patient to more prolonged risk and lengthens the diagnostic process. Rechallenge will establish the cause, but should only be done where there is a major need for the medication, as there is a risk of more serious reactions such as exfoliative dermatitis or nephritis.

When a drug is identified as causing fever, the patient should be informed and the reaction documented in the record so future administration is avoided.

MANAGEMENT

Discontinuation of the drug is discussed under diagnosis. Rarely, the drug cannot be discontinued because it is vital and no alternative medication exists. The major risk to continuation is end-organ damage, especially exfoliative dermatitis, hepatitis, interstitial nephritis, and vasculitis. Fever may be suppressed by salicylates, acetaminophen, steroids, and, possibly, antihistamines. Suppression of fever does not eliminate the risk of damage to other organs and the patient should be closely monitored.

Pneumonia

EPIDEMIOLOGY

Pneumonia remains a major cause of postoperative morbidity and mortality, representing 10–20% of all nosocomial infections. The mortality rate of nosocomial pneumonia is high at 20–30% (141). Due to the high morbidity rate, pneumonia is the leading postoperative infection contributing to death on the surgical services. The risk of pneumonia is increased with general anesthesia, intubation, ICU, altered level of consciousness, atelectasis, aspiration, advanced age, debilitation, malnutrition, immunosuppression, prior steroids, antacids/H_2-blocks, antibiotic use, congestive heart failure, and chronic lung disease (19, 243–244, 327). The risk of pneumonia may be increased by prior or prophylactic antibiotic use, but this remains unproven.

Data on the bacteriology of postoperative pneumonia derive mainly from all nosocomial pneumonias (231–238, 241). Of aerobic organisms, gram-positives represent 20–35% gram-negatives 40–80%. Anaerobes account for about 35%. (232–235, 241). Multiple organisms have been found in 35–50%. Careful anaerobic cultures have not been systematically done in a series of postoperative pneumonias. Immunosuppressed or debilitated hosts may acquire unusual bacterial or fungal organisms (236).

Aspiration of oropharyngeal bacteria is the principal mechanism of acquisition (237), though inhalation from respiratory equipment and hematogenous spread both play a role. Airborne transmission in the hospital is unimportant. Normal throat flora of hospitalized patients will convert to gram-negative colonization similar to fecal flora in 27% of patients not on antibiotics and 47% of those on antibiotics (238). In severely ill individuals, the colonization is rapid and approaches 75% in the first few days. Combining the high colonization rates of potential pathogens with any of the risk factors explains the hospitalized patient's susceptibility to pneumonia.

Endogenous gram-negative aerobic bacilli *(Klebsiella, E. coli, Pseudomonas, Enterobacter, Proteus serratia)* cause 40–80% of nosocomial pneumonias. While direct aerosol spread may occur, endogenous colonization with subsequent bronchial aspiration is the most common mechanism. Contamination of respiratory equipment contributes to colonization. Other organisms are transmitted through direct personal hand contact.

Staphylococcus aureus accounts for 10–30% of nosocomial pneumonias (241). The reservoir of *S. aureus* is the nasal vestibule, and some hospital employees are persistent carriers. Contact transmission and colonization of the nasopharynx with subsequent aspiration is the main acquisition route, though hematogenous spread from peripheral sites such as intravenous catheters contributes to pneumonia due to staphylococci.

The pneumococcus is responsible for 2–10% of nosocomial pneumonias from aspiration from the upper respiratory tract. Group A *Streptococcus* contributes another 0–5% of cases. A wide variety of other organisms cause sporadic cases. *Haemophilus influenzae* is another re-

ported agent in a small number of patients. Nosocomially acquired *Legionella pneumophila* pneumonia has a suggestive clinical presentation and should be considered in any pneumonia of uncertain etiology (222). Mild cough despite extensive consolidation, multiple rigors, profound malaise, diarrhea, relative bradycardia, hypophosphatemia, and abnormal liver function tests are clues to *Legionella* infection. Other causes of nosocomial "pneumonia" include viruses, mycobacteria, and fungi.

DIAGNOSTIC ACTIVITIES

Criteria for the diagnosis of pneumonia include fever, purulent bronchial secretions, leukocytosis, consistent gram stain, and a new or progressive chest infiltrate developing after surgery. Cultures are required to identify the type and antibiotic susceptibility of organisms seen on gram stain.

In the postoperative patient already producing sputum, a reliable sign of pneumonia is increased purulence of the sputum and number of white cells seen on gram stain (239).

Transtracheal aspirates, pleural fluid, and blood cultures correlate best with the correct pathogen. Needle lung aspiration and protected brush bronchoscope may yield more accurate diagnoses but are more invasive.

Sputum cultures are of limited value because of oropharyngeal contamination. Sputum cultures are more reliable if the gram stain on the same specimen shows few epithelial cells and a predominant organism. Transtracheal aspirates are indicated if the gram stain is not diagnostic, sputum cannot be obtained by other measures, or the clinical picture is complex.

Additional tests in compromised hosts or in suggestive clinical circumstances include serology for *Legionella* pneumonia, cytomegalovirus, and influenza; cultures and stain for fungi, and tuberculosis.

The differential diagnosis of postoperative pneumonia includes atelectasis, pulmonary embolism, aspiration, and, occasionally, pulmonary edema. Signs and symptoms suggestive but not diagnostic of pneumonia include a new or progressive infiltrate on x-ray, an increase in fever, leukocytosis, and changes in the character, amount, or microscopic appearance of sputum.

Pulmonary superinfection occurs with variable frequency depending on the series. Tillotson and Finland (239) reported 149 patients with bacterial pneumonia in whom 24 developed superinfections. Onset is usually 4–7 days after the initial infection and is suggested most reliably by new fever after 2 afebrile days, increased purulence of the sputum or white cells on gram stain, and new infiltrate on x-ray. Early recognition is important because morbidity is high.

MANAGEMENT

Antimicrobial agents should be begun in the ill or toxic patient pending outcome of cultures. The initial antimicrobial agent should be selected based on gram stain results and the clinical circumstances. If the gram stain does not show a predominant organism, a penicillinase-resistant penicillin and aminoglycoside are reasonable empirical coverage. If witnessed aspiration has occurred, clindamycin or a cephalosporin with anaerobic activity should be given in addition to an aminoglycoside. Third generation cephalosporins with anti-pseudomonal activity, such as ceftazidine, may be used in place of an aminoglycoside. The most commonly recommended empirical agents for gram-negative pneumonias are third-generation cephalosporins, aminoglycosides, or a combination of both, until definitive therapy can be based on sensitivity results.

Colonization, defined as a change in organism cultured without other signs of pneumonia, is not an indication for a change in antibiotics.

Pulmonary toilet has increased importance in the surgical patient who does not cough well due to pain and narcotics. Useful modalities include incentive spirometry, backclapping, and postural drainage.

Prevention of pneumonia and superinfection depends on good pulmonary toilet, prevention of aspiration in high-risk patients, and avoidance of multiple antibiotic regimens.

Pulmonary Aspiration

The potential aspiration of gastric or oropharyngeal secretions represents a significant risk to the postoperative patient. Most retrospective reviews (245–247) exclude those with only suspected aspiration and, thus, the clinical spectrum is undoubtedly much wider than that reported in the literature. The challenge is to recognize aspiration early and distinguish it from other postoperative pulmonary complications.

Epidemiology. The mean interval from operation to aspiration is 1½ days, though episodes occur up to 30 days postoperatively. The clinical course of gastric acid aspiration follows one of three patterns: (*a*) a rapidly progressive acute course to death within 24 hours; (*b*) clinical and radiological improvement over 2–16 days after initial aspiration; or (*c*) initial improvement followed in 2 or more days by clinical deterioration associated with signs and symptoms of superimposed nosocomial pneumonia. It must be emphasized that infection is not thought to be part of the initial process of gastric aspiration. Infection develops secondarily, probably as a result of chemical damage, or more insidiously, associated with aspiration of small amounts of colonized oropharyngeal secretions.

The less fulminant form is seldom witnessed and may present insidiously days to weeks later with clinical deterioration, putrid sputum, and pulmonary cavitation or abscess. After witnessed aspiration, infection may not develop for 1–2 days, with over half occurring in 3–5 days; and some infections occurring as late as 2 or more weeks. The risk of bacterial infection after acid aspiration is 25–40% within the first week (248).

BACTERIOLOGY

The bacteriology of hospital aspiration is complex, depending largely on colonization of the oropharynx. Normal oropharyngeal colonization may be replaced by gram-negative organisms in the hospital, especially with antibiotics or intubation. The three studies summarized in Table 16.38 indicate the number of multiple pathogens present in many patients (249–251).

DIAGNOSTIC ACTIVITIES

Indicators of infection after aspiration include new or increased fever, leukocytosis, purulent sputum, new or extending pulmonary infiltrate appearing more than 48 hours after aspiration (progression of x-ray findings 36–48 hours after witnessed aspiration usually indicates superimposed infection), increased hypoxia,

Table 16.38. Bacteriology of Aspiration Pneumonia

	Total Patients		
	54[a]	32[b]	28[c]
Bacteroides			
Melaninogenicus	23	11	3
Fragilis	9	5	3
Oralis	8	5	
Fusobacterium nucleatum	18	8	4
Peptostreptococcus	16	11	5
Peptococcus	7	4	
Other anaerobes	31		2
Streptococcus pneumoniae	7	4	1
Staphylococcus aureus	8	8	4
Klebsiella	6	5	
Pseudomonas	6	5	8
Escherichia coli	6	4	5
Enterobacter	4	3	
Proteus			6

[a] Bartlett JG, Gorbach SL, Finegold SM: The bacteriology of aspiration pneumonia. *Am J Med* 56:202, 1974.
[b] Bartlett JG, Gorbach SL: The triple threat of aspiration pneumonia. *Chest* 68:560, 1975.
[c] Lorber B, Swenson RM: Bacteriology of aspiration pneumonia. *Ann Intern Med* 81:329, 1974.

a consistent gram stain, unexplained deterioration, and positive cultures. Cultures must be interpreted with caution because colonization alone is not indicative of infection.

The predictability of the bacteriology of community acquired aspiration pneumonia makes invasive procedures indicated only in selected cases. In the postoperative patient, the bacteriology is less predictable due to colonization by hospital-acquired organisms. Transtracheal aspiration or protected brush bronchoscope for bacteriology are sometimes needed.

MANAGEMENT

There is inadequate data in the literature to document a superior antibiotic regimen for aspiration pneumonia. Although theoretically antibiotics should not be given until infection is documented, this is not done clinically because of the degree of illness and the precarious situation of most patients who aspirate. The decision to begin and the selection of antibiotics is based on the degree of clinical illness, severity of aspiration, gram stain results, the underlying illness, and general condition of the patient. For most postoperative patients, this means starting antibiotics for all but minor aspirations.

Although therapy should be guided by the clinical situation, gram stain, and culture results, these are often not diagnostic early in nosocomial aspiration. Antibiotics should cover anaerobes and gram-negative organisms. Staphylococci are significant causes of nosocomial pneumonia, but are uncommon after aspiration. A reasonable empiric choice would be clindamycin and an aminoglycoside.

Other important aspects of therapy are pulmonary toilet and prevention of repeated episodes of aspiration.

Atelectasis

Atelectasis is the most common cause of early postoperative fever and represents up to 90% of postoperative pulmonary complications. The incidence of atelectasis is about 10–20% in abdominal surgery. Atelectasis is more common (20–30%) in surgery of the upper abdomen. The contribution of atelectasis to the febrile response is variable, and may be clinically difficult to interpret in the individual patient. Livelli (191) noted segmental or subsegmental atelectasis in 62% of febrile patients and 54% of non-febrile patients 6 days after cardiac surgery.

Axioms on atelectasis include the following: (a) clinical and x-ray findings of various degrees of atelectasis should cautiously be considered the cause of early fever; (b) fever does not necessarily correlate with the extent of atelectasis and should gradually decline as treatment proceeds unless complications arise; (c) auscultation may detect atelectasis earlier than x-ray and rales often precede decreased breath sounds; (d) atelectasis with fever but normal x-ray and physical findings can occur; (e) infection is not thought to be present in early atelectasis, though unrecognized aspiration could be a common cause of postoperative atelectasis; (f) atelectasis could be due to other processes, i.e., subdiaphragmatic abscess or pulmonary infarction.

Thus, while treatment for atelectasis proceeds, a constant awareness of other febrile conditions must be maintained (258). Atelectasis in the febrile postoperative patient remains common, but is in part a diagnosis of exclusion; one must avoid ending the search for other causes.

MANAGEMENT

See page 60.

Thrombophlebitis and Pulmonary Embolism

Thrombophlebitis and pulmonary embolism are discussed in Chapter 8. In the postoperative setting, these entities are often in the differential diagnosis of fever. Fever, up to 102°F, may occur in deep vein thrombosis, and rarely up to 104°F with pulmonary embolism. The frequency of fever in thrombophlebitis is difficult to quantitate. Fever alone may be the sole presenting feature of deep venous thrombosis, and further investigations are required for diagnosis.

In a review of fever and pulmonary embolism, Murray (259) reported fever in 64% of angiographically proven cases. Fever was more common with pulmonary infarction. Temperatures to 40°C are noted early in the course and may persist for more than 1 week. The persistence of (rectal) temperatures of 38.5°C after 4 days or 38°C after 6 days were uncommon and should not be attributed solely to emboli unless evidence for reembolization exists. Only one patient in the series had hectic fever spikes. The findings of leukocytosis in the range of 10,000–20,000 WBCs/mm^3 (occasionally up to 40,000/mm^3) and empyema-like pleural fluid make these unreliable indicators of infection versus infarction. No patient in this series had shaking chills, although rigors have been reported with pulmonary embolism previously.

Thrombophlebitis and pulmonary embolism should be considered in all postoperative febrile patients. However, the fever itself provides no substantial clues and diagnosis must rely on other parameters.

Urinary Tract Infection

See also page 177.

EPIDEMIOLOGY

Infections of the urinary tract constitute the largest single source of nosocomial infection, and one closely related to catheterization. Urinary tract infections (UTI) are generally recognized as the most common nosocomial infection (30–40%), the most common cause of gram-negative bacteremia (30–40%), and the second or third most common cause of postoperative fever. Approximately 15% of hospitalized patients receive indwelling urinary catheters, and the rate of infection varies from 10–25%. The rate of infection varies from 53% of catheterized patients in orthopaedics and the surgical intensive care unit to 0–2% for ophthalmology and otolaryngology. Common morbidity includes asymptomatic bacteriuria, cystitis, pyelonephritis, and bacteremia. Rarely, complications include perinephric abscess, epididymitis, orchitis, and vertebral osteomyelitis.

The most important etiologic factor is urethral catheterization. In addition to urethral catheterization, surgical instrumentation of the urinary tract and fistulas produced from surgery in adjacent structures result in urinary infections. The risk of infection is increased by lack of meticulous technique in catheter insertion and care. Lack of hand washing by physicians and nurses causes cross-contamination between catheter and patients. Risk of infection is related to the duration of catheterization (greater than 48–72 hours). Additional risk factors are age, the presence of chronic asymptomatic bacteriuria before catheterization, the severity of underlying illness, structural and functional abnormalities of the urinary tract, and the proximity of other patients with catheters (260, 262–263).

BACTERIOLOGY

Nearly all studies of nosocomial urinary infections concur that *E. coli* is the most frequent pathogen, ranging from 30–50% of isolates. Other frequent pathogens are *Klebsiella-Enterobacter* (13–15%), *Pseudomonas* (10–20%), *Proteus* (3–13%), *Enterococci* (2–10%), and *Candida*. Patients with surgical instrumentation catheters and prior antibiotics tend to have a greater incidence of *Pseudomonas, Serratia, Providentia, Citrobacter, Acinetobacter,* and *Candida albicans.* The selective pressure of antibiotics within a given hospital will contribute to the distribution of bacteria colonizing the susceptible patient. Knowledge of the most frequent organisms causing nosocomial urinary infections in an individual hospital is important.

DIAGNOSTIC ACTIVITIES

In the uncatheterized patient, the typical symptoms of frequency, urgency, dysuria, and suprapubic discomfort are early clues but may also be caused by or obscured by mechanical or chemical irritants in the postoperative period. Fever, flank pain and tenderness, and chills suggest upper tract infection. In the catheterized patient, manifestations may include blood-tinged or turbid urine, bladder spasms with leakage around the meatus, fever, chills, flank pain, and signs of sepsis and shock. In the postoperative patient, fever alone may be the sole clinical clue, and usually begins at least 48–72 hours after surgery or time of catheterization.

Pyuria is nonspecific, but 5–10 WBCs/HPF of a spun urine are suggestive; up to 30% of specimens with 10^5 bacteria/ml do not have significant pyuria. A rapid, reliable, presumptive diagnosis of infection can be made by observing one or more bacteria per oil immersion field in a gram-stained, uncentrifuged specimen, as this correlates highly (>90%) with 10^5 bacteria/ml on culture. The absence of bacteria in several fields mitigates against infection. Culture of 10^2 organisms/ml is diagnostic when obtained from a suprapubic bladder puncture or properly obtained catheterized specimen. Patients currently on antibiotics may have fewer than 10^5 colonies/ml on culture in the presence of infection.

It is generally accepted that 10^5 bacteria/ml indicate infection. However, less than 10^5 organisms may be a significant cause of infection in a catheterization or suprapubic tap specimen in the presence of antibiotics and for certain organisms. It must be stressed that finding 10^5 organisms/ml in the urine is not a guarantee that this is the source of the patient's fever. Because asymptomatic bacteriuria is common, the diagnosis should be based on the clinical situation, culture, and careful follow-up.

MANAGEMENT

The therapy of urinary tract infection depends on the clinical illness and whether a Foley catheter remains in place.

Uncatheterized patients should be treated if symptomatic. For seriously ill patients, an aminoglycoside and ampicillin should be used until the sensitivities of the organism are known. Less ill patients can be treated with a second or third generation cephalosporin or trimethoprim-sulfamethoxazole. Patients with mild symptoms can be treated with other antibiotics if resistance is not common in the specific hospital. Asymptomatic bacteriuria needs to be treated only if occurring after instrumentation or in the pregnant patient.

Patients with indwelling Foley catheters should be treated for symptomatic or febrile urinary infections. The urine should be routinely cultured when or shortly after the catheter is removed and infection treated, even if asymptomatic. Routine cultures in the catheterized patient should not usually be treated because of the emergence of resistant organisms.

Once culture results are available, less toxic and expensive antibiotics to which the organism is sensitive may be used. Treatment should be continued for 10–14 days for upper tract infections and 7 or fewer days for lower tract.

Repeat cultures should be obtained after 2–3 days and after completion of antibiotics in seriously ill patients.

The incidence of infection can be reduced by proper catheter care as detailed elsewhere (260). The most important measures are avoiding unnecessary catheterization, use of closed one-way drainage system, proper insertion and daily care, and avoidance of cross-contamination by hospital personnel.

SPECIAL CONSIDERATIONS: CANDIDURIA

The report of a urine culture positive for *Candida albicans* frequently prompts consultation. The spectrum of infections include asymptomatic candiduria, urethritis, cystitis, primary renal candidiasis, and systemic disease (265–266). Candiduria can coexist with bacterial infections.

The majority of urine cultures containing *Candida* represent either contamination or colonization related to the use of indwelling catheters, antibiotics, and steroids. The significance of candiduria depends on the presence of infection with tissue invasion, upper urinary tract disease, or systemic illness. The problem of assessing the significance of candiduria relates to the difficulty in proving tissue invasion or upper tract involvement.

A urine culture positive for *Candida* should not be ignored. If the patient is asymptomatic, the culture is repeated to minimize contamination and reconfirm candiduria. Some data suggest that if less than 10,000 colonies/ml are present in a midstream urine, renal *Candida* is unlikely. The significance of colony counts is controversial, and colony counts cannot be used in the chronically catheterized patient. Culture of the sediment of 10 cc of centrifuged urine will detect more candiduria than uncentrifuged specimens.

In the asymptomatic patient, predisposing factors should be removed if possible, including Foley catheters and antibiotics.

Even candiduria that has been present for a prolonged time may clear with removal of predisposing factors.

Tissue invasion usually occurs in compromised hosts, debilitated patients, or patients extremely ill from other causes. Some authorities advocate treating high-risk patients with candiduria with amphotericin bladder washes or 5-flucytosine. Bladder irrigation can be done with amphotericin B, 50 mg 1N 1,000 cc D5W as a continuous irrigation over 24 hours for 3–5 days, using a closed triple lumen catheter (38).

The presence of invasive *Candida* infection is difficult to demonstrate but may be shown by positive blood culture, skin or eye findings, or intravenous pyelogram. Unreliable indicators of invasion are pyuria, pseudohyphae, and serologic tests. Systemic or invasive renal candidiasis require intravenous amphotericin; 5-flucystosine may be used in addition. The oral antifungal agent ketoconazole is not significantly excreted in the urine and is usually ineffective in urinary candidiasis. A newer analog fluconazole is more promising.

PERINEPHRIC ABSCESS

Perinephric abscesses are uncommon infections and typically difficult to diagnose. Seventy to ninety percent follow an upper urinary tract infection with rupture of a parenchymal abscess into the perinephric space. The rest result from hemotogenous spread, usually from the skin. However, in only about one-quarter of patients can a history of urinary or skin infection be obtained. Renal abscess is more common in the presence of diabetes. Causative bacteria are usually enteric gram-negative pathogens or *Staphylococcus*. Urine cultures are positive in up to 80% of patients and usually contain the same organism as the abscess. Blood cultures are positive in about one-half of cases.

Most patients have fever (90%), unilateral flank pain (73%), or abdominal pain (60%), and are initially thought to have upper urinary tract infection (167, 168). The physical exam, maximum temperature, white count, and urinary findings do not discriminate between those with pyelonephritis and perinephric abscess, unless a flank mass is palpated. Abdominal masses may be palpated in only a minority of patients. A useful diagnostic clue is that patients with acute pyelonephritis are usually not febrile more than 4 days after the initiation of appropriate antibiotics.

Patients with perinephric abscess are often febrile after 5 or more days of antibiotic therapy, and often remain febrile until surgical drainage. Abdominal x-rays may show obliterated psoas shadows and loss of renal borders. An intravenous pyelogram may show a perinephric mass, but may be mistaken for a pseudocyst from the tail of the pancreas. Ultrasonography, computerized axial tomography, gallium scanning, and arteriography have revealed abscesses when other studies were negative or equivocal.

In the postoperative period, most patients seen will have been on antibiotics for suspected pyelonephritis. If a patient with a urinary tract infection has been febrile without other cause after 5 days of appropriate antibiotic therapy, perinephric abscess should be sought.

The usual treatment is antibiotics and drainage, usually surgically. Some cases of renal carbuncle, which do not extend into the perinephric space, have been treated successfully with antibiotics alone without surgical drainage.

Wound Infection

The surgeon will appropriately manage postoperative wound infections; however, the internist must be aware of selected aspects of wound infections to assist in evaluation of the febrile patient.

BACTERIOLOGY

S. aureus (19%) and *E. coli* (11%) remain the most common pathogens in wound infections; (25) however, percentages of these and other pathogens vary between hospitals. Gram-negative pathogens are increasing in frequency, and unusual bacteria and fungi continue to be uncommon but persistent problems. Anaerobes constitute a small but probably underreported percentage. Multiple pathogens are found in a variable percentage of cases. Candida is found in a small percentage of cases.

DIAGNOSTIC ACTIVITIES

The diagnosis of wound infection is made clinically. Purulent drainage from a wound site defines infection, whether or not the culture is positive. This excludes stitch abscesses, unless they involve the wound. In general, induration, erythema, tenderness, and drainage are found. Although much overlap occurs in the appearance of wound infections by different organisms, some clinical differences between organisms are useful. Staphylococcal infections usually appear in 4–6 days with a localized area of induration, cellulitis, and thick, odorless, creamy, yellow pus. If there is not drainage, throbbing local pain, redness and swelling with fever and leukocytosis generally occur. With deep invasion, systemic symptoms appear. Aerobic streptococcal infections usually occur within the first several days postoperatively with a rapidly progressing cellulitis. Early toxic symptoms may be present, indicative of the invasive nature of the infection.

Gram-negative infections are more indolent and the signs more subtle. The incubation period is generally more than 1 week, but can be as long as a month, especially if the patient has been on antibiotics. Deep or obscure abscesses are a particular problem with gram-negative wound infections.

Anaerobic streptococcal infections caused by peptostreptococcus may be recognized by a thick grayish pus with a fetid odor.

MANAGEMENT

Surgical drainage remains the cornerstone of therapy. When needed, antibiotics can be rationally chosen based upon the gram stain, clinical appearance of the wound, and state of the patient. Antibiotics may be started before the wound is drained or debrided but after appropriate specimen for stain and culture are taken. Rare, distant hematogenous complications of wound infections include pneumonitis, meningitis, endocarditis, and major organ abscess (liver, kidney, spleen).

Special Considerations

Several types of *necrotizing infections of soft tissue* (skin, subcutaneous tissue, fascia, muscle) may rarely be seen in postoperative patients, but prompt recognition is critical. All have in common the formation of subcutaneous gas. The classification and terminology of these diseases vary widely; the classification of Finegold as modified by Swartz (4) is used here. All of these syndromes may follow surgery or be seen in trauma patients.

Clostridial anaerobic cellulitis is an infection of subcutaneous tissue, usually not involving deep fascia and muscle (as contrasted to the more well known clostridial gas gangrene). Onset is gradual. Skin is minimally discolored and moderately swollen; systemic toxicity is absent.

Nonclostridial anaerobic cellulitis is a similar illness to clostridial anaerobic cellulitis, but is caused by other anaerobic bacteria, often in a mixed infection with multiple gram-positive and gram-negative anaerobes. Onset may be gradual or abrupt. Skin appearance is similar to clostridial cellulitis; some systemic toxicity may be present. Differentiation can only be made by gram stain.

Necrotizing fasciitis involves the superficial and deep fascia; it is caused by a mixed flora of anaerobes, gram-positive, and gram-negative organisms. Onset is abrupt. Skin is erythematous and markedly swollen. Systemic toxicity is present and may be marked.

Fournier's syndrome is considered a subcategory of necrotizing fasciitis, involving the perineum. It is discussed in more detail below.

Synergistic necrotizing cellulitis is considered a subcategory of necrotizing fascitis, but involves the skin and muscle as well as fascia. The bacteria include mixed anaerobes and gram negatives. Onset is abrupt. Skin has scattered areas of necrosis; swelling is significant. Characteristic "dishwater pus" may be present. Systemic toxicity is marked.

Gas gangrene is a disease mainly of muscle. Onset is usually abrupt. Pain is early and marked (moderate pain can be seen with necrotizing fascitis and synergistic necrotizing cellulitis, but is usually not as early and dramatic). Skin is edematous and white early on, followed by yellowish-bronze discoloration; bullae and necrosis may be present. Systemic toxicity is marked and dramatic. Gas gangrene should be contrasted to clostridial anaerobic cellulitis, which is caused by the same species of organism but involves subcutaneous tissues. The lack of systemic toxicity, severe pain, and minimal discoloration of the skin differentiate clostridial cellulitis from gangrene clinically (see below).

Infected vascular gangrene is a mixed bacterial infection of devascularized muscle, most commonly due to arteriosclerosis. It involves the devascularized muscle and usually does not spread to more proximal muscle. This is easily separated clinically from the other entities.

Despite the differences in clinical presentation listed above, differentiation of these entities clinically is often difficult, because of overlapping clinical pictures, subtle early presentations, and (fortunately) the inexperience of most physicians in dealing with these infections. Needle aspiration of subcutaneous tissue with stat gram stain is helpful in differentiating clostridial from mixed infections, but failure to obtain pus or a negative gram stain does *NOT* exclude infection. X-rays are helpful in establishing the presence of subcutaneous air. The differentiation of muscle involvement often must be made at surgery. This is critical, because entities involving muscle require more extensive surgery to be lifesaving.

Treatment is appropriate antibiotics and immediate, *adequate* surgical drainage or amputation. Antibiotics of choice are penicillin for clostridial infections and combinations of penicillin, clindamycin, and an aminoglycoside for mixed infections (pending final culture results). In our experience the physicians caring for these patients are often reluctant to undertake surgery without a trial of antibiotics or to perform adequate surgical debridement; this is mandatory if the patient is to be saved. The degree of surgical debridement varies with the different entities (4), depending on the involvement of deep fascia and muscle. Tetanus immunization (a different clostridium) should not be forgotten.

Fournier's syndrome is a rare but dramatic syndrome following surgical procedures involving the perineal area; some authors do not distinguish it from other syngergistic necrotizing infections (272). A mixed aerobic-anaerobic infection with *E. coli*, *Proteus*, or *Enterococcus* with *Bacteroides fragilis* causes an obliterative endarteritis and acute dermal gangrene.

The syndrome follows herniorrhaphy, hydrocele repair, circumcision, orchiectomy, hemorrhoidectomy, vasectomy, or transrectal prostatic biopsy. The syndrome has an acute onset of genital itching, pain, erythema, swelling, and subcutaneous gas accompanied by chills, fever, prostration, and toxicity. Involvement may rapidly progress to gangrene and spread to the entire abdominal wall.

Aggressive surgical debridement and antibiotics directed against *B. fragilis* and enteric gram-negative rods are essential in preventing a high rate of morbidity and mortality. This infection emphasizes the need to examine the skin and soft tissues of the perineal and genital areas in postoperative patients with fever.

Tuberculous, mycotic, and viral infections do occasionally cause wound infections and should be searched for with unresponsive infections. *Candida* is a frequent colonizer of wounds. Distinguishing colonization from wound infection with *Candida* is difficult. Demonstration of hyphal forms in biopsy tissue is the best single criterion of infection.

Toxic shock syndrome may present a difficult diagnostic problem postoperatively, because of the lack of localizing, diagnostic symptoms, its rarity, and the similarity of its symptoms with other causes of postoperative or postpartum sepsis (273). It is included in this section, because most cases have their origin in wound "infection" with *Staphylococcus aureus* producing the toxin. A high degree of suspicion is needed to make the diagnosis. The rash is diagnostic, but is late and may be subtle. Other findings suggestive of toxic shock are extremely high temperature (over 104) without an obvious source, pharyngeal or conjuctival injection, sore throat, strawberry tongue, severe myalgias ("respiratory symptoms"), vomiting *and* diarrhea, mental status change, and multiple organ dysfunction (kidney, liver, blood, muscle, CNS). The onset may occasionally be insidious initially but there is an abrupt worsening or abrupt onset, with multiple organ system dysfunction and profound shock. The occurrence of abrupt shock accompanied by multiple organ system dysfunction, possibly including some of the findings above atypical for surgical sepsis (respiratory symptoms, watery diarrhea), in the absence of any source of sepsis, should raise the possibility of postoperative toxic shock syndrome. The wound may appear to be benign. Diagnosis is made by criteria listed elsewhere (4) and isolation of staphylococci, usually from the surgical wound. Therapy includes mandatory adequate drainage, antistaphylococcal antibiotics (PSRP, vancomycin), and complex supportive care, beyond the scope of this text (4).

Pelvic Infections

Gynecologists usually manage proven pelvic infections. Consultation is requested for questions of antibiotic management, persistent fever, and differentiation from other sources of fever.

Puerperal endometritis is the most serious febrile complication of delivery. Diagnosis is clinical, based on the presence of fever, uterine or parametrial tenderness, and abnormal lochia. The leukocyte count is less helpful, unless very high, as the postpartum patient may have a moderately elevated white count with a left shift as a normal finding. Other common causes of febrile morbidity in the postpartum cesarean patient are urinary and wound infections. Penicillin and an aminoglycoside are used for endometritis. Clindamycin should be added if there is no improvement in 48 hours; some authorities recommend clindamycin-aminoglycoside as initial therapy.

In the postoperative gynecologic patient (Table 16.39), infection can be classified as endometritis (uterine tender-

Table 16.39.   Management of Soft Tissue Pelvic Infections without Abscess[a]

Initial Therapy
1. *Regimen A:* Doxycycline 100 mg IV or PO every 12 hours and cefoxitin 2.0 gm IV every 6 hours.
   or
2. *Regimen B:* Clindamycin 600 mg IV every 6 hours and gentamicin 2 mg/kg IV initial dose followed by 1.5 mg/kg IV every 8 hours (adjusted to renal function).
3. Either *Regimen A or B* should be continued for minimum of 4 days and at least 48 hours after the patient improves. Then, either doxycycline 100 mg PO every 12 hours (or alternatively clindamycin 450 mg PO 5 times daily) to complete 10–14 total days of therapy.

No Response over 48–72 hours
1. Reexamine to rule out need for surgical drainage; ultrasound.

Still No Response Over Next 24–72 hours
1. Reexamine to rule out need for surgical drainage.
2. Trial of heparin intravenously for suspected diagnosis of septic pelvic thrombophlebitis.

[a]From "1989 STD Treatment Guidelines" *MMWR* 38 (S–8): 31–33, 1989. Treatment of sexually transmitted diseases. *Medical Letter* 32:5–10, 1990. Sweet RL: Pelvic infection. *Obstet Gynecol Annu* 9:99, 1980 (protocol outline).

ness), salpingitis (adnexal tenderness), or peritonitis (by cul de sac aspiration). In the first 24 hours, infection from group A *Streptococcus,* non-group A *Streptococcus, Clostridia,* or less commonly, gram-negative rods, may produce a rapid toxic picture. Gram stain for *Clostridia* is important at this stage, and if not seen, therapy with either penicillin or clindamycin and an aminoglycoside is begun.

With fever beginning after 48–72 hours, the diagnosis may be endometritis, vaginal cuff abscess, pelvic cellulitis or abscess, peritonitis, or tubo-ovarian abscess. Pelvic exam identifies the location of the infection and whether drainage is required. Not all masses represent abscesses, as matted omentum and bowel may be mistaken for large abscesses. A clue to an abscess is a positive culture that is sensitive to the antibiotic being used. If no improvement is seen in 48–72 hours of antibiotic treatment, clindamycin is added to the regimen.

With continuous fever and coverage for anaerobes, septic pelvic thrombophlebitis or other sources of fever should be considered. Ultrasound or computerized tomography of the pelvis are helpful in detecting localized fluid collection. Differentiation from sterile, postoperative fluid collection or matted omentum may require aspiration.

Septic pelvic thrombophlebitis represents 1–2% of presumed pelvic infections and presents with persistent spiking fever despite appropriate antibiotics (278). Pain and pelvic findings may be minimal or vague. The diagnosis is made by exclusion. A therapeutic trial of heparinization should produce rapid defervescence within 24–48 hours. The use of heparin is controversial in the absence of septic pulmonary emboli. Failure to defervesce should prompt further search for abscess or other sources of fever.

Trauma

Trauma is responsible for a large number of admissions to general hospitals.

Infections occur with variable frequency, related to underlying host factors, site of trauma, extent of the traumatic injury, and the degree of contamination. For example, in a series of 600 cases of penetrating chest trauma, there were only two infectious complications: one subphrenic abscess and one empyema. The rates of infection in abdominal trauma are much higher.

Infections following abdominal trauma are clearly related to perforation of the bowel distal to the ileocecal valve and to the number of organs damaged, with rates of wound infection and abscess formation to 20–40% before the use of effective antibiotics (282–287).

Abdominal infection after penetrating injury begins with an acute peritonitis due to gram-negative enteric bacilli followed by abscess formation secondary to anaerobic bacteria (1). Other risk factors include age or degree of injury (290). Polymicrobial infection is the rule and abdominal abscesses are the result of aerobic-anaerobic synergism. Other traumatic injuries associated with infectious complications include compound fractures, soft tissue trauma, skull and facial fractures, and penetrating eye trauma (282). The late infectious complications of a series of severely traumatized patients are listed in Table 16.40.

Principles of antimicrobial treatment follow general rules for "contaminated" and "dirty" surgical cases. Antimicrobials in trauma patients represent treatment (not prophylaxis), since bacteria are introduced before antimicrobial agents (see p. 378). Antibiotics are warranted when the gastrointestinal tract is involved, when the wound enters a joint space or involves a tendon, when a compound fracture exists, when clostridial infections are likely, and when the wound is grossly contaminated. Treatment is continued for 48–72 hours followed by observation, except in cases of abdominal trauma with gross contamination, in which case a course of 7–14 days is given. Continued use of an-

Table 16.40.   Sites of Infection in Severely Traumatized Patients[a]

	Infections (No.)	Bacteremia No.	%
Primary bacteremia	4	4	(12)
Vascular			
Artery	5	3	(9)
Vein	10	6	(18)
Central nervous system	6	1	(3)
Surgical wound	6	2	(6)
Intraabdominal	5	3	(9)
Urinary tract infection	30	1	(3)
Lower respiratory			
Pneumonia	19	7	(21)
Empyema	12	7	(21)
Upper respiratory	9	0	(0)
Osteomyelitis	2		

[a] From Caplan ES, Hoyt N, Cowley RA: Changing patterns of nosocomial infections in severely traumatized patients. *Am Surg* 45:204, 1979.

tibiotics may mask the late development of an abscess, and their use should not be prolonged without justification.

Fever in the first few days following major trauma is common and does not necessarily indicate infection. Late fever (>3 days) has the same significance as any postoperative fever. Pulmonary embolism should be included in the differential diagnosis of fever in the trauma patient.

The use of antibiotics in penetrating chest trauma remains controversial, because reported rates of infection after trauma range from 1–20% (286). The recommended antibiotic is a cephalosporin; clindamycin or penicillinase-resistant penicillin are alternatives.

The combination of clindamycin and an aminoglycoside is used for abdominal trauma; an alternative regime is cefoxitin alone or with an aminoglycoside. Treatment will be prolonged 10–14 days or more if gastrointestinal perforation has occurred; treatment for 48 hours or less is sufficient in the absence of gastrointestinal perforation, genitourinary trauma, or external contamination.

Diarrhea (Clostridium Difficile)

Clostridium difficile diarrhea (pseudomembranous colitis) is a frequent reason for postoperative consultation, either because of a diagnostic dilemma or questions about therapy. The etiology is a toxin-mediated diarrhea caused by *C. difficile*. Predisposing factors are antibiotic therapy and presence of *C. difficile* in the hospital environment (epidemics have occurred) (331). Almost all antibiotics have been associated with *C. difficile*.

Presenting symptoms include diarrhea, abdominal pain, discomfort or distention, and fever. Atypical presentations in the surgical patient causing diagnostic problems are fever of uncertain etiology, ileus *without* marked diarrhea, and abdominal pain.

Diagnosis is made by identification of *C. difficile* toxin in the stool by laboratory assay and sigmoidoscopy/colonscopy with biopsy. Diagnostic difficulties are posed by the fact that *C. difficile* can colonize the colon (up to 2–10% of patients in some hospitals) with positive assays, but not be the cause of the patient's symptoms, and by the nonspecific appearance of the colon, requiring biopsy for diagnosis. The diagnosis should be made by a combination of findings including prior antibiotic use, compatible clinical picture, *and* toxin assay, endoscopic or biopsy results; *and* exclusion of other similar diseases. Differential diagnosis includes other causes of postoperative diarrhea or abdominal symptoms, nonspecific antibiotic-related diarrhea, and nosocomial infectious diarrhea.

Treatment includes either metronidazole or vancomycin orally (274); neither drug reaches optimal levels in the colon when given intravenously. Postoperative patients unable to take medication by the oral or nasogastric route pose a difficult therapeutic problem; intravenous metronidazole is generally preferred, supplemented by oral drug to the extent that the patient can take it. Cholestyramine can be used for symptomatic relief. Cholestyramine can provide symptomatic relief by binding the toxin; it is not a definitive therapy. The effectiveness of vancomycin or metronidazole may be reduced because of binding to the cholestyramine resin. Staggering antibiotic and cholestyramine doses may help but does not totally eliminate this problem. The inciting antibiotic should be stopped or changed; all antibiotics should be stopped when possible.

Vertebral Osteomyelitis and Disc Space Infection

EPIDEMIOLOGY

In the postoperative setting, vertebral osteomyelitis is an uncommon infection following genitourinary instrumentation, urinary tract infection, pelvic surgery, back surgery, or a septic process. If unrecognized, vertebral osteomyelitis may extend to produce a retroperitoneal abscess. The offending organism reflects the initial site of infection and may be bacterial, fungal, or mycobacterial.

Disc space infection usually follows back surgery. *Staphylococcus aureus* is the most common organism.

DIAGNOSTIC ACTIVITIES

Symptoms usually do not appear until after the first or second postoperative week and the diagnosis is often delayed or missed. Clinical clues include fever; acute, subacute, or insidious back pain; paravertebral soft tissue mass; or localized vertebral tenderness. If the onset is insidious, fever may be absent, with anorexia, malaise, and weight loss predominating.

The sedimentation rate is elevated but there may or may not be leukocytosis. When the diagnosis is suspected, cultures of blood, urine, or other infected sites should be obtained. X-rays, including tomograms, should include tender areas by physical examination and surgical site. If x-rays are negative, bone scan may be positive. Computerized tomography and magnetic resonance imaging scanning may also be diagnostic if other radiologic studies are not. Aggressive attempts should be made to obtain the organism, as antibiotic therapy is curative in nearly all cases. If fluoroscopic percutaneous aspiration or biopsy is unsuccessful, open biopsy may be required.

MANAGEMENT

Intravenous antibiotics for 6 weeks are successful in most cases. Until the organism is defined, a penicillinase-resistant penicillin and an aminoglycoside are appropriate for vertebral osteomyelitis. A penicillinase-resistant penicillin is adequate for initial treatment of disc space infection.

Special Considerations

Osteitis pubis is the painful inflammation of the bone, cartilage, periosteum, and ligamentous structures of the anterior pelvic girdle. Osteitis pubis is a rare complication of prostatectomy, urinary incontinence procedures, pyelonephritis, and abortion (293).

Symptoms begin 2–12 weeks after surgery and last weeks to months without treatment. The symptoms are characteristic and consist of suprapubic pain with radiation to the inner thighs, worsened by abduction of the legs and by walking. Findings include intermittent fever in nearly all cases, leukocytosis in 50%, tenderness over the symphysis pubis, and x-ray evidence of bone destruction and separation of the symphysis.

Most cases are due to infection, most commonly *Escherichia coli* or *Pseudomonas,* but occasionally the process is sterile. Diagnosis requires either needle aspiration or biopsy of the bone, since treatment will fail if the specific organism is not identified.

Management consists of 4–6 weeks of intravenous antibiotics and surgical debridement in selected cases.

Decubitus Ulcers

EPIDEMIOLOGY

Sepsis is a well-recognized complication of decubitus ulcers (294). The incidence is unknown and is not related to any specific surgical procedure.

BACTERIOLOGY

A wide variety of aerobic and anaerobic organisms are cultured from decubiti. While aerobes are more prevalent in the ulcer, the resultant bloodstream isolates are more frequently anaerobic, with *B. fragilis* being most common. Group D *streptococcus* is frequently isolated from the wound but is rarely a cause of the bacteremia. Polymicrobial isolates are frequently found in the blood.

DIAGNOSTIC ACTIVITIES

Most patients present with signs of and symptoms of sepsis. Many have recurrent or persistent fever despite antibiotics, either because the infection develops during treatment of an unrelated infection or because of inadequate surgical debridement.

Blood cultures are required. Bacteremia will often persist without adequate debridement. The size of the ulcer has no bearing, but there is usually marked tissue necrosis. Gram stain of the ulcer is of limited usefulness in documenting the organism causing sepsis.

MANAGEMENT

Adequate antibiotics, surgical debridement, and further preventive measures are important. Antibiotics should include coverage for gram-negative rods and anaerobes. Clindamycin or ampicillin-sulbactam and an aminoglycoside are recommended, although other regimens are acceptable.

Adequate local care and nutritional support are required for healing of the decubitus ulcer.

Postoperative Parotitis

EPIDEMIOLOGY

Postoperative parotitis is an acute unilateral or bilateral swelling of the parotid glands that occurs in the postoperative patient. The incidence of parotitis has been estimated to be 1:1000 postoperative patients (296).

Common predisposing conditions are age over 60, debility, dehydration, use of anticholinergics, and alcoholism. The involved parotid gland is infected, usually with *Staphylococcus aureus*.

A non-infectious swelling of the parotid gland may also occur in the immediate few hours postoperatively (297). Organisms can not be cultured from the parotid gland and the etiology is uncertain.

DIAGNOSTIC ACTIVITY AND APPROACHES

The usual presentation is unilateral parotid swelling, although bilateral swelling may occur in up to 20% of cases. The swelling is painful, although the patient may not complain of pain because of debility or pain medication. Postoperative parotitis usually occurs in elderly, very debilitated, malnourished, and dehydrated patients.

Fever is present in some cases. On examination, the parotid gland is swollen, firm to hard, and tender. Pus may be seen, from Stenson's duct, but is absent in many cases where the duct is totally obstructed.

A gram stain and culture should be obtained from the drainage from Stenson's duct. Gentle massage of the parotid gland may produce pus where none is apparent. Plain x-rays should be obtained to look for stones in Stenson's duct and subcutaneous air.

The major differential diagnosis is benign postoperative parotid swelling ("anesthesia mumps"). Postoperative benign non-infectious swelling usually occurs in the first few hours postoperatively, whereas infectious parotitis occurs 1–6 days postoperatively. Pus is not present in benign swelling and culture of drainage shows only normal flora.

MANAGEMENT

Patients with postoperative parotitis should be treated aggressively, because of the high mortality. An antibiotic active against penicillin-resistant *Staphylococcus* should be administered and modified by gram stain and culture results. The patient should be hydrated with intravenous fluids; lozenges should be administered every 2–3 hours in order to promote drainage.

If drainage is not seen coming from Stenson's duct within the first 24 hours, otolaryngological consultation should be obtained since surgical drainage may be needed.

Drugs promoting thick secretions should be avoided, especially parasympathomimetic agents.

Benign postoperative parotid swelling can be treated with hydration and lozenges. It does not require surgical drainage or antibiotics.

Starch Peritonitis

The potential for starch peritonitis exists in every abdominal surgical procedure, but occurs rarely, for unknown reasons. Surgical gloves contain a cornstarch derivative treated with epichlorohydrin and 2% magnesium oxide, and this lubricant poses a shedding hazard during surgery, even if the gloves are washed and wiped. Cornstarch is used because of its supposed innocuous nature, though many reports of granulomas and peritonitis exist. Talc is well known to cause granulomatous reactions, and has not been used as a *primary* agent in surgical gloves for many years. Talc has recently been found in minute quantities in a majority of gloves, and its contribution to "starch" peritonitis is thus unknown.

Inadvertently shed particles cause an inflammatory reaction, which presents clinically in 2–3 weeks after surgery with cramping, migratory, diffuse abdominal pain, nausea, diarrhea, and low-grade fever (298–299). Temperatures to 39.4°C have occurred. The patient is usually not toxic. Diffuse abdominal tenderness is usually present. Rarely, an abdominal mass (adhesions or indurated omentum) is palpated and may be confused with an abscess. Diagnosis may be possible by paracentesis or abdominal lavage, revealing starch particles by polarized microscopy, but often exploration becomes necessary to rule out abscess or other abdominal diseases. Conservative treatment with steroids or indomethacin has been successful.

Intravenous Cannula Infections

EPIDEMIOLOGY

Purulent thrombophlebitis is a common iatrogenic nosocomial infection. Infection of 0.2% of patients with intravenous lines seems low, but the large number of patients receiving intravenous fluids creates a significant problem (Table 16.41). The case fatality rate of up to 30% for cannula-related septicemia makes its early recognition important. Intravenous infusion-associated infections may arise from contaminated cultures, tubing, and fluids.

In most infections, skin organisms migrate along the cannula and a small fibrin-platelet clot develops. The clot can then be contaminated by migrating skin bacteria, hematogenously from remote sites, or by contaminated infusions.

Plastic cannulas are associated with higher rates of infection than steel needles. Additional risk factors are use of catheters for more than 72 hours, cutdowns or central (versus peripheral) cannulas, use of lower extremity veins, placement under emergency conditions, and improper catheter care. Infections are decreased with the use of intravenous teams and iodine-containing ointments; change of the catheter every 48–72 hours is controversial.

BACTERIOLOGY

Staphylococcus aureus is the most important organism (33%), followed by gram-negative rods, *Candida,* and *Enterococcus. Candida* is more common with total parenteral nutrition than peripheral catheters. Intravenous infusion infections are more likely to be from *Klebsiella, Enterobacter,* and *Serratia.*

Table 16.41. Summary of Selected Literature on IV Cannula-associated Septicemia[a]

	Number of Studies	Number of Cannulations	Septicemia Episodes	Percent with Septicemia
Plastic cannulas				
Percutaneous				
Peripheral	17	7618[b]	36	0.5
Subclavian	4	393	15	3.8
Umbilical	6	374	8	2.1
Cutdowns	6	248	16	6.5
Steel needles	4	577	1	0.2
TPN[c]	15	1162[d]	139[e]	12.0

[a] From Rahme FS, Make DG, Bennett JU: In Bennett JU, Brachman PS (eds): *Hospital Infections.* Boston, Little, Brown & Co. 1979, p 437. Used with permission.
[b] Includes at least 100 cutdowns.
[c] Total parenteral nutrition (see text).
[d] Number of patients.
[e] In 10 studies that identified pathogens, 46% of 90 pathogens were *Candida albicans.*[a]

DIAGNOSTIC ACTIVITIES

Infection at a cannula site should be suspected when erythema, tenderness, induration, or frank pus is noted around the intravenous site.

Fever of uncertain origin may be the only symptom and the cannula site may appear normal in the presence of infection. Patients on antibiotics may develop persistent fever, clinical deterioration, or positive blood cultures with no findings at the site. The site of a previously removed cannula may be at fault and is frequently overlooked on examination.

In a recent review of intravenous cannula infections, 83% had pain at the site, 44% had fever, 37% had swelling, and pus was recognized in only 9%. High fever (to 104°–106°F) was noted in one-third of the patients and in one-half there was a delay in diagnosis because of the benign-appearing nature of the site (300).

Differentiation of septic thrombophlebitis from non-bacterial inflammation may be difficult. Septic thrombophlebitis is usually suggested by clinical sepsis, positive blood cultures, leukocytosis or fever, or pus at the catheter site.

MANAGEMENT

When an infection is suspected, the cannula area should be cleaned with alcohol and a 5-cm portion of the catheter tip cultured. Quantitative cultures on plates help to differentiate colonization from infection. If pus is not evident after catheter removal, the vein should be vigorously "milked" or aspirated by needle. Pus may be aspirated from fluctuant areas or a cutdown site may be opened. Gram stain should be performed on all aspirates, as well as culture. Positive blood culture or lack of improvement in 24–48 hours is an indication for surgical exploration and vein excision (Table 16.42).

Antibiotics are based on the gram stain; empirical antibiotics should be directed against *Staphylococcus* and gram-negative rods.

Intravenous Infusion Infections

A brief febrile reaction to blood is common and results from leukoagglutins, platelet agglutinins, or from transfused antigens. The temperature is usually less than 102°F and the patient is not toxic, though flushing and headache may be present. Bacterial contamination is rare but the temporal association of transfusion with the onset of high fever, headache, vomiting, hypotension, and toxicity suggest the diagnosis. Hemolytic transfusion reaction is an important differen-

Table 16.42.   Prevention and Management of Septic Phlebitis[a]

Prevention	Diagnosis	Treatment
1. Use scalp vein needles when possible.	1. Culture catheter tip if phlebitis develops.	1. Apply heat and elevate the involved area.
2. Place polyethylene catheters with strict aseptic technique.	2. Maintain a high index of suspicion in febrile, septic patients with intravenous catheters.	2. Use appropriate antibiotics.
3. Dress catheters with antibiotic ointment: change dressing daily.	3. Massage or aspirate the involved vein for pus.	3. If no response to above in 24 hours, excise the involved vein (completely).
4. Change catheter site every 48 to 72 hours.	4. Perform local exploration and venotomy if necessary.	4. Leave the wound open and perform delayed primary closure when feasible.
5. Remove catheters inserted in the emergency department as soon as possible.		
6. Remove catheters when phlebitis, infiltration, or unexplained fever develops.		

[a] From Baker CC, Peterson SR, Sheldon GF: Septic phlebitis. *Am J Surg* 138:97, 1979, with permission.

tial diagnosis. Organisms are usually gram-negative bacilli. Platelet transfusion and albumin infusions have transmitted infection, mostly in outbreaks of *Salmonella* and *Enterobacter*.

Intravenous fluid therapy is associated with infection from the cannula (see p. 430) from in-use contamination and from contamination during manufacture. Infusion-related sepsis may present dramatically several hours after infusion or may be masked in a critically ill patient by coexisting disease. Recognition that intrinsic or in-use contamination is the source of septicemia may be difficult or impossible. Because the entire infusion set is suspect, both the cannula and a specimen of infusion fluid should be cultured (4).

Unusual gram-negative bacteria and fungi are occasionally involved. Recovery of multiple or unusual organisms from blood cultures should raise the suspicion of intravenous contamination. Patients with unexplained fever and intravenous devices should have both the catheter and fluid cultured.

Antibiotics should be given to critically ill and immunosuppressed patients, and those with vascular prostheses. If the patient appears well, bacteremia may clear with discontinuation of the infusion, although antibiotics are indicated with positive blood cultures or persistent fever. Antimicrobials effective against *Staphylococcus* and drug-resistant gram-negative bacilli should be used.

Procedure and Device-related Infections

Increasingly invasive diagnostic tests, monitoring devices, and therapeutic procedures pose a considerable infection risk to the postoperative patient. The common portals of infection are the urinary tract catheters, intravascular catheters, and respiratory devices, but other specialized procedures or devices are less frequently causes of infection or bacteremia (301). For example, arterial pressure catheters produced local infection in 18% of patients and caused septicemia in 4% of patients in one study (301).

Infection has been caused by contami-

Table 16.43.   Source of Infection from Procedures and Devices

Procedures	Devices
Intravenous therapy	Urinary catheters
Transfusion	Arterial catheters
Nasotracheal intubation	Nasogastric tube
Bronchoscopy	Tracheal tubes
Gastrointestinal/diagnostic procedures	Intravenous cannulas
Urologic procedures	Pressure transducers (CSF)
Manipulation of septic foci	Vascular grafts/valves
	Hemodialysis shunts
	Prosthetic orthopaedic implants
	Skin grafts
	Lens implants

nated skin grafts, porcine valves, prosthetic devices, and intraocular lenses. Whenever a fever or bacteremia is present without explanation, careful consideration must be given to prostheses inserted during surgery and monitoring equipment. Bacteremia after procedures is usually transient and may go unnoticed. A partial list of procedures and devices demonstrated to cause bacteremia or infection is shown in Table 16.43. No estimate of risk of bacteremia is given because of the wide variation in the literature. The actual incidence of established infection after bacteremia is unknown.

Aspiration of a prosthesis or removal with culture of the device may help prove the source of infection. Empirical antibiotic selection depends on the device and clinical situation, but usually includes a penicillinase-resistant penicillin and aminoglycoside.

Prosthetic Graft Infections

EPIDEMIOLOGY

The internist is likely to encounter many patients with prosthetic vascular grafts undergoing unrelated surgery. Primary graft infection rates vary from 1.3–6% and usually occur in aortofemoral or lower extremity grafts; however, carotid and autogenous graft infections do occur. The most common organisms are staphylococci and gram-negative aerobes.

Late infections do occur secondary to other infections such as diverticulitis, sepsis, and, rarely procedures involving contaminated areas (98, 99).

DIAGNOSTIC ACTIVITIES

Clinical manifestations depend on the pathologic features. Most graft infections present as infection (with fever) or graft breakdown with fistula. An aortoprosthetic fistula involves the aorta and a hollow viscus, almost always the fourth part of the duodenum. The most common symptom is gastrointestinal bleeding. A paraprosthetic fistula involves a duodenal erosion with gastrointestinal bleeding, nonspecific, but persistent, abdominal pain and signs of low-grade infection. An aortoparaprosthetic fistula involves a more extensive virulent infection, and sepsis is the main presenting feature (302–303).

Symptoms of graft infection are quite variable. Presentations include gastrointestinal bleeding, fever, distal embolization, local bleeding, and inflammation at the operative site.

Physical findings suggestive of infection are distal emboli, petechial rash or skin infarction, local inflammation, and pulsatile mass.

Blood cultures should be obtained prior to antibiotic therapy. Blood cultures may be commonly negative, unlike other intravascular infections. The number required is not documented, but six cultures are recommended. Arterial cultures distal to the graft are occasionally positive when venous cultures are negative.

Arteriography and/or endoscopy are helpful in excluding other sources of bleeding and defining the status of the graft.

MANAGEMENT

Massive bleeding requires immediate surgery without further diagnostic workup. Most infections require eventual surgery to remove the infected prosthesis. Surgery is required for suture line infections, bleeding, thrombosis, distal embolization, pseudoaneurysm formations, and fistula.

Initial empirical antibiotic selection is similar to recommendations for endocarditis: a semisynthetic penicillin, penicillin, and an aminoglycoside. The antibiotic regimen should be modified for the organisms isolated from blood and graft cultures once culture and sensitivity results are available.

Prosthetic Valve Endocarditis

Prosthetic valve endocarditis is classified as early (<60 days) or late (>60 days). Late infections up to 15 years are now being recognized with increased frequency. Infection acquired following unrelated surgery usually occur as "late" endocarditis. The incidence of prosthetic valve infection varies from 0.2–9.5% and should be considered in the febrile postoperative patient with a prosthetic valve. Organisms responsible include streptococci (50%), staphylococci (25%), gram-negative bacilli (15%), and miscellaneous bacteria (including *Staphylococcus epidermidis,* diptheroids, *Candida,* and *Aspergillus*). Risk factors include those procedures producing bacteremia and infections at distant sites.

Recognition of prosthetic valve endocarditis is facilitated by the appearance of fever, a regurgitant murmur or congestive failure, the disappearance of the prosthetic valve click, or echocardiographic or fluoroscopic demonstration of valve dysfunction. Other findings are similar to those in patients without prosthetic valves.

Adequate blood cultures should be obtained before therapy is begun. Empirical therapy in the critically ill patient should include penicillin, a penicillinase-resistant semisynthetic penicillin, and an aminoglycoside (4, 314).

Prosthetic Joint Infections

Large number of prosthetic joints continue to be implanted. Hip prostheses will be specifically addressed because of the more extensive literature; experience with infected prosthesis in other locations is limited. The orthopaedist will manage all early infections, but the internist must be aware of late infections and the risks from bacteremia from distant infections or unrelated surgery (see p. 383).

EPIDEMIOLOGY

The incidence of infection after total hip arthroplasty averages 2.1% while rates of up to 6% have been reported in total knee replacements. Bacteremic infection from distant sites has been well-documented, especially from the urinary tract (136, 139).

BACTERIOLOGY

Staphylococcus aureus, S. epidermidis, and gram-negative rods comprise over 90% of pathogens in deep-wound infections. In late infections, *S. aureus* and *S. epidermidis* each represent 40% and gram-negatives 10%. Late infections are caused both by operative contamination and by hematogenous seeding from other sites. In the series by Fitzgerald, those with postoperative urinary infections had a higher rate of infected prosthesis, but there was poor correlation with the organism found in the wound and urine (136, 139).

DIAGNOSTIC ACTIVITIES

Superficial wound infection is more common than deep wound sepsis immediately following surgery. The manifestations of superficial infection are wound erythema, induration, or drainage.

Prosthetic infections can be separated into three groups based on clinical behavior. The early, acute, fulminating infections begin with a spontaneously draining hematoma or a superficial wound infection during the first 2–5 days. These present with fever, leukocytosis, local inflammatory signs, and frequently with drainage of pus. If an early infection is superficial to the fascia lata, decompression and antibiotics may prevent deep extension. If loosening or dislocation of the device occurs, the prosthesis is involved. A second group has an indolent infection recognized in the first 2 years; and the third, probably from hematogenous sources, often later than 2 years.

The primary late symptoms are pain in the hip either at rest or with weight bearing, loosening of the prosthesis, and fever. Spontaneous drainage occurs in some. The sedimentation rate is elevated above 40 in most patients, but the WBC count is variable. Fever occurs less than half the time. The diagnosis may be suggested by x-ray and/or arthrogram. Aspiration or synovial biopsy are necessary for bacteriological diagnosis. Radionucleide scans are occasionally helpful.

Any patient with a skeletal prosthesis should have the joint carefully examined during the evaluation of postoperative fever as hematogenous seeding from another infected site can occur at any time. The absence of pain or loosening of the prosthesis make infection less likely. However, any indication of infection should prompt orthopaedic consultation and consideration of aspiration (321).

Initial treatment depends on the organism suspected clinically and by gram stain.

Prevention includes prompt treatment of distant infections, especially of the genitourinary tract. The use of prophylactic antibiotics during unrelated surgery is controversial but recommended for gastrointestinal and genitourinary procedures with a high risk of bacteremia (see p. 472).

ACQUIRED IMMUNE DEFICIENCY SYNDROME (AIDS)

The extensive literature on the many problems posed by the acquired immune deficiency syndrome in the surgical patient is beyond the scope of this book, but is reviewed elsewhere (324). Three issues occur frequently enough to require comment.

Questions on *precautions for the health care providers* caring for the AIDS patient are becoming more frequently asked of medical consultants. The Centers for Disease Control (CDC) has published a set of recommendations called "Universal Precautions" (Table 16.44) (322–325). These should be applied to all patients, not just known AIDS cases, because of the significant incidence of human immunodeficiency virus (HIV) positivity unknown to health care providers in some health care settings (e.g., 3% in one emergency room) (324).

Screening for HIV positivity in surgical patients is covered in Chapter 23 (p. 634). At the time this text was written, most authorities were not recommending universal screening of all surgical patients, but recommendations have been frequently updated (324).

Performing surgery that is unrelated to AIDS and its complications on the patient with HIV infection poses a difficult decision; there are no generally accepted guidelines (337–338). In addition to multiple procedures for their primary disease, patients with asymptomatic HIV infection and symptomatic AIDS may require surgery for unrelated urgent conditions (e.g., cholecystitis) or elective reasons (e.g., hip replacement).

The general guidelines for decision making given in Chapter 3 would seem to remain applicable with the following additional considerations. Patients with HIV infection represent a wide spectrum, from the asymptomatic HIV positive patient with good laboratory prognostic factors who may have a mean life expectancy of many years, to the preterminal patient with multiple malignancies and opportunistic infections. These two hypothetical patients represent very different problems. Decision making should therefore be individualized based on: (a) the status of the patient's HIV infection (asymptomatic, AIDS related complex [ARC],

Table 16.44.   Universal Precautions for Prevention of Transmission of Human Immunodeficiency Virus (HIV) [a,b,c]

1. *NEEDLES/SHARPS:* Take care when handling scapels and other sharp instruments after procedures. Needles/sharps should be handled with extreme care. *Needles should not be recapped, cut, bent or broken. All sharps should be disposed of promptly in an impervious container, located as close as possible to the area of use.*
2. *GLOVES:* Use for handling blood, blood-containing fluids, mucous membranes, and non-intact skin of patients. Also use for venipuncture, items/surfaces contaminated with blood or body fluids. Promptly replace torn glove during procedure.
3. *MASKS/PROTECTIVE EYEWEAR:* Use for procedures likely to generate airborne droplets.
4. *GOWNS/APRONS:* Use if splashing of blood or body fluids is anticipated.
5. *HANDWASHING:* Wash immediately and thoroughly following contamination with blood or body fluids.
6. *CPR:* Use mouth pieces, resuscitation bags, or similar devices available to limit need for mouth-to-mouth resuscitation.
7. *SPILLS OF BLOOD AND BODY FLUIDS:* Immediately clean and disinfect, using approved procedures and gloves.
8. *INVASIVE PROCEDURE:* Take barrier precautions including mask and gloves for all procedures; eyewear, gowns per listed recommendations.
9. *MISC.:* Health care workers with weeping or exudative skin lesions—refrain from patient care and handling patient care equipment (until the condition resolves).

---

[a] Adapted from Bur, S: Communicable Disease Bulletin, Dept. of Health & Mental Hygiene, State of Maryland, Feb. 1989. (See also references 322, 324–325.)
[b] Applies to *ALL* patients, not just HIV-positive or known AIDS patients.
[c] Body fluids include blood, any fluid possibly contaminated with blood, semen, vaginal fluid, cerebrospinal fluid, synovial, pleural, peritoneal, pericardial, and amniotic fluid.

symptomatic AIDS), the patient's mean life expectancy, and the patient's wishes and desires, and (b) the indications for surgery, the benefit of surgery to the patient during his life expectancy (versus normal life expectancy for a patient of the same age), and the increased risks posed by immune deficiency.

READINGS

General

1. Bennett JV, Brachman PA (eds): *Hospital Infections.* Boston, Little, Brown & Co., 1979.
1a. Jarvis WR, White JW, Munn VP, et al.: Nosocomial infection surveillance, 1983. *MMWR* 33(2SS):9SS–21SS, 1984.
2. Gantz NM, Gleckman RA: *Manual of Clinical Problems in Infectious Disease.* Boston, Little, Brown & Co., 1979.
3. Alexander JW (ed): Surgical infections. *Surg Clin North Am* 60: February, 1980.
4. Mandell GL, Douglas RG Jr, Bennett JE (eds): *Principles and Practice of Infectious Diseases.* New York, John Wiley & Sons, 1985.
5. Grieco MH (ed): *Infections in the Abnormal Host.* New York, Yorke Medical Books, 1980.
6. Kunin CM, Efron HY: Guidelines for peer review veterans administration ad hoc interdisciplinary advisory committee on antimicrobial drug usage. *JAMA* 237:1001–1008, 1977.
7. Flynn NM, Lawrence RM: Antimicrobial prophylaxis. *Med Clin North Am* 63:1225–1244, 1979.
8. Brachman PS, Dan BB, Haley RW, et al.: Nosocomial surgical infections: Incidence and cost. *Surg Clin North Am* 60:15, 1980.
9. Gross PA, Neu HC, Aswapokee P, et al.: Deaths from nosocomial infections: Experience in a university hospital and a community hospital. *Am J Med* 68:219, 1980.
10. Daschner F, Nadjem H, Langmaack H, et al.: Surveillance, prevention and control of hospital-acquired infections. III. Nosocomial infections as cause of death: retrospective analysis of 1,000 autopsy reports. *Infection* 6:261, 1978.
11. McGowan JE Jr, Barnes MW, Finland M: Bacteremia at Boston City Hospital: Occurrence and mortality during 12 selected years (1935–1972), with special reference to hospital-acquired cases. *J Infect Dis* 132:316–335, 1975.
12. Spengler RF, Greenough WB III, Stolley PD: A descriptive study of nosocomial bacteremias at The Johns Hopkins Hospital, 1968–1974. *Johns Hopkins Med J* 142:77–84, 1978.
13. McGowan JE Jr, Parrott PL, Duty VP: Nosocomial bacteremia potential for prevention of procedure-related cases. *JAMA* 237:2727–2729, 1977.
14. Harris AA, Levin S, Trenholme GM: Selected aspects of nosocomial infections in the 1980s. *Am J Med* 76:3–10, 1984.
15. National Academy of Sciences-National Research Council: Postoperative wound infections: The influence of ultraviolet irradiation of the operating room and of various other factors. *Ann Surg* 160:122–125, 1964.
15a. Cruse PJE: Surgical wound sepsis. *CMA J* 102:251–258, 1970.
16. Cruse PJE: Incidence of wound infection on the surgical services. *Surg Clin North Am* 55:1269–1275, 1975.
17. Cruse PJE, Foord R: The epidemiology of wound infection: A 10-year prospective study of 62939 wounds. *Surg Clin North Am* 60:27–40, 1980.

18. Garner JS, et al.: *Guideline for Prevention of Surgical Wound Infections, 1985.* Atlanta, CDC, 1985.

19. Graybill JR, Marshall LW, Charache P, et al.: Nosocomial pneumonia: A continuing major problem. *Am Rev Resp Dis* 108:1130–1140, 1973.

20. Price DJE, Sleigh JD: Control of infection due to klebsiella aerogenes in a neurosurgical unit by withdrawal of all antibiotics. *Lancet* 2:1213–1215, 1970.

21. Simmons HE, Stolley PD: This is medical progress? Trends and consequences of antibiotic use in the United States. *JAMA* 227:1023–1028, 1974.

22. Shapiro M, Townsend TR, Rosner B, et al.: Use of antimicrobial drugs in general hospitals: Patterns of prophylactics. *N Engl J Med* 301:351–355, 1979.

23. Burke JF: Preventive antibiotic management in surgery. *Annu Rev Med* 24:289–294, 1973.

24. Burke JF: The effective period of preventive antibiotic action in experimental incisions and dermal lesions. *Surgery* 50:161–168, 1961.

25. Howard RJ, Simmons RL: *Surgical Infectious Diseases.* Norwalk (Conn.), Appleton & Lange, 1988.

26. Davidson AIG, Clark C, Smith G: Postoperative wound infection: A computer analysis. *Br J Surg* 58:333–337, 1971.

27. Berger SA, Nagar H, Weitzman S: Prophylactic antibiotics in surgical procedures. *Surg Gynecol Obstet* 146:469–475, 1978.

28. Chodak GW, Plaut ME: Use of systemic antibiotics for prophylaxis in surgery: A critical review. *Arch Surg* 112:326–334, 1977.

29. McGowan JE Jr, Finland M: Usage of antibiotics in a general hospital: Effect of requiring justification. *J Infect Dis* 130:165–168, 1974.

30. Moody ML, Burke JP: Infections and antibiotic use in a large private hospital, January 1971. Comparisons among hospitals serving different populations. *Arch Intern Med* 130:261–266, 1972.

31. Jacoby I, Mandell LA, Weinstein L: The chemoprophylaxis of infection. A brief review of recent studies. *Med Clin North Am* 62:1083–1093, 1978.

32. Alexander JW, Altemeier WA: Penicillin prophylaxis of experimental staphylococcal wound infections. *Surg Gynecol Obstet* 120:243–254, 1965.

33. Roberts NJ Jr, Douglas RG Jr: Gentamicin use and pseudomonas and serratia resistance effect of a surgical prophylaxis regimen. *Antimicrob Agents Chemother* 13:214–220, 1978.

34. Quintiliani R, Klimek J, Nightingale CH: Penetration of cephapirin and cephalothin into the right atrial appendage and pericardial fluid of patients undergoing open-heart surgery. *J Infect Dis* 139:348–352, 1979.

35. The choice of antimicrobial drugs. *Med Letter* 30:33–40, 1988.

36. Antimicrobial prophylaxis in surgery. *Med Letter* 31:105–108, 1989.

37. *Handbook of Antimicrobial Therapy.* New Rochelle, *Medical Letter,* 1986.

38. Sanford JP: *Guide to Antimicrobial Therapy, 28. 1989.* Bethesda, MD, 1989.

39. Guglielmo BJ, Hohn DC, Koo PH, et al.: Antibiotic prophylaxis in surgical procedures. *Arch Surg* 118:943–955, 1983.

40. DiPiro JT, Bowden TA, Hooks VH: Prophylactic parenteral cephalosporins in surgery: Are the newer agents better? *JAMA* 252:3277–3279, 1984.

41. Platt R: Antibiotic prophylaxis in surgery. *Rev Infect Dis* 6:S880–S886, 1984.

42. Conte JE, Jacob LS, Polk HC: *Antibiotic Prophylaxis in Surgery.* Philadelphia, JB Lippincott, 1984.

43. DiPiro JT, Cheung RPF, Bowden TA, et al.: Single dose systemic antibiotic prophylaxis of surgical wound infections. *Am J Surg* 152:552–559, 1986.

44. Symposium: Prophylactic use of antibiotics. *South Med J* 70:1–71, 1977.

45. Bartha M, Fry DE, Neu HC: Symposium: efficacy and cost implications of the new cephalosporins. *Am J Surg* 155(5A):1–110, 1988.

46. Moellering RC: Symposium on ceftriaxone. *Am J Surg* 148(4A):1–43, 1984.

47. Jones RN, Wojeski W, Bakke J, et al.: Antibiotic prophylaxis of 1,036 patients undergoing elective surgical procedures. *Am J Surg* 153:341–346, 1987.

48. Nichols RL: Prevention of infection in high risk gastrointestinal surgery. *Am J Med* 76(5A):111–119, 1984.

Studies on Prophylactic Antibiotics

Pneumonia

49. Feeley TW, Du Moulin GC, Hedley-Whyte J, et al.: Aerosol polymyxin and pneumonia in seriously ill patients. *N Engl J Med* 293:471–475, 1975.

50. Klick JM, Du Moulin GC, Hedley-Whyte J, et al.: Prevention of gram-negative bacillary pneumonia using polymyxin aerosol as prophylaxis: II. Effect on the incidence of pneumonia in seriously ill patients. *J Clin Invest* 55:5–519, 1975.

51. Thulbourne T, Young MH: Prophylactic penicillin and postoperative chest infections. *Lancet* 2:907–909, 1962.

52. Petersdorf RG, Curtin JA, Hoeprich PD, et al.: A study of antibiotic prophylaxis in unconscious patients. *N Eng J Med* 257:1001–1009, 1957.

Appendectomy

53. Magarey CJ, Chant ADB, Rickford CRK, et al.: Peritoneal drainage and systemic antibiotics after appendectomy: A prospective trial. *Lancet* 2:179–182, 1971.

54. Wilson RG, Taylor EW, Dreghaorn C, et al.: A comparative study of cefotetan and metronidazole against metronidazole alone to prevent infection after appendectomy. *Surg Gynecol Obstet* 164:447–451, 1987.

Biliary Surgery

54a. Keighley MRB, Baddeley RM, Burdon DW, et al.: A controlled trial of parenteral prophylactic gentamicin therapy in biliary surgery. *Br J Surg* 62:275–279, 1975.

55. Sone HH, Hooper CA, Kolb LD, et al.: Antibiotic prophylaxis in gastric, biliary and colonic surgery. *Ann Surg* 184:443–450, 1976.

56. Strachan CJL, Black J, Powis SJA, et al.: Prophylactic use of cephazolin against wound sepsis after cholecystectomy. *Br Med J* 2:1254–1256, 1977.

57. Morran C, McNaught W, McArdle CS: Prophylactic co-trimoxazole in biliary surgery. *Br Med J* 3:462–464, 1978.

58. Chetlin SH, Elliott DW: Preoperative antibiotics in biliary surgery. *Arch Surg* 107:319–323, 1973.

59. Lewis RT, Goodall RG, Marien B, et al.: Biliary bacteria, antibiotic use, and wound infection in surgery of the gallbladder and common bile duct. *Arch Surg* 122:44–47, 1987.

60. Crenshaw CA, Glanges E, Webber CE, et al.: A prospective, randomized, double blind study of preventive cefamandole therapy in patients at high risk for undergoing cholecystectomy. *Surgery* 153:546–552, 1981.

61. Kaufman Z, Engelberg M, Eliashin A, et al.: Systemic prophylactic antibiotics in elective biliary surgery. *Arch Surg* 119:1002–1004, 1984.

Upper Gastrointestinal

62. Evans C, Pollock AV: The reduction of surgical wound infections by prophylactic parenteral cephaloridine. *Br J Surg* 60:434–437, 1973.

63. Stone HH, Haney BB, Kolb LD, et al.: Prophylactic and preventive antibiotic therapy: Timing, duration and economics. *Ann Surg* 189:691–698, 1979.

64. Polk HC Jr, Lopez-Mayor JF: Postoperative wound infection: A prospective study of determinant factors and prevention. *Surgery* 66:97–103, 1969.

65. Lewis RT: Wound infection after gastroduodenal operations: A 10-year review. *Can J Surg* 20:435–440, 1977.

65a. Nichols RL, Webb WR, Jones JW, et al.: Efficacy of antibiotic prophylaxis high risk gastroduodenal operations. *Am J Surg* 143:94–97, 1982.

Colon

66. Clarke JS, Condon RE, Bartlett JG, Gorbach SL, Nichols RL, Ochi S: Preoperative oral antibiotics reduce septic complications of colon operations: Results of prospective, randomized, double-blind clinical study. *Ann Surg* 186:251–258, 1977.

67. Condon RE, Bartlett JG, Nichols RL, Schulte WJ, Gorbach SL, Ochi S: Preoperative prophylactic cephalothin fails to control septic complications of colorectal operations: Results of controlled clinical trial. *Am J Surg* 137:68–74, 1979.

68. Willis AT, Ferguson IR, Jones PH, Phillips KD, Tearle PV, Fiddian RV, Graham DF, Harland DHC, Hughes DFR, Knight D, Mee WM, Pashby N, Rothwell-Jackson SRL, Sachdevor AK, Sutch I, Kilbey C, Edwards D: Metronidazole in prevention and treatment of bacteriodes infections in elective colonic surgery. *Br Med J* 1:607–610, 1977.

69. Goldring J, Scott A, McNaught W, Gillespie G: Prophylactic oral antimicrobial agents in elective colonic surgery. *Lancet* 2:997–999, 1975.

70. Nichols RL, Broido P, Condon RE, Gorbach SL, Nyhus LM: Effect of preoperative neomycinerythromycin intestinal preparation on the incidence of infectious complications following colon surgery. *Ann Surg* 178:453–459, 1973.

71. Hughes ESR, Hardy KJ, Cuthbertson AM, Rubbo SD: Chemoprophylaxis in large bowel surgery: I. Effect of intravenous administration of penicillin on incidence of postoperative infection. *Med J Aust* 1:305–308, 1970.

72. Washington JA II, Dearing WH, Judd ES, Elveback LR: Effect of preoperative antibiotic regimen on development of infection after intestinal surgery: Prospective, randomized, double-blind study. *Ann Surg* 180:567–572, 1974.

73. Rosenberg IL, Graham NG, de Dombal FT, Goligher JC: Preparation of the intestine in patients undergoing major large-bowel surgery, mainly for neoplasms of the colon and rectum. *Br J Surg* 58:266–269, 1971.

74. Burdon JW, Morris PJ, Hunt P, Watts JM: A trial of cephalothin sodium in colon surgery to prevent wound infection. *Arch Surg* 112:1169–1173, 1977.

75. Keighley MRB, Arabi Y, Alexander-Williams J, Youngs D, Burdon DW: Comparison between systemic and oral antimicrobial prophylaxis in colorectal surgery. *Lancet* 1:894–897, 1979.

76. Altemeier WA, Hummel RP, Hill EO: Prevention of infection in colon surgery. *Arch Surg* 93:226–233, 1966.

77. Sellwood RA, Burn JI, Waterworth PM, Welbourn RB: A second clinical trial to compare two methods for preoperative preparation of the large bowel. *Br J Surg* 56:610–612, 1969.

78. Nichols RL, Condon RE: Preoperative preparation of the colon. *Surg Gynecol Obstet* 132:323–337, 1971.

79. Eykyn SJ, Jackson BT, Lockhart-Mummery HE, Phillips I: Prophylactic preoperative intravenous metronidazole in elective colorectal surgery. *Lancet* 2:761–764, 1979.

80. Bornside GH, Cohn I Jr: Intestinal antisepsis. Stability of fecal flora during mechanical cleansing. *Gastroenterology* 57:569–573, 1969.

81. Karl RC, Mertz JJ, Veith FJ, Dineen P: Prophylactic antimicrobial drugs in surgery. *N Eng J Med* 275:305–308, 1966.

82. Griffiths DA, Shorey BA, Simpson RA, Speller DCE, Williams NB: Single-dose preoperative antibiotic prophylaxis in gastrointestinal surgery. *Lancet* 2:325–328, 1976.

83. Bernard HR, Cole WR: The prophylaxis of surgical infection: The effect of prophylactic antimicrobial drugs on the incidence of infection following potentially contaminated operations. *Surgery* 56:151–157, 1964.

84. Ketcham AS, Bloch JH, Crawford DT, Lieberman JE, Smith RR: The role of prophylactic antibiotic therapy in control of staphylococcal infections following cancer surgery. *Surg Gynecol Obstet* 114:345–353, 1962.

85. Ketcham AS, Lieberman JE, West JT: Antibiotic prophylaxis in cancer surgery and its value in staphylococcal carrier patients. *Surg Gynecol Obstet* 117:1–6, 1963.

86. Pollock AV, Tindal DS: The effect of a single-dose parenteral antibiotic in the prevention of wound infection. A controlled trial. *Br J Surg* 59:98–99, 1972.

87. Stokes EJ, Waterworth PM, Franks V, Watson B, Clark CG: Short-term routine antibiotic prophylaxis in surgery. *Br J Surg* 61:739–742, 1974.

88. Stone HH, Hester TR Jr: Incisional and peritoneal infection after emergency celiotomy. *Ann Surg* 177:669–678, 1973.

89. Suri PK, Johnston DWB: Prophylactic role of cephaloridine in surgical wounds. *Can J Surg* 18:361–363, 1975.

90. Polk HC Jr, Trachtenberg L, Finn MP: Antibiotic activity in surgical incisions. The basis for prophylaxis in selected operations. *JAMA* 244:1353–1354, 1980.

91. Azar H, Drapanas T: Relationship of antibiotics to wound infection and enterocolitis in colon surgery. *Am J Surg* 115:209–217, 1968.

92. Brass C, Richards GK, Ruedy J, Prentis J, Hinchey EJ: The effect of metronidazole on the incidence of postoperative wound infection in elective colon surgery. *Am J Surg* 135:91–96, 1978.

93. Bröte L, Gillquist J, Höjer H: Prophylactic cephalothin in gastrointestinal surgery. *Acta Chir Scand* 2:238–245, 1976.

94. The Norwegian Study Group: Should antimicrobial prophylaxis in colorectal surgery include agents effective against both anaerobic and aerobic microorganisms? *Surgery* 97:402–407, 1985.

95. Portnoy J, Kagan E, Gordon PH, Mendelson J: Prophylactic antibiotics in elective colorectal surgery. *Dis Colon Rectum* 26:310–313, 1983.

Vascular Surgery

96. Kaiser AB, Clayson KR, Mulherin JL Jr, Roach AC, Allen TR, Edwards WH, Dale WA: Antibiotic prophylaxis in vascular surgery. *Ann Surg* 188:283–289, 1978.

97. Hasselgren P, Ivarsson L, Risberg B, Seeman R: Effects of prophylactic antibiotics in vascular surgery. *Ann Surg* 200:86–92, 1984.

98. Szilagyi DE, Smith RF, Elliott JP, et al.: Infection in arterial reconstruction with synthetic grafts. *Ann Surg* 176:321–333, 1972.

99. Bunt TJ: Synthetic vascular graft infections. *Surgery* 93:733–746, 1983.

100. Sonne-Holm S, Boeckstyns M, Menck H, Sinding A, et al.: Prophylactic antibiotics in amputation of the lower extremity for ischemia. *J Bone Jt Surg* 67A:800–803, 1985.

Hysterectomy

101. Swartz WH, Tanaree P: T-tube suction drainage and/or prophylactic antibiotics: a randomized study of 451 hysterectomies. *Obstet Gynecol* 47:665–670, 1976.

102. Bivens MD, Neufeld J, McCarthy WD: The prophylactic use of keflex and keflin in vaginal hysterectomy. *Am J Obstet Gynecol* 122:169–175, 1975.

103. Bolling DR Jr, Plunkett GD: Prophylactic antibiotics for vaginal hysterectomies. *Obstet Gynecol* 41:689–692, 1973.

104. Breeden JT, Mayo JE: Low-dose prophylactic antibiotics in vaginal hysterectomy. *Obstet Gynecol* 43:379–385, 1974.

105. Glover MW, van Nagell JR Jr: The effects of prophylactic ampicillin on pelvic infection following vaginal hysterectomy. *Am J Obstet Gynecol* 126:385–388, 1976.

106. Grossman JH III, Adams RL, Hierholzer WJ Jr, Andriole VT: Endometrial and vaginal cuff bacteria recovered at elective hysterectomy during a trial of antibiotic prophylaxis. *Am J Obstet Gynecol* 130:312–316, 1978.

107. Harralson JD, van Nagell JR Jr, Roddick JW Jr, Sprague AD: The effect of prophylactic antibiotics on pelvic infection following vaginal hysterectomy. *Am J Obstet Gynecol* 120:1046–1049, 1974.

108. Ledger WJ, Sweet RL, Headington JT: Prophylactic cephaloridine in the prevention of postoperative pelvic infections in premenopausal women undergoing vaginal hysterectomy. *Am J Obstet Gynecol* 115:766–774, 1973.

109. Ledger WJ, Gee C, Lewis WP: Guidelines for antibiotic prophylaxis in gynecology. *Am J Obstet Gynecol* 121:1038–1045, 1975.

110. Mendelson J, Portnoy J, De Saint Victor JR, Gelfand MM: Effect of single and multidose cephradine prophylaxis on infectious morbidity of vaginal hysterectomy. *Obstet Gynecol* 53:31–35, 1979.

111. Ohm MJ, Galask RP: The effect of antibiotic prophylaxis on patients undergoing vaginal operations. I. The effect on morbidity. *Am J Obstet Gynecol* 123:590–596, 1975.

112. Chodak GW, Plaut ME: Wound infections and systemic antibiotic prophylaxis in gynecologic surgery. *Obstet Gynecol* 51:123–127, 1978.

113. Grossman HJ III, Greco TP, Minkin MJ, Adams RL, Hierholzer WJ Jr, Andriole VT: Prophylactic antibiotics in gynecologic surgery. *Obstet Gynecol* 53:537–544, 1979.

114. Jennings RH: Prophylactic antibiotics in vaginal and abdominal hysterectomy. *South Med J* 71:251–254, 1978.

115. Ohm MJ, Galask RP: The effect of antibiotic prophylaxis on patients undergoing total abdominal hysterectomy. I. Effect on morbidity. *Am J Obstet Gynecol* 125:442–447, 1976.

116. Allen JL, Rampone JF, Wheeless CR: Use of prophylactic antibiotic in elective major gynecologic operations. *Obstet Gynecol* 39:218–224, 1972.

117. Forney JP, Morrow CP, Townsend DE, Disaia PJ: Impact of cephalosporin prophylaxis on conization-vaginal hysterectomy morbidity. *Am J Obstet Gynecol* 125:100–103, 1976.

118. Hirsch HA, Prophylactic antibiotics in obstetrics and gynecology. *Am J Med* 78:170–176, 1985.

119. Shapiro M, Munoz A, Tager IB, Schoenbaum

SC, et al.: Risk factors for infection at the operative site after abdominal or vaginal hysterectomy. *N Engl J Med* 307:1661–1666, 1982.

Transurethral Prostectomy

120. Plorde JJ, Kennedy RP, Bourne HH, Ansell JS, Petersdorf RG: Course and prognosis of prostatectomy. With a note on the incidence of bacteremia and effectiveness of chemoprophylaxis. *N Engl J Med* 272:269–277, 1965.
121. Morris MJ, Golovsky D, Guinness MDG, Maher PO: The value of prophylactic antibiotics in transurethral prostatic resection: A controlled trial, with observations on the origin of postoperative infection. *Br J Urol* 48:479–484, 1976.
122. Matthew AD, Gonzalez R, Jeffords D, Pinto MH: Prevention of bacteriuria after transurethral prostatectomy with nitrofurantoin macrocrystals. *J Urol* 120:442–443, 1978.
123. Gibbons RP, Stark RA, Correa RJ Jr, Cummings KB, Mason JT: The prophylactic use or misuse of antibiotics in transurethral prostatectomy. *J Urol* 119:381–383, 1978.
124. Wear HB Jr, Haley P: Transurethral prostatectomy without antibiotics. *J Urol* 110:436–440, 1973.
125. Miller AL Jr, Scott FB, Scott R Jr: An evaluation of antibiotics prior to prostatectomy. *J Urol* 92:711–713, 1964.
126. McGuire EJ: Antibacterial prophylaxis in prostatectomy patients. *J Urol* 111:794–798, 1974.
127. Lacy SS, Drach GW, Cox CE: Incidence of infection after prostectomy and efficacy of cephaloridine prophylaxis. *J Urol* 105:836–839, 1971.
128. Genster HG, Madsen PO: Urinary tract infections following transurethral prostatectomy: With special reference to the use of antimicrobials. *J Urol* 104:163–168, 1970.
129. Landes RR, Medenbach K, Lee RE: Effect of preoperative antibiotic therapy on bacterial prostatitis after transurethral prostatectomy. *Urology* 8:352–356, 1976.
130. Hills NH, Bultitude MI, Eykyn S: Co-trimoxazole in prevention of bacteriuria after prostatectomy. *Br Med J* 2:498–499, 1976.
131. Gonzalez R, Wright R, Blackard CE: Prophylactic antibiotics in transurethral prostatectomy. *J Urol* 116:203–205, 1976.
132. Murphy DM, Falkiner FR, Carr M, et al.: Septicemia after transurethral prostatectomy. *Urology* 22:133–135, 1983.
133. Goldwasser B, Bogokowsky B, Nativ O, et al.: Prophylactic antimicrobial treatment in transurethral prostatectomy. *Urology* 22:136–138, 1983.
134. Grabe M: Antimicrobial agents in transurethral prostatic resection. *J Urol* 138:245–252, 1987.

Orthopaedics

135. Boyd RJ, Burke JF, Colton T: A double-blind clinical trial of prophylactic antibiotics in hip fractures. *J Bone Jt Surg* 55A:1251–1258, 1973.
136. Cruess RL, Bickel WS, vonKessler KLC: Infec-

tions in total hips secondary to a primary source elsewhere. *Clin Orthop* 106:99–101, 1975.
137. Derian PS, Green BM: Postoperative wound infections. 5-year review of 1163 consecutive operative orthopedic patients. *Am Surg* 32:388–390, 1966.
138. Ericson C, Lidgren L, Lindberg L: Cloxacillin in the prophylaxis of postoperative infections of the hip. *J Bone Jt Surg* 55A:808–813, 1973.
139. Irvine R, Johnson BL Jr, Amstutz HC: The relationship of genitourinary tract procedures and deep sepsis after total hip replacements. *Surg Gynecol Obstet* 139:701–706, 1974.
139a. Ainscow DA, Denham RA: The risk of haematogenous infection in total joint replacements. *J Bone Jt Surg* 66-B:580–582, 1984.
140. Olix ML, Klug TJ, Coleman CR, Smith WS: Prophylactic penicillin and streptomycin in elective operations on bones, joints, and tendons. *Surg Forum* 10:818–819, 1959.
141. Patzakis MJ, Harvey P Jr, Ivler D: The role of antibiotics in the management of open fractures. *J Bone Jt Surg* 56A:532–541, 1974.
142. Pavel A, Smith RL, Ballard CA, Larsen IJ: Prophylactic antibiotics in clean orthopaedic surgery. *J Bone Jt Surg* 56A:777–782, 1974.
143. Pollard JP, Hughes SPF, Scott JE, Evans MJ, Benson MKD: Antibiotic prophylaxis in total hip replacement. *Br Med J* 1:707–709, 1979.
144. Schonholtz GJ, Borgia CA, Blair JD: Wound sepsis in orthopaedic surgery. *J Bone Jt Surg* 44A:1548–1552, 1962.
145. Visuri T, Antila P, Laurent LE: A comparison of dicloxacillin and ampicillin in the antibiotic prophylaxis of total hip replacement. *Ann Chir Gynaecol* 65:58–61, 1976.
146. Gatell JM, Riba J, Lozano ML, et al.: Prophylactic cefamandole in orthopaedic surgery. *J Bone Jt Surg* 66A:1219–1222, 1984.
147. Doyon F, Evrard J, Mazas F, et al.: Long-term results of prophylactic cefazolin versus placebo in total hip replacement. *Lancet* I 860, 1987.
148. Hill C, Mazas F, Flamant R, et al.: Prophylactic cefazolin versus placebo in total hip replacement. *Lancet* 1:795–797, 1981.

Thoracic Surgery

149. Truesdale R, D'Alessandri R, Manuel V, et al.: Antimicrobial vs. placebo prophylaxis in noncardiac thoracic surgery. *JAMA* 241:1254–1256, 1979.
150. Grover FL, Richardson JD, Fewel JG, et al.: Prophylactic antibiotics in the treatment of penetrating chest wounds. A prospective double-blind study. *J Thorac Cardiovasc Surg* 74:528–536, 1977.
151. Kvale PA, Ranga V, Kopacz M, et al.: Pulmonary resection. *South Med J* 70:64–68, 1977.

Neurosurgery

152. Klastersky J, Sadeghi M, Brihaye J: Antimicrobial prophylaxis in patients with rhinorrhea or otorrhea: A double-blind study. *Surg Neurol* 6:111–114, 1976.
153. Ignelzi RJ, VanderArk GD: Analysis of the treatment of basilar skull fractures with and

without antibiotics. *J Neurosurg* 43:721–726, 1975.

154. MacGee EE, Cauthen JC, Brackett CE: Meningitis following acute traumatic cerebrospinal fluid fistula. *J Neurosurg* 33:312–316, 1970.

155. Hoff JT, Brewin A, Sang UH: Antibiotics for basilar skull fracture. *J Neurosurg* 44:649, 1976.

156. Wright RL: A survey of possible etiologic agents in postoperative craniotomy infections. *J Neurosurg* 25:125–132, 1966.

157. Hand WL, Sanford JP: Posttraumatic bacterial meningitis. *Ann Intern Med* 72:869–874, 1970.

158. Savitz MH, Malis LI: Prophylactic clindamycin for neurosurgical patients. *N Y State J Med* 76:64–67, 1976.

158a. Slight PH, Gundling K, Plotkin SA, et al.: A trial of vancomycin for prophylaxis of infections after neurosurgical shunts. *N Engl J Med* 312:921, 1985.

159. Shulman ST, et al.: Prevention of bacterial endocarditis. *Circulation* 70:1123A–1127A, 1984.

160. Durack DT, Kaplan EL, Bisno AL: Apparent failures of endocarditis prophylaxis. *JAMA* 250:2318–2322, 1983.

161. Brooks SL: Survey of compliance with American Heart Association guidelines for prevention of bacterial endocarditis. *JADA* 101:41–43, 1980.

162. Baltch AL, Pressman HL, Schaffer C, et al.: Bacteremia in patients undergoing oral procedures. *Arch Intern Med* 148:1084–1088, 1988.

Bacterial Endocarditis

163. Sipes JN, Thompson RL, Hook EW: Prophylaxis of infective endocarditis: A re-evaluation. *Annu Rev Med* 28:371–391, 1977.

164. Everett ED, Hirschmann JV: Transient bacteremia and endocarditis prophylaxis: A review. *Medicine* 56:61–77, 1977.

165. Weinstein L, Schlesinger J: Treatment of infective endocarditis—1973. *Prog Cardiovasc Dis* 16:275–302, 1973.

166. Petersdorf RG: Antimicrobial prophylaxis of bacterial endocarditis. Prudent caution or bacterial overkill? *Am J Med* 65:220–223, 1978.

167. Durack DT, Petersdorf RG: Chemotherapy of experimental streptococcal endocarditis. I. Comparison of commonly recommended prophylactic regimens. *J Clin Invest* 52:592–598, 1973.

168. Parrillo JE, Borst GC, Mazur MH, et al.: Endocarditis due to resistant viridans streptococci during oral penicillin chemoprophylaxis. *N Engl J Med* 300:296–300, 1979.

169. Ayoub EM, Gordis L, Kaplan EL, et al.: Prevention of bacterial endocarditis. *Circulation* 46:3–6, 1972.

170. Harvey WP, Capone MA: Bacterial endocarditis related to cleaning and filling of teeth. With particular reference to the inadequacy of present day knowledge and practice of antibiotic prophylaxis for all dental procedures. *Am J Cardiol* 7:793–798, 1961.

171. Authors: Dentists found to skimp on penicillin. *J Am Dent Assoc* 100:13–14, 1980.

172. Karchmer AW, Dismukes WE, Buckley MJ, et al.: Late prosthetic valve endocarditis. Clinical features influencing therapy. *Am J Med* 64:199–206, 1978.

173. Sande MA, Johnson WD Jr, Hook EW, et al.: Sustained bacteremia in patients with prosthetic cardiac valves. *N Engl J Med* 286:1067–1070, 1972.

174. Mostaghim D, Millard HD: Bacterial endocarditis: A retrospective study. *Oral Surg Oral Med Oral Path* 40:219–234, 1975.

175. Hook EW, Kaye D: Prophylaxis of bacterial endocarditis. *J Chronic Dis* 15:635–646, 1966.

176. Glaser RJ, Dankner A, Mathes SB: Effect of penicillin on the bacteremia following dental extraction. *Am J Med* 4:55–63, 1948.

177. Oakley CM, Darrell JH: Antibiotic prophylaxis for bacterial endocarditis. *Am J Cardiol* 46:1073–1074, 1980.

178. Engeling ER, Eng BF, Sullivan-Sigler N, et al.: Bacteremia after sigmoidoscopy: Another view. *Ann Intern Med* 85:77–78, 1976.

179. LeFrock JL, Ellis CA, Turchik JB, et al.: Transient bacteremia associated with sigmoidoscopy. *N Engl J Med* 289:467–469, 1973.

180. Watanakunakorn C: Infective endocarditis as a result of medical progress. *Am J Med* 64:917–919, 1978.

181. Pace NL, Horton W: Indwelling pulmonary artery catheters. Their relationship to aseptic thrombotic endocardial vegetations. *JAMA* 233:893–894, 1975.

182. Greene JF Jr, Fitzwater JE, Clemmer TP: Septic endocarditis and indwelling pulmonary artery catheters. *JAMA* 233:891–892, 1975.

182a. Dugrue D, Blake S, Troy P, et al.: Antibiotic prophylaxis against infective endocarditis after normal delivery—Is it necessary? *Br Heart J* 44:499–502, 1980.

183. Rovenstine EA: Postoperative respiratory complications: Occurrence following 7874 anesthesias. *Am J Med Sci* 191:807–812, 1936.

184. Naito H, Toya S, Shizawa H, et al.: High incidence of acute postoperative meningitis and septicemia in patients undergoing craniotomy with ventriculoatrial shunt. *Surg Gynecol Obstet* 137:810–812, 1973.

185. Dellinger P: Perioperative antibiotics in urologic surgery. *Urol Clin North Am* 3:323–331, 1976.

186. Lorian V (ed): *Significance of Medical Microbiology in the Care of the Patient.* Baltimore, Williams & Wilkins, 1977.

Postoperative Problems

187. Cranston WI: Central mechanisms of fever, abstracted. *Fed Proc* 38:49–51, 1979.

188. Musher DM, Fainstein V, Young EJ, et al.: Fever patterns: Their lack of clinical significance. *Arch Intern Med* 139:1225–1228, 1979.

189. Weinstein L, Fields BN: Fever of obscure origin. *Semin Infect Dis* 1:1–33, 1978.

190. Dykes MHM: Unexplained postoperative fever: Its value as a sign of halothane sensitization. *JAMA* 216:641–644, 1971.

191. Livelli FD, Johnson RA, McEnany MT, et al.:

Unexplained in-hospital fever following cardiac surgery. *Circulation* 57:968–975, 1978.

192. Bell DM, Goldmann DA, Hopkins CC, et al.: Unreliability of fever and leukocytosis in the diagnosis of infection after cardiac valve surgery. *J Thorac Cardiovasc Surg* 75:87–90, 1978.

193. Roe CF: Surgical aspects of fever. *Curr Probl Surg* November 1978.

194. Weinstein MP, Reller LB: Clinical importance of breakthrough bacteremia. *Am J Med* 76:175–180, 1984.

195. Wilson RF: Special problems in the diagnosis and treatment of surgical sepsis. *Surg Clin North Am* 64:965–990, 1985.

196. Hinsdale JG, Jaffe BM: Re-operation for intra-abdominal sepsis. *Ann Surg* 199:31–36, 1984.

197. Machiedo GW, Tikellis J, Lee BC, et al.: Re-operation for sepsis. *Am Surg* 51:149–154, 198.

198. Craven DE, Kunches LM, Lichtenberg DA, et al.: Nosocomial infections and fatality in medical and surgical intensive care unit patients. *Arch Intern Med* 148:1161–1168, 1988.

199. Stone HH: Infection in postoperative patients. *Am J Med* 81:39–44, 1986.

200. Martin LF, Max MH, Polk HC: Failure of gastric pH control by antacids or cimetidine in the critically ill: A valid sign of sepsis. *Surgery* 88:59–67, 1980.

201. Harris RL, Musher DM, Bloom K, et al.: Manifestations of sepsis. *Arch Intern Med* 147:1895–1906, 1987.

202. Maki DG: Risk factors for nosocomial infection in intensive care. *Arch Intern Med* 149:30–35, 1989.

203. Altemeier WA, Culberstson WR, Fullen WD, et al.: Intra-abdominal abscesses. *Am J Surg* 125:70–78, 1973.

204. Altemeier WA, Alexander JW: Retroperitoneal abscess. *Arch Surg* 83:512–524, 1961.

205. Wang SMS, Wilson SE: Subphrenic abscess: The new epidemiology. *Arch Surg* 112:934–936, 1977.

206. Deck KB, Berne TV: Selective management of subphrenic abscesses. *Arch Surg* 114:1165–1168, 1979.

207. Finegold SM: *Abdominal and Perineal Infections in Anaerobic Bacteria in Human Disease.* New York, Academic Press, 1977, p 257.

208. Rubin RH, Swartz MN, Malt R: Hepatic abscess: Changes in clinical, bacteriologic, and therapeutic aspects. *Am J Med* 57:601–610, 1974.

209. Camer SJ, Tan EGC, Warren KW, et al.: Pancreatic abscess: A critical analysis of 113 cases. *Am J Surg* 129:426–431, 1975.

210. Chun CH, Raff MJ, Contreras L, et al.: Splenic abscess. *Medicine* 59:50, 1980.

211. Polk HC Jr, Shields CL: Remote organ failure: A valid sign of occult intra-abdominal infection. *Surgery* 81:310–313, 1977.

212. Fry DE, Pearlstein L, Fulton RL, et al.: Multiple system organ failure. The role of uncontrolled infection. *Arch Surg* 115:136–140, 1980.

213. Milligan SL, Luft FC, McMurray SD, et al.: Intra-abdominal infection and acute renal failure. *Arch Surg* 113:467–471, 1978.

214. Haaga Jr, Alfidi RJ, Havrilla TR, et al.: CT detection and aspiration of abdominal abscess. *Am J Roentgenol* 128:465–474, 1977.

215. Biello DR, Levitt RG, Melson GL: The roles of gallium-67 scientigraphy, ultrasonography, and computed tomography in the detection of abdominal abscesses. *Semin Nucl Med* 9:58–65, 1979.

216. McNeil BJ, Sanders R, Alderson PO, et al.: A prospective study of computed tomography, ultrasound, and gallium imaging in patients with fever. *Radiology* 139:647–653, 1981.

217. Korobkin M, Callen PW, Filly RA, et al.: Comparison of computed tomography, ultrasonography, and gallium-67 scanning in the evaluation of suspected abdominal abscess. *Radiology* 129:89–93, 1978.

218. Kreger BE, Craven DE, Carling PC, et al.: Gram-negative bacteremia: III. Reassessment of etiology, epidemiology, and ecology in 612 patients. *Am J Med* 68:332–343, 1980.

219. Kreger BE, Craven DE, McCabe WR: Gram-negative bacteremia: IV. Re-evaluation of clinical features and treatment in 612 patients. *Am J Med* 68:344–355, 1980.

220. Musher DM, McKenzie SO: Infections due to *Staphylococcus aureus. Medicine* 56:383–409, 1977.

221. Shah M, Watamakunakorn C: Changing patterns of *staphylococcus aureus* bacteremia. *Am J Med Sci* 278:115–121, 1979.

222. Kirby BD, Snyder KM, Meyer RD, et al.: Legionnaires' disease: Report of sixty-five nosocomically acquired cases and review of the literature. *Medicine* 59:188–205, 1980.

223. Harris JA, Cobbs GC: Persistent gram-negative bacteremia. Observations in twenty patients. *Am J Surg* 125:705–717, 1973.

224. McHenry MD, Gavan TL, Hawk WA, et al.: Gram-negative bacteremia of long duration. *Cleve Clin Q* 40:47–56, 1973.

225. Stone HH, Kolb LD, Currie CA, et al.: Candida sepsis: Pathogenesis and principles of treatment. *Ann Surg* 179:697–110, 1974.

226. Klein JJ, Watanakunakorn C: Hospital-acquired fungemia: Its natural course and clinical significance. *Am J Med* 67:51–58, 1979.

227. Walker AM, Jick H, Porter J: Drug-related superinfection in hospitalized patients. *JAMA* 242:1273–1275, 1979.

228. Kerkering TM, Espinel-Ingroff A, Shadomy S: Detection of *candida* antigenemia by counterimmunoelectrophoresis in patients with invasive candidiasis. *J Infect Dis* 140:659–664, 1979.

229. Harvey RL, Myers JP: Nosocomial fungemia in a large community teaching hospital. *Arch Intern Med* 147:2117–2120, 1987.

230. Lipsky BA, Hirschmann JV: Drug fever. *JAMA* 245:851–854, 1981.

231. Sanford JP, Pierce AK: Lower respiratory tract infections, in Bennett JV, Brachman PS (eds): *Hospital Infections.* Boston, Little, Brown & Co., 1979, pp 255–286.

232. Tuazon CU: Gram-positive pneumonias. *Med Clin North Am* 64:343–361, 1980.

233. Reyes MP: The aerobic gram-negative bacil-

lary pneumonias. *Med Clin North Am* 64:363–383, 1980.

234. Lerner AM: The gram-negative bacillary pneumonias, in Dowling HF, et al (eds): *Disease-A-Month*. Chicago, Year Book Medical Publishers, 1974.

235. Pierce AK, Sanford JP: Aerobic gram-negative bacillary pneumonias. *Am Rev Respir Dis* 110:647–658, 1974.

236. Ramsey PG, Rubin RH, Tolkoff-Rubin NE, et al.: The renal transplant patient with fever and pulmonary infiltrates: Etiology, clinical manifestations, and management. *Medicine* 59:206–222, 1980.

237. Johanson WG Jr, Pierce AK, Sanford JP, et al.: Nosocomial respiratory infections with gram-negative bacilli: The signifance of colonization of the respiratory tract. *Ann Intern Med* 77:701–706, 1972.

238. LeFrock JL, Ellis CA, Weinstein L: The impact of hospitalization on the aerobic fecal microflora. *Am J Med Sci* 277:269–274, 1979.

239. Tillotson JR, Finland M: Bacterial colonization and clinical superinfection of the respiratory tract complicating antibiotic treatment of pneumonia. *J Infect Dis* 119:597–624, 1969.

240. Shulman JA, Phillips LA, Petersdorf RG: Errors and hazards in the diagnosis and treatment of bacterial pneumonias. *Ann Intern Med* 62:41–58, 1965.

241. Bartlett JG, O'Keefe P, Tally FP, et al.: Bacteriology of hospital-acquired pneumonia. *Arch Intern Med* 146:868–871, 1986.

242. Karnad A, Alvarez S, Berk SL: Pneumonia caused by gram-negative bacilli. *Am J Med* 79(Suppl 1A):61–67, 1985.

243. Driks MR, Craven DE, Celli BR, et al.: Nosocomial pneumonia in intubated patients given sucralfate as compared with antacids or histamine type-2 blockers. *N Engl J Med* 317:1376–1382, 1987.

244. Craven DE, Kunches LM, Kilinsky V, et al.: Risk factors for pneumonia and fatality in patients receiving continuous mechanical ventilation. *Am Rev Respir Dis* 133:792–796, 1986.

245. Bynum LJ, Pierce AK: Pulmonary aspiration of gastric contents. *Am Rev Respir Dis* 114:1129–1136, 1976.

246. Cameron JL, Mitchell WH, Zuidema GD: Aspiration pneumonia: Clinical outcome following documented aspiration. *Arch Surg* 106:49–59, 1973.

247. Tinstman TC, Dines DE, Arms RA: Postoperative aspiration pneumonia. *Surg Clin North Am* 53:859–862, 1973.

248. Murray HW: Antimicrobial therapy in pulmonary aspiration. *Am J Med* 66:188–190, 1979.

249. Bartlet JG, Gorbach SL: The triple threat of aspiration pneumonia. *Chest* 68:560–566, 1975.

250. Bartlett JG, Gorbach SL, Finegold SM: The bacteriology of aspiration pneumonia. *Am J Med* 56:202–207, 1974.

251. Lorber B, Swenson RM: Bacteriology of aspiration pneumonia. *Ann Intern Med* 81:329, 1974.

252. Wynne JW, Modell JH: Respiratory aspiration of stomach contents. *Ann Intern Med* 87:466–474, 1977.

253. Zavala DC: The threat of aspiration pneumonia in the aged. *Geriatrics* 32:46–51, 1977.

254. Stewardson RH, Nyhus LM: Pulmonary aspiration: An update. *Arch Surg* 112:1192–1197, 1977.

255. Toung T, Cameron JL: Cimetidine as a preoperative medication to reduce the complications of aspiration of gastric contents. *Surgery* 87:205–208, 1980.

256. Schlenker JD, Hubay CA: The pathogenesis of postoperative atelectasis. A clinical study. *Arch Surg* 107:846–850, 1973.

257. Latimer RG, Dickman M, Day WC, et al.: Ventilatory patterns and pulmonary complications after upper abdominal surgery. Detection by pre- and post-operative computerized spirometry and blood gas analysis. *Am J Surg* 122:622–632, 1971.

258. Schmidt GB: Prophylaxis of pulmonary complications following abdominal surgery, including atelectasis, ARDS, and pulmonary embolism. *Surg Annu* 9:29–73, 1977.

259. Murray HW, Ellis GC, Blumenthal DS, Sos TA: Fever and pulmonary thromboembolism. *Am J Med* 67:232–235, 1979.

260. Kunin CM: Urinary tract infections, in Bennett JV, Brachman PS (eds): *Hospital Infections*. Boston, Little, Brown & Co., 1979, pp 239–254.

261. Siroky MB, Moylan RA, Austen G Jr, et al.: Metastatic infection secondary to urinary tract sepsis. *Am J Med* 61:351–360, 1976.

262. Andriole VT: Hospital-acquired urinary infections and the indwelling catheter. *Urol Clin North Am* 2:451–469, 1975.

263. Fincke BG, Friedland G: Prevention and management of infection in the catheterized patient. *Urol Clin North Am* 3:313–321, 1976.

264. Kunin CM: New developments in the diagnosis and treatment of urinary tract infections. *J Urol* 113:585–594, 1975.

265. Michigan S: Genitourinary fungal infections. *J Urol* 116:390–397, 1976.

266. Kozinn PJ, Taschdjian CL, Goldberg PK, et al.: Advances in the diagnosis of renal candidiasis. *J Urol* 119:184–187, 1978.

267. Thorley JD, Jones SR, Sanford JP: Perinephric abscess. *Medicine* 53:441–451, 1974.

268. Truesdale BH, Rous SN, Nelson RP: Perinephric abscess: A review of 26 cases. *J Urol* 118:910–911, 1977.

269. Altemeier WA: Surgical infections: Incisional wounds, in Bennett JV, Brachman PS (eds): *Hospital Infections*. Boston, Little, Brown & Co., 1979, pp 287–306.

270. Anderson CB, Marr JJ, Ballinger WF: Anaerobic infections in surgery: Clinical review. *Surgery* 79:313–324, 1976.

271. Baxter CR: Surgical management of soft tissue infections. *Surg Clin N Am* 52:1483–1499, 1972.

272. Jones RB, Hirschmann JV, Brown GS, et al.: Fournier's syndrome: Necrotizing subcutaneous infection of the male genitalia. *J Urol* 122:279–282, 1979.

273. Bartlett P, Rengold AL, Graham DR, et al.: Toxic shock syndrome associated with surgical wound infections. *JAMA* 247:1448–1450, 1982.

274. Teasley DC, et al.: Prospective randomized trial of metronidazole versus vancomycin for *Clostridium difficile*-associated diarrhea and colitis. *Lancet* 2:1043–1045, 1983.

275. Green SL, Sarubbi FA: Risk factors associated with post-cesarean section febrile morbidity. *Obstet Gynecol* 49:686–690, 1977.

276. Levin S, Jupa JE: Principles of antibiotic usage in obstetrics and gynecology. *Obstet Gynecol Annu* 5:293, 1976.

277. Sweet RL: Pelvic infection. *Obstet Gynecol Annu* 9:77–107, 1980.

278. Josey WE, Staggers SR Jr: Heparin therapy in septic pelvic thrombophlebitis: A study of 46 cases. *Am J Obstet Gynecol* 120:228–233, 1974.

279. Wenger DR, Gitchell RG: Severe infections following pudendal block anesthesia: Need for orthopedic awareness. *J Bone Jt Surg* 55A:202–207, 1973.

280. Hibbard LT, Snyder EN, McVann RM: Subgluteal and retropsoal infection in obstetric practice. *Obstet Gynecol* 39:137–150, 1972.

281. Svancarek W, Chirino O, Schaefer G Jr, et al.: Retropsoas and subgluteal abscesses following paracervical and pudendal anesthesia. *JAMA* 237:892–894, 1977.

282. Cushing RD: Antibiotics in trauma. *Surg Clin North Am* 57:165–177, 1977.

283. Allgöwer M, Dürig M, Wolff G: Infection and trauma. *Surg Clin North Am* 60:133–144, 1980.

284. Caplan ES, Hoyt N, Cowley RA: Changing patterns of nosocomial infections in severely traumatized patients. *Am Surg* 204–210, 1979.

285. Thadepalli H: Principles and practice of antibiotic therapy for post-traumatic abdominal injuries. *Surg Gynecol Obstet* 148:937–951, 1979.

286. Pankey GA: Post-traumatic antibiotic management. *Bull NY Acad Med* 55:272–283, 1979.

287. Thadepalli H, Gorback SL, Broido PW, et al: Abdominal trauma, anaerobes, and antibiotics. *Surg Gynecol Obstet* 137:270–276, 1973.

288. Gleckman RA: Fever of unknown origin: An approach, in Gantz NM, Gleckman RA (eds): *Manual of Clinical Problems in Infectious Disease.* Boston, Little, Brown & Co., 1979, pp 240–247.

289. Nichols RL: Empiric antibiotic therapy for intra-abdominal infections. *Rev Infect Dis* 5(Suppl 1):S90–S97, 1983.

290. Nichols RL, Smith JW, Klein DB, et al.: Risk of infection after penetrating abdominal trauma. *N Engl J Med* 311:1065–1070, 1984.

291. Genster HG, Andersen MJF: Spinal osteomyelitis complicating urinary tract infection. *J Urol* 107:109–111, 1972.

292. Musher DM, Thorsteinsson SB, Minuth JN, et al.: Vertebral osteomyelitis: Still a diagnostic pitfall. *Arch Intern Med* 136:105–110, 1973.

293. Bouza E, Winston DJ, Hewitt WL: Infectious osteitis pubis. *Urology* 12:663–664, 1978.

294. Galpin JE, Chow AW, Bayer AS, et al.: Sepsis association with decubitus ulcers. *Am J Med* 61:346–350, 1976.

295. Petersdorf RG, Forsyth BR, Bernanke D: Staphylococcal parotitis. *N Engl J Med* 259:1250–1254, 1958.

296. Travis LW, Hecht DW: Acute and chronic inflammatory diseases of the salivary glands: Diagnosis and management. *Otolaryngol Clin North Am* 10:329–338, 1977.

297. Sarr MG, Frey H: A unique case of benign postoperative parotid swelling. *Johns Hopkins Med J* 146:11–12, 1980.

298. Sternlieb JJ, McIlrath DC, van Heerden JA, et al.: Starch peritonitis and its prevention. *Arch Surg* 112:458–461, 1977.

299. Kirshen EJ, Naftolin F, Benirschke K: Starch glove powders and granulomatous peritonitis. *Am J Obstet Gynecol* 118:799–804, 1974.

300. Baker CC, Petersen SR, Sheldon GF: Septic phlebitis: A neglected disease. *Am J Surg* 138:97–102, 1979.

301. Stamm WE: Infections related to medical devices. *Ann Intern Med* 89:764–769, 1978.

302. O'Mara C, Imbembo AL: Paraprosthetic-enteric fistula. *Surgery* 81:556–566, 1977.

303. Kleinman LH, Towne JB, Bernhard VM: A diagnostic and therapeutic approach to aortoenteric fistulas: Clinical experience with 20 patients. *Surgery* 86:868–878, 1979.

304. Cohen PS, Maguire JH, Weinstein L: Infective endocarditis caused by gram-negative bacteria: A review of the literature, 1945–1977. *Prog Cardiovasc Dis* 22:205–242, 1980.

305. Pelletier LL Jr, Petersdorf RG: Infective endocarditis: A review of 125 cases from the University of Washington Hospitals, 1963–1972. *Medicine* 56:287–313, 1977.

306. Watanakunakorn C, Baird IM: Staphylococcus aureus bacteremia and endocarditis associated with a removable infected intravenous device. *Am J Med* 63:253–256, 1977.

307. Cannady PB, Sanford JP: Negative blood cultures in infective endocarditis: A review. *South Med J* 69:1420–1424, 1976.

308. Ellner JJ, Rosenthal MS, Lermer PI, et al.: Infective endocarditis caused by slow-growing, fastidious gram-negative bacteria. *Medicine* 58:145–158, 1979.

309. Rubinstein E, Noriega ER, Simberkoff MS, et al.: Fungal endocarditis: Analysis of 24 cases and review of the literature. *Medicine (Baltimore)* 54:331–344, 1975.

310. Hutter AM Jr, Moellering RC: Assessment of the patient with suspected endocarditis. *JAMA* 235:1603–1605, 1976.

311. Weinstein L: "Modern" infective endocarditis. *JAMA* 233:260–263, 1975.

312. Gleckman R: Culture negative bacterial endocarditis: Confirming the diagnosis. *Am Heart J* 94:125–126, 1977.

313. Pesanti EL, Smith IM: Infective endocarditis and negative blood cultures. An analysis of 52 cases. *Am J Med* 66:43–50, 1979.

314. Sande MA, Scheld WM: Combination antibiotic therapy of bacterial endocarditis. *Ann Intern Med* 92:390–395, 1980.

315. Stinson EB: Surgical treatment of infective endocarditis. *Prog Cardiovas Dis* 22:145–168, 1979.

316. Duma RJ (ed): *Infections of Prosthetic Heart Valves and Vascular Grafts: Prevention, Diagnosis, and Treatment.* Baltimore, University Park Press, 1977.

317. Weinstein L: Infective endocarditis, in Braunwald E (ed): *Heart Disease, A Textbook of Cardiovascular Medicine.* Philadelphia, WB Saunders, 1980, pp 1187–1190; 1208–1210.

318. Jung JY, Saab SB, Almond CH: The case for early surgical treatment of left-sided primary infective endocarditis: A collective review. *J Thorac Cardiovas* 70:590–518, 1975.

319. Karchmer AW, Dismukes WE, Buckley MJ, et al.: Late prosthetic valve endocarditis. Clinical features influencing therapy. *Am J Med* 64:199–206, 1978.

320. Fitzgerald RH, Nolan DR, Ilstrup DM, et al.: Deep wound sepsis following total hip arthroplasty. *J Bone Jt Surg* 59:847–855, 1977.

321. Hughes PW, Salvati EA, Wilson PD Jr, et al.: Treatment of subacute sepsis of the hip by antibiotics and joint replacement criteria for diagnosis with evaluation of twenty-six cases. *Clin Orthop* 141:143–157, 1979.

322. Update: Universal precautions for prevention of transmission of Human Immunodeficiency Virus. *MMWR* 37:377–387, 1988.

323. Marcus R, et al.: Surveillance of health care workers exposed to blood from patients infected with the Human Immunodeficiency Virus. *N Engl J Med* 319:1118–1123, 1988.

324. DeVita VT, Hellman S, Rosenberg SA: *AIDS: Etiology, Diagnosis, Treatment And Prevention.* Philadelphia, JB Lippincott, 1988.

325. Recommendations for prevention of HIV transmission in health-care settings. *MMWR* 36(2S):15, 1987.

326. Finegold SM, *Anaerobic Bacteria in Human Disease.* New York, Academic Press, 1977.

327. Garibaldi RA, Britt MR, Coleman ML, et al.: Risk factors for postoperative pneumonia. *Am J Med* 70:677–680, 1981.

328. Solomkin JS, et al.: Design and conduct of antibiotic trials: A report of the scientific studies committee of the surgical infection society. *Arch Surg* 122:158–164, 1987.

329. Coppa GF, Eng K: Factors involved in antibiotic selection in elective colon and rectal surgery. *Surgery* 104:853–858, 1988.

330. Haley RW, Culver DH, Morgan WM, et al.: Identifying patients at high risk of surgical wound infection. *Am J Epid* 121:206–215, 1985.

331. McFarland LV, Mulligan ME, Kwok RY, et al.: Nosocomial acquisition of *Clostridium difficile* infection. *N Engl J Med* 320:204–210, 1989.

332. Christou NV, Nohr CW, Meakins JL: Assessing operative site infection in surgical patients. *Arch Surg* 122:165–169, 1987.

333. Bunt TJ: Non-directed relaparotomy for intra-abdominal sepsis: a futile procedure. *Am Surg* 52:294–298, 1986.

334. Dobrin PB, et al.: Radiologic diagnosis of an intra-abdominal abscess: Do multiple tests help. *Arch Surg* 121:41–46, 1986.

335. Rutledge R, Mandel SR, Wild RE: *Candida* species: Insignificant contaminant or pathogenic species. *Am Surg* 52:299–302, 1986.

336. Wey S, et al.: Risk factors for hospital-acquired candidemia. *Arch Intern Med* 149:2349–2353, 1989.

337. LaRaja RD, et al.: The incidence of intra-abdominal surgery in acquired immunodeficiency syndrome. *Surgery* 105:175–179, 1989.

338. Robinson G, Wilson SE, Williams RA: Surgery in patients with acquired immunodeficiency syndrome. *Arch Surg* 122:170–175, 1987.

339. Platt R, Zaleznik DF, Hopkins CC, et al.: Perioperative antibiotic prophylaxis for herniorrhaphy and breast surgery. *N Engl J Med* 322:153–160, 1990.

17

Dermatology

Donald P. Lookingbill

The skin, the most visible organ of the body is, paradoxically, often the one most overlooked. As a result, a dermatologic sign of a systemic process may be missed. One of the purposes of this chapter is to review some of the important skin expressions of systemic diseases. Such skin signs are not common, but they can be very important. Occasionally, a skin eruption provides a diagnostic clue to a treatable, life-threatening disease. The second purpose of this chapter is to discuss the diagnosis and treatment of skin disorders that result from hospitalization.

For consultation purposes, skin findings will be classified into one of three categories:

1. The disorder is purely a cutaneous one and bears no relationship to the reasons for the patient's hospitalization, nor has it resulted from any complication of the hospitalization. These skin findings are merely incidental. Most skin lesions fit into this category. Examples include nevi, seborrheic keratoses, senile hemangiomas, psoriasis (usually), eczema, etc. It is not the purpose of this chapter to provide a text in general dermatology to discuss these common skin disorders.

2. The skin finding is a sign of a systemic disease, including the disease for which the patient is hospitalized.

3. The skin disorder represents a cutaneous complication of the hospitalization. This category includes postoperative skin problems.

The remainder of the chapter will describe skin disorders in the last two categories. Dermatologic therapy will also be briefly discussed.

SKIN SIGNS OF SYSTEMIC DISEASE

The skin might be involved in a systemic process in one of four ways:

1. A primary skin disorder is the origin for the systemic process. Examples include cellulitis and tumors of skin origin, especially malignant melanoma and lymphoma.

2. The skin finding is a secondary expression of some primary systemic process. Examples include septicemia, skin signs of AIDS or malignancy, hypersensitivity reactions, and cutaneous expressions of metabolic diseases.

3. The skin is involved in a multisystem disease by the same pathologic process as are the internal organs. Examples are collagen vascular diseases, vasculitis, disseminated intravascular coagulation, and granulomatous diseases such as sarcoidosis.

4. The skin disease is severe enough to cause systemic complications.

PRIMARY SKIN DISORDERS RESULTING IN SYSTEMIC DISEASE

Infectious and malignant etiologies predominate in this category and are important to recognize for obvious reasons.

Infection

Cellulitis is the most common skin infection with systemic ramifications.

Though common, it is not always easy to diagnose. It may sometimes be confused with superficial thrombophlebitis or even with stasis or contact dermatitis. To help differentiate, one should remember that with cellulitis, all the cardinal clinical signs of inflammation are present: redness, swelling, warmth, and tenderness. In addition, two other features are often present: fever and leukocytosis.

The diagnosis of cellulitis is more secure when an organism is recovered. This is more easily said than done. Blood cultures are sometimes rewarding. The classic method of recovering bacteria from the skin is to inject non-bacteriostatic saline into the affected area and to culture the aspirate (5). In some cases with negative aspirates, bacteria have been recovered by culturing the tissue from a deep 4-mm punch biopsy of the affected area. But even this method is not always successful, and the diagnosis of cellulitis then remains presumptive, a presumption that is reinforced by a prompt response to antibiotic therapy.

In otherwise healthy adult patients, cellulitis is thought to be caused by gram-positive cocci, either Group A beta-hemolytic streptococcus or, less commonly, *Staphylococcus aureus.*

Patients with recurrent cellulitis frequently have tinea pedis ("athlete's foot"), and the macerated fissures in the toe webs serve as portals of entry for pathogenic bacteria. The saphenous venectomy legs in coronary bypass surgery patients seem particularly predisposed to this process (6). Diagnosis and treatment of tinea pedis may help prevent further recurrences of the cellulitis.

It is critical to remember that unusual organisms may cause cellulitis in the hospitalized or postsurgical patient. In immunosuppressed or otherwise debilitated patients, a wide variety of gram-negative organisms can cause cellulitis, which may be clinically indistinguishable from the gram-positive variety. In the same setting, *Cryptococcus* infection can also present with a cellulitis.

Malignancy

Two important primary skin tumors have a particular propensity for metastasis.

MYCOSIS FUNGOIDES

This is an inappropriately named lymphoma arising in, and peculiar to, the skin. The clinical course is highly variable. When it metastasizes, the lymph nodes are usually the first to be involved. Mycosis fungoides is usually first diagnosed in the plaque stage where the diagnosis is suspected because the plaques are: irregular in shape, peculiar in color (red-brown or violaceous or "orangish"), and asymmetrical in distribution. **A bizarre or "atypical" dermatosis should raise the suspicion of mycosis fungoides.** If possible, dermatologic consultation should be obtained. Multiple biopsies, over time, may be necessary to confirm the diagnosis.

MALIGNANT MELANOMA

This is easily the skin tumor most demanding of early diagnosis. The point to be made is that for the vast majority of these lesions, early diagnosis is possible and consequent surgical cure achievable. The most common type of melanoma is the **superficial spreading melanoma.** Seventy per cent of all melanomas fall into this category. Diagnostically, the key word is irregularity as expressed in the following "ABCD" features:

A—asymmetry with one half of the lesion unlike the other half;

B—border irregularity with a scalloped or notched border;

C—color variation, sometimes including the colors of the American flag—red, white and especially, **blue;**

D—diameter, with melanomas usually being greater than 6 mm.

Nodular melanoma is the next most common type of melanoma and often appears as a blue-black nodule in the skin. Deep invasion in nodular melanoma often occurs early. A third type of melanoma, lentigo maligna melanoma, usually occurs in sun-exposed skin of elderly patients. Superficial spreading melanomas and lentigo maligna melanomas may be present for years before becoming deeply invasive; therefore, **a diagnosis of melanoma should not be excluded on the basis of long-standing duration.**

The reader is encouraged to consult a color atlas on melanoma in order to become fully familiar with the diagnostic features of this important skin tumor (10).

SKIN SIGNS AS A SECONDARY EXPRESSION OF A PRIMARY SYSTEMIC DISEASE

Though not primarily involved, the skin may show signs of an underlying systemic disease process. Four general categories will be considered: (*a*) infection; (*b*) malignancy; (*c*) hypersensitivity reactions; and (*d*) metabolic diseases.

Infection: Rash and Fever

Of all the skin signs of systemic disease, the skin manifestations of sepsis require the most urgent recognition. This includes not only signs of bacterial sepsis but also skin findings in septicemia due to fungal, rickettsial, treponemal, and viral organisms.

BACTERIAL SEPSIS

With bacteremia, the basic lesion is one of a necrotizing vasculitis originating from septic emboli and/or associated immune complexes. The clinical expression of a necrotizing vasculitis is a purpuric papule, i.e., palpable purpura. **Sepsis must always be ruled out when purpuric lesions occur in the setting of fever.** Septic skin lesions occur most commonly with bacteremias due to the following organisms: *Neisseria meningitidis, Neis-*

seria gonorrhoeae, Streptococcus viridans, Staphylococcus aureus, and *Pseudomonas aeruginosa.*

Purpuric papules frequently occur in patients with meningococcemia and are often important diagnostic findings. In an acutely ill, febrile patient, even a few purpuric papules on the extremities should raise the suspicion of meningococcemia. Meningitis is usually, but not always present.

The triad of fever, polyarthralgia/arthritis, and specific skin lesions characterize the syndrome of gonococcemia. Tenosynovitis may also be present. The skin lesion is a **hemorrhagic pustule.** There are usually only a handful of such lesions located in a peripheral distribution; hands, feet, and distal extremities. Although the skin lesions are the result of septic emboli to the skin, the organism often cannot be cultured from the pustule. If the patient has been symptomatic for more than 2 days, blood cultures are also often negative. The organism usually can be recovered from the body orifice that is the primary site of infection.

Staphylococcal septicemia can result in a variety of purpuric lesions in the skin, ranging from petechiae, to purpuric papules, to hemorrhagic bullae. Subungual splinter hemorrhages may also be seen, though they are by no means specific for endocarditis and, in fact, are more commonly encountered in a noninfectious setting.

Skin lesions of pseudomonas sepsis can also be expressed in several ways, such as petechiae, hemorrhagic bullae, and less commonly, cellulitis. The lesion specifically associated with pseudomonas sepsis is **ecthyma gangrenosa,** a round, indurated, ulcerative lesion in which the depressed center is covered with a black eschar. This lesion is most frequently found in the axillary or anogenital region. The organism may sometimes be cultured from this lesion. As with the other bacteremias in which skin lesions appear, blood cultures and early therapy are essential.

FUNGAL SEPTICEMIA: DISSEMINATED CANDIDIASIS

With a growing population of immuno-suppressed individuals, the incidence of systemic fungal infections has been increasing. Skin manifestations may occur with most of these infections (for example, cellulitis in disseminated crypto-coccosis) but are uncommon with the exception of disseminated candidiasis. This infection is a particular problem in patients with hematologic malignancies. The responsible organism is usually either *Candida tropicalis* or *Candida albicans*. Associated septic skin lesions occur in a sizable minority (13%) of infected patients (12). Lesions are usually multiple and occur on the trunk and proximal extremities. They have most frequently been described as "maculonodules," a contradiction in terms used to define an indurated papule within an erythematous macular base. The lesions are less than 1 cm in size and often have a pale center. Unless the patient is thrombocytopenic, the lesions are not purpuric. Thus, this lesion, along with the "rose spots" of typhoid fever, represent two exceptions to the rule that septic skin lesions are purpuric. **In disseminated candidiasis, a skin biopsy can be particularly useful** in that the organism can often be cultured from the skin tissue, as well as seen on pathology sections specially stained for fungus.

TREPONEMAL SEPTICEMIA: SYPHILIS

Syphilis still exists. Treponemal septicemia occurs in the secondary form of the disease and results in a systemic disorder with protean manifestations. The skin rash of secondary syphilis sometimes, but not always, involves the palms and soles. Palmar and plantar involvement is not peculiar to secondary syphilis, however. For example, the palms and soles can be involved with purpuric lesions in Rocky Mountain spotted fever or with erythematous macules in viral exanthemas and drug eruptions. But with secondary syph-

ilis, the palmar and plantar lesions often have a peculiar copper or red-brown color and, additionally, may be indurated and/or scaling. The generalized lesions are usually scaling papules and plaques, sometimes misdiagnosed as "atypical pityriasis rosea." In any patient with a systemic febrile disease in whom an accompanying "atypical" rash is present, a serologic test for syphilis should be done.

VIREMIAS

A generalized erythematous exanthem is a common skin expression of a viral illness and is often clinically indistinguishable from a cutaneous drug reaction. Viral exanthems are more frequent in children, resolve spontaneously, and seldom pose a threat to the patient or a serious diagnostic problem to the clinician. Disseminated herpes infection can be an exception. Infections from herpes viruses seldom cause a serious problem in the normal host, but in the immunosuppressed, they can be fatal. Disseminated herpes simplex sometimes occurs without skin lesions; disseminated herpes zoster and disseminated varicella are always accompanied by skin involvement. The skin lesions in herpetic infections appear as multiple vesicles. A definitive diagnosis of a herpes infection can be immediately established with the **Tzanck smear.** This involves opening a vesicle, scraping the base, smearing the contents on a glass slide, and staining with Wright's, Giemsa's or toluidine blue stain. Under the microscope, multinucleated giant cells are visualized. This finding is diagnostic for herpes infection but does not specify the type. Precise viral identification can be subsequently confirmed with viral cultures.

Skin Signs of AIDS

Skin manifestations are common in the acquired immunodeficiency syndrome (AIDS) and frequently are the presenting sign (13). Because of their immuno-suppression, AIDS patients are susceptible to a wide range of mucocutaneous infections. **Oral candidiasis** can be the initial manifestation of AIDS, as can herpes zoster in young adults who are otherwise apparently healthy. Chronic herpes simplex also occurs in AIDS patients and appears as a chronic ulcerative process particularly in the perianal area. Widespread molluscum contagiosum and warts may also occur but are not specific. Atypical mycobacterial infections may involve the skin and often present as abscesses.

Other mucocutaneous manifestations of AIDS include: Kaposi's sarcoma, oral "hairy" leukoplakia, and seborrheic dermatitis. **Kaposi's sarcoma** was the first cutaneous manifestation to be described in AIDS patients; it is present in about 1/2 of homosexual AIDS patients at the time of their initial diagnosis. Kaposi's sarcoma is probably derived from endothelial cells, and the skin lesions therefore have a vascular appearance. These red or purple macules or papules are often benign in appearance and are easily misdiagnosed as hemangiomas or bruises. The lesions may be single or multiple and can be located anywhere on the skin surface. Kaposi's sarcoma has been described mainly in homosexual AIDS patients. Any new red or purple macule, papule, plaque or nodule on a homosexual man should be biopsied. If it shows Kaposi's sarcoma, a diagnosis of AIDS is virtually certain.

Oral "hairy" leukoplakia appears as a white, roughened, thickening of the lateral margin of the tongue. It is commonly found in homosexuals with AIDS and is probably due to Epstein-Barr virus infection.

Seborrheic dermatitis is also a common skin finding in patients with AIDS and frequently appears early in the course of the disease. In one survey, 46% of AIDS patients had seborrheic dermatitis versus 5% of patients without AIDS. Seborrheic dermatitis appears as severe "dandruff" of the scalp accompanied by scaling of the face, particularly in the eyebrows and na-solabial folds. Proliferation of the yeast organism *Pityrosporon ovale* has been implicated in seborrheic dermatitis, and the immunosuppression present in AIDS patients may allow this organism to flourish. This theory is supported by the improvement of the eruption with ketoconazole therapy.

Skin Signs of Malignancy

Skin signs of malignancy are uncommon. Although remote effects of cancers can be expressed in the skin, such reactions are few and distinctly uncommon. Many of these skin reactions are idiopathic in nature, but their frequent occurrence with an underlying malignancy has established a relationship. Table 17.1 is a partial list of uncommon idiopathic skin disorders frequently associated with an internal malignancy.

Direct tumor infiltration is the most common, and certainly the most unequivocal way in which an internal malignancy is reflected in the skin. Metastatic carcinoma, melanoma, and myeloma, as well as lymphoma and leukemia, can all infiltrate the skin. The infiltrates almost always present as firm to hard nodules in the skin, either single or multiple and

Table 17.1. Idiopathic Skin Signs of Internal Malignancy

Skin Sign	Tumor Type
1. Acanthosis nigricans	Carcinoma
2. Dermatomyositis, adult-onset	Carcinoma
3. Erythema gyratum repens	Carcinoma
4. Hypertrichosis lanugosa ("malignant down")	Carcinoma
5. Ichthyosis, adult-onset	Lymphoma
6. Necrolytic erythema migrans	Glucagonoma
7. Acrokeratosis paraneoplastica (Bazex syndrome)	Carcinoma (upper respiratory tract)
8. Eruptive keratoses (Leser-Trélat)	Carcinoma (GI tract)
9. Multiple sebaceous neoplasms (Torre's syndrome)	Carcinoma (GI tract)

sometimes "purplish" in color. Occasionally, the skin involvement is the presenting sign.

For any nodule in the skin, a specific diagnosis is usually not possible on clinical grounds alone. The cardinal rule is that **for undiagnosed, firm nodules in the skin, a tissue diagnosis is necessary.** This can be achieved either with an excisional or deep punch biopsy.

Hypersensitivity Reactions: The Erythemas

Vascular reactions sometimes occur in the skin as presumed hypersensitivity responses to some underlying systemic process. Erythema marginatum, the non-pruritic, annular eruption associated with acute rheumatic fever, is seldom seen in adults. Erythema multiforme, erythema nodosum, and urticaria are more common.

Urticaria

Urticaria is more easily recognized than described. It is helpful to remember that with urticaria, individual lesions seldom last longer than 24 hours. Also, itching is often a prominent symptom. Often a cause for an urticarial reaction cannot be determined; but in hospitalized patients, drugs should be prime suspects. Urticaria is not usually a marker of an underlying systemic disease unless it is accompanied by fever. Then, systemic processes should be considered, including: (a) the hepatitis prodrome in which fever, arthralgias, and urticaria occur, and (b) serum sickness, which can occur in response to drugs as well as serum and is characterized by fever, arthralgias, lymphadenopathy, and urticaria. Urticaria may be symptomatically treated with diphenhydramine or hydroxyzine given on a routine (not a "prn") basis. Twice daily doxepin may be even more effective.

Erythema Multiforme

Compared to urticaria, erythema multiforme is a more severe type of a hypersensitivity vascular reaction. Its most severe form is called the Stevens-Johnson syndrome. Unlike urticaria, the lesions persist for many days and often weeks.

As the name implies, in erythema multiforme a variety of skin lesions may occur, including the following: erythematous plaques, blisters, mucous membrane involvement, and/or **target lesions.** Sometimes, urticarial wheals are confused with target lesions. The distinction is that an urticarial wheal has no more than two zones of color, a central pale area surrounded by an erythematous halo; whereas to meet the criteria for a target lesion, three zones must be present: a central dark area, surrounded by a pale zone, surrounded by a peripheral rim of erythema.

One can find tables in textbooks that list innumerable "causes" for erythema multiforme. Most are poorly substantiated with the exception of the following three: (a) herpes simplex infection, (b) mycoplasma infection, and (c) drugs. **Recurrent erythema multiforme is most frequently associated with recurrent herpes simplex.**

Erythema Nodosum

As the name implies, this reaction is characterized by tender erythematous nodules. They are usually located in the pretibial areas. Erythema nodosum may be associated with any of the following: (a) drugs, (b) streptococcal infection, (c) sarcoidosis, (d) deep fungal infections (coccidiomycosis and histoplasmosis), (e) tuberculosis, (f) infectious colitis secondary to Yersinia enterocolitica, and (g) inflammatory bowel disease. Appropriate history and a few simple tests can screen for these. Sometimes no specific etiology can be determined. The course is self-limited and usually requires no therapy. If not contraindicated, a short course of systemic steroids results in rapid involution of the lesions in patients severely affected.

Metabolic Disorders

A number of metabolic conditions can be expressed in the skin.

ENDOCRINE

Skin changes have been associated with dysfunction of most endocrine glands. Examples include:

1. Pituitary. The skin changes associated with acromegaly can best be described as "dermatomegaly" - i.e., the skin and its appendages are hypertrophied and hyperfunctioning, resulting in skin thickening, increased sweating, and increased oiliness. Acanthosis nigricans can also be associated with acromegaly as well as other pituitary disorders, including tumors. In a young, obese person, however, acanthosis nigricans is usually not related to any systemic disease. **In an older, slender patient, an underlying internal malignancy should be sought.**

2. Thyroid. Most physicians are aware of the skin and hair changes occurring with hyperthyroidism (warm, moist skin and fine textured hair) and hypothyroidism (dry, cool, "doughy" skin with coarse hair and loss of lateral third of the eyebrows). Diffuse scalp hair loss can occur in both conditions.

3. Adrenal. Addisonian pigmentation has a predilection for sun-exposed areas, skin creases, and oral mucosa. Affected patients often do not lose their tans from one summer to the next. It should be remembered that patients with ACTH-producing pituitary tumors can also develop Addisonian pigmentation along with Cushingoid features.

4. Diabetes Mellitus. Of the many skin signs that have been associated with diabetes mellitus, **necrobiosis lipoidica diabeticorum** is both the most distinctive and most awkward to pronounce. Mature lesions appear as erythematous, indurated, often depressed lesions with a distinct orange coloration. Through an atrophic epidermis, dilated tortuous blood vessels are frequently seen. The lesions are usually located on the pretibial areas. They are not very common, being found only in three per thousand of diabetic patients. A minority of patients with this skin disorder have no associated diabetes. Diabetic dermopathy, or "shin spots," are depressed brown atrophic scar-like lesions located in the pretibial areas, and are commonly found in diabetics.

HYPERLIPIDEMIAS

In the hyperlipidemic disorders, a variety of associated xanthomas can occur in the skin, including planar, tuberous, tendon, and eruptive. **Tendon xanthomas are stony hard nodules** found most commonly on the Achilles tendons and extensor tendons over the dorsal aspect of the hands. They are associated with hypercholesterolemia. **Eruptive xanthomas are associated with very high serum levels of triglycerides,** and appear as red-yellow papules often located on the trunk. They not only erupt abruptly but can disappear just as quickly, often within weeks, with lowering of the triglycerides to normal levels. Xanthelasma are relatively common "yellowish" plaques confined to the eyelids. It is appropriate to screen for hyperlipidemia in patients with xanthelasma, but normal values will be found in about 50%.

PORPHYRIA

Acute intermittent porphyria is the only type of porphyria without skin manifestations. All other types have associated skin lesions which are usually related to the photosensitizing effects of the elevated porphyrins present in the skin. For example, in porphyria cutanea tarda, blisters and increased skin fragility are seen on the backs of patients' hands.

MULTISYSTEM DISEASE WITH SKIN INVOLVEMENT

In the following examples, the skin is involved by the same pathologic process as the internal organs.

Necrotizing Vasculitis

Confusion reigns in the characterization and classification of vasculitis. Strictly speaking, any inflammation of blood vessels could be termed a "vasculitis." More commonly, the term vasculitis is used to describe a leukocytoclastic necrotizing reaction in blood vessels. When the skin is affected, the clinical appearance is **palpable purpura.** This is to be distinguished from the macular, nonpalpable, non-inflammatory purpura seen with bleeding disorders. One cause for nonpalpable purpura is increased capillary fragility as is seen in the common, but benign, "senile" purpura, or in the less common, but more important purpura associated with amyloidosis. In the former, the purpura is confined to the lower arms; in the latter, it is more widespread. Purpura associated with coagulation disorders is also of the nonpalpable variety. With thrombocytopenia, the lesions are small—i.e., petechial.

Because of the inflammation in and around the affected dermal blood vessels, the purpuric lesions from vasculitis are elevated, at least initially. Later, if the process has been extensive or if large vessels have been involved, skin necrosis may occur. Vasculitis is thought to be immune complex-initiated and complement-mediated, and can occur in a variety of settings. Sepsis has already been discussed. Other conditions include: collagen vascular disease (particularly lupus erythematosus and rheumatoid arthritis), cryoglobulinemia, drug reactions, and occasionally malignant lymphoma. **Whenever purpuric papules appear in the skin, necrotizing vasculitis should be strongly suspected.** If desired, confirmation can be simply obtained with a skin biopsy. When necrotizing vasculitis is diagnosed in the skin, a search should be carried out for: (*a*) the underlying cause and (*b*) any extracutaneous involvement. Concomitant renal involvement is particularly common. Sometimes, necrotizing vasculitis is confined to the skin, but this is a diagnosis of exclusion. One final clinical point: the palpability of vasculitis lesions in the skin may be transient. Surprisingly, within a day, a new lesion may have flattened out and already begun to fade.

Disseminated Intravascular Coagulation

This is the other pathological setting in which palpable purpura can occur in the skin. Other hemorrhagic cutaneous signs can occur in this condition as well. These include: petechiae, non-palpable purpura, hemorrhagic bullae, purpura fulminans, acral cyanosis, dissecting hematomas, and prolonged bleeding from wound sites (16). Histologically, fibrin thrombi are found in the blood vessels. In contrast to the findings in vasculitis, only a minimal inflammatory infiltrate is present. The cutaneous lesions may be the presenting signs for this systemic process in which sepsis is a frequent cause. Skin biopsy findings may suggest the diagnosis; coagulation tests will be confirmatory.

Collagen Vascular Disease

Skin involvement occurs in most of the collagen vascular diseases and is often diagnostically extremely helpful. Skin manifestations are prevalent in the American Rheumatism Association diagnostic criteria for lupus. Included in these criteria are: 1) malar rash, 2) discoid rash, 3) photosensitivity, and 4) oral or nasopharyngeal ulcers. In the malar rash of lupus, telangiectasis are often present, but scaling usually is not. These features will help in differentiating lupus from seborrheic dermatitis, a red scaling rash of the face. **Seborrheic dermatitis is the most common cause of a "butterfly rash"** and often develops in hospitalized patients with a history of dandruff. In the laboratory evaluation of lupus, serologic tests are of most diagnostic value, but a skin biopsy can provide further information. In patients with systemic lupus, immunoglobulins are deposited at the dermal-epidermal junction of clinically involved and uninvolved skin. Immunofluorescent staining of a skin biopsy from the extensor surface of the forearm will be positive in over 50% of patients with systemic lupus.

Sarcoidosis

Two types of skin involvement occur in patients with sarcoidosis: (a) erythema nodosum, a hypersensitivity response already discussed, and (b) granulomatous infiltration of the skin. The skin infiltration can take several forms, depending in part on the race of the patient. In black patients, flesh-colored papules and annular lesions may be present, often on the face. In whites, papules and nodules are often brownish-red in color. When the red color is blanched out with pressure, an apple jelly coloration remains ("diascopy test"). A positive test is strongly suggestive of granulomatous infiltration. In sarcoidosis, histologic confirmation will be desired, and when it is involved, the skin provides a convenient source of tissue. But it must be remembered that the histologic findings of non-caseating granulomas in a single tissue supports, but does not establish, the diagnosis of sarcoidosis.

SYSTEMIC COMPLICATIONS CAUSED BY SKIN DISEASE

Most skin disorders are relatively limited in extent and accordingly do not interfere with function. Two notable exceptions are: (a) exfoliative erythroderma, and (b) extensive blistering disorders. Another potential complication of skin disease relates to dermatologic therapy, i.e., the systemic effect of topically applied steroids.

Exfoliative Erythroderma

In exfoliative erythroderma, the total skin surface is, by definition, red and desquamating. Three etiologic categories should be considered: (a) drugs; (b) generalization of a pre-existing dermatosis, most commonly psoriasis or atopic dermatitis; and (c) malignancy, specifically the Sezary syndrome, a variant of mycosis fungoides. Systemic effects are manifested when the total skin surface is erythematous. Heat and fluid losses occur, and with maximally dilated cutaneous blood vessels, a high output cardiac state can develop which might result in congestive heart failure in patients with preexisting heart disease. Heat loss can be marked enough to drop the body's core temperature, leading to shaking chills. The heat subsequently generated from the shaking can "overshoot" the body's thermostat and hyperthermia can result. With chills and fever, infection should be sought, but is seldom found. The scaling and erythema of the skin also result in increased transcutaneous loss of water and protein. Erythrodermic patients will often be thirsty and dehydrated. Also, most patients will be hypoalbuminemic, attributable in part to the transcutaneous protein loss. Finally, these patients often have reactive lymphadenopathy, so that large lymph nodes in the setting of erythroderma do not necessarily indicate a malignant condition. Sometimes, however, lymph node biopsy is needed in order to distinguish between benign dermatopathic lymphadenopathy and malignant lymphadenopathy.

Blistering Diseases

Extensive primary blistering disorders of the skin are fortunately rare. The most dramatic example is **pemphigus,** a widespread blistering disease of skin and mucous membranes which, before the days of antibiotics and systemic steroids, was usually fatal. As with burn patients, patients with extensive pemphigus are prone to problems with nutrition and infection. **Bullous pemphigoid** is another primary blistering disorder of the skin, usually occurring in an older population, and usually less severe than pemphigus. In both of these diseases, immunoglobulins can be found deposited in the skin in the region of the blister formation. Therefore, a skin biopsy done at the border of an active lesion and specially processed with **immunofluorescent staining techniques** is diagnostically helpful. In patients with pemphigus and pemphigoid, the responsible autoantibodies may also be found in the circulation.

Patients with widespread blistering diseases such as pemphigus, pemphigoid, and the Stevens-Johnson syndrome are subject to the same systemic complications as are erythrodermic patients. In addition, the denuded areas are highly susceptible to bacterial infection. These patients may need to be managed in much the same fashion as burn patients. Acutely, systemic steroids form the mainstay of systemic therapy for the blistering process.

Occasionally, blisters are seen in comatose, drug-overdose patients. Often these blisters are not noted until the second day of hospitalization. At one time they were thought to be specific for barbiturate overdosage. It is now clear that they simply represent blisters located over the bony prominences which were subjected to pressure during the comatose period.

Systemic Effects of Topically Applied Steroids

It has been repeatedly shown that topically applied steroids are absorbed. This absorption can be enhanced if the steroids are used under plastic occlusion. Even without plastic occlusion, adrenal suppressive doses of corticosteroids can be absorbed from the application of a moderate strength topical steroid applied to **total body inflamed skin,** or from the application of one of the newer "superpotent" steroids (Diprolene®, Temovate®) to more limited areas. For preoperative purposes, patients chronically using large amounts of topical steroids should be managed in the same way as patients who have been on systemic suppressive doses of steroids (see Chapter 13).

CUTANEOUS COMPLICATIONS OF HOSPITALIZATION

Circumstances associated with hospitalization sometimes result in cutaneous reactions. The following categories will be considered: (*a*) drug eruptions; (*b*) contact dermatitis; (*c*) skin infections; and (*d*) skin manifestations of nutritional deficiencies.

Drug Eruptions

This is easily the most common cutaneous condition for which consultation is requested. In one large hospital survey, cutaneous reactions to drugs were found to occur in 2.2% of hospitalized patients (18). This study included only morbilliform eruptions, hives, and generalized itching. Other manifestations of drug reactions include vasculitis, erythema multiforme, and erythema nodosum as described previously. Certain drugs can also be responsible for lichen planus-like reactions, photosensitivity eruptions, and blistering disorders such as toxic epidermal necrolysis. **Drugs should be considered in the differential diagnosis of any type of skin rash of uncertain etiology.** The extensive tables in Fitzpatrick's general dermatology text list the different types of drug eruptions with the drugs most commonly responsible.

The most common type of cutaneous drug reaction is the morbilliform or so-called "maculopapular" eruption. This is a generalized eruption, comprised of erythematous macules and papules that tend to be confluent in large areas. The eruption usually starts proximally and proceeds distally; the legs are usually the last to be involved and likewise the last to clear. The erythema is often bright red, a feature which may clinically help to distinguish a drug reaction from a viral exanthem, which it can sometimes mimic. The presence of eosinophilia may also be helpful in this regard. In adults, viral exanthems are a much less common cause for morbilliform eruptions than are drug reactions.

Unfortunately, there is no clinical method or laboratory test to identity which drug is responsible. Since the average hospitalized patients receives eight drugs, this poses a problem. To try to implicate a particular drug, two variables can be considered: (a) the timing of the eruption in relationship to the initiation of the drug, and (b) the incidence of reactions to specific drugs. Most (but not all) drug eruptions occur within several days of initiating the medication. The drug rash incidence rates developed by Arndt and Jick can be used as guidelines in assessing the statistical likelihood for a given drug to cause a rash. From their data, some of the most common offending agents are listed in Table 17.2.

It is not always possible to implicate a specific drug for a suspected drug rash. Under these circumstances, it is advisable to reduce the number of administered drugs to the absolute minimum and to change the most likely drug or drugs to alternative ones if possible.

What happens if you guess wrong? That is, what are the risks of continuing on with a drug in the face of a cutaneous reaction caused by that drug? These risks need to be considered also when one cannot discontinue a suspected drug because it is essential to the patient's therapy. The risks are mainly two: (a) cutaneous, and (b) renal. The cutaneous risk is progression of the inflammatory reaction to an exfoliative erythroderma or toxic epidermal necrolysis with complications as already described. Such progression seldom occurs, and so drug therapy may sometimes be continued in the face of a drug eruption if it is essential to the patient's therapy. The renal risk is allergic interstitial nephritis, a rare complication most commonly associated with the penicillins and cephalosporins. In addition to the rash, many of these patients have fever and eosinophilia. The finding of eosinophils in the urine is a valuable diagnostic clue. The condition is usually reversible with discontinuance of the offending agent.

Acute anaphylaxis is **not** a hazard in the continued administration of the drug thought to be responsible for a drug rash. Anaphylaxis *is* a consideration in re-administering a drug to a patient with a history of a cutaneous reaction to that drug, particularly if the eruption was urticarial. In this regard, predictive testing in patients with a history of penicillin allergy can be carried out with penicilloyl-polylysine and minor determinant skin tests. A serum radioallergosorbent test (RAST) is also available. There appears to be a reasonably good correlation between positive tests and penicillin hypersensitivity, but both false-positive and false-negative results occur (Table 17.3). Penicillin is the only drug for which these tests are available.

Drug eruptions clear after discontinuation of the drug. The time course is important to keep in mind. Drug eruptions usually take 1–2 weeks to clear completely. In fact, the eruption may worsen for several days after the suspected offending agent has been discon-

Table 17.2. Drug Rash Incidence Rates[a]

Drug	Reaction Rate (Reactions/100 Recipients)
Trimethoprim-sulfamethoxazole	5.9
Ampicillin	5.2
Semisynthetic penicillins	3.6
Blood, whole human	3.5
Erythromycin	2.3
Sulfisoxazole	1.7
Penicillin G	1.6
Gentamycin sulfate	1.6
Cephalosporins	1.3
Quinidine	1.2

[a] From Arndt KA, Jick H: Rates of cutaneous reactions to drugs. A report from the Boston collaborative drug surveillance program. *JAMA* 235:918–923, 1976.

Table 17.3.   Predicting Allergic Reactions to Penicillin and Cephalosporin[a]

(a) Type of reaction by history	Positive skin test to PPL and/or penicillin G (%)
Anaphylaxis	46
Angioedema or urticaria	17
Maculopapular rash	7
(b) PPL[b] and/or penicillin G skin test	Reaction to penicillin challenge (%)
Negative	3
Positive	67
(c) History of prior penicillin reaction	Reaction to cephalosporins (%)[c]
Negative	5%
Positive	18%

[a] From Green GR, Rosenblum AH, Sweet LC: Evaluation of penicillin hypersensitivity: Value of clinical history and skin testing with penicilloyl-polylysine and penicillin G. *J Allerg Clin Immunol* 60:339–345, 1977.
[b] PPL, penicilloyl-polylysine.
[c] Data from Thoburn R, Johnson JE III, Cluff LE: Studies on the epidemiology of adverse drug reactions: IV. The relationship of cephalothin and penicillin allergy. *JAMA* 198:345–348, 1966.

tinued. Explaining this to the patient should help to alleviate anxiety when the rash does not clear overnight.

The final aspect of allergic cutaneous drug reactions is what to tell the patient about his "allergy." This may be difficult when the reaction was relatively mild and/or a single drug could not be implicated with certainty. However, patients should be advised, and their charts should be appropriately labeled, if a cutaneous reaction occurred in which either: (*a*) a specific drug was identified with relative certainty, no matter what the nature of the cutaneous reaction, or (*b*) a serious (e.g., vasculitis, erythroderma, or extensive blistering reaction) or potentially serious (e.g., urticaria) reaction occurs and one drug is implicated as being the most likely cause.

Contact Dermatitis

ALLERGIC CONTACT DERMATITIS

In allergic contact dermatitis, an offending substance comes in contact with the skin of a sensitized individual and results in a delayed hypersensitivity reaction involving the epidermis, as well as the underlying dermal blood vessels. Clinically, the epidermal reaction is characterized by vesicles in the acute phase and by poorly demarcated areas of confluent, superficial, glistening small papules in the subacute phase. **Itching is invariably present.**

Poison ivy is the prototypic contact allergen. Unless the delivering florist has unusual taste, poison ivy is unlikely to be encountered in a hospital setting. Tape, local antiseptics, and other topically applied medications are frequently encountered in a hospital, however, and sometimes these can induce a contact dermatitis in a sensitized individual. The configuration and distribution of the dermatitis often provide the clues leading to the diagnosis. For example, square- and rectangular-shaped areas of dermatitis might lead to the suspicion of a tape allergy; a large area of dermatitis over the abdomen with streaks extending along the flanks in a postlaparotomy patient should suggest a contact dermatitis to the solution used in prepping for surgery. When localized, contact dermatitis can satisfactorily be treated with cool soaks followed by a topical steroid cream and a systemic antihistamine for the itching. The process usually takes a week or more to resolve.

MILIARIA

Miliaria ("heat rash") is a form of externally induced dermatitis seen on the backs of patients confined to a supine position for extended periods of time. Orthopaedic patients trapped in various devices are frequently affected. The eruption appears as multiple individual erythematous papules or crystal-clear vesicles over the back. Sometimes, an allergy to the bed linen is incorrectly implicated. "Sheet allergy" is uncommon, though uncommonly an irritant reaction to the detergent remaining in the laundered sheets may occur. Accordingly, many hospitals provide "hypoallergenic sheets" simply by passing the sheets through the rinse cycle an extra time. The skin lesions in miliaria result from occlusion of the sweat ducts followed by retention of sweat in the skin. Treatment simply involves increased air exposure and the problem resolves spontaneously.

Superficial Skin Infections

The most common hospital-acquired superficial skin infections are of fungal and herpetic etiology (see p. 449 for herpes infections).

CANDIDIASIS

Of the superficial fungal infections, candidiasis is the most common. Two factors predispose to *Candida albicans* infection: (*a*) antibiotic therapy, which may suppress the normal bowel flora and allow *Candida* to thrive, with resultant perianal, oral, and esophageal infection and, (*b*) increased heat and moisture in the perineal and perianal areas of bedfast patients, providing a more attractive environment for the growth of the organism. Clinically, candidiasis appears as a **beefy red eruption** with poorly demarcated borders but with **satellite papules and pustules.** It occurs most commonly in the groin and perianal areas, but in bedfast patients, the lesions may extend up the back as well. A diagnosis can be confirmed with a potassium hydroxide preparation of a scraping of superficial pus or scale. Under the microscope, hyphae or pseudohyphae are seen; spores are not

diagnostic. Local therapy with a topical agent such as nystatin, clotrimazole, or miconazole applied twice daily is usually satisfactory. Widespread or resistant disease can be treated with oral ketoconazole. Procedures to promote dryness of the skin in the susceptible areas are helpful as well.

Skin Manifestations of Nutritional Deficiencies

Patients with severe malabsorption can develop a variety of mucocutaneous abnormalities, presumably on a nutritional basis. Glossitis, stomatitis, dermatitis, alopecia, and increased pigmentation all can occur.

The early use of total parenteral nutrition resulted in several specific deficiency states. Essential fatty acid deficiency causes an erythematous, desquamating eruption that usually begins in the body folds but can become generalized. The use of fat emulsions has largely obviated this problem. Alopecia and a seborrheic dermatitis-like skin eruption have been related to zinc deficiency in some patients on parenteral nutrition. These lesions resolve with zinc replacement (see also Chapter 5).

DERMATOLOGIC THERAPY

Dermatologic therapy is most frequently aimed at infection or inflammation. Skin infections can often be treated topically. Topical imidazoles (for example, clotrimatole, miconazole, and ketoconazole) are effective for both candida and tinea infections; topical acyclovir can be used for localized herpes simplex; and topical antibiotics are helpful for superficial bacterial infections. Systemic therapy is used for more severe or widespread disease.

Noninfected inflammatory skin conditions are most often treated with a topical steroid. The bewildering array of preparations that are available can be divided into categories according to potency (see Table 17.4). The selection of an agent

Table 17.4. Topical Steroid Potency[a]

	Brand	Generic	%
Strong	Halog	Halcinonide	0.1
	Lidex	Fluocinonide	0.5
	Diprosone	Betamethasone dipropionate	0.5
	Topicort	Desoximetasone	0.25
Medium	Valisone	Betamethasone valerate	0.1
	Aristocort, Kenalog	Triamcinolone acetonide	0.1
	Synalar	Fluocinolone acetonide	0.025
	Westcort	Hydrocortisone valerate	0.2
Weak	Hytone, Carmol HC	Hydrocortisone	1.0

[a]From Lookingbill DP, Marks JG: Dermatologic therapy, *Principles of Dermatology*, Philadelphia, W. B. Saunders, 1986.

depends upon the type of disease and its location. In general, **the weakest effective preparation should be employed.** For example, seborrheic dermatitis can (and should) be treated with a mild steroid such as hydrocortisone; whereas, psoriasis will respond best to stronger preparations. However, the more potent topical steroids should not be used on "sensitive" skin such as the face, genitalia, and flexural folds; hydrocortisone is the steroid of choice for these locations. These sensitive skin areas are more susceptible to local adverse effects which include steroid acne (particularly on the face), and skin atrophy, which sometimes results in skin breakdown. The occurrence of these local side effects increases with the potency of the topical steroid.

Topical steroids are available in several vehicles, including creams, ointments, lotions, and solutions. Creams are most commonly employed and are easy to use since they are in a water base and are not "greasy." Ointments are in an oil base and are therefore more occlusive and more effective. They are particularly useful for dry, scaly conditions. Lotions are sometimes employed when large areas of the skin are involved. Solutions are used for conditions in the scalp. Plastic wrap occlusion will increase the potency of topical steroids tenfold; but wraps are awkward

to use and increase the risk of local and systemic side effects, so they are not generally recommended.

READINGS

1. Lookingbill DP, Marks JG: *Principles of Dermatology*. Philadelphia, WB Saunders, 1986.
2. Fitzpatrick TB, Eisen AZ, Wolff K, et al. (eds): *Dermatology in General Medicine*. 3rd ed. New York, McGraw-Hill, 1987.
3. Moschella SL, Hurley HJ: *Dermatology*. 2nd ed. Philadelphia, WB Saunders, 1983.
4. Braverman IM: *Skin Signs of Systemic Disease*. 2nd ed. Philadelphia, WB Saunders, 1981.
5. Uman SJ, Kunin CM: Needle aspiration in the diagnosis of soft-tissue infections. *Arch Intern Med* 135:959–961, 1975.
6. Baddour LM, Bisno AL: Recurrent cellulitis after coronary bypass surgery. Association with superficial fungal infection in saphenous venectomy limbs. *JAMA* 251:1049–1052, 1984.
7. Fleisher G, Ludwig S, Campos J: Cellulitis: Bacterial etiology, clinical features, and laboratory findings. *J Pediatr* 97:591–593, 1980.
8. Broder S, Bunn PA: Cutaneous T-cell lymphomas. *Semin Oncol* 7:310–331, 1980.
9. Lamberg SI, Green SB, Byar DP, et al.: Clinical staging for cutaneous T-cell lymphomas. *Ann Intern Med* 100:187–192, 1984.
10. Sober AJ, Fitzpatrick TB, Mihm MC, et al.: Early recognition of cutaneous melanoma. *JAMA* 242:2795–2799, 1979.
11. Holmes KK, Counts GW, Beaty HN: Disseminated gonococcal infection. *Ann Intern Med* 74:979–993, 1971.
12. Grossman ME, Silvers DN, Walther RR: Cutaneous manifestations of disseminated candidiasis. *J Am Acad Dermatol* 2:111–116, 1980.
13. Kaplan MH, Sadick N, McNutt NS, et al.: Dermatologic findings and manifestations of acquired immunodeficiency syndrome (AIDS). *J Am Acad Dermatol* 16:485–506, 1987.

14. Thiers BH: Dermatologic manifestations of internal cancer. *CA-A Cancer Journal for Clinicians.* 36:130–148, 1986.

15. Gilliam JN, Smiley JD: Cutaneous necrotizing vasculitis and related disorders. *Ann Allergy* 37:328–339, 1976.

16. Robboy SJ, Mihm MC, Colman RW, et al.: The skin in disseminated intravascular coagulation. *Br J Dermatol* 88:221–229, 1973.

17. Jablonska S, Beutner EH, Michel B, et al.: Uses for immunofluorescence tests of skin and sera. Utilization of immunofluorescence in the diagnosis of bullous diseases, lupus erythematosus, and certain other dermatoses. *Arch Dermatol* 111:372–381, 1975.

18. Bigby M, Jick S, Jick H, et al.: Drug-induced cutaneous reactions: A report from the Boston Collaborative Drug Surveillance Program on 15 438 consecutive inpatients, 1975 to 1982. *JAMA* 256:3358–3363, 1986.

19. Wintroub BU, Stern R: Cutaneous drug reactions: Pathogenesis and clinical classification. *J Am Acad Dermatol* 13:167–179, 1985.

20. Green GR, Rosenblum AH, Sweet LC: Evaluation of penicillin hypersensitivity: Value of clinical history and skin testing with penicilloyl polylysine and penicillin G. *J Allerg Clin Immunol* 60:339–345, 1977.

21. Maibach HI, Stoughton RB: Topical corticosteroids. *Med Clin North Am* 57:1253–1264, 1973.

22. Arndt KA: *Manual of Dermatologic Therapeutics with Essentials of Diagnosis.* 4th ed. Boston, Little, Brown & Co., 1988.

18

Orthopaedics and Rheumatology

John W. Burnside

The purpose of this chapter is to focus on the medical evaluation of patients requiring bone and joint surgery and in addition, to focus on patients requiring other surgery who have concomitant joint disease. Special risk factors pertaining to these two groups and focal points to minimize morbidity and mortality will be discussed.

HIP FRACTURES

Surgical repair of a fractured hip is among the five most common procedures performed in medicare beneficiaries. Seventy per cent of these operations are done for patients over the age of 70. Most commonly the patient is a white osteoporotic woman, osteoporosis being much less frequent in blacks and men.

Twenty per cent of patients operated on for hip fractures will die within 3 months. This high mortality is due to the combination of preexisting disease and concomitant acute medical problems superimposed on the fracture. This figure may, however, be declining in recent years, owing in part to more comprehensive multidisciplinary management through the perioperative period.

Certain patient characteristics define a particularly high-risk group (Table 18.1). Each of the following at least doubles the mortality risks: (*a*) age over 70, (*b*) male, (*c*) non-ambulatory prior to fracture, (*d*) uncompensated congestive heart failure, (*e*) 24–48 hour delay between injury and hospitalization, and (*f*) malnutrition. Deaths are unusual in the immediate perioperative period, but begin to occur in

Table 18.1. Hip Fractures: Risk Factors for Mortality[a]

1. Age > 70 yr
2. Male
3. Non-ambulatory prior to fracture
4. 24–48-hr delay from injury to admission
5. Uncompensated congestive heart failure
6. Inanition, malnutrition

[a]Each factor at least doubles expected mortality rate.

Table 18.2. Hip Fractures: Causes of Mortality

1. Pneumonia	40%
2. Congestive heart failure	20%
3. Pulmonary emboli	15%
4. Myocardial infarction	10%
5. Cerebrovascular accident	5%
6. Sepsis (any source)	10%

the first postoperative week, and peak in weeks 2 to 4.

A review of the causes of death suggests that a prudent preoperative evaluation and intensive postoperative follow-up may influence postoperative morbidity and mortality. The three major causes of mortality are pneumonia, heart failure, and pulmonary emboli (Table 18.2).

Preoperative Evaluation

Begin the assessment with an inquiry regarding the accident. Hip fractures generally occur because of a fall and one should determine why the patient fell. If a history of seizure or syncopy emerges, pursue the usual cardiac and neurologic causes. A full evaluation can usually be deferred to the postoperative period with the exception of obvious arrhythmia or

Table 18.3. Hip Fractures: Concomitant Medical Diseases

1. Heart disease	
a. Congestive heart failure	20% (10% decompensated)
b. Ischemic heart disease	20%
c. Hypertension-uncontrolled	10%
2. Anemia	20%
3. Chronic lung disease	10%
4. Urinary tract infection	15%
5. Diabetes mellitus	10%
6. Central nervous system disorder	10%

myocardial infarction. Twenty-five percent of patients will report feeling dizzy prior to the fall.

Certain aspects of the history and physical deserve special attention (Table 18.3). Assess volume status. A full test for orthostatic hypotension is not possible, but a blood pressure change from supine to sitting might be detected. Skin turgor is unreliable in the elderly. A urine-specific gravity at admission is a fair test of both volume and renal-concentrating ability, since associated hemorrhage will call into play aldosterone and antidiuretic hormone. Blood (500–1500 cc) will be lost into the thigh. The thirst mechanism of the elderly often does not function well. Adequate replacement, either self-induced or by intravenous fluid, results in hematocrit values of about 30%.

A careful neurologic examination is important. The spectrum of postoperative confusion, fat emboli, or cerebral vascular accident is most accurately evaluated if a good baseline has been recorded.

The old lung provides good soil for pathogens. Properly performed, the best preoperative test of pulmonary function is the maximum breathing capacity since it tests not only volumes but the entire mechanical willingness of the lungs and the patient's ability to generate an effective cough. A value of less than 40 liters per minute almost surely predicts trouble. Measurement of arterial blood gases is mandatory in elderly or debilitated patients. If the patient is a chronic bronchitic or is producing any sputum, gram stain or culture may guide subsequent antibiotic therapy if pneumonia appears.

In addition to examining for congestive heart failure by physical and chest x-ray, a long rhythm strip with a standard lead cardiogram is important. Note carefully the presence/absence of peripheral pulses, again for subsequent reference.

Most patients are well served by bladder catheterization for evaluation of fluid volumes and comfort. Initial specimens should be cultured even if the total amount of organisms is small. Sepsis and urinary tract infections are frequent enough to merit this, but scrupulous care of the catheter is also demanded.

Rotten teeth may break with intubation. Full stomach contents might wind up in the airways. If preoperative nasogastric suction is required, give some antacids prior to the procedure so that "lung burn" will be avoided if gastric contents are aspirated.

Whether and When to Operate

There are no good data on matched patients treated surgically and treated conservatively. The mortality of the non-operated group is alleged to be higher, but this is probably because other serious conditions precluded surgery. In some cases, a conservative approach is fully justified.

There probably is an optimum time for surgery. This is not an emergency procedure. In fact, mortality is higher in patients taken directly from the emergency room to the surgical suite. Surgery from 24–48 hours after admission allows sufficient time to correct volume status, digitalize if necessary, and stabilize diabetes or other medical problems.

Operative Care

The choice of anesthesia is, of course, a decision for the anesthesiologist. The conventional wisdom of regional anesthesia as the safest may not be true. Hypotension is probably more common, agitation and anxiety may be greater, and pulmonary toilet is much more difficult.

The only common intraoperative complication is hypotension. Adequate volume replacement with colloid and crystalloid is the best prophylaxis.

There is evidence now that prophylactic antibiotics are effective in reducing the incidence of **wound infections.** Nafcillin 500 mg intravenously preoperatively and every 6 hours for 2 days has been recommended. There is no documented beneficial effect on mortality or for morbidity other than wound infection (9).

Low-dose heparin as thromboembolic prophylaxis is ineffective. Clot begins to form shortly after the fracture, and there is far too much activated Factor X to be influenced by the inhibitor stimulated by low-dose heparin. Full anticoagulation has not been shown to be effective in this group and the attendant bleeding complications suggest that this should not be done as a routine measure.

Postoperative Care

Fifty per cent of the patients will develop a fever. Half of these will be pyogenic. All absolutely unnecessary drugs should be avoided from the outset to minimize the confusion with drug reactions. The next most common cause is blood transfusions.

The common pneumonia often has few clinical signs other than fever. Sputum examination offers the best diagnostic hope.

Pulmonary emboli cause 15–30% of the deaths and are present in 50% or more of the autopsied cases of hip fracture. Vigilance and early ambulation remain the best approach (Table 18.4).

A relaxation of clinical scrutiny sets in after the first week. In fact, this is the most dangerous time. The conscientious medical consultant will reexamine the patient with particular care at this time.

Table 18.4.   Hip Fracture: Postoperative Complications

1. Fever (all sources)	50%
2. Intra- and immediate postoperative hypotension	20%
3. Altered mentation	14%
4. Infection: lung, bladder, wound	16%
5. GI bleeding	6%
6. Acute renal failure	4%
7. Congestive heart failure (uncompensated)	2%
8. Pulmonary embolism (clinically evident)	2%

JOINT REPLACEMENTS

Approximately 90,000 total hip replacements (THR) will be performed this year. This major surgical advance regularly yields a high quality, functional result. The primary indications are pain, diminished range of motion, and altered mechanics, producing disability and damage to other joints. Major complications of the procedure are thromboembolic disease, sepsis, dislocation of the prosthesis, and heterotropic ossification (particularly in patients with ankylosing spondylitis). Surgical success has been assisted by prudent management of concomitant medical problems. Still, one-fourth of these patients will have medical complications during hospitalization (Table 18.5). Unlike fractured hips, young patients with THR seem to have higher morbidity than the old (65% of patients with complications are under 60 and 35% over 60; perhaps proof that advanced years testify to

Table 18.5.   Medical Complications of Total Hip Replacement

Urinary retention and/or infection	22%
Thrombophlebitis (clinically evident)	13%
Pneumonia/atelectasis	10%
Pulmonary embolus (clinically evident)	6%
GI bleeding	4%
Myocardial infarction	1.6%
Wound infection	1.3%
Death	1.0%

durability, although many of the younger THR patients have chronic systemic diseases, i.e., rheumatoid arthritis, or trauma).

Flushed with success with hip surgery, our orthopaedic colleagues now replace knees and less often ankles, shoulders, elbows, wrists, and fingers. As the techniques improve, these will become more frequent.

With all of these procedures, it is well to recall that none are emergency or even urgent. All are elective. There is no magic point beyond which a hip cannot be replaced. Utilization review and surgical schedules notwithstanding, there is no excuse for allowing surgery on a poorly prepared patient.

The mortality of THR, unlike hip fracture surgery, is low (0.5–2.8%). Not surprisingly, pulmonary embolus leads the list of fatal complications (1%). There are few clinical predictors of this complication. Obesity and previous thrombophlebitis correlate with the development of phlebitis but not with pulmonary embolus. Osteoarthritis (rather than rheumatoid arthritis), age over 60, and congestive heart failure are factors that increase risk (Table 18.6).

No group of medical specialists is more concerned with embolic prophylaxis than orthopaedic surgeons. Espousal and disavowal of various prophylactic anticoagulation programs is emphatic and it is unlikely that you will influence the surgeon's personal choice of program. The combination of heparin and dihydroergotamine is supported by studies from Great Britain (12). Low-molecular-weight dextran interferes with platelet function and fibrin bridging. In our experience, dextran causes the highest postoperative bleeding (16%), and full-dose heparin or warfarin combined with aspirin or dextran also caused excessive bleeding (15–25%). Full warfarin dosage provided the best protection and fewest bleeding episodes in our institution. Hydroxychloroquin has also been used in Great Britain

Table 18.6. Correlation of Selected Factors in THR Patients with Pulmonary Embolism (PE), Thrombophlebitis (T), and Medical Morbidity (MM)[a]

	Correlates	Does not Correlate
Age > 60	PE	T, MM
Weight (>20% above ideal)		T, PE, MM
Smoking		PE
Venous varicosities		PE, T
Previous pulmonary embolism		T, PE
Previous thrombophlebitis	T, MM	PE
Abnormal BUN and creatinine	MM	PE

[a] From Anderson L, Kammerer WS, Greer RB: *Clin Orthop Relat Res* 141:53, 1979. Used with permission.

with apparent success. In one series of over 2000 total hip replacements, hydroxychloroquin provided statistically significant improvement over low-dose heparin or low-molecular-weight dextran (see Chapter 9).

A recent randomized controlled study of low-molecular-weight heparin showed significant reduction of proximal vein thrombosis compared to placebo controls. In addition there was no increase in bleeding complications (11).

Total knee replacements are also complicated by thrombosis. Because the procedure includes the application of a tourniquet, thrombosis below the knee is almost the rule (57% of those receiving heparin prophylaxis and 72% of those treated only with aspirin) (10). It has been concluded in several studies that prophylaxis is indicated but that full anticoagulation postoperatively is only for those with clots extending into the thigh.

An undocumented portent of danger of pulmonary embolism is an abnormally short prothrombin time and/or short partial thromboplastin time detected preoperatively. Patients in congestive heart failure should be optimally compensated prior to surgery to help reduce the risk of emboli.

Superficial wound infection occurs in 1.3% of patients. Local measures and appropriate antibiotics are effective within 7 days. Prophylaxis with perioperative antibiotics reduces the risk of deep wound infection and the effects of ultra-clean air are additive (9).

Deep wound sepsis occurs in 1% of total hip replacements. Curiously, half of these appear between 3 months and 2 years of surgery, strongly implicating hematogenous seeding. Of the 87 cases of prosthetic joint infection reported since 1975, 52 had established infections elsewhere, generally in the urinary and respiratory tract. The majority of pathogens were *Staphylococcus,* few of which were sensitive to penicillin. The usual prophylactic program recommended for patients with valvular heart disease may be inadequate. Europeans enjoy success with gentamicin-impregnated methyl methacrylate (the bone cement for the prosthesis), but this has not yet been approved by the Food and Drug Administration (FDA).

Infections will occur in 12% of patients. The most common site is the urinary tract. Prolonged postoperative bladder infection may provide the source of sepsis for the hip. No patient should go to the operating room with an untreated urinary tract infection. Bladder catheterization causes most postoperative genitourinary tract infections. Three-way catheter systems are effective but resisted because of staff time required. Preoperative prostatism presages postoperative obstruction. Too many patients enter the hospital to have a hip replacement and leave, having not only a prosthetic hip but also a transurethral prostatectomy. Better to have a planned sequence.

An important indicator of medical morbidity is an elevated blood urea nitrogen (BUN) or creatinine. Such patients have more (but not specific) complications of surgery.

Myocardial infarctions or congestive heart failure will occur in 2% of patients. A previous myocardial infarction within 3-6 months is cause to postpone surgery since the risk of a perioperative myocardial infarction (MI) is 6%. The average intraoperative blood loss is 1500 ml and this needs to be adequately replaced. The intake and output sheet assumes great importance in both the patient with cardiac or renal disease.

Prosthetic joints attract infectious agents just as do damaged or prosthetic heart valves. Patients admitted to the hospital for potentially "dirty" surgery require prophylaxis to avoid late joint infection. The generally suggested program differs somewhat from heart valve prophylaxis (Table 18.7).

Table 18.7.   Antibiotic Prophylaxis for Patients with Prosthetic Joints

---

I. Oropharyngeal Procedures
   A. Procaine penicillin G 1.2 million units IM 30–60 min prior to procedure then penicillin V 500 mg PO q 6 hr × 8
   B. If allergic to penicillin, use clindamycin 1.2 gm IM 60 min prior to surgery, then 300 mg PO q 4 hr × 8
II. Genitourinary or gastrointestinal procedures (1st dose 1 hr before procedure)
   A. Ampicillin 1.0 gm IM/IV q 8 hr × 3, plus gentamicin 1.0 mg/kg (not to exceed 80 mg) q 8 hr × 3 or streptomycin 1.0 gm q 12 hr × 3
   B. If allergic to penicillin, use vancomycin 1.0 gm IV q 8 hr × 3 plus streptomycin as above
III. Procedures on infected tissue (variable depending on anticipated pathogens). For *Staphylococcus aureus,* 1st dose 1 hr before procedure
   A. Nafcillin 2.0 gms IM/IV, then dicloxacillin 500 mg PO q 6 hr × 8
   B. Or Cefazolin 1.0 gm IM/IV, then cephalexin 500 mg PO q 6 hr × 8
   C. Or Clindamycin 1.2 gm IM/IV, then 300 mg PO q 6 hr × 8

OUTPATIENT EVALUATION

The emphasis on shortened hospital stays has moved much of the preoperative evaluation for elective surgery to the outpatient office. In addition to any special studies dictated by the particular circumstances, attention should focus on:

A. Indolent infection, particularly urinary tract
B. Renal function
C. Hematologic parameters, especially clotting studies and prior history of deep vein thrombosis (DVT)
D. Cardiovascular compensation
E. Drug review, particularly **estrogen.**

Operating room schedules and scheduled admission dates notwithstanding, total joint replacement is a totally elective procedure.

FAT EMBOLIZATION

Fractures of long bones, burns, and rapid decompression sickness predispose to fat embolism. Perhaps 5% of deaths from multiple trauma are caused by fat embolism. When recognized clinically, this syndrome carries a 15% mortality.

The usual clinical picture consists of rapidly progressive respiratory embarrassment, trunkal and retinal petechiae, fat globules in the blood and urine, a rising serum lipase, and electrocardiographic changes of acute right heart strain. Thrombocytopenia, anemia, and pyrexia soon follow. Central nervous system changes ranging from confusion to stupor are common. The most consistent clinical findings include tachycardia, tachypnea, pyrexia, central nervous system changes, and significant hypoxemia (pO_2 below 50 mm Hg).

The mainstay of therapy consist of respiratory support to ensure adequate oxygenation. Corticosteroids are used to reduce cerebral edema, to preserve platelets, and to blunt the effect of vasoactive substances on the lungs. Alcohol, heparin, and dextran have all been shown to be ineffective and may even be contraindicated.

RHEUMATOLOGY CONSIDERATIONS IN SURGICAL PATIENTS

Drugs

Almost all patients with rheumatic diseases will be admitted to hospital taking at least one drug. Perioperative problems with corticosteroids are covered in Chapter 13.

The analgesics and anti-inflammatory drugs share certain characteristics worth remembering in dealing with surgical patients. Almost all have an effect on prostaglandins and may thereby alter renal function with resultant fluid accumulation. Congestive heart failure may be the unhappy consequence.

These drugs also have variable effects on the clotting scheme. It is best to consult standard references regarding particular agents and their interference with coumadin use and their effects on platelets (see also Chapter 13).

Most of these drugs are unavailable in parenteral form, and their use is therefore precluded in the patient who can have nothing by mouth (NPO).

The only available rheumatic medications for parenteral use are corticosteroids, gold, and colchicine. Parenteral analgesics may be used to control pain but will not provide anti-inflammatory effect.

There is no unanimity of opinion regarding the effect of prolonged bedrest on patients with rheumatic diseases. Although the potential for stress-induced flare in any particular joint may be decreased, the known effects of calcium loss from bone, flexion contractures, and muscle wasting are clearly detrimental. If prolonged post-operative bedrest is anticipated, early involvement of the physical therapy department should be part of the preoperative planning. Range of motion exercise devices and splints are available to maintain muscle tone and delay or prevent contractures.

Postoperative acute flares of arthritis may be infectious in etiology. It is unwise to assume that they are always the result of the underlying arthritis. This especially pertains to contaminated surgery, where an abnormal or artificial joint provides the same attractiveness to circulating bacteria as a diseased or artificial heart valve. Compounding the diagnostic dilemma of infection in a joint (or elsewhere) is the frequent state of immunosuppression that exists in patients with long-standing rheumatic diseases treated with corticosteroids and/or cytotoxic agents.

Recent studies conclude that 17% of patients taking at least eight aspirin a day for 3 months or more will have **gastric ulcers** and 40% will have gastric erosions. The treacherous fact is that fully one-third of the ulcers will be asymptomatic. The risk, then, of upper gastrointestinal bleeding with the additional stress from a surgical procedure becomes a real concern. The role of cimetidine in such patients (i.e., not diagnosed as having a lesion, but at risk for it) has not been established. Antacid therapy is prudent.

One of the fatal complications of rheumatoid arthritis is atlanto-occipital subluxation. Surgical procedures requiring hyperextension of the neck, such as rigid bronchoscopy, may be hazardous because of instability of the atlantoaxial joint. Preoperative neck films (lateral views in flexion and extension) should be part of the preoperative evaluation in such patients. Similarly, endotracheal intubation may prove difficult in patients with ankylosing spondylitis who have become fused in the cervical spine. Respiratory insufficiency may occur due to rheumatoid lung disease or restricted mobility of the rib cage. In addition, several other anatomic and physiologic changes of rheumatoid arthritis, as summarized in Table 18.8, can complicate perioperative and anesthetic management. The anesthesiologist is well served when alerted to these potential problems.

Crystal-induced Arthritis

Surgery has long been recognized as a precipitant for acute gout. Likewise, the acute inflammation of pseudogout (chondrocalcinosis) may appear in the postoperative period. We have found that the event is more likely to occur 5–7 days after surgery.

The definitive diagnostic procedure is examination of synovial fluid, with attention to the presence of birefringent crystals characteristic of the disease: weakly positive blunt rods and rhomboids of calcium pyrophosphate or strongly negative birefringent needles of sodium urate crystals. The synovial analysis is also important to exclude septic arthritis.

Colchicine may be used as a diagnostic test if synovial fluid is not available. Two milligrams intravenously will provide prompt (24 hours) relief from gout. It may have a mild effect on pseudogout. Thereafter, the treatment of choice for either disorder in the acute phase is indomethacin.

The most important therapy is prophylaxis. For most patients with this problem there is an appropriate past history. Medications stopped for surgery are often forgotten postoperatively and the attack occurs.

Felty's Syndrome

Patients with rheumatoid arthritis may display this syndrome of splenomegaly and granulocytopenia. As a group, they are susceptible to infection but the correlation between the level of depression of white cells and that risk is poor. The best guide in evaluating the individual patient is the past history. A low white count with no history of recurrent infection should not call for extra measures (e.g., splenectomy, prophylactic antibiotics) through pregnancy or surgery. However, those with frequent infections re-

Table 18.8.   Anaesthetic Hazards in Patients with Rheumatoid Arthritis[a]

Respiratory	
Airway	Ventilation
Hypoplastic mandible	Rheumatoid nodules in lung
Temperomandibular ankylosis	Chronic diffuse interstitial fibrosis
Restriction cervical spine motion	Caplan's syndrome
Atlantoaxial subluxation	Costovertebral joints
Low cervical subluxation	Thoracic vertebrae flexion deformity
Cricoarytenoid arthritis	Tuberculous lung
Laryngeal tissue damage	

Cardiovascular
Pericardial, myocardial, coronary arteries
Aortic valve-regurgitation
Arrhythmias
Disseminating necrotizing arteritis

Haemopoietic, Hepatic, and Renal
Anemia
Leukopenia
Bleeding tendency (decreased platelets)
Renal amyloidosis

Posture
Skin fragility
Postoperative chest complications
Multiple joint disease
Recent surgical site healing

[a] Adapted from Jenkins and McGraw (11) by permission.

quire very careful culture techniques, prophylactic antibiotics, and may respond to splenectomy, although the leukopenia may recur. The predictability of success with splenectomy for any one individual, however, is not great enough to justify the additional surgical risk of performing a splenectomy at the time of other indicated surgery, even if it is associated with a high incidence of infection.

Shoulder Hand Syndrome

This is the most common reflex neurovascular dystrophy. Twenty per cent of these cases occur after myocardial infarction and 20% are complications of cervical spine disease. The onset may be insidious or acute and is characterized by marked vasomotor instability with variable pallor, erythema, livedo reticularis, and swelling. The pain is diffuse and poorly localized and is shortly followed by rapid, significant osteoporosis of the bones of the upper extremity. The best treatment is vigorous physical therapy, analgesics for pain, and occasionally neural blockade. Corticosteroids or indocin are also frequently of great help.

READINGS

1. Coventry MB, Beckenbaugh RD, Nolan DR, et al.: 2,012 total hip arthroplasties: A study of postoperative course and early complications. *J Bone Joint Surg* 56A:273–284, 1974.
2. Dines DE, Burgher LW, Okazaki H: The clinical and pathologic correlation of fat embolism syndrome. *Mayo Clinic Proc* 50:407–411, 1975.
3. Fitzgerald RH: Laboratory diagnosis of postoperative sepsis of the musculoskeletal system. *Orthop Clin North Am* 10:361–374, 1979.
4. Harris WH: Total joint replacement. *N Engl J Med* 297:650–651, 1977.
5. Jenkins LC, McGraw RW: Anaesthetic management of the patient with rheumatoid arthritis. *Can Anaesth Soc J* 16:407–415, 1969.
6. Lattimer GL, Keblish PA, Dickson TB, et al.: Hematogenous infection in total joint replacement. Recommendations for prophylactic antibiotics. *JAMA* 242:2213–2214, 1979.
7. Liang MH, Cullen KE, Poss R: Primary total hip or knee replacement: Evaluation of patients. *Ann Int Med* 97:735–739, 1982.
8. Lyon LJ, Nevins MA: Non-treatment of hip fractures in senile patients. *JAMA* 238:1175–1176, 1977
9. Norden CW: Prevention of bone and joint infections. *Am J Med* 78(Sup B):229–234, 1985.
10. Stulberg BN, Insall JN, Williams GW, et al.: Deep-vein thrombosis following total knee replacement. *J Bone Joint Surg* 66(2):194–201, 1984.
11. Turpie AGG, Levine MN, Hirsh J, et al.: A randomized controlled trial of a low-molecular-weight heparin (enoxaparin) to prevent deep-vein thrombosis in patients undergoing elective hip surgery. *N Engl J Med* 315:925–929, 1986.
12. Kakkar VV, Fok PJ, Murray WJG, et al.: Heparin and dihydroergotamine prophylaxis against thrombo-embolism after hip arthroplasty. *J Bone Joint Surg* 67B:538–542, 1985.

19

Neurologic Conditions in the Perioperative Setting

Lourdes C. Corman

Internists are often asked to evaluate patients preoperatively who give a history of prior stroke or transient ischemic attacks (TIA), or in whom an incidental cervical bruit is identified prior to the surgical procedure. Patients with epilepsy, dementia, myasthenia gravis, and other neurologic illnesses also present for preoperative evaluation. Surgical risk in these patients, as in others, is best defined by the patient's overall health; their cardiac and respiratory status; the type, extent, and urgency of the surgical procedure; the quality of operative and perioperative care; and the patient's age. In addition, the neurologic condition may increase perioperative risks and merit special precautions or considerations. In the postoperative period, new onset of seizures, altered mental status, stroke, or a peripheral nerve palsy may develop even in patients without prior neurologic findings. This chapter will focus on the identification and management of these conditions in the perioperative period.

PREOPERATIVE EVALUATION AND PERIOPERATIVE RISKS OF PATIENTS WITH PREEXISTING NEUROLOGIC CONDITIONS

Risks Associated With Cerebrovascular Disease

The diagnosis of cerebrovascular disease is apparent in the patient with a permanent hemiparesis or some other obvious result of cerebral infarction. More commonly, cerebrovascular disease may be present but silent. In these instances, its presence may only be surmised by a history suggestive of a prior stroke or TIA, or an associated marker like a cervical bruit. In any patient with signs or symptoms of cerebrovascular disease presenting for elective surgery, the most important questions to answer are similar to those posed by any non-neurologic condition. These include (*a*) How stable is the patient's clinical condition? (*b*) Can it be further stabilized or improved prior to the scheduled surgery? (*c*) What changes need to be made in the patient's surgical and anesthetic care? (*d*) What postoperative complications are most likely to occur? Can they be prevented? (*e*) If a TIA or stroke is present, What is the most likely cause, and therefore, the best treatment? and (*f*) How long should a patient with a recent stroke wait before undergoing surgery?

Patients with cerebrovascular disease by definition, are considered at risk for stroke even in the absence of any surgical intervention. When undergoing surgery, their postoperative risks are likewise related to their widespread atherosclerosis. Cerebral or myocardial infarction, or death from either, are the most dreaded postoperative complications. Although other postoperative neurologic complications are discussed later in this chapter, perioperative stroke might best be discussed in the context of perioperative risks in patients with known or suspected cerebrovascular disease. These patients must also be carefully evaluated and treated for cardiovascular disease since these two conditions *always* coexist. In fact, a history of prior stroke has been reported as one of five independent risk factors for the development of postoperative cardiac complications (1).

PERIOPERATIVE STROKES

Perioperative strokes occur in two distinct time periods: early (within 5 days of surgery) or late (5 days to 2 years after the operation). Most early strokes are reported within the first 2–5 days after surgery rather than during the surgical procedure (2, 3). However, others have described 70% of all early strokes as occurring in the intraoperative period (4, 5). These discrepancies may reflect intercontinental methodologic differences in collection of data, patient population, surgical technique and/or reporting. Early strokes are usually embolic and only rarely secondary to occlusion or hypoperfusion of the extracranial carotid arteries (2, 6, 7). The mortality of early postoperative stroke has been reported as high as 29% in retrospective reviews (5), probably because only patients with major deficits are identified retrospectively.

Patients undergoing peripheral vascular reconstructive surgery or coronary artery bypass surgery may also develop a stroke during the 2 years following the procedure. These late strokes are more likely a result of widespread atherosclerotic disease present in these patients than due to the earlier surgery.

The incidence of early postoperative stroke in patients who survive the surgical procedure is reviewed in Table 19.1. Only series published after 1979 are included (5, 8–16). It is well to remember that most of these figures are generated from the patients who survived the procedure. Therefore, the combined overall stroke morbidity and mortality may be as much as 1–2% higher than the values quoted in Table 19.1, depending on the surgical center. As can be seen, postoperative stroke is uncommon in association with nonvascular surgery, even in the elderly (8). Among all surgical procedures, carotid artery surgery and cardiac valvular replacement have the highest risk

Table 19.1.   Incidence of Early Postoperative Stroke Among Survivors

Series Author/Year		Type of Surgery (reported mortality)	# of Patients	% Stroke (*includes TIAs)
Goldman 1979	P[a]	general and vascular, excluding cardiac, carotid, and neurologic	617	0.16
Turnipseed 1980	P	peripheral vascular,	160	3.1
		coronary	170	4.7
Barnes 1981	P	vascular or coronary, excluding carotid (mortality = 2.2%)	449	1.1
Ropper 1982	P	general and vascular, excluding carotid, coronary, and neurologic	568	0
		coronary	167	3.0
Bojar 1983	R	coronary (mortality 2.8%)	3,206	1.0
Coffey 1983	R	coronary	1,669	0.8
Breuer 1983	R	coronary	421	5.2*
Jones 1984	R	coronary plus carotid (mortality = 3%)	132	1.6
		coronary only (mortality = 0.6%)	167	0.6
Parker 1985	R	coronary	893	0.9
Taylor 1987	P	coronary (mortality = 2.4%)	453	2.2
Reed 1988	R	coronary	5,915	0.9

[a]P = prospective study; R = retrospective study. Postoperative period is defined as duration of hospitalization or the first 31 days in the postoperative period.

of neurologic complications including stroke (15). Patients with valvular heart disease are at a higher risk of stroke even in the absence of surgery because of the high prevalence of arrhythmias and intracardiac thrombi associated with the valvular disease, so it is not surprising that their postoperative risk of stroke is also higher.

Stroke following peripheral arterial surgery has been reported as low as 0 (11) and as high as 4.3% (9) and is probably less than 1% (see Table 19.1). **Stroke in association with coronary bypass** has ranged from 4.7% (9) to as low as 0.6% in otherwise well patients (13). It is most likely between 0.5 and 3.0%. Among patients undergoing less invasive procedures, 0.2% had a stroke following **percutaneous transluminal coronary angioplasty** (16). Patients with aortic stenosis undergoing **balloon aortic valvuloplasty** had a hospital mortality rate of 3.5% and a stroke rate of 0.6% (17). Among **patients over age 80 undergoing open heart surgery** for coronary or valvular disease, 3% developed a stroke and two of the three patients died (18). Overall early mortality was 29%. These findings confirm the high risk of open heart surgery in this age group and the low but definite risk of stroke and associated high mortality in survivors.

Risk factors for perioperative stroke included older age, presence of a carotid bruit, and extent of grossly obvious atheromatous disease of the ascending aorta at the time of aortic cannulation in a retrospective study of patients undergoing coronary artery bypass grafting. Diabetes, hypertension, and prior neurological symptoms were not (13). In Breuer's prospective study of over 400 patients, on the other hand, none of the several hundred variables, including those listed above, were found to be risk factors (19). **Cardiopulmonary bypass in and of itself appears to be a major risk factor for perioperative stroke.** Embolization of polyvinyl tubing, silicone, or air

(introduced by the machine) have been found at autopsy (20) Atherothrombotic emboli from the cross-clamped aorta has been thought a bigger culprit than the similarly affected carotid artery (7). As one might have expected from this data, improvements in surgical and anesthetic techniques, and technical modifications of the cardiopulmonary bypass unit have greatly improved outcome and contributed to the lower incidence of stroke in recent series.

CERVICAL BRUIT AND THE RISK OF POSTOPERATIVE STROKE

A cervical bruit was first described by C.M. Fisher in the early 1950s as indicative of increased flow over the artery contralateral to an occluded carotid. Since then, the presence of a cervical bruit has been correctly viewed as a marker for increased risk of future stroke. In adult populations, the prevalence of a cervical bruit is close to 5%, and appears to increase with increasing age in women, and in persons with hypertension (21). Among adults in the fourth decade or older, the incidence of cervical bruits increases when the underlying carotid is stenosed or occluded, but the reported frequencies of underlying abnormalities of the vessels vary greatly. In fact, the presence of a cervical bruit by itself is *not* a reliable indicator of occlusive disease of the ipsilateral or contralateral carotid arteries (22).

The natural history of asymptomatic cervical bruits has been clarified since the last edition of this book. Sixteen hundred residents of Evans County, Georgia over age 45 (without prior stroke) were followed prospectively. The incidence of stroke was 31.9% among subjects with bruits compared to 3.4% among subjects without a bruit (21). However, the stroke was ipsilateral to the bruit in only one-third of the cases, and the presence of a bruit was as good (or better) a marker for cardiac morbidity. This role of the cervical bruit as a marker of ischemic cardiac disease has been confirmed in several studies (23–25). In the Framingham cohort, the presence of a carotid bruit was an indicator of increased risk for stroke, myocardial infarction, and death, rather than an indicator of ipsilateral arterial stenosis leading to cerebral infarction (25).

Another recent study followed 500 asymptomatic patients with cervical bruits with clinical and Doppler ultrasonographic assessments. At 1 year, the incidence of cardiac ischemic events and death were 7% and 4% respectively, and that of TIA plus stroke 6%. The overall incidence of stroke at 1 year was 1.7%, and these usually occurred after warning TIAs. The degree of carotid artery stenosis at initial presentation and the rate of progression of stenosis of the carotid artery were powerful predictors of neurologic sequelae. However, less than half of those in whom the stenosis progressed to complete occlusion became symptomatic (24). Again, what was most striking was that cardiac ischemic events, cardiac death, and sudden death were even more common than TIA or stroke in this population. From this data, it has been estimated that the risk of disabling stroke occurring without prior warning TIAs is less than 2% (21, 24, 26). Given this knowledge, there is no rationale for the recommendation of carotid endarterectomy to treat asymptomatic patients with cervical bruits. Even in the best of hands, the incidence of mortality and stroke associated with endarterectomy is around 2%. To this, one must add the risk of angiography, which also hovers at 0.5–2% (27, 27a), although Duplex ultrasound is probably more accurate (28), and may eventually eliminate the need for angiography.

The contribution of a cervical bruit in asymptomatic patients to the risk of postoperative stroke is reviewed in Table 19.2. As can be seen, a cervical bruit may be associated with a minimal to no increased risk of stroke (29). In the most recent retrospective case control study reported, the absolute risk of postoperative stroke associated with presence of a bruit was small, while the odds ratio was 3.9. This odds ratio was higher than had been shown earlier in two other retrospective studies (5, 30). In contrast, the odds ratio in prospective studies were 0.7, 1.5, and 1.5 (9, 11, 19). Prophylactic endarterectomy in this group of patients is unlikely to prevent strokes and is much more likely to cause them.

Evidence of obstruction of the cervical carotid by Doppler sonogram identifies a

Table 19.2.   Incidence of Early Postoperative Stroke Among Survivors With or Without a Cervical Bruit

Series Author/Year		Surgery	% Stroke			
			Bruit	Present	Bruit	Absent
Turnipseed 1980 P[c]		vascular or coronary	6	(6/98)	4.3	(10/232)
		vascular only	5.6	(4/70)	3.3	(3/90)
		coronary only	7.1	(2/28)	4.0	(7/142)
Barnes 1981	P	vascular or coronary	?	(0/28)[a]	?	(0/92)[a]
Breslau 1981	P	coronary	?	(0/18)[a]	3	(2/72)
Martin 1982	R	coronary	7.0	(1/14)	3	(7/245)
Ropper 1982	P	vascular or coronary	2.7	(1/37)[b]	3.1	(4/130)
		all surgery	1.0	(1/104)	0.6	(4/631)
Jones 1984	R	coronary	3.3	(2/60)	unstated	

[a]True incidence is indeterminate.
[b]Some patients with bruits were symptomatic.
[c]P = prospective studies; R = retrospective studies; postoperative period is defined as duration of hospitalization or the first 31 days in the postoperative period.

group of patients at higher risk of perioperative stroke (3.5%) and death (10.6%) compared to patients without a cervical bruit or with a cervical bruit but with a normal sonogram (stroke 0.5%, death 0.3%) (31). However, even in patients thus identified, there was no evidence that prophylactic endarterectomy would improve outcome, since only one patient developed a stroke in the territory corresponding to the obstruction, and this occurred following cardiac arrest during induction of anesthesia for coronary surgery (31). In actuality, even confirmed extracranial carotid stenosis that is asymptomatic fails to increase the risk of ipsilateral perioperative stroke (7).

In patients undergoing coronary artery bypass surgery, the risk of early and late strokes is considered high, and prophylactic carotid endarterectomy has been advocated in this setting as well. Protocols calling for carotid endarterectomy prior to scheduled coronary bypass have been associated with prohibitive morbidity and mortality from postoperative myocardial infarction (31). The current trend in some centers is to perform simultaneous coronary bypass and carotid endarterectomy in all patients with cervical bruits scheduled for coronary surgery. In other centers, this approach is limited to patients with symptoms or findings (by non-invasive means) of significant stenosis of the extracranial carotid arteries. The data to support either of these practices is exceedingly weak. Most postoperative strokes are embolic and unrelated to disease of the carotid arteries (2). Studies of cerebral blood flow have shown that neither the percent stenosis nor the residual lumen is a reliable indicator of the hemodynamic status of the cerebral circulation (32). This is most likely the reason why preoperative non-invasive screening was not found helpful by Breslau et al. (33). As noted earlier, combined cardiac and carotid surgery only succeeds in adding the short-term risk of stroke and death from carotid endarterectomy to

the risks of death and stroke associated with coronary bypass (13). Since most patients with strokes have warning TIAs, close follow-up of patients after their vascular or coronary surgery appears to be the best approach. Carotid endarterectomy should be reserved for patients who develop neurovascular symptoms that appear due to lesions of the cervical carotid.

THE PATIENT WITH PREVIOUS STROKE OR TIA

The postoperative stroke risk in patients with a previous stroke or TIA may be higher than in those without (11, 13, 30), as can be seen in Table 19.3, but this has not always been confirmed (9, 19).

Establishing the cause or source of the prior stroke or TIA is helpful in identifying the most appropriate treatment. In a postoperative setting, new onset of atrial fibrillation is associated with increased risk of stroke (30). In a nonsurgical setting, multiple processes may result in a stroke, but the most common etiology is thromboembolic infarction secondary to atherosclerosis and hypertension (34). Classification of the stroke as thrombotic, embolic, or lacunar helps define the prognosis and treatment. For example, a lacunar infarction usually involves small areas in the deep substance of the brain, occurs in patients with hypertension, should be treated by vigorous control of the blood pressure, and as a rule, is associated with good recovery. Embolism from a cardiac source in association with abnormal heart rhythms or valvular disease requires evaluation to determine the need for antiarrhythmic medication, anticoagulation, and/or valvular replacement, and prognosis is more serious. Strokes secondary to intracerebral bleeding account for approximately one-fifth of all strokes and are usually catastrophic. On the other hand, embolism from an atheromatous plaque in the cervical carotid, or a transient neurologic deficit occurring in association with stenosis or occlusion of the ipsilateral artery has a varied prognosis. In this setting,

Table 19.3. Incidence of Early Postoperative Stroke in Survivors With or Without a History of Prior Stroke, TIA, or Carotid Endarterectomy (CE)

Series Author/Year		Surgery	% Postoperative Stroke	
			+ History	− History
Turnipseed 1980	P[a]	vascular or coronary excluding carotid	2.7 (3/108)	5.9 (13/222)
Ropper 1982	P	non-neurologic or vascular excluding carotid	3 (1/32)	0.6 (4/703)
Jones 1984	R	coronary	8.6[b]	0.9[c]
		coronary (prior CE)	(5.1)[d]	

[a]P = prospective studies; R = retrospective studies; postoperative period is defined as duration of hospitalization or the first 31 days in the postoperative period.
[b]Stroke incidence in 70 patients with a history of stroke or TIA.
[c]Stroke incidence in 5,675 patients. Some of the 51 patients who developed a stroke had a prior neurological symptom.
[d]Stroke incidence in 39 patients with a history of prior carotid endarterectomy. Indication for endarterectomy not given.

carotid endarterectomy may be indicated although its efficacy is not firmly established.

In the patient with a known prior stroke, there are no definitive data available establishing how long to wait after the stroke before proceeding with nonneurologic surgery. It is reasonable to expect that delaying nonemergency surgery should result in a more clinically stable patient population that, by definition, would include only those patients well enough to stabilize and survive the acute stroke. An acceptable waiting period is 6–12 weeks since the clinical condition has often been established by then. However, this can (and should) be modified as necessary for each patient, depending on the type of surgery contemplated and how urgently it is needed.

Therapy for postoperative stroke appears to have little impact on final outcome, and consists mainly of treating any associated conditions like arrhythmias. Although heparin started within 48 hours of the onset of stroke symptoms in a nonsurgical setting has not been helpful, in postoperative strokes it may be useful if started early since the pathogenesis of these strokes is often embolic (7). Unfor-

tunately, its use would be limited by the risk of bleeding from the surgical wound. Other therapeutic modalities may yet emerge for acute perioperative stroke, including calcium channel blockers, and hemodilution (35), but in general, meticulous anesthetic, surgical, and medical management in the intra- and perioperative period offer the best treatment. Our recommendations for the perioperative care of patients with cerebrovascular disease are summarized in Table 19.4

Patients on antiplatelet therapy with aspirin and/or dipyridamole, or on warfarin for TIAs may require discontinuation of treatment 1 week prior to their scheduled elective surgery, if the scheduled surgery is associated with a high risk of bleeding in a critical anatomic site. Otherwise antiplatelet therapy is best continued until 2–3 days prior to surgery. Warfarin may also be discontinued 24–48 hours before surgery, and its anticoagulation effect can be reversed by oral or parenteral vitamin K.

In symptomatic patients, or those with a cervical bruit that you wish to evaluate further, Duplex ultrasound is the preferred method of evaluation. It is a combination of pulsed echo or B-mode ultra-

Table 19.4. Recommendations for the Perioperative Management of Patients with Cerebrovascular Disease

1. In a patient with recent stroke or TIA, establish the most likely etiology and treat appropriately. Whenever possible, delay elective surgery until the neurologic status has stabilized and maximum recovery of function has occurred. This usually means a minimum of 6–12 weeks.
2. For patients with stroke-in-evolution, postpone surgery and institute appropriate medical treatment until stable.
3. Patients with an asymptomatic cervical bruit should be assessed for evidence of generalized atherosclerosis. Prophylactic carotid endarterectomy prior to scheduled surgery is not indicated.
4. There is no evidence to support the common practice of simultaneous or staged carotid endarterectomy and coronary artery bypass graft in asymptomatic patients.
5. Bedridden patients or patients who are likely to be confined to bed postoperatively should receive appropriate prophylactic anticoagulation or intermittent external pneumatic calf compression to prevent deep venous thrombosis, unless specific contraindications exist.

sound and pulsed Doppler ultrasound. It is considered more accurate and useful than angiography because it provides information about the atherosclerotic plaque and the vessel wall, and has virtually no complications (28). Its sensitivity and specificity are 85% and close to 90% respectively, and it can distinguish high-grade stenosis from occlusion. Whether the findings should be followed by prophylactic carotid endarterectomy before the contemplated noncarotid surgery is unsettled at this time. This writer favors reserving endarterectomy for symptomatic patients with ipsilateral or severe bilateral carotid disease. Results from an ongoing prospective multicenter trial should be very helpful in delineating who might benefit from carotid endarterectomy (36).

Seizure Disorders

It has been estimated that up to 0.5% of the general population have suffered from some form of epilepsy or seizure disorder at some time in their lives. Although many seizures never recur, a history of seizures or ongoing seizure activity is a common reason for consulting internists in the preoperative period. The most important questions to answer when seeing these patients are (*a*) How recent are the seizures? (*b*) What are they due to? and (*c*) How well controlled are they?

A seizure disorder does not require **any special anesthetic management,** but good seizure control is important to decrease morbidity from breakthrough seizures in the perioperative period. The extent and force of involuntary muscle contraction during seizures can disturb the surgical wound. In addition, cerebral anoxia, and aspiration during the seizure can markedly impair recovery (37).

Only 25% of patients with recurrent seizures have an identifiable cause. Drugs, neoplasms, vascular injury, metabolic derangements, and trauma are the most commonly identified causes. Drugs can cause seizures either as a toxic effect from large doses (i.e., meperidine, lidocaine, penicillin, propoxyphene, etc.), or secondary to acute withdrawal after previous excessive use (i.e., alcohol, diazepam, chlordiazepoxide, barbiturates, etc.) (38). As a rule, focal seizures are due to structural lesions, but in nonketotic hyperglycemia 75% of motor seizures are focal. Most patients with recurrent seizures have idiopathic epilepsy. Once diagnosed, treatment of epilepsy is guided by the type of epileptic syndrome manifested by the patient.

In alcoholics, "rum fits" are a common cause for consultation. These seizures usually occur within 48 hours of stopping alcohol intake and consist of one or two generalized tonic-clonic seizures without lateralizing signs. "Rum fits" do not recur except in the setting of withdrawal and do not require anticonvulsant medication. **Continuing seizure activity** suggests a structural lesion of the central nervous system and should be evaluated further. Patients at risk for "rum fits" are also at high risk of injury, and a subdural hematoma should be excluded. In addition, they may also abuse other drugs that can produce seizures. A drug screen is worth obtaining when seizures persist or are difficult to control. This is the same population that may also develop delirium tremens. Tranquilizers (i.e., chlordiazepoxide, benzodiazepines), beta blockers, and clonidine have been advocated for management. In some settings, intravenous alcohol has also been used (39). **Co-morbidity is common in alcohol abusers.** Alcohol-induced hepatic disease of varying degree often coexists. These patients are usually chronic heavy smokers and may have previously unrecognized chronic obstructive pulmonary disease. Impairment of lung and/or hepatic function may require modifications in intra- and postoperative care. Finally, their nutritional status is often borderline and we recommend administration of parenteral thiamine 100 mg a day for a week plus supplementation with other B vitamins at the time of admission.

Patients with well-controlled seizures should be continued on their anticonvulsant regimen through the morning of surgery, and have their medications resumed immediately following surgery. Table 19.5 reviews the doses and routes of

Table 19.5.   Some Commonly Used Anticonvulsant Drugs: Effective Blood Levels, Route of Administration, and Serum Half-Lives

	Usual Daily Dose	Route	Serum Half-Life in Hours	Therapeutic Blood Levels (mg/l)
Phenytoin[a] (Dilantin)	300–400 mg qd (3–5 mg/kg)	Oral or IV	24 + 12	10–20
Phenobarbital	120–250 mg qd (3–5 mg/kg)	Oral or IV	96 + 12	15–35
Primidone (Mysoline)	250 tid (to 1500 mg qd)	Oral	12 + 6	6–12
Carbamazepine (Tegretol)	200 mg bid or tid (to 1200 mg qd)	Oral	15 + 2	6–12
Ethosuximide (Zarontin)	750 mg qd (to 2000 mg qd)	Oral	60 + 6	40–100
Sodium Valproate (Depakene)	500 mg bid (to 1000 mg tid)	Oral	6 + 20	50–100
Diazepam (Valium) (used only in status epilepticus)	10 mg, may repeat q 20 min for two doses	IV (Must be given slowly at 1–2 mg/min)	24–48	—

[a] Intramuscular administration is erratic and not recommended. When starting therapy by the intravenous route, give a loading dose of 100 mg at a rate below 50 mg/min. Phenytoin should be dissolved in saline *not* glucose solution. Given too rapidly it can produce cardiovascular collapse and/or CNS depression. When given orally, the loading dose is given in divided doses to improve gastric tolerance.

Table 19.6. **Recommendations for the Perioperative Management of Patients with a Seizure Disorder**

1. Establish the diagnosis.
2. Assess the degree of seizure control preoperatively.
3. If seizures are controlled, continue the same medications through the morning of surgery and resume in the postoperative period. If drugs must be given parenterally, intravenous phenytoin and/or phenobarbital and/or diazepam may be used.
4. If seizures are poorly controlled, postpone elective procedures until seizures are controlled. Control is achieved by monitoring anticonvulsant blood levels and modifying the dose as needed.
5. Identify drug and alcohol users at the time of admission to prepare for withdrawal seizures. In alcoholics, an ethanol drip may be instituted to avoid seizures and delirium (39). Atenolol and clonidine have also been used in the prevention and treatment of delirium with some success. Make certain there are no other causes for the seizures/delirium (i.e., subdural hematoma).
6. If improved seizure control is desired within 6–12 hr, phenytoin may be given orally in a loading dose of 1000 mg followed by 300 mg daily. A similar loading dose may be given by the intravenous route diluted in saline at a rate less than 50 mg/min and a daily maintenance dose of 300 mg. If preferred, intravenous diazepam at a dose of 2 mg/min to a maximum of 20 mg may be used instead for rapid seizure control. However, the patient will continue to need phenytoin for ongoing seizure control.
7. When giving diazepam intravenously, you must be ready to support ventilation, especially in patients with known or suspected chronic obstructive airway disease.

administration for these drugs. If the patient's epilepsy is poorly controlled, therapy should be started or optimized prior to the scheduled surgery, and the procedure should be delayed if possible (40).

Women of childbearing age with idiopathic seizures requiring anticonvulsant treatment may also be referred for consultation. Careful control of the serum level is usually needed because of changes in protein binding and metabolism of these drugs during pregnancy. The relative risk of fetal malformation in this population is increased 2–3 times above that of the general population, but the risk of recurrent seizures poses greater risks to mother and unborn child than the possible increased risk of teratogenicity. Epileptic mothers are at no greater risk of toxemic seizures than normal women. A megaloblastic anemia responsive to folic acid may develop after long-term treatment with hydantoin. Newborn children of women on anticonvulsants are at risk of bleeding secondary to deficiency of vitamin K-dependent clotting factors induced by some of these drugs, especially hydantoin, phenobarbital, and primidone. A summary of recommendations for the perioperative evaluation and treatment of seizure patients is listed in Table 19.6.

Dementia (Organic Brain Syndrome)

Dementia is a syndrome characterized by chronic, progressive failure of intellectual function severe enough to interfere with normal social and work activities. It may occur at any age and may be caused by over 60 different disorders. Demented persons have diminished survival compared to age-matched controls. The dementia syndrome can be classified into two major categories depending on the neuroanatomical areas affected. Cortical dementia is the most common and is typified by Alzheimer's disease. In this syndrome, aphasia, amnesia, apraxia, cognitive impairment, and abnormalities in visual-spatial relationships occur early. Abnormalities of gait and movement do not occur until quite late in the illness. In contrast, subcortical dementias manifest dysarthria, hypophonic speech, abnormal posture, tremor and gait disturbance. Subcortical dementias occur in association with Parkinson's disease, progressive supranuclear palsy, Huntington's disease, normal pressure hydrocephalus, etc. (41). Multi-infarct dementia presents features of cortical and subcortical disease.

Potentially correctable causes need

to be excluded whenever signs or symptoms of dementia are identified. Mild dementias may go unrecognized until the patient is stressed, as occurs with hospitalization and surgery. Changes mimicking dementia can be caused by drugs, even drugs like digoxin, which are not often recognized as having a central neural effect, and even in therapeutic doses. Multi-infarct dementia is potentially treatable when diagnosed early, and so are many of the less common causes of dementia like vitamin deficiencies and endocrinopathies. Depression and other affective disorders can also mimic idiopathic dementia but respond to medications (42). Unfortunately, it appears that the prevalence of potentially reversible causes of dementia were overestimated earlier (43, 44).

The most common cause of dementia is Alzheimer's disease. The prevalence of Alzheimer's disease increases with age and has been estimated at 15% in the over age 65 population (10% with mild dementia, 4–5% with severe symptoms (45)). In patients who appear otherwise normal, Alzheimer's disease is suspected in the presence of amnesia, or if the patient is unable to compose and write a sentence, and/or in the presence of frontal release signs like the snout and grasp reflexes. Mild disorientation is not specific enough to diagnose dementia. A variety of neuropsychological tests are available for more formal testing.

A multitude of pharmacologic agents are presently under consideration for the treatment of dementia (46). Alzheimer's disease has been consistently associated with diminished levels of acetycholine and other substances like somatostatin in the cortical areas of the brain. Trials with large doses of acetylcholine precursors in the form of lecithin, in conjunction with administration of centrally acting acetylcholinesterase inhibitors like tetrahydroaminoacridine, appear encouraging (47) but await further testing.

Operative risks in demented persons are comparable to those in nondemented persons. However, the underlying cause for the demented state may introduce a risk specific to that condition. For example, a patient with dementia due to unrecognized hypothyroidism may develop myxedema coma in the postoperative period. On the other hand, the procedure used for treatment of the dementia may carry a high risk of morbidity, as occurs with shunting procedures for normal pressure hydrocephalus. Mortality and morbidity in this setting are reported between 10–40%. Inability of the patient to cooperate may also impair recovery. In general, recommendations for the perioperative care of demented persons are straightforward, and are summarized in Table 19.7.

Myasthenia Gravis

Myasthenia gravis is a disorder of neuromuscular function. It is characterized by the sudden or insidious onset of muscle weakness associated with exertion. The bulbar and ocular muscles are preferentially affected, but any muscle group can be involved (48). Diagnosis is confirmed by electromyographic demonstration of a decremental response in muscle action potentials, by the resolution of muscle weakness within 30–60 seconds following parenteral administration of edrophonium (Tensilon), and by increased levels of antibodies to the acetylcholine receptor. The prevalence of the disease is 33 per million population. It can occur at any age but appears most commonly in young females and older males. Among younger females, lymphocyte typing has revealed an over-representation of HLA-B8. Patients with myasthenia gravis often have findings suggestive of auto-immunity. **Antibodies to the acetylcholine receptor** of skeletal muscle are present in 80–90% of patients with generalized myasthenia (48, 49), 20% have antinuclear antibodies, and 30% antibodies to common antigens pres-

Table 19.7.   Recommendations for the Perioperative Management of Patients with Dementia

1. Any member of the health care team addressing the patient should identify her or himself, and if necessary review the surgical procedure done, the length of hospitalization to date, and other information that helps orient the patient.
2. Remember that elderly demented patients require smaller doses of most medications, and that medications may worsen an already compromised intellect.
3. Acute anxiety, restlessness, agitation, and/or combative behavior in the postoperative period should *always* be considered secondary to a correctable cause rather than to the underlying demented state. Any infection, drugs, water, acid-base, or electrolyte imbalance, hypoxemia, hypercarbia, impaired cardiac output, urinary retention, shock, and sepsis can worsen the demented state and should be identified and corrected.
4. After all correctable causes for the altered behavior have been evaluated and ruled out, therapy with psychotropic agents may be indicated. This is more likely to occur in patients who required these drugs preoperatively. The same drug in an equivalent oral or parenteral dose should be given. In others, haloperidol (Haldol) 0.5–1 mg orally or 1 mg intramuscularly every 8–12 hr can be helpful. Remember that any of these drugs may produce paradoxical agitation, insomnia, and anticholinergic and extrapyramidal side effects. For insomnia, diphendydramine, 50 mg orally or IM, or the newer short-acting hypnotics in very low doses can be tried.

ent in skeletal muscle, gastric mucosa, and thymus. Thymoma occurs in 10–15% of myasthenics and thymic hyperplasia in over 50%. Hyperthyroidism occurs in 5%. Systemic lupus erythematosus and other rheumatic diseases of probable auto-immune etiology have also been reported to occur in these patients more commonly than expected.

Drug therapy depends on drugs that inhibit acetylcholinesterases, and on steroids and/or cytotoxic drugs. Thymectomy is recommended mostly in young adults when the response to anticholinesterases is unsatisfactory. **Myasthenic "crisis"**, manifested by sudden onset of difficulty breathing severe enough to require mechanical ventilatory support, occurs in up to 25% of these patients. **Overtreatment** with cholinesterase inhibitors can cause weakness, so careful titration of the dose of neostigmine or pyridostigmine is important. Steroid therapy is generally initiated with low doses and under careful medical supervision in order to minimize the worsening of symptoms often seen during the first days of therapy. Steroid-resistant patients or those with high morbidity from this hormone have been managed successfully with azathioprine or cyclophosphamide. Plasmapheresis has also been advocated and may provide lim-

ited improvement (48). A milder form of the disease limited to the ocular muscles is easier to treat and has a better prognosis.

Anesthesia and surgery should be performed by a team experienced in the care of myasthenic patients. The major risks are pulmonary complications, including apnea, prolonged need for mechanical ventilatory support, and excessive secretions. Preoperative sedation, induction with thiopental, tracheal intubation, succinyl-choline in conventional doses, and nitrous oxide or halothane anesthesia have been given without any adverse effects. Management is aimed at reducing the risk of inadequate ventilation and avoiding drugs or conditions that may worsen the neuromuscular abnormalities. The number of drugs that can produce, worsen, or mimic myasthenia gravis continues to grow. Table 19.8 lists those identified to date (50).

The following clinical features have been suggested as predictive of postoperative complications: long-standing disease, coexistent pulmonary disease, high maintenance dose of acetylcholinesterase inhibitors, and low preoperative vital capacity. Unfortunately, other studies have failed to confirm the ability of these features to predict which patients are likely

Table 19.8. **Drugs Associated With the Onset, Worsening, or Development of Myasthenia Gravis or a Myasthenic-Like Syndrome (50)**

1. Induce myasthenia gravis through the formation of antibodies to the acetylcholine receptor: D-penicillamine, phenytoin.
2. Aggravate symptoms in myasthenia gravis patients: curare, choloroquine, kanamycin, streptomycin, phenytoin, trimethadione, propanolol, timolol, lidocaine, procainamide, quinidine, quinine, ACTH, thyroid hormones, corticosteroids.[a]
3. Interfere with neuromuscular transmission and produce myasthenic symptoms in normal individuals: curare, streptomycin, beta-blockers, D-carnitine.[b]
4. Enhance the action of muscle relaxants and/or anesthetic agents and produce myasthenic symptoms in normal individuals: colistin, gentamicin, kanamycin, lincomycin, neomycin, polymyxin B, streptomycin, tobramycin, lidocaine, quinidine, trimethaphan, lithium salts, phenelzine, promazine, clindamycin.[c]

[a] (only during initial therapy).
[b] L-carnitine does not have this effect.
[c] Drugs must likely to aggravate myasthenia gravis include: quinidine, procainamide, and aminoglycoside antibiotics.

to develop complications (51). Recommendations for the perioperative management of these patients is outlined in Table 19.9.

The Extrapyramidal Disorders: Parkinson's Disease

The extrapyramidal disorders are characterized by a combination of abnormal involuntary movements, altered muscle tone, and impaired postural reflexes. They include the parkinsonian syndromes, the dystonias, choreas, hemiballism, and athetosis. The parkinsonian syndromes are by far the most common of the extrapyramidal syndromes, with a prevalence in the United States of 1% in the population over age 60, and a yearly incidence of 50,000 new cases. The prevalence in the United States is estimated as affecting over 1 million people. Most cases are idiopathic, but there are several primary causes of the syndrome, among them carbon monoxide or heavy metal (manganese especially) poisoning, as a late consequence of the epidemic of encephalitis lethargica in 1918 (possibly due to influenza A virus), trauma, hypoparathyroidism and associated calcifications of the basal ganglia, and cerebral arteriosclerosis. In addition, a parkinsonian syndrome and tardive (or late onset) dyski-

Table 19.9. **Recommendations for the Perioperative Management of Patients with Myasthenia Gravis**

1. Assess thyroid function to exclude associated thyroid abnormalities. Identify any coincident autoimmune disorder and treat appropriately.
2. Obtain preoperative vital capacity. Postoperatively, follow the patient with bedside spirometry to monitor peak flow rates.
3. Continue cholinesterase inhibitors through the day prior to surgery, and discontinue on the day of surgery to avoid muscarinic side effects (increased secretions, facilitated cardio-inhibitory reflexes, etc.).
4. If the patient is currently, or has recently been, on steroids, "cover" with parenteral corticosteroids on the day of surgery as recommended in Chapter 13.
5. Be prepared to continue mechanical ventilation postoperatively for as long as necessary.
6. Withhold cholinergic therapy until patient's condition stabilizes (i.e., fever subsides), then begin at one-half the preoperative dose before extubating. If the drug is given parenterally, give one-tenth of the oral dose intramuscularly, or one-thirtieth of the oral dose intravenously.
7. Drugs with a known potential for aggravating neuromuscular blockade (see Table 19.8) should be avoided unless absolutely required (see also Chapter 4).
8. If the patient is on cholinergic medication, avoid stimuli that would further exacerbate cardio-inhibitory vagal reflexes (i.e., enemas and Valsalva maneuver).

Table 19.10. Recommended Dosages in the Treatment of Parkinson's Disease

Benztropine (Cogentin):
  0.5–6.0 mg per day, orally, given as one dose or divided into 2–4 doses per day.
Trihexyphenidyl (Artane):
  1–8 mg per day, orally, in four equally divided doses before or after meals. Rarely, the total daily dose needed may be as high as 15 mg.
Diphenhydramine (Benadryl):
  25–200 mg per day, orally, given in 2–4 equally divided doses.
Carbidopa/Levodopa (Sinemet):
  10/100 or 25/100, one tablet given 2–4 times per day. Dose is increased by one tablet every 2–3 days until a response is achieved.

nesias occur in patients on neuroleptic drugs and similar medications. In younger adults with slow onset of parkinsonian symptoms, Wilson's disease must be excluded.

Major advances in our current understanding of Parkinson's disease developed from the observation (52) that severe acute symptoms resulted from ingestion of synthetic heroin contaminated with a toxin. The toxin MPTP (1-methyl-4-phenyl-1,2,5,6-tetrahydropyridine) exerts its damage by selective killing of the substantia nigra cells by its oxidation product MPP^{++}. In an experimental model in primates, damage can be prevented by administration of selegiline (Deprenyl), a selective inhibitor of monoamine oxidase B (MAO-B). A multicenter trial is underway to evaluate the usefulness of this drug and of vitamin E as an anti-oxidant in the treatment of this disease. Another breakthrough in our understanding of the role of toxins in this disease is the recent discovery of the pathogenesis of a similar syndrome in Guam. Chronic exposure to small amounts of a nonphysiologic amino acid present in a local food staple produced a parkinsonian syndrome, while higher doses of the same product over shorter periods produced a syndrome similar to amyotrophic lateral sclerosis (53).

Several classes of drugs are available to treat the Parkinsonian syndrome (54), and recommended dosages are listed in Table 19.10. The major toxic side effects for these drugs are dry mouth, blurring of vision secondary to cycloplegia, urinary and fecal retention, worsening of glaucoma, confusion, and hallucinations. Because of marked variation in individual responsiveness, the dose range is wide. Since the advent of levodopa (L-dopa), most patients sooner or later have this drug added as the mainstay of therapy (55). Prior to the advent of levodopa, disability occurred in 90% of Parkinson's disease patients affected longer than 15 years, and mortality was three times higher than in a matched control population. The major causes of death were aspiration pneumonia and respiratory insufficiency secondary to inability to swallow secretions and to rigidity of the chest wall musculature. Generalized rigidity and associated immobility continue to be a common prelude to death.

Treatment with L-dopa, although ineffective in preventing progression of the disease, has improved the quality of life and prolonged survival by 3 or more years in the 80% of patients who respond to the drug. The dramatic response of muscle rigidity to this drug, and the decrease in cardiovascular and gastrointestinal side effects when combined with the peripheral dopa decarboxylase inhibitor carbidopa, as in Sinemet, gave rise to an enthusiastic era in the treatment of Parkinson's disease. Unfortunately, side effects of central origin, including mental aberrations, tardive dyskinesias, and hypotension, were not eliminated by adding carbidopa. As treatment progresses, a greater number of patients develop these side effects. For example, after 2 years, abnormal movements are noted in 70% of patients. "On-off" phenomenon, a very disabling side effect, occurs after chronic therapy with L-dopa, with or without carbidopa, in 50% of patients. Limiting protein intake to suppertime, variation in the time of dosing, and slow reduction of the daily dose to the minimum effective level, although of some benefit, have not eliminated the occurrence or severity of these attacks. Lithium salts and estrogens have also been tried. "Drug holidays", popular for a while, appear to worsen patients with severe disease. Gradual reduction of dose and combination therapy with other dopaminergic agents like bromocriptine appear more useful (55).

Optimal therapeutic benefit from L-dopa occurs in the first 3 years of therapy and declines, often to pretreatment levels, over the next 3–4 years. Initial response to levodopa is independent of the duration of severity of the disease or the age of the patient. Transplantation of autogenous adrenal medulla to the neostriatum (56)

is probably of limited use, while administration of selective MAO-B inhibitors or anti-oxidants may be shown to improve the outcome for these patients.

Postoperative complications are common in untreated patients with Parkinson's disease because of widespread muscle rigidity. Involvement of the chest muscles ("wooden chest") may lead to secondary ventilatory insufficiency. Rigidity of the muscles of deglutition prevents normal swallowing of food and saliva, often leading to aspiration. Rigidity of other muscle groups prevents frequent changes of position and normal gastrointestinal and urinary emptying. Optimal use of drugs in the perioperative period and anesthetic management were reviewed recently (57). In addition, patients with Parkinson's disease have a markedly increased risk of confusion and hallucinations in the postoperative period (57a). As far as the internist's role, the major concern is to improve the patient's condition prior to surgery as much as possible. A recommended approach to these patients is outlined in Table 19.11. Parenteral levodopa preparations are not currently

Table 19.11.   Recommendations for the Perioperative Management of Patients with Parkinsonism

1. Establish the etiology of the syndrome looking for reversible causes.
2. When the condition is secondary to a currently administered drug, discontinue the offending drug. If necessary, treat with a centrally acting anticholinergic or antihistamine. Choose one preparation only, start at a low dose, and increase at 2–5 day intervals as necessary.
3. Patients with muscular rigidity severe enough to interfere with postoperative ventilation should be treated. Treatment should be started with amantadine (Symmetrel) 100 mg postoperatively b.i.d. Maximal response to amantadine occurs within a week and decays within 6–8 weeks of continuous treatment, so surgery should be planned during this grace period.
4. If the patient is already on levodopa or Sinemet, continue therapy to within 6–8 hours prior to anesthesia and resume as soon as possible. Levodopa has a very variable, relatively short, plasma half-life of 1–2 hr, but its effectiveness lasts 3–4 days. Increasing problems with muscle rigidity, diminished ventilation, and peristalsis are most likely to surface on the 2nd or 3rd postoperative day.
5. Worsening of rigidity during the postoperative period can be managed with benztropine mesylate (Cogentin), 1–2 mg intravenously or intramuscularly if oral intake is not possible. Partial relief should occur within a few minutes, and the dose can be repeated every 10–12 hr as needed until oral medications can be resumed.
6. Arrhythmias and hypotension developing during the intraoperative period are probably related to anesthetic and surgical manipulations rather than to levodopa or other anti-Parkinsonian drugs.
7. Avoid drugs containing droperidol (a butyrophenone) and fentanyl (a synthetic opioid), e.g., Innovar, as they may induce or aggravate a parkinsonian syndrome.
8. Aggressive postoperative physical therapy emphasizing ambulation, deep breathing, and cough should be instituted at the earliest opportunity.

available. Other drugs usually less effective remain the mainstay of parenteral therapy for patients unable to take oral medications.

Myotonic Dystrophy

Myotonic Dystrophy and some of the limb girdle dystrophies are the only dystrophies that present during adulthood. Myotonic dystrophy is an autosomal dominant multisystem disease with highly variable clinical expression. Patients with myotonic dystrophy are at a very high risk of complications in the perioperative period (58, 59). Myotonia is a characteristic finding and may be the only clue to the presence of the disease in undiagnosed patients. Muscle weakness and atrophy, cardiac and endocrine abnormalities, cataracts, testicular atrophy, mental deterioration, and frontal baldness, singly, or in combination, may complete the clinical picture. Abnormalities in membrane function leading to repetitive depolarization is responsible for myotonia and weakness (59). The condition is worsened by cold and may improve with continued muscular activity. A beneficial effect from Class I anti-arrhythmic agents like procainamide, phenytoin, and quinidine, as well as calcium channel blockers has been reported.

Perioperative complications tend to occur in the intraoperative and immediate postoperative periods due to adverse reactions to drugs. Delayed complications occur in proportion to the severity of the disease (58). Depolarizing neuromuscular blockers like succinylcholine and decamethonium should be avoided, while nondepolarizing drugs like curare appear to be tolerated. As with other preexisting neurologic illnesses, making the diagnosis prior to surgery is the best way to avoid complications.

POSTOPERATIVE NEUROLOGIC COMPLICATIONS

Multiple factors contribute to neurologic morbidity in the postoperative pe-

Table 19.12.   Postoperative Neurologic Complications

1. Localized ischemic injury to the cental nervous system (strokes).
2. Altered mental status, delirium, and coma.
3. Seizures of new onset.
4. Cauda equina syndrome.
5. Peripheral nerve palsies.

riod. General, spinal, and local anesthesia can all result in transient or permanent neurologic deficits (60, 61). In addition, the surgical procedure itself, or the trauma or condition necessitating the surgery may produce neurologic sequelae. Drugs used in the perioperative period may also contribute to alterations in nervous system function. Finally, the stress associated with the underlying illness and its resulting hospitalization and surgery can affect mentation. Some of the more common or devastating postoperative neurologic complications are listed in Table 19.12.

Localized ischemia of the central nervous system leading to strokes in the perioperative period was discussed earlier. In summary, early postoperative strokes occur within the first days after surgery. Intraoperative hypotension and secondary decrease in cerebral blood flow is rarely the mechanism for perioperative stroke. Therefore, attempts to "protect" the brain by performing prophylactic carotid endarterectomy prior to the necessary surgery only adds to the total morbidity and mortality (2). Most postoperative strokes are embolic, although hypercoagulability associated with surgical manipulation of certain tissues may also play a role. Prevention is the best treatment for postoperative stroke. This is best done by treating arrhythmias, and preventing contamination of the blood with air, clots, or foreign substances during cardiopulmonary bypass. Postoperative institution of prophylactic anticoagulation for deep venous thrombosis with low-dose heparin may have a beneficial effect in preventing postoperative stroke.

Altered mental status, delirium, and

coma in the postoperative period should always be considered due to a complication of drug therapy, a metabolic abnormality, or sepsis. Persistent treatment with neuroleptics is not advised, except as a temporary measure, while further diagnostic studies are underway. In the elderly, overmedication with "usual" doses of analgesics can lead to apnea. In the obese, delayed recovery from anesthesia due to continued slow release of fat-soluble inhalational agents accumulated in fatty depots is common. Underlying mild or unrecognized liver or kidney impairment can precipitate the altered mental status. In patients with recent trauma, fat emoblism should be considered, especially if associated with fractures of long bones. Altered mentation secondary to global ischemia is common in patients undergoing valvular or other cardiac surgery. Symptoms usually clear prior to discharge but may be long-lived (4, 15). (See also Chapter 20)

Seizures of new onset in the postoperative period may occur secondary to alcohol, from drug withdrawal in unrecognized abusers, or from abnormalities in fluid or electrolytes. When associated with acute hyponatremia from excessive administration of hypotonic fluids, mortality and severe morbidity approach 100% in women (62, 63). Grand mal seizures develop 2–3 days postoperatively in association with serum sodium values of less than 110 mmol/liter, and other laboratory evidence of inappropriate secretion of antidiuretic hormone (ADH). Rapid correction of the serum sodium restores normal brain function for only a few hours or days. Recurrence of seizures, coma, and death or irreversible brain damage then ensue. The syndrome has been variously ascribed to too long a period of hyponatremia, too fast correction of hyponatremia, or to attainment of too high a sodium level. Amid the current controversy, prompt identification of hyponatremia and cautious treatment with normal saline is recommended. Since this syndrome is, at least in part, iatrogenic, prevention should be the cornerstone of treatment of this devastating and unnecessary complication.

Cauda equina syndrome secondary to ischemic injury of the spinal cord presents with bowel and bladder difficulties, sensory abnormalities, and autonomic dysfunction. It is uncommon but occurs in association with aortic/cardiac surgery in the elderly or from local trauma due to spinal or epidural anesthesia. Patients with a history of poliomyelitis, disc disease, or other diseases of the central nervous system may be at higher risk of complications from spinal anesthesia (60).

Peripheral nerve palsies can result from prolonged pressure or stretching of a peripheral nerve which produces ischemia. When the ischemic episode is short-lived, paresthesias result. During sleep, these sensations allow us to shift position to avoid pressure damage to the nerve. Under anesthesia, prolonged pressure on a peripheral nerve can occur and result in axonal degeneration (axonotmesis) or in death of the axon and the Schwann cells that envelop the axon (neuromesis). While axonal degeneration is slowly reversible, neuromesis can be irreversible (64). Patients with underlying neuropathy, particularly diabetics, are at higher risk for this complication.

Certain nerves are at particularly high risk of injury. These include the cranial nerves, the brachial plexus, and some nerves to the limbs. The optic nerve can be permanently injured when undue pressure is applied around the orbit leading to increased intraocular pressure and ischemia. If the ischemic episode lasts longer than four minutes, blindness results. Reversible damage to the superficial branches of the trigeminal nerve can occur from a tight-fitting anesthesia face mask. Retainers to hold the mask in place can compress the facial nerve at the lower edge of the mandibular rami and produce palsy. The sciatic nerve is injured most often from intramuscular injections in the buttocks outside of the recommended upper outer quadrants. Malposition of the legs or arms can result in foot drop and sensory deficits, or ulnar and radial nerve palsies (65).

Damage to the brachial plexus is the single most common serious injury seen in the postoperative period. It occurs following open heart surgery and was reported in 5% of patients studied prospectively at the Cleveland Clinic (66). Several different mechanisms may cause the injury. Direct compression, excessive depression of the shoulder girdle in the Trendelenburg position, hyperabduction of the arm, cannulation of the internal jugular vein, and plexus penetration by a fractured first rib from the sternotomy have all been implicated. *Injury of peripheral nerves is best treated by prevention.* This is best achieved by meticulous attention to positioning of all body parts throughout the surgery to avoid direct pressure on the nerve. In summary, most postoperative neurologic complications can be avoided with due attention to detail in intra- and postoperative care.

READINGS

Cerebrovascular Disease

1. Cooperman M, Pflug B, Martin EW Jr, et al.: Cardiovascular risk factors in patients with peripheral vascular disease. *Surgery* 84:505–509, 1978.
2. Hart R, Hindman B: Mechanisms of perioperation infarction. *Stroke* 13:766–773, 1982.
3. Reed GL III, Singer DE, Picard EH, et al.: Stroke following coronary-artery bypass surgery. *N Engl J Med* 319:1246–1250, 1988.
4. Shaw PJ: Neurological complications of cardiovascular surgery: II. Procedures involving the heart and thoracic aorta. *Int Anesthesiol Clin* 24:159–200, 1986.
5. Coffey CE, Massey EW, Roberts KB, et al.: Natural history of cerebral complications of coronary artery bypass graft surgery. *Neurology* 33:1416–1421, 1983.
6. Rowed DW (Toronto Cerebrovascular Study Group): Risks of carotid endarterectomy. *Stroke* 17:848–852, 1986.
7. Furlan AJ, Brewer AC: Central nervous system complications of open heart surgery. *Stroke* 15:912–915, 1984.
8. Goldman L, Caldera DL: Risks of general anesthesia and elective operation in the hypertensive patient. *Anesthesiology* 50:285–292, 1979.
9. Turnipseed WD, Berkoff HA, Belzer FO: Postoperative stroke in cardiac and peripheral vascular disease. *Ann Surg* 192:365–368, 1980.
10. Barnes RW, Liebman PR, Marszalek PB, et al.: The natural history of asymptomatic carotid disease in patients undergoing cardiovascular surgery. *Surgery* 90:1075–1083, 1981.
11. Ropper AH, Wechsler LR, Wilson LS: Carotid bruit and the risk of stroke in elective surgery. *N Engl J Med* 307:1388–1390, 1982.
12. Bojar RM, Najafi H, DeLaria GA, et al.: Neurological complications of coronary revascularization. *Ann Thorac Surg* 36:427–432, 1983.
13. Jones EL, Craver JM, Michalik RA, et al.: Combined carotid and coronary operations: When are they necessary? *J Thorac Cardiovasc Surg* 87:7–16, 1984.
14. Parker FB, Marvasti MA, Bove EL: Neurologic complications following coronary artery bypass. The role of artherosclerotic emboli. *Thorac Cardiovasc Surg* 33:207–209, 1985.
15. Sotaniemi KA, Mononen H, Hokkanen TE, et al.: Long-term cerebral outcome after open-heart surgery—a five-year neuropsychological follow-up study. *Stroke* 17:410–416, 1986.
16. Galbreath C, Salgado ED, Furlan AJ, et al.: Central nervous system complications of percutaneous transluminal coronary angioplasty. *Stroke* 1986; 17:616–619, 1986.
17. Safian RD, Berman AD, Diver DJ, et al.: Balloon aortic valvuloplasty in 170 consecutive patients. *N Engl J Med* 319:125–130, 1988.
18. Edmunds LH Jr., Stephenson LW, Edie RN, et al.: Open-heart surgery in octogenarians. *N Engl J Med* 319:131–136, 1988.
19. Breuer AC, Furlan AJ, Hanson MR, et al.: Central nervous system complications of coronary artery bypass graft surgery: Prospective analysis of 421 patients. *Stroke* 14:682–687, 1983.
20. Orenstein JM, Sato N, Aaron B, et al.: Microemboli observed in deaths following cardiopulmonary bypass surgery: Silicone antifoam agents and polyvinyl chloride tubing as sources of emboli. *Hum Pathol* 13:1082–1090, 1982.
21. Heyman A, Wilkinson WE, Heyden S, et al.: Risk of stroke in asymptomatic persons with cervical arterial bruits: A population study in Evans County, Georgia. *N Engl J Med* 302:838–841, 1980.
22. Corman LC: The preoperative patients with an asymptomatic bruit. *Med Clin North Am* 63:1335–1340, 1979.
23. Ford CS, Frye JL, Toole JF, et al.: Asymptomatic carotid bruit and stenosis—a prospective follow-up study. *Arch Neurol* 43:219–222, 1986.
24. Chambers BR, Norris JW: Outcome in patients with asymptomatic neck bruits. *N Engl J Med* 315:860–865, 1986.
25. Wolf PA, Kannel WB, Sorlie P, et al.: Asymptomatic carotid bruit and risk of stroke: The Framingham study. *JAMA* 245:1442–1445, 1981.
26. Bogousslavsky J, Despland PA, Regli F: Asymptomatic tight stenosis of the internal carotid

artery: Long-term prognosis. *Neurology* 36:861–863, 1986.

27. Allen GS, Preziosi TJ: Carotid endarterectomy: A prospective study of its efficacy and safety. *Medicine* 60:298–309, 1981.

27a. Cebul RD, Whisnant JP: Carotid endarterectomy. *Ann Intern Med* 111:660–670, 1989.

28. Feussner JR, Matchar DB: When and how to study the carotid arteries. *Ann Intern Med* 109:805–818, 1988.

29. Martin WRW, Hashimoto FA: Stroke in coronary bypass surgery. *Canadian J Neurol Sci* 9:21–26, 1982.

30. Taylor GJ, Malik SA, Colliver JA, et al.: Usefulness of atrial fibrillation as a predictor of stroke after isolated coronary artery bypass grafting. *Am J Cardiol* 60:905–907, 1987.

31. Barnes RW: Asymptomatic carotid disease in patients undergoing major cardiovascular operations: Can prophylactic endarterectomy be justified? *Ann Thorac Surg* 42 supplement: S36–S40, 1986.

32. Powers WJ, Press GA, Grubb RL Jr, et al.: The effect of hemodynamically significant carotid artery disease on the hemodynamic status of the cerebral circulation. *Ann Intern Med* 106:27–35, 1987.

33. Breslau PJ, Fell G, Ivey PD, et al.: Carotid arterial disease in patients undergoing coronary artery bypass operations. *J Thorac Cardiovas Surg* 82:765–767, 1981.

34. Mohr JP, Caplan LR, Melski JW, et al.: The Harvard Cooperative Stroke Registry: A prospective registry. *Neurology* 28:754–763, 1978.

35. Meyer FB, Sundt TM Jr, Yanagihara T, et al.: Focal cerebral ischemia: Pathophysiologic mechanisms and rationale for future avenues of treatment. *Mayo Clin Proc* 62:35–55, 1987.

36. Hobson RSII, Towne J: Carotid endarterectomy for asymptomatic carotid stenosis. *Stroke* 20:575–576, 1989.

Epilepsy

37. Roizen MF: Anesthetic implications of concurrent disease. In Miller RD (ed): Anesthesia, 2nd ed. New York, Churchill Livingstone, 1986, vol 1. p. 255–357.

38. Messing RO, Simon, RP: Seizures as a manifestation of systemic disease. *Neurologic Clin* 4:563–584, 1986.

39. Hansbrough JF, Zapata-Sirventm RL, Carroll WJ, et al.: Administration of intravenous alcohol for prevention of withdrawal in alcoholic burn patients. *Am J Surg* 142:266–269, 1984.

40. Leppik IE: Status epilepticus. *Neurologic Clin* 4:633–643, 1986.

Dementia

41. Foster JB: Subcortical dementia. *Br Med J* 292:1035–1036, 1986.

42. Van Horn G: Dementia. *Am J Med* 83:101–110, 1987.

43. Barry PP, Moskowitz MA: The diagnosis of reversible dementia in the elderly: A critical review. *Arch Intern Med* 148:1914–1918, 1988.

44. Clarfield AM: The reversible dementias: Do they reverse? *Ann Intern Med* 109:476–486, 1988.

45. Katzman R: Alzheimer's Disease. *N Engl J Med* 314:964–973, 1986.

46. Klawans HL, Genovese N: Pharmacology of dementia. *Neurologic Clin* 4:459–467, 1986.

47. Summers WK, Majovski LV, Marsh GM, et al.: Oral tetrahydroaminoacridine in long-term treatment of senile dementia, Alzheimer type. *N Engl J Med* 315:1241–1245, 1986.

Myasthenia Gravis

48. Seybold ME: Myasthenia gravis—a clinical and basic science review. *JAMA* 250:2516–2521, 1983.

49. Drachman DB: Present and future treatment of myasthenia gravis. *N Engl J Med* 316:743–745, 1987.

50. Kaeser H: drug-induced myasthenic syndromes. *Acta Neurol Scand* 70(suppl 100):39–47, 1984.

51. Eisenkraft JB, Papatestas AE, Kahn CH, et al.: Predicting the need for postoperative mechanical ventilation in myasthenia gravis. *Anesthesiology* 65:79–82, 1986.

Parkinson's Disease

52. Lewin R: Trail of ironies to Parkinson's Disease. *Science* 224:1083–1085, 1984.

53. Anonymous: A poison tree. *Lancet* ii:948–948, 1987.

54. Anonymous: Drugs for Parkinsonism. *Med Lett Therapeutics* 28:62–64, 1986.

55. Lees AJ: L-dopa treatment and Parkinson's Disease. *Quart J Med* 59:535–547, 1986.

56. Moore RY: Parkinson's Disease—a new therapy? *N Engl J Med* 316:872–873, 1987.

57. Severn AM: Parkinsonism and the anaesthetist. *Br J Anaesth* 61:761–770, 1988.

57a. Golden WE, et al.: Acute postoperative confusion and hallucinations in Parkinson disease. *Am Intern Med* 111:218–222, 1989.

Myotonic Dystrophy

58. Aldridge LM: Anaesthetic problems in myotonic dystrophy. *Br J Anaesth* 57:119–130, 1985.

59. Anonymous: Treatment of Myotonia. *Lancet* i:1242-1244, 1987.

Postoperative Neurologic Complications

60. Vandam L: Neurological sequelae of spinal and epidural anesthesia. *Int Anesthesiol Clin* 24:231–255, 1986.

61. Seibert CP: Recognition, management and prevention of neuropsychological dysfunction after operation. *Int Anesthesiol Clin* 24:39–58, 1986.

62. Arieff AI: Hyponatremia, convulsions, respiratory arrest, and permanent brain damage after elective surgery in healthy women. *N Engl J Med* 314:1529–1535, 1986.

63. Stem RH, Riggs JE, Schochet SS Jr: Osmotic demyelination syndrome following correction of

hyponatremia. *N Engl J Med* 314:1535–1542, 1986.

64. Narins RG: Therapy of hyponatremia. Does haste make waste? *N Engl J Med* 314:1573–1575, 1986.

65. Dornette WHL: Compression neuropathies: Medical aspects and legal implications. *Int Anaesthesiol Clin* 24:201–229, 1986.

66. Hanson MR, Brever AC, Furlan AJ, et al.: Mechanism and frequency of brachial plexus injury in open-heart surgery: A prospective analysis. *Ann Thorac Surg* 36:675–679, 1983.

20

Psychiatry

Janet Woodcock

CONSULTATION TO PSYCHIATRY

The consulting internist will encounter patients with psychiatric symptoms and those who take psychotropic medications in many settings. The purpose of this chapter is to provide the information necessary to take these factors into account when making recommendations about patient care.

The initial part of the chapter deals with medical consultation to psychiatric services. The first section discusses psychiatric symptoms that can result from physical disorders, and how to sort out the contribution of physical factors. This is followed by a discussion of the evaluation and treatment of medical problems in patients with psychiatric disorders. For example, the significance of an abnormal endocrine test result in a patient who is depressed may need to be clarified, or medical clearance for electroconvulsive therapy may be requested.

The second part of the chapter deals with psychiatric issues in consultation to surgical services and includes a discussion of the differential diagnosis of postoperative delirium.

Finally, there is an overview of the pharmacology and medical effects of psychotropic drugs, including overdosage. To facilitate communication with psychiatric colleagues, the medical consultant who deals frequently with their patients should become familiar with *DSM-III-R* [*Diagnostic and Statistical Manual of Mental Disorders,* ed. 3, revised, American Psychiatric Association, Washington, DC, 1987] which establishes diagnostic criteria for psychiatric disorders.

The internist must learn to feel comfortable interacting with patients who display psychiatric symptoms, while maintaining an open and unprejudiced attitude toward their evaluation.

THE PATIENT WITH PSYCHIATRIC SYMPTOMS: EVALUATION FOR CAUSATIVE PHYSICAL ILLNESS

Mental symptoms are frequently caused by physical illness. While in most cases the organic disease will be apparent, occasionally, the underlying process will be occult, rare, or difficult to detect, and the patient will be assigned a primary psychiatric diagnosis. The consequences of misdiagnosis can be profound. Once a patient has been given a psychiatric "label," further medical workup may not be pursued, even when new symptoms develop and potentially treatable diseases progress. For this reason, **the possibility of an organic syndrome should be investigated in any patient presenting with the new onset of psychiatric symptoms.**

Many psychiatrists do not feel comfortable performing detailed medical evaluations, both because of doctor-patient relationship issues, and because of their different areas of expertise. Thus, the internist is often part of the team assessing the psychiatric patient. Since not only traditional medical disease, but also self-prescribed drugs, illicit substances, toxic

This chapter was written by Janet Woodcock in her private capacity. No official support or endorsement by the Food and Drug Administration is intended or should be inferred.

occupational exposures, and even environmental pollutants can cause psychiatric syndromes, a thorough knowledge of the differential diagnosis will enhance medical input. The following discussion is an approach to the diagnosis of causative physical disorders in the patient with psychiatric symptoms.

Epidemiology

Estimates of the frequency of undetected causative physical illness in psychiatric patients have ranged from 5–42%, depending on the population (1–3). For example, when 658 psychiatric outpatients in a suburban setting were screened, about 9% were found to have a causative physical disease. Although physically ill patients tended to be older (mean age 57), 26% were under age 30 (4). Even more striking results have been found in hospitalized patients. Hall et al. (5) evaluated 100 patients on a psychiatric research ward. Most of the patients, who were from lower socioeconomic classes, had presented to a city hospital emergency room, and would ordinarily have been admitted (or committed) to a state psychiatric hospital for treatment. Seventy-six percent of patients were psychotic at the time of admission. In this relatively young group (69% between the ages of 18 and 30), 46% had physical illnesses felt to be highly contributory to their mental symptoms. In 28%, there was rapid resolution of psychiatric symptoms with treatment of the underlying disease.

While the incidence of causative physical disease undoubtedly varies greatly, depending on the population studied, detection of these diseases is a challenge for internists and psychiatrists alike.

Diagnosis

A good medical history and general physical examination is essential in every psychiatric patient. In addition, special attention should be given to specific aspects of the presentation that provide clues to organicity. Clues in the medical history include: abrupt onset, older patient with no previous psychiatric history, family history of late-onset psychosis, concomitant medical illness, recent trauma (for subdural hematoma), recent medication change.

Table 20.1 summarizes the spectrum of organic syndromes that may cause psychiatric symptoms. The findings on care-

Table 20.1. The Spectrum of Organic Syndromes That May Present as Psychiatric Disorders

Syndrome	With Marked Disturbance of Cognitive Function Characteristics
1. Dementia	Gradual onset of diminished higher cortical function
2. Delirium	Acute to subacute clouding of consciousness
3. Catatonic syndrome	Organic syndrome can closely resemble catatonic schizophrenia
4. Amnestic syndromes	Primary memory deficits
5. Aphasias	Primary communication deficit
6. Drug intoxication/withdrawal	Variable

Syndrome	With Predominant Neuropsychiatric Symptoms Characteristics
1. Organic hallucinosis	Isolated visual or auditory hallucinations
2. Organic delusional syndrome	Paranoid delusions most frequent
3. Organic mood syndromes	
Mania	Classic manic symptoms
Depression	Absence of previous depressive episode suggestive in older patient
4. Organic personality syndrome	Emotional lability, poor judgment, poor impulse control, indifference, paranoia

ful mental status examination distinguish two major groups. Psychiatric patients with marked disturbance of level of consciousness or of cognitive function have a high probability of underlying or concomitant physical illness and should be investigated thoroughly. Patients whose sensorium is clear, but who exhibit classic psychiatric symptoms such as hallucinations, delusions, or mood change, may also, less commonly, have causative physical disease. Thus, specific attention to mental status, as well as review of the patient's psychiatric symptoms, may alert the clinician that an underlying physical disorder is present.

Mental Status

The mental status examination is an important tool in evaluating patients with psychiatric complaints. For use in medical consultation, however, the standard methods are time-consuming and suffer from poor interobserver reproducibility. The following streamlined procedure is recommended:

1. The patient's level of consciousness and degree of agitation are assessed and recorded. Extreme disorganization or somnolence makes further formal testing futile.
2. Cognitive abilities—orientation, attention, memory, calculation, language—are tested next. Several short questionnaires for assessing cognitive function are available in the literature. These employ numerical scoring to detect organically based cognitive deficits in medical or psychiatric patients. A low score, relative to the patient's socioeconomic and educational background, suggests that delirium, dementia, or other organic process may be present. Recent studies suggest, however, that these tests have poor predictive value (6, 7).
3. Content of thought—hallucinations,

delusions, and suicidal, violent, or inappropriate ideation—is recorded.
4. A note is made of general affect.

PATIENTS WITH MARKED DISTURBANCE IN COGNITIVE FUNCTION

Patients who have both psychiatric symptoms and changes in the sensorium are challenging diagnostic problems. Confusing nomenclature frequently complicates the situation.

Acute Psychotic Illness

"Acute psychosis" is a purely descriptive term implying a distortion of the thinking process which has placed the patient completely or partially out of touch with reality. "Acute" implies a time span of hours to weeks. Although frequently applied exclusively to psychiatric illnesses, the term "psychotic" does not imply etiology: both delirium tremens and schizophrenia cause "acute psychoses." **When a patient presents with an acute psychosis, all possible organic causes must be ruled out.**

DELIRIUM

"Delirium" is an acute, organically based psychosis, caused by disturbances in brain metabolism, and chartacterized by deficits in arousal and cognitive function. Secondary symptoms such as hallucinations, delusions, and agitation frequently accompany this syndrome. Delirium appears to be a nonspecific final common pathway of expression for numerous types of insults to cerebral function. Little is known about pathophysiology. During delirium, cerebral metabolism is altered and oxygen uptake diminished.

Clinical characteristics help distinguish delirium from functional psychosis. Delirium is characterized by a constellation of mental status changes often referred to as "confusion," "clouding of consciousness," or "a clouded sensorium." Quantifiable criteria (Table 20.2) should

Table 20.2.   Delirium

Characteristics of delirium
1. Abrupt onset
2. Fluctuation in the state of consciousness
3. Disturbed sleep/arousal patterns
4. Disorientation
5. Disordered attention
6. Changes in perception: illusions, delusions, hallucinations
7. Global impairment of cognitive function
8. Abnormal psychomotor activity
9. Neurologic signs: tremor, asterixis, multifocal myoclonus
10. Diffuse slowing on EEG

Common etiologic factors in delirium

1. Drugs (see Table 20.6)	Anticholinergics
	Anticonvulsants
	Antihypertensives
	Anti-arrhythmics
	Narcotics
	Drug withdrawal states
2. Infection	Any site
3. Metabolic disorders	Hypo-, hyperglycemia
	Thiamine deficiency (Wernicke's encephalopathy)
	Electrolyte abnormalities
	Hypoxemia
4. Major organ dysfunction	Hepatic insufficiency
	Renal failure
	Cardiac failure
	Pulmonary disease
	Pulmonary embolism
5. Endocrinopathies	Thyrotoxicosis
	Hypothyroidism
	Adrenal insufficiency
6. Central nervous system pathology	Infection
	Embolism
	Vasculitis
7. Nonspecific contributory factors	Sleep deprivation
	Pain
	Unfamiliar surroundings
	Sensory deprivation

be used instead of these rather vague descriptive terms:

1. *Onset.* Delirium often begins abruptly (e.g., hours to days), whereas a prodromal period of unusual behavior, melancholia, or euphoria usually precedes frank psychosis in psychiatric illnesses.

2. *Fluctuation.* Variation in the state of consciousness is a hallmark of delirium. Observers encountering the patient at different times may form widely varying opinions of mental status. Periods of somnolence or obtundation in a psychiatric patient point toward an organic cause.

3. *Disturbed sleep/arousal patterns.* Abnormal sleep and arousal patterns in delirium are felt to reflect metabolic dysfunction in the brainstem. Hypervigilant or hypersomnolent states of consciousness, or both, may be seen. A disordered sleep cycle, combining diminished normal sleep with nocturnal confusion ("sundowning") is a harbinger of frank delirium. In severe delirium, as well as in acute functional psychosis, normal sleep may be absent.

4. *Disorientation.* Orientation to time and place is lost in more advanced stages of delirium. Patients with functional psychosis are usually oriented unless such data are part of a delusional system (e.g., "I'm on Mars"). Loss of personal identity is uncommon in delirium and points toward functional illness, especially dissociative ("hysterical") states.

5. *Disordered attention.* Many of the cognitive and perceptual deficits seen in delirium result from a loss of ability to focus attention. The patient may show intense, inappropriate interest in a spot on the bedclothes, but be unable to follow a simple question.

6. *Changes in perception.* Patients with delirium have difficulty identifying and integrating environmental stimuli. Sensory data may be misinterpreted: illusions and frank hallucinations may occur. Attempts to explain these phenomena can result in delusions. For example, a hospitalized patient may believe he is being

held prisoner and tortured. Delusional beliefs in delirium usually have a shifting, fragmentary quality when compared with the more fixed delusional systems seen in psychiatric illness.

7. *Impaired cognition.* Subtle impairment of higher cortical function is an early sign of delirium and may be the only clue that an organic process is present. Although the deficit may be slight, the cognitive dysfunction is global, affecting all areas of rational thinking. This lack of specificity contrasts with the profile found in functional psychosis, in which, for example, memory and calculation abilities are usually relatively intact.

8. *Abnormal psychomotor activity.* Behavior of delirious patients usually reflects the level of consciousness. In hypervigilant states such as delirium tremens, patients are frequently agitated and combative. Repetitive purposeless movements are characteristic.

9. *Neurologic signs.* Tremor and asterixis are common findings. Occasionally, multifocal myoclonus is seen. Emergence of further neurologic finds such as the Babinski sign, hemiplegia, seizures, or coma indicates progression beyond delirium (e.g., hepatic encephalopathy, hyperosmolar state).

10. *Diffuse slowing of the EEG during delirium.* This finding reflects disturbances in cerebral metabolism. It also helps to confirm the diagnosis of delirium in an acutely psychotic patient. Psychiatric disorders do not cause EEG changes. In early delirium, however, the EEG may be normal.

The presence of all the aforementioned characteristics indicates florid delirium. In the early stages of the syndrome, delusions and hallucinations may be prominent, and the underlying cognitive deficits inapparent, unless specific mental status assessment is made. Often, definitive mental status testing is not immediately possible in the acutely psychotic patient. In these cases, life-threatening organic diseases should be ruled out, and further testing performed when the patient is more cooperative.

The presence of delirium requires a complete medical evaluation for causative factors. Almost any systemic medical illness can cause this syndrome. Often, etiology is multifactorial. Elderly patients, and those with preexisting cortical dysfunction (alcoholism, cerebrovascular disease, brain damage) become delirious with relatively less physiologic stress. Drug intoxications and withdrawal states are the most common causes of delirium. Other important causes are listed in Table 20.2. See page 518 for a discussion of therapy.

CATATONIA

Catatonia is an acute psychotic illness that is occasionally caused by organic disease. Catatonic symptoms include muscular rigidity, stupor, negativism, mutism, catalepsy, posturing, and bizarre mannerisms. Patients with affective disorders or schizophrenia may demonstrate these symptoms at some point in their illness. Catatonic stupor with profound immobility and rigidity can lead to fatal medical complications, such as hyperthermia, aspiration, thromboembolism, or sepsis. For these reasons, rapid diagnosis and treatment are essential. The psychiatric causes of catatonia usually respond to psychotropic drugs or electroconvulsive therapy (ECT). **This treatment is ineffective for the life-threatening disorders that have been reported in organically based catatonia** (Table 20.3). High-potency neuroleptic drugs can cause a catatonic syndrome, the "neuroleptic malignant syndrome" (page 522). This disorder requires withdrawal of antipsychotic drugs, and thus must be differentiated from other types of catatonia.

Several other organic syndromes may

Table 20.3. Medical Illnesses That May Present as Specific Psychiatric Syndromes

Catatonia	
Ketoacidosis	Stroke
Porphyria	Brain tumor
Hypercalcemia	Encephalitis
Exogenous steroids	Subdural hematoma
Pellagra	Subarachnoid hemorrhage
Neurosyphilis	Lupus cerebritis

Organic Hallucinosis	
Drug abuse:	Sensory deprivation
Alcohol	Subclinicial delerium
Hallucinogens	Psychomotor epilepsy
Amphetamines	

Organic Delusional Syndrome	
Encephalopathies:	Drugs:
B$_{12}$ deficiency, pellagra	Isoniazid
Acute intermittent	
porphyria	Sympathomimetics
Endocrinopathies	Amphetamines
Cerebral emboli	Bromides
Lupus cerebritis	Neurosyphilis
Alcoholism	Huntington's chorea
Wilson's disease	HIV disease

Mania	
Drugs:	Hyperthyroidism
Sympathomimetics,	Neurosyphilis
cocaine, ampheta-	
mines	
Tricyclic antidepres-	
sants	
MAO inhibitors	
Isoniazid	
Procarbazine	

Depression	
Cushing's syndrome	Parkinsonism
Hypercalcemia	Sleep apnea
Apathetic hyperthyroid-	Cardiac/renal/hepatic
ism	insufficiency
Hypothyroidism	Drugs:
Hepatitis; mononucleosis	Exogenous steroids
Anemia; iron deficiency	Benzodiazepines
Carbon monoxide poison-	Antihypertensives
ing	L-Dopa

Polymyalgia rheumatica:
temporal arteritis
Paraneoplastic syn-
dromes: pancreatic
carcinoma

Episodic Anxiety Attacks	
Stimulant drug use	Arrhythmia
Drug withdrawal state	Mitral valve prolapse
Hyperparathyroidism	Asthma, emphysema
Insulinoma, hypogly-	Autonomic or psychomo-
cemia	tor epilepsy
Pheochromocytoma	Multiple sclerosis
Acute intermittent por-	Vertebrobasilar insuffi-
phyria	ciency
Electrolyte disorder	Meniere's disease

precipitate or mimic acute psychosis. Hallucinogenic drug intoxication is a ubiquitous example. Patients with grand mal epilepsy may experience prolonged postictal periods (twilight states) that resemble delirium. Uncontrolled psychomotor epilepsy can closely resemble a psychiatric illness. Patients with neurologic disorders such as amnestic syndromes (e.g., Korsakoff's psychosis) or aphasia may appear psychotic because of apparent confusion. Formal cognitive testing will reveal selective deficits in these cases.

Nomenclature of longstanding mental status derangements is more widely accepted. "Dementia" refers to a chronic (stable or gradually deteriorating) loss of higher cortical function. In contrast to delirium, consciousness or state of arousal is usually unimpaired until very late in the disease. Cognitive deficits do not fluctuate. The diagnosis of dementia can usually be established by: *(a)* a low score on cognitive function tests; *(b)* historical data confirming existence of a deficit over time; and *(c)* absence of the noncognitive aspects of delirium.

OTHER ORGANIC BRAIN SYNDROMES

While the sensorium is clear and general intellectual functioning is not markedly impaired, **content of thought** is markedly abnormal in these disorders. They closely resemble, and are easily mistaken for, functional psychiatric illnesses; however, certain aspects of the presentation can suggest organic etiology.

HALLUCINATIONS

Hallucinatory experiences occur in a variety of physical conditions and intoxications. Visual hallucinations are common in organic deliria. Hall et al. (4), screening psychiatric outpatients with a symptom checklist, found that 20% of patients with primary organic disease reported visual hallucinations or illusions, compared with only 0.5% of patients in whom no physical disorder could be found. The authors suggest that **a history of visual hallucinations is a clue to possible organic etiology.**

Auditory hallucinations occur in a number of organic states. Various noises can be heard as a part of psychomotor seizures. Patients with delirium may hear voices; however, these patients are usually distinguishable by their confused state. "Echo de pensee," the experience of hearing one's own thoughts as if spoken aloud, is felt to be pathognomonic of schizophrenia when occurring in a clear sensorium.

Tactile hallucinations (e.g., insects crawling on the skin), should raise a suspicion of underlying medical illnesses, such as cocaine or amphetamine abuse, or delirium tremens. The delusional belief that insects are throughout one's body (somatic zoopathy) has been reported in a number of organic states, as well as in functional psychosis. Olfactory hallucinations may result from a variety of central nervous system (CNS) diseases.

The designation "organic hallucinosis" refers to physically based syndromes in which hallucinations are the predominant feature (Table 20.3). By definition, the patients have a clear sensorium, and delusions, if present, relate only to the presence or content of the hallucinations. Alcoholic hallucinosis is the best-known example of this syndrome; however, current or previous (flashbacks) ingestion of hallucinogenic drugs, amphetamine toxicity, and certain seizure disorders can present this way. Sensory deprivation, such as in postoperative bandaging of the eyes, can also cause vivid hallucinations (black patch psychosis).

Organic Delusional Syndromes

The patient presenting with delusions should be evaluated carefully for physical disease. Abrupt onset of delusional thinking suggests delirium. Paranoia is characteristic in organically based delusions, and patients may display a classic paranoid syndrome: jealousy, suspiciousness, sullenness, litigiousness, persecutory delusions, and ideas of reference. A wide variety of serious medical illnesses may present as a paranoid syndrome.

ORGANIC AFFECTIVE SYNDROMES

Disturbances of *mood* that resemble psychiatric mood disorders but are caused by physical disease are known as organic affective syndromes.

MANIA

Behavioral characteristics of mania include elation, hyperactivity, flight of ideas, grandiosity, push of speech, and decreased sleep. Patients typically lack judgment and are easily distracted. Normally, mania occurs as part of the spectrum of a bipolar affective disorder. However, less commonly, certain other illnesses and drugs can cause manic symptoms (Table 20.3). Krauthammer and Klerman (16) mention space-occupying lesions of the central nervous system, psychomotor epilepsy, and drugs, including steroids, INH, procarbazine, levodopa, and bromides. Other authors have reported mania presumed secondary to sympathomimetic agents (phenylephrine, ephedrine, isophedrine), which are frequently used in over-the-counter cold remedies. Euphoriant drugs such as amphetamines and cocaine may cause manic symptoms with acute intoxication. Monoamine oxidase (MAO) inhibitors and tricyclic antidepressants can precipitate mania in patients with manic-depressive illness.

DEPRESSION

Few features distinguish endogenous depression from that caused by an occult physical illness. The absence of a previous personal or family history of depression is suggestive. Awareness of drug reactions and medical illnesses that can masquerade as depressive episodes will aid in screening patients (Table 20.3).

NONSPECIFIC PSYCHIATRIC SYMPTOMS

Vague personality changes may be the presenting symptom of dementing illnesses. The diagnosis "organic personality syndrome" can be applied to patients who have marked behavioral changes involving emotional lability, poor impulse control, apathy, or paranoia, when these symptoms are associated with physical illness. Frontal or temporal lobe disease is the usual cause.

Excessive anxiety is a frequent psychiatric symptom. In organic disease, anxiety may be an appropriate response to a physical derangement, or a direct physiologic expression of the disease, as in pheochromocytoma. Mitral valve prolapse appears to be associated with an anxiety syndrome that responds to adrenergic blocking agents.

MEDICAL ILLNESSES THAT CAN PRESENT AS PSYCHIATRIC DISORDERS

Awareness of diseases frequently presenting with psychiatric symptoms will increase the yield of medical evaluation. Most systemic disorders can cause mental changes, and **evolution of psychiatric symptoms in a patient with known medical illness should always prompt a search for complications of the disease or its therapy.** For example, abrupt behavioral changes in a patient with lung cancer are overwhelmingly more likely to be due to some complication—cerebral metastases, syndrome of inappropriate anti-diuretic hormone (SIADH), sepsis—than to new psychiatric problems.

In patients without preexisting illness, commonplace rather than exotic organic etiologies predominate. Endocrinopathies, especially thyroid disease, should always be suspected. Since lists of causative illnesses read like a compendium of internal medicine practice, most disorders should not pose diagnostic difficulties for the consultant, once they are suspected. Appendix A is a partial listing of illnesses that can present with predominant psychiatric symptoms. Further aspects are discussed below.

Endocrinopathies

Thyroid dysfunction can mimic a number of psychiatric disorders. In addition to the "nervousness" and agitation often seen in hyperthyroidism, subtle cognitive dysfunction and personality changes can appear at higher hormone levels. Patients may show neurotic trends on personality profiles, and have impairment of memory and concentration, so that they are unable to do simple mental arithmetic. These changes revert to normal with treatment. Paranoid ideation, illusions, and visual hallucinations have been found when carefully sought in hyperthyroid patients who do not display overt psychopathology. When these symptoms are prominent, patients may be misdiagnosed as having paranoid schizophrenia and treated inappropriately. **Hyperthyroid patients are especially vulnerable to the extrapyramidal effects of high-potency antipsychotic agents.** Bulbar symptoms may develop, and death has been reported from aspiration. Mental changes, combined with absence of classic hyperthyroid signs, can lead to the diagnosis of agitated or psychotic depression in patients with "apathetic" hyperthyroidism.

Cognitive deficits are even more prominent in patients with hypothyroidism. The paranoia, delusions, and hallucinations that occur ("myxedema madness") reflect increasing degrees of delirium with general disorganization of thinking. Hypothyroid patients are more vulnerable to the systemic effects of antipsychotic agents, such as hypotension and hypothermia. Less agitated hypothyroid patients usually appear depressed. Thyroid function screening is of value in virtually all types of psychiatric patients; however, test results should be interpreted with caution (page 507).

Parathyroid disorders cause mental changes related to alterations in the serum calcium. Hypercalcemia often initially causes depressive symptoms of anxiety along with fatigue and reduced ability to concentrate. With higher calcium levels, a confusional state with paranoia, hallucinations, and delusions may occur before stupor intervenes. Patients with idiopathic or surgical hypoparathyroidism may present with anxiety, agitation, depersonalization, paresthesias, or organic delirium before seizures or other dramatic manifestations begin.

Depression is the most common mental symptom in endogenous hypercortisolism. However, almost any type of psychiatric disturbance may be seen, including mania, paranoid states, and psychosis. Cognitive dysfunction is usually not prominent. The fatigue, lassitude, and weight loss seen in adrenal insufficiency can be mistakenly attributed to depression. More marked behavioral changes may also occur.

Profound (e.g., blood glucose <35 mg%) hypoglycemia, from any cause, may lead to purely psychiatric symptoms. **If the rate of fall of blood glucose is not precipitous, autonomic symptoms such as anxiety, tachycardia, hunger, and sweating may not be triggered.** Instead, the individual will show symptoms of cerebral glycopenia such as emotional lability, bizarre behavior, irritability, and mental slowing. These are often misdiagnosed as acute intoxications, personality disorders, or psychosis. With repetitive neuroglycopenic episodes, such as result from insulinoma, the patient develops a chronic dementia which may be accompanied by paranoid features. Reversibility diminishes with duration of the illness.

Other endocrine disorders may result in psychiatric syndromes (Appendix A). Personality changes can accompany both hypopituitarism and pituitary tumors. Schizophrenia-like disorders have been reported. Pheochromocytoma should be suspected in a hypertensive patient who has episodic anxiety attacks.

Nervous System Disease

It is not surprising that diseases affecting the central nervous system may present with psychiatric symptoms. Chronic meningeal infiltration or infection from a variety of agents may present initially with vague neuropsychiatric complaints and headache. Parkinsonism is often mistaken for endogenous depression in cases where tremor is not prominent. Patients with early demyelinating, neuromuscular, or myopathic disease frequently appear to suffer from anxiety or hypochondriasis.

Approximately 50% of patients with Huntington's chorea display psychiatric symptoms before chorea or other neurologic signs predominate. Early symptoms include personality changes, irritability, violence, and antisocial behavior. Anxiety and depression or paranoid delusions may occur.

Metabolic Disorders

Because of its treatable nature, every effort should be made to diagnose Wilson's disease early. A significant percentage of these patients first come to medical attention because of behavioral abnormalities. Absolutely any type of emotional disorder may appear, including sociopathy, bizarre behavior (voyeurism, episodic violence), mania, and various psychotic states. Manifestations usually occur in late adolescence, but onset may be delayed up to age 40. In the absence of active liver disease, liver function tests can be normal; however, serum copper and ceruloplasmin are decreased. Any psychiatric patient with liver disease, cerebellar ataxia, or extrapyramidal signs of unknown etiology should be investigated for Wilson's disease. Kayser-Fleischer rings are pathognomonic, but not always present early.

Patients with porphyria often display psychiatric symptoms. Between attacks, depression or vague complaints can persist. During acute porphyria, behavioral abnormalities ranging from severe anxiety to delirium and frank psychosis may obscure concurrent abdominal pain or neurologic signs. **Because of the onset in young adulthood, patients with psychotic episodes are sometimes thought to have schizophrenia.** Infections, alcohol, barbiturates, or sulfonamides precipitate acute porphyria in some patients. Diagnosis is confirmed by an erythrocyte uroporphyrinogen I synthetase level.

Deficiency Diseases

It is not widely appreciated that central nervous system manifestations including mood swings, hallucinations, delusions, and delirium can accompany the peripheral signs of pernicious anemia. Confusional states can also occur in Wernike's encephalopathy, chronic zinc depletion, and pellagra. In addition, the latter two illnesses, as well as pyridoxine and possibly folate deficiency, may present as a depressive disorder. The diagnosis should be suspected in patients who have a history of nutritional inadequacy (alcoholism, bowel disease, food faddism, hyperalimentation), who take drugs that may dispose them to vitamin deficiency (oral contraceptives, dilantin, isoniazid), or who have systemic signs of deficiency diseases (rashes, megaloblastic anemia, neuropathy).

Drugs

Drug toxicity is a major source of behavioral changes. Often, careful questioning is required to obtain a complete drug history including over-the-counter medications, drugs that the patient takes as needed or has taken habitually for years, home remedies, and drugs of abuse. Drug intoxication is not the only mechanism for producing psychiatric symptoms. The following must be considered as sources of possible behavioral drug reaction:

1. *Drug abuse.* Acute psychotic states can result from deliberate use of alcohol, cannabis, cocaine, amphetamines, and any of the hallucinogens. Patients may deny ingestion.
2. *Drug withdrawal.* Abrupt discontinuation of narcotics, sedative-hypnotic, caffeine, alcohol, or benzodiazepines in the habituated subject causes distinctive abstinence syndromes.
3. *Intoxications.* Drugs such as lidocaine, digoxin, anticonvulsants, sympathomimetics, or anticholinergics commonly cause mental symptoms at high blood levels. Intoxication can be iatrogenic or patient-induced (abuse of diet pills or caffeine; overdose of anticholinergic sleeping pills.)
4. *Reported effect.* Usual doses of propranolol, disulfiram, indocin, dapsone, and many other drugs will occasionally cause an acute psychosis. Prediction of susceptible patients is difficult. Other drugs such as ketamine, reserpine, or corticosteroids are known to cause psychiatric symptoms in a significant number of patients.
5. *Physiologic drug effects.* Insulin-induced hypoglycemia and hypokalemia caused by carbenicillin are examples of predictable drug actions that can lead to behavioral changes.
6. *Atropinic delirium.* A wide range of drugs and over-the-counter preparations have anticholinergic effects, including belladonna derivatives, scopol-

amine, antihistamines, antispasmodics, proprietary sleeping medications, low-potency antipsychotics, and tricyclic antidepressants. Used in high doses, or in combination, they can cause delirium with hallucinations, delusions, and paranoia. Patients may pick at the bedclothes or attempt to grab at objects in the air. Peripheral signs of cholinergic blockade are usually, but not always, prominent.

7. *Topically applied medication.* Unusual routes of drug exposure must also be considered. Eye drops can cause atropinic delirium, as can transdermal scopolamine. Hallucinations, paranoia, and mania have been reported with overuse of sympathomimetic nasal sprays. Skin exposure to organophosphate insecticides causes a confusional state as well as cholinergic signs.

8. *Drugs for psychiatric conditions.* These are discussed in later sections.

Table 20.4 is a partial list of commonly encountered nonpsychiatric drugs that have been reported to cause psychiatric symptoms.

Infections

A high percentage of patients infected with HIV will eventually develop CNS disease. A subacute encephalitis, the AIDS dementia complex, is directly related to virus infection of the CNS. Some patients will present with neuropsychiatric symptoms as the initial manifestation of disease, and a subset of these may not develop systemic signs of immunodeficiency [21, 22]. Presenting symptoms usually include mental slowing and behavioral disturbances, which may be interpreted as

Table 20.4.   Drugs Causing Psychiatric Symptoms

	Symptoms	Comments
Antibiotics		
Amphotericin B	Delirium	
Penicillin	Depersonalization	High doses
Procaine penicillin	Delirium, agitation	Possibly 2° to procaine
Nalidixic acid	Delirium, agitation	
Anticholinergics		
Atropine	Delirium with disorientation, agitation, visual and tactile hallucinations, paranoia. Also see dry skin and mucosa, cutaneous flush, fever and tachycardia with poorly reactive dilated pupils.	Responds to physostigmine
OTC cold, asthma, migraine, headache, insomnia remedies		
Transdermal scopolamine		
Anticonvulsants		
Carbamazepine	Acute confusional states, hallucinations, depression, paranoia.	Usually represents intoxication
Phenytoin		
Primidone		
Antihypertensives		
Aldomet	Depression, confusional state	
Clonidine	Hallucinations	
Propranolol	Psychotic behavior, delirium	Can occur at low dosages
Reserpine	Depression	Can be severe
Antiinflammatory agents		
Ibuprofen	Delirium	Patients with connective tissue disorders
Indomethacin	Paranoia, psychotic behavior, depersonalization, nightmares	CNS reaction common in this group of drugs
Sulindac		

Table continues next page

Table 20.4.   Drugs Causing Psychiatric Symptoms (*continued*)

	Symptoms	Comments
Antiparasitic drugs		
Chloroquine	Delirium, agitation, personality change	May be an acute reaction
Quinacrine		
Thiabendazole	Delirium, anxiety Hallucinations	
Antitubercular drugs		
INH	Psychosis, hallucinations, delirium, euphoria	
Rifampin	Confusional state	
Cardiac drugs		
Digoxin	Delirium, visual hallucinations, confusion	
Lidocaine	Disorientation, illusions	
Disopyramide	Hallucinations, agitation	
Drugs interacting with dopaminergic systems		
Levodopa	Confusion, hallucinations, euphoria, paranoia	
Amantadine	Psychosis Lilliputian hallucinations	Also has anticholinergic effects
Bromocriptine	Hallucinations, delusions, mania	
Narcotics		
Butorphanol tartrate (Stadol)	Confusion	
Nalbuphine Hcl (Nubain)	Hallucinations	
Pentazocine Hcl (Talwin)	Delusions	
Propoxyphen (Darvon)	Confusional state	
Meperidine (Demerol)	Hallucinations, excitation	Normeperidine, a stimulating metabolite, may be responsible
Sympathomimetics		
Anorectics	Mania, psychosis, auditory hallucinations, anxiety	May cause amphetamine-like toxicity at high doses
Decongestants: phenylephrine pseudoephedrine ephedrine phenylpropylamine		
Miscellaneous		
Amicar	Delirium	
Aminophylline	Anxiety	
Birth control pills	Depression	
Cimetidine	Paranoia, hallucinations, psychosis, delirium	Elderly, renal failure, may also see signs of neurotoxicity
Caffeine	Anxiety state	
Dapsone	Anxiety, psychotic reaction	
Corticosteroids	Euphoria to frank mania, catatonia, paranoia, delirium, hallucinosis	
Disulfuran	Delirium, depression	Independent of ethanol reaction
Metrizamide (Amipaque)	Hallucinations, confusional state	Especially with contrast material above foramen magnum
Lioresol (Baclofen)	Mania, hallucinations	

depressive symptoms. Organic psychosis with hallucinations and delusions may also be seen. The majority of patients have cerebrospinal fluid (CSF) abnormalities and have serum antibody to HIV, so that diagnosis is relatively straightforward once the possibility of HIV disease has been considered. However, there are a few reports of seronegative patients with documented HIV infection of the CNS (23). Appendix A summarizes other infections that may present with psychiatric symptoms.

APPROACH TO THE PATIENT

Table 20.5 presents a format for the orderly medical investigation of psychiatric patients. **Every patient with the new onset of psychiatric symptoms should have a baseline medical evaluation, including laboratory studies.** Patients with serious illnesses such as

acute psychosis require more detailed screening studies. Thyroid function tests are useful in all patient subsets; however, results must be interpreted with caution (see page 507). The role of CT scanning in the evaluation of psychiatric patients has not been clearly delineated. It is not cost-effective as a screening test. An atypical psychiatric presentation and/or findings on history, physical examination, or laboratory tests may suggest the need for further evaluation by CT scanning of the brain (25). In a series of 156 cases, the finding of mental status impairment or focal neurologic signs correlated with an abnormal CT scan; however, neither finding had good predictive value (26).

MANAGEMENT OF CONCOMITANT MEDICAL ILLNESS IN THE PSYCHIATRIC PATIENT

There is a higher incidence of medical illness in psychiatric patients than in the

Table 20.5. Format for Medical Evaluation of Psychiatric Patients

History Points to Stress in Addition to General Medical History	If History Suggestive

1. Drug history
    Prescribed?
    Over-the-counter, topical?
    Home remedies, herbal teas, caffeine?
    Vitamins, tonics?
    Tranquilizers, nerve pills?
    Illicit drugs?
	Evaluate for toxicity

2. Potential toxin exposure
    Occupational: mining, metals, plastics, other industry, paints, mercury
    Hobbies: lead (ceramics), metals, hydrocarbons
    Home: cleaning fluids, space heaters (carbon monoxide)
	Evaluate for toxicity

3. Family history
    Neurologic disease?
    Wilson's disease? (liver disease?)
    Porphyria?
    Huntington's chorea?	

4. Dietary history
    Alcoholism, chronic vomiting?
 	
    Bizarre diet
	Administer thiamine
	Consider deficiency diseases
	Consider deficiency diseases

5. Psychiatric history
    Abrupt onset?
    Visual hallucinations only?
	Evaluate for delirium
	Suspect organic cause

Table continues next page

Table 20.5. Format for Medical Evaluation of Psychiatric Patients (*continued*)

History Points to Stress in Addition to General Medical History	If History Suggestive
Psychiatric symptoms accompanied by multiple somatic symptoms in older patient?	Probable organic disease
History of changes in consciousness, memory losses, fugue states, repetitive episodes?	Evaluate for psychomotor epilepsy

Physical Examination: Emphasize in Addition to General Exam	If Positive Findings
1. Mental status	
Altered state of consciousness, obtundation?	Evaluate for delirium and serious medical illnesses
Cognitive function decreased?	Suspect delirium or dementia, consider formal psychometric testing
2. Neurologic examination	
Tremor, asterixis?	Suspect delirium
Myoclonus about face and neck?	Almost pathognomonic for delirium
Hard neurologic findings, focal deficits?	Evaluate appropriately for neurologic disease
Peripheral neuropathy?	Consider vitamin deficiency, diabetes, lead poisoning, alcoholism
Standard screening tests	
CBC with differential	
Sedimentation rate	
Urinalysis	
Blood chemistries, including: electrolytes	
calcium	
renal function	
liver function	
glucose	
Thyroid function tests	
Serologic test for syphilis	
When appropriate: HIU antibody	

Physical Examination: Emphasize in Addition to General Exam	If Positive Findings
Further evaluation	
Acute psychosis	
1. Send urinary and blood drug screens	
2. In older patient: EKG, chest x-ray	
3. EEG	
4. In appropriate clinical situation: screen for porphyria, Wilson's disease	
Delirium	
1. Anticholinergic signs: flushing, fever, tachycardia, dilated pupils?	
2. If alcoholism, chronic vomiting: administer thiamine	
3. Chest x-ray	
EKG	
Blood gases and carboxyhemoglobin level	
Urine and blood drug screen	
EEG	
4. If EEG shows diffuse slowing, treat supportively for delirium and investigate further for underlying disease	
5. Lumbar puncture	

general population. Chronic disease itself frequently leads to depression. Existing psychiatric problems can be exacerbated by concomitant physical disorders such as hypothyroidism, heart failure, and emphysema, or by drug therapy. On the other hand, emotional turmoil may cause noncompliance, neglect, or even self-destructive sabotage of medical treatment. Because of these interactions, optimal therapy addresses all aspects of the patient's illness. Several common clinical situations requiring an integrated approach to management are discussed below.

The Hypertensive Patient

Because of its high prevalence in the general population, hypertension is a commonly encountered medical problem in psychiatric patients. Certain points should be kept in mind during diagnostic evaluation of hypertensive psychiatric patients.

1. Antipsychotics, tricyclic antidepressants and acute manic states elevate plasma catecholamines. Screening tests for pheochromocytoma must be interpreted with care.
2. Tricyclics (and some antipsychotics) can "unmask" occult pheochromocytoma by virtue of inhibiting re-uptake of norepinephrine. Hypertension of hypotension (secondary to beta stimulation with alpha blockade) can be seen, as well as flushing and tachycardia (27).
3. Hypersecretion of cortisol may occur in depression (see below). This abnormality, which is reversible with therapy, must be distinguished from laboratory evidence of Cushing's disease.

Hypertension and Depression

Drug interactions complicate the treatment of the patient with both hypertension and depression (Table 20.6). Since certain depressions are thought to result from depletion of (or insensitivity to) brain amines, and antihypertensive therapy is often directed at blocking peripheral adrenergic action, pharmacologic goals can conflict. **In depressed patients already on blood pressure medication, the possibility of drug-induced depression should be investigated.** Reserpine and alpha-methyl dopa commonly cause depression. In some patients, beta blockers contribute to depression by causing fatigue and loss of energy. Selective agents with low central nervous system penetration may be better tolerated than propranolol. Patients may temporally relate the onset of depression to drug use. Unless depression is severe, a change to an alternate antihypertensive agent is satisfactory therapy.

Concomitant antihypertensive/antidepressant therapy is frequently necessary. In patients taking tricyclic antidepressants, severe orthostatic hypotension may limit antihypertensive therapy. Changing to a tricyclic causing less orthostatic drop may solve the problem. If good blood pressure levels are not achieved, further therapy must be individualized with consideration of the interactions summarized in Table 20.6.

Diuretics can precipitate lithium toxicity by decreasing renal excretion of the ion. Frequent lithium level monitoring must be initiated when beginning diuretic therapy. Enhanced central nervous system toxicity has been occasionally reported in patients taking both lithium and alpha-methyl dopa; nonetheless, these drugs may usually be used together safely. Calcium channel blockers used with lithium may result in neurotoxicity.

Patients on Antipsychotics

In evaluating the psychotic hypertensive patient, consider a drug reaction, especially in the elderly. Clonidine can cause delirium and hallucinations. Beta-blockers, alpha-methyl dopa, and hydralazine have been reported to cause mental symptoms. Propranolol and chlorpromazine in-

Table 20.6.   Drug Therapy in the Psychiatric Patient with Hypertension

| Antihypertensive Drug | Interactions with Psychiatric Agents | | | Psychiatric Effects |
	Tricyclic Antidepressants	Lithium	Antipsychotic Agents	
ACE inhibitors	None	None	None	Improved quality of
Alpha-methyl dopa	Diminished tricyclic efficacy possible; not usually clinically significant	Enhanced lithium CNS toxicity (rare)	Delirium reported with combined therapy (rare)	Depression Delirium
Beta-blockers	May decrease efficacy of tricyclics: Clinical relevance not clear	None	Metabolic interaction with phenothiazines results in increased blood levels of both	1. Energy loss, fatig may enhance depression 2. Hallucinations, delirium (rare)
Calcium channel blocker	Possible orthostatic hypertension	Neurotoxicity	Possible orthostatic hypotension	Low incidence depressive effects
Clonidine	Antihypertensive effects partially antagonized. May interfere with tricyclic therapy. Enhanced rebound hypertension.	None	Hypotension (occasional) Delirium reported with combined therapy (rare)	Delirium Depression
Diuretics	Increased orthostatic hypotension	Alter renal excretion	Increased orthostatic hypotension	Hypokalemia may cause depressive syndrome
Guanethidine	Antihypertensive effects blocked	None	Antihypertensive effect blocked	Depression
Vasodilators, Prazosin	Increased orthostatic hypotension	None	Increased orthostatic hypotension	None

terfere with each other's metabolism, potentiating the effects of both agents. In addition, antipsychotics block the effects of guanethidine and may result in hypotension when used with clonidine.

The Cardiac Patient

THE DEPRESSED CARDIAC PATIENT

A substantial body of experience has been accumulated on the use of tricyclic antidepressants in patients with cardiac disease (30). **In the majority of cases, tricyclics may be used safely if patients receive careful initial evaluation and are monitored during therapy.** In addition, two new tricyclic-related antidepressant agents, trazodone and fluoxetine, which have fewer cardiovas-

cular effects, are now available. Fluoxetine does not appear to increase heart rate or cause significant orthostatic hypotension and has no effect on cardiac conduction (32). Trazodone has a first-dose hypotensive effect and also does not appear to cause cardiac conduction disturbances (33), but may occasionally result in increased ventricular ectopy. The role of these agents in patients with heart disease is currently being explored.

The following points should be considered before initiating tricyclic or related antidepressant therapy in the patient with heart disease:

1. Prior to starting therapy, the patient's cardiovascular status should be evaluated with emphasis on the presence of angina, orthostatic hypotension,

congestive heart failure, conduction disturbances, and arrhythmias.

2. Postural hypotension from tricyclics is likely to be accentuated in patients with cardiovascular disease (30). Patients with angina or cerebrovascular disease are especially vulnerable to sudden decreases in arterial pressure. Lying and standing blood pressures should be monitored frequently (see also Table 20.16).

3. Tricyclics have some myocardial depressant effect in overdose, but do not generally appear to depress myocardial function at therapeutic levels (30, 34). Patients with heart failure, and also those with fixed valvular obstruction, may be unable to tolerate drug-induced tachycardia. Such patients may require daily observation at the start of therapy and after dosage increases.

4. Electrocardiogram (EKG) changes should be observed carefully.

  a. Caution should be used in patients with conduction disturbances on EKG. Tricyclics prolong AV conduction times. In normal individuals taking therapeutic doses of tricyclics, the PR and QT_c intervals are often increased compared with pretreatment. Occasionally, bundle-branch block or complete heart block is precipitated in the patient with underlying conduction system disease.

  b. The effect of tricyclics on arrhythmias is unpredictable. The supraventricular tachyarrhythmias that are occasionally seen may be related to anticholinergic effects. Tricyclics also have quinidine-like actions. In some patients, ventricular extrasystoles will be less frequent during tricyclic therapy. Imipramine has been used experimentally with some success as an anti-arrhythmic for resistant ventricular ectopy. However (similar to quinidine), during tricyclic overdose and rarely at therapeutic plasma levels, ventricular tachycardia and ventricular fibrillation have been reported. These arrhythmias are postulated to result from differential slowing of distal conduction which facilitates re-entrant rhythms. In patients with known cardiac disease, the QRS and QT_c interval should be monitored during tricyclic therapy. Because of the similar cardiac effects, toxicity can result when a tricyclic is used in patients taking Class I antiarrhythmic agents (e.g., disopyramide, quinidine, procainamide).

5. Low initial dosage, with small increments, is preferable in the presence of cardiac disease. Amitriptyline and imipramine should be avoided. Preliminary experience with trazodone and fluoxetine suggests a lower incidence of cardiac toxicity. Because of the variability of drug absorption and metabolism, use of plasma drug levels, if available, is recommended in the cardiac patient.

6. Watch for drug interactions in the cardiac patient taking tricyclics. Tricyclics potentiate oral anticoagulants. Administration of epinephrine or other vasoconstrictors during procedures can result in acute hypertension. Atropine with tricyclics can cause delirium.

7. Use of tricyclics in patients with severe cardiac disease is controversial. Many authors feel these drugs are contraindicated in the immediate post-myocardial infarction (MI) period, and recommend ECT as an alternative. In profound, life-threatening depression after myocardial infarction, however, use of a tricyclic under monitored conditions in the hospitalized patient may be preferable to ECT, which requires brief anesthesia (see below).

The use of lithium is difficult in patients with congestive heart failure who are salt restricted or taking diuretics.

Lithium should not be used until the patient is stabilized and diuretic dosage is constant. Levels must be monitored frequently. Because ventricular ectopy or conduction disturbances can occur, an EKG should be obtained after the initiation of therapy.

THE CARDIAC PATIENT REQUIRING ANTIPSYCHOTIC THERAPY

High-potency antipsychotic agents are the drugs of choice in the psychotic patient with cardiac disease. Haloperidol, which has little cardiac interaction, a low incidence of orthostatic hypotension, and minimal anticholinergic effects, is probably the best available agent. Although haloperidol is a relatively safe drug in the cardiac patient, complications, including hypotension and arrhythmias, have occurred. Extreme caution is warranted in the elderly.

The Patient with Renal Disease

Psychotropic drugs must be used cautiously in the patient with renal insufficiency. These agents (with the exception of lithium) are metabolized by the liver (Table 20.7); however, potentially active metabolites may accumulate in the presence of renal failure. Also, the potential for drug interactions and adverse effects is high.

Renal disease is not a contraindication to tricyclic antidepressant therapy. If a small initial dose is well tolerated, dosage may be increased in a stepwise fashion. Because lithium is known to cause changes in renal function, its use in patients with underlying kidney disease is controversial. There have been several reports of the use of lithium in patients on hemodialysis; the lithium is given as a single oral dose after each dialysis (36).

The presence of concomitant cardiovascular or neurologic disease should dictate the choice of antipsychotic agent in the patient with renal insufficiency. High-potency agents, while generally preferable, have a higher potential for neurologic side effects in the patient with underlying CNS disease. An acute delirium has been reported in patients with chronic renal failure treated with phenothiazines (chlorpromazine or promethazine) (37).

Table 20.7.   Use of Common Psychotropic Drugs in Renal Failure

Drug		Usual Route of Metabolism	Dosage Adjustment for Renal Failure
Sedative-Hypnotics			
Barbiturates	Pentobarbital	Nonrenal	No change
	Secobarbital		
	Phenobarbital	1/3 renal	Double-dose interval for GFR < 10
Benzodiazepine	Fluorazepam		
	Diazepam		None
	Chlordiazepoxide	Hepatic	
	Lorazepam		None
	Oxazepam		
Antipsychotic agents			
Phenothiazines		Hepatic	Caution indicated[a]
Haloperidol		Hepatic	No
Antidepressants			
Tricyclics		Hepatic	Caution indicated[a]
Tetracyclics		Hepatic	No
Lithium		Renal	Yes[b]

[a] Active metabolites may accumulate, e.g., glucuronides.
[b] Used only with extreme caution in renal failure—see text.

Endocrine Disturbances in the Psychiatric Patient

THYROID SCREENING TESTS

Thyroid function tests are useful in psychiatric patients. **However, up to 20% of newly admitted psychiatric patients will have some abnormality on the initial thyroid screen.** Most of these values will revert to normal if the test is repeated after 2 weeks (38, 39). In the absence of clinical signs of thyroid dysfunction, minor abnormalities in routine thyroid function tests should be interpreted with caution and verified by repeating after several weeks. Both amphetamine abuse and acute schizophrenia can cause transient hyperthyroxinemia.

ENDOCRINE ABNORMALITIES IN DEPRESSION

With the advent of sophisticated neuroendocrinologic testing, interesting abnormalities have been uncovered in patients with affective disorders. Many of the behavioral aspects of depression suggest a hypothyroid state. Additionally, numerous studies have demonstrated that a small daily dose of T3 potentiates the antidepressant action of tricyclics in some patients. However, standard measures of thyroid function, including ankle reflex time, and plasma T3, T4, and TSH levels, are usually normal in depressed patients who are clinically euthyroid.

Abnormalities of the hypothalamic-pituitary-adrenal axis are also found in depression. The finding that some depressed patients hypersecrete cortisol, with loss of the normal circadian secretory patterns, led to the use of the dexamethasone suppression test (DST) in psychiatry (42). Patients are given 1 mg of dexamethasone orally at 11 p.m., and plasma cortisol levels are drawn at 8 a.m., 4 p.m., and 11 p.m. the following day. In normal patients, cortisol levels are suppressed for 24 hours after dexamethasone. Failure of suppression, especially later in the day, occurs in approximately 50% of severely depressed patients. During recovery from depression, the DST normalizes. Al-

though marked cortisol hypersecretion may occur in extreme depression, such patients do not develop the physical signs of Cushing's syndrome.

These neuroendocrinologic findings suggest that at least some types of depression have a definable biochemical substrate. As the distinction between "medical" and "psychiatric" disease is blurred, the internist will have increasing involvement in the evaluation of patients with affective disorders.

Medical Problems in Anorexia Nervosa

A constellation of secondary medical abnormalities is found in patients with anorexia nervosa. **While the primary treatment of this disorder is psychiatric, with the goal of increasing voluntary food intake, life-threatening complications may require medical intervention.**

The typical patient with anorexia nervosa does not complain of weight loss or of poor appetite. Decreased food intake in this disorder results from refusal to eat rather than "anorexia" in the usual sense. Amenorrhea is a usual feature; other symptoms include cold intolerance, constipation, and abdominal pain. Bulimia (binge eating) can occur in anorexia nervosa. On examination, in addition to cachexia, the anorectic patient may have sallow, scaly skin covered with lanugo hair, acrocyanosis, hypotension, hypothermia, bradycardia, and ankle edema. If present prior to disease onset, axillary and pubic hair are usually preserved. Occasionally, bilateral parotid enlargement is seen.

Diagnosis is usually not difficult. Although medical illnesses causing weight loss should be ruled out, **the anorectic should not be subjected to a prolonged series of medical tests prior to psychiatric therapy.** An elevated serum carotene level, found in three-quarters of patients with anorexia nervosa, but not present in other types of weight loss, is a useful distinguishing factor when present (43). Other distinctive laboratory abnormalities are found in this disorder:

1. *Endocrinologic findings.* Although characteristic hypothalamic-pituitary abnormalities occur in anorexia nervosa, they are not usually of clinical relevance. The adrenal axis is unimpaired, with normal or somewhat increased baseline cortisol levels, and a normal response to ACTH stimulation. Serum T4 and TSH levels are usually in the low normal range; however, serum T3 (by RIA) may be decreased. This probably reflects diminished conversion of T4 to T3, similar to that seen in chronic disease states and in starvation. With these findings, frank hypopituitarism, hypothyroidism, and Addison's disease may be ruled out.

2. *Renal and electrolyte disturbances.* Self-induced vomiting, as well as diuretic and/or laxative abuse, are weight control measures for some anorectics. Evidence for volume depletion is frequently found, and prerenal azotemia may be severe. Acute tubular necrosis is a rare complication. Chloride-responsive hypokalemic metabolic alkalosis is the most common electrolyte abnormality. Primary respiratory alkalosis, as well as metabolic acidoses, are also seen. Profound degrees of hypokalemia should be corrected prior to beginning refeeding. Hypomagnesemia may complicate the picture. Magnesium levels should be determined in patients with other electrolyte abnormalities. Oral salt and potassium repletion is usually adequate.

   Renal alterations in anorexia nervosa include decreased glomerular filtration rate (GFR), diminished renal concentrating capacity, and decreased ability to excrete a free water load. These abnormalities make the patient more vulnerable to iatrogenic electrolyte disorders.

3. *Hematologic changes.* Hematologic findings in anorexia are similar to those seen in starvation. Mild normochromic normocytic anemia is common; a very low hematocrit suggests a complicating disease or deficiency. Abnormalities of red blood cell morphology such as spur cells or acanthocytes are frequent. The serum iron is low or low normal, with low total iron binding capacity, in the presence of adequate marrow iron stores. Subclinical folate depletion is common, while serum B_{12} levels are generally normal. Bone marrow examination characteristically shows a hypocellular marrow in which fat is replaced by mucopolysaccharide ground substance (46). During refeeding of the anorectic patient, an initial sharp drop in hematocrit may occur, due to changes in plasma volume. Frank iron or folate deficiency may develop during the recovery period.

   Varying degrees of leukopenia and thrombocytopenia are observed. Abnormal peripheral granulocyte distribution, with normal bone marrow reserves, may account for the apparent neutrophil depletion. Although neutropenia may be profound and prolonged, there is no evidence for increased incidence of infection except in very late stages of this disorder. Similarly, the thrombocytopenia of anorexia nervosa does not result in bleeding problems.

4. *Cardiac findings.* Repolarization abnormalities in EKG, including ST depression and diffuse T wave flattening or inversion, may be seen in anorectic patients in the absence of hypokalemia or known heart disease. An increased incidence of ventricular arrhythmias has been reported.

Physical changes in the heart in anorexia are similar to those seen in other types of starvation. There are reductions in cardiac mass, wall thickness, and intracardiac volumes, which are roughly proportional to weight loss. These cardiac dimensions increase with nutritional repletion. Although bradycardia and diminished cardiac volumes result in a lowered cardiac output, myocardial contractility does not appear to be affected in anorexia. The ejection fraction is normal, increases appropriately with exercise, and is unchanged after weight gain.

HAZARDS OF NUTRITIONAL THERAPY IN THE ANORECTIC

The vast majority of patients with anorexia nervosa can be treated successfully with psychiatric techniques, including behavioral modification, individual psychotherapy, and family therapy. However, an occasional patient will be refractory to such interventions, or will not seek medical aid until seriously ill. Patients with severe electrolyte disturbances, loss of more than 40% of normal body weight, loss within 3 months of more than 30% of normal body weight, or a life-threatening complication, require enteral or parenteral therapy if they will not eat voluntarily. Interestingly, these patients often develop a more favorable psychologic outlook when significant weight gain is affected by alimentation. While both enteral and parenteral feeding have been shown to be effective in anorexia, each has its drawbacks. **A substantial number of reported deaths in this illness have been caused by iatrogenic complications incurred during refeeding of the severely cachectic patient.** The targeted rate of weight gain should be restricted to less than ½ lb. per day.

Enteral alimentation via tube is the preferred route, although patients may sabotage therapy by removing the tube or by vomiting. During starvation, atrophy of the gastrointestinal mucosa occurs. In addition, hypokalemia, psychotropic drugs, and other unknown factors appear to decrease gut motility in anorexia. Aspiration, ileus, acute gastric dilatation, and fatal gastric rupture have been reported after enteral alimentation in anorexia. Pancreatitis has also occurred. To avoid such problems, initial volumes of feedings should be small (e.g., 500 cc/day) with gradual increments. For those patients

with gastric emptying disturbances, metaclopramide may be helpful (51).

Parenteral alimentation has been used successfully in anorexia. Some degree of patient cooperation is necessary since hemorrhage or air embolism may result from manipulation of the catheter. Peripheral vein hyperalimentation techniques should be considered in resistant patients.

Since electrolyte and osmotic disturbances are common during the early phases of alimentation in anorectics, careful monitoring is required. Severe hypokalemia, hypomagnesemia, or hypophosphatemia can develop. Because of diminished renal compensatory mechanisms, attention to salt and water balance is mandatory. Echocardiographic studies of cachectic patients, including anorectics, have shown that intracardiac volumes normalize promptly and that cardiac output and metabolic rate may rise above the normal range under conditions of rapid nutritional repletion. On the other hand, left ventricular mass is repleted slowly (over 4–6 weeks). This discrepancy in recovery may explain the occurrence of clinical heart failure during enteral or parenteral hyperalimentation in anorexia nervosa (52).

Medical Evaluation for Electroconvulsive Therapy

Electroconvulsive therapy (ECT) has been shown to be an efficacious and rapid treatment for severe depression, including cases that are resistant to tricyclics and other therapy (53). The typical candidate for ECT is an older patient with a serious depression that may have psychotic features. In this age group, concurrent medical problems are frequent, and the question of eligibility for ECT often arises (54).

ECT administered in a standard fashion is a relatively safe procedure with a mortality rate of less than 0.03%. The patient is premedicated with an anticholinergic, and light anesthesia is induced with a short-acting barbiturate given intravenously. After muscle paralysis with succinylcholine, oxygen is administered by mask, and an electric shock is delivered via electrodes on the head. The patient is then ventilated by positive-pressure bag until spontaneous breathing begins.

The predominant morbidity of ECT is its effect on memory. The procedure may induce retrograde amnesia as well as deficits in memory function which tend to resolve over time (months). The long-term effect of ECT on memory function is controversial. Modern techniques, which include brief-pulse stimuli and unilateral electrode placement, are believed to minimize effects on cognition; however, they may be less efficacious (53).

Cardiac events are the major source of mortality reported from ECT. The onset of electrical convulsive activity in the brain results in a diffuse autonomic discharge. In the absence of cholinergic blockade, severe bradycardia and even asystole may be seen. In atropinized subjects, heart rate, blood pressure, and plasma catecholamines increase markedly in the immediate post-ictal period. Holter monitoring during ECT in atropinized patients with normal cardiovascular systems showed an increase in heart rate of 40 beats per minute, but no increase in arrhythmias (55).

Cardiovascular evaluation of the pre-ECT patient should focus on the presence of hypertension, angina, heart failure, or arrhythmias. If these disturbances are well controlled, the patient with cardiac disease may undergo ECT. Hypertensives are prone to have an exaggerated blood pressure rise in the post-ictal period, and should have careful blood pressure monitoring. If an unacceptable rise does occur, prophylactic beta-blockade is usually adequate. In extreme cases, successful use of vasodilators such as nitroprusside during the procedure have been reported. Beta-adrenergic blockade may also be warranted in patients with angina, to prevent catecholamine-induced exacerbation, or prophylactically for patients who have developed atrial tachyarrhythmias or ventricular ectopy in the post-ictal period. Intravenous lidocaine may be used *after* the cerebral seizure activity has taken place.

An implanted cardiac pacemaker is not a contraindication for ECT; however, certain precautions should be observed (56). Pacer function must be documented by EKG prior to therapy. Wire placement and structural integrity should be verified by x-ray. The electrical discharges during ECT will not affect an intact pacemaker. However, muscle potentials during the seizure may be sensed as cardiac activity by demand pacemakers, resulting in suppression. An external magnet to convert demand to fixed mode should be immediately available during ECT in patients with demand pacemakers. The most serious threat to patients with pacemakers is from inadvertent myocardial shock via inadequately grounded monitoring equipment. Patients with known broken or damaged pacer wires, in which insulation may be defective, should not undergo ECT. A battery-powered cardiac monitor should be used, or an EKG machine which is plugged in after the shock is delivered.

The use of ECT in patients with severe cardiovascular disease requires clinical judgment (57). The impact of psychiatric illness on the patient's well-being must be balanced against risks of the procedure. ECT (in the presence of a resuscitation team) has been done in the immediate post-MI period when a psychiatric condition such as mania or psychotic depression has endangered the patient's life. Caution is indicated in patients with large aneurysms.

Patients with respiratory diseases are at increased risk of morbidity from ECT. Those with ventilatory compromise—morbid obesity, advanced emphysema, secretion problems, or chest wall deformities—may not tolerate the brief apneic period; and CO_2 retainers may have compromise of the hypoxic drive.

Animal studies have demonstrated a transient rise in intracranial pressure during ECT, and a subsequent increase in cerebrovascular permeability. The technique should not be used in patients with raised intracranial pressure.

CONSULTATION TO SURGICAL SERVICES: PSYCHIATRIC ISSUES

Undergoing surgery stresses both body and mind. The medical consultant must determine if surgery will deplete the patient's physiologic reserves, and must plan to compensate for any deficiencies in organ function. Mental dysfunction causes significant postoperative morbidity. Patients with previously compromised mental function are at hish risk for delirium. Individuals with diminished emotional reserves may develop postopertive psychiatric illnesses which severely compromise rehabilitation. Frequently, these problems are precipitated by medical conditions such as infection or organ failure. There is a high incidence of both psychiatric illness and organic brain syndrome in patients with chronic medical disease. Because of the complex interrelationships of mind and body, the internist will have an important role in the evaluation of altered mental status in surgical patients. It is essential that all physicians who do preoperative evaluations be aware of the psychological risk factors for surgery.

PSYCHIATRIC ASPECTS OF PREOPERATIVE EVALUATION

General Psychological Risk Factors for Surgery

EPIDEMIOLOGY

Numerous studies have demonstrated the profound emotional impact of surgery, as well as the contribution of psychological factors to surgical outcome. An elective procedure in the emotionally precar-

ious patient may result in a technically cured but psychologically devastated person. Severe depression or anxiety preoperatively is predictive of increased surgical morbidity and prolonged hospital stay. Unfortunately, these psychological risk factors are often overlooked. **Because of its contribution to the physical and emotional risks of surgery, a rough determination, at least, of the psychological state of the patient is an essential part of good preoperative management.**

RISK FACTORS

Most individuals fare well after surgery, and there is no need for a detailed psychiatric profile on every patient. If the clinician is sensitive to possible problem areas, sufficient data can be gathered in the course of ordinary history taking and examination. It is important to realize that a past history of psychiatric illness or treatment is not an invariable predictor of postoperative problems. Conversely, the absence of such a history does not guarantee lack of psychological risk. Rather, in patients without known psychiatric illness, the clinician should be alert for the following potential problems (Table 20.8).

1. *Panic states.* Occasionally, a patient will develop extreme and incapacitating anxiety prior to surgery. This can

Table 20.8. Preoperative Psychological Evaluation

Psychological risk factors in preoperative evaluation
  1. Panic states or extreme anxiety
  2. Absence of anxiety
  3. Major depression
  4. "Hidden agenda" for surgery:
        Munchausen syndrome
        Somatization disorder ("Briquet syndrome")
        Psychogenic pain disorder
  5. Prior adverse psychological reaction to surgery
  6. Organic brain syndrome
  7. Drug-dependency states
Preoperative risk factors in the psychiatric patient
  1. Acute psychosis
  2. Inability to coooperate
  3. Treatment with MAO inhibitor

occur in the habitually anxious person, or as a result of individual circumstances (e.g., patient's relative died during similar surgery, or patient does not understand procedure). Usually, panic states resolve quickly after reassurance from the physician. The individual's control over events should be emphasized. Attempts to pressure the patient are unwise, as they will magnify his/her sense of powerlessness. Benzodiazepines are helpful if necessary. Brief delays in surgery are advisable if required for the management of the acutely frightened patient.

2. *Absence of anxiety.* Anxiety about surgery is a normal phenomenon. Most ostensibly unconcerned patients are using a mechanism of denial to avoid thinking about potential dangers. While this is a useful coping mechanism, it can mask an underlying panic state. In other patients, lack of anxiety signals that a "hidden agenda" is being carried out (59). Seriously depressed patients may calmly accept surgery as a form of suicide; these patients are at high risk for postoperative mortality.

3. *Severe depression.* Major depression increases the risk of surgical morbidity and mortality. The depression referred to here is not the chronic, unhappy state experienced by some people ("depressive neurosis") or a reaction secondary to physical illness. A major depressive episode consists of severely depressed mood combined with symptoms such as decreased appetite, crying spells, sleep disturbance, and fatigue, persisting for more than 2 weeks. Depression of this magnitude is an indication for psychiatric evaluation prior to elective surgery. Postponement of surgery may be recommended to allow for psychiatric treatment. If the need for surgery is urgent, immediate psychiatric consultation should be obtained postoperatively. Suicide is a more frequent complication of severe depression in the physically ill; suicide precautions should be used pending psychiatric assessment.

4. *The "hidden agenda" for surgery.* Some patients seek operations for psychological reasons which are at variance from the stated surgical goals. Frequent unnecessary surgery is a complication of Munchausen's syndrome, somatization disorder (Briquet's syndrome), and psychogenic pain disorder, among others. Clues such as: *(a)* a history of multiple previous surgical procedures for vague indications; *(b)* the patient's stated dissatisfaction with all previous health providers; or *(c)* immediate disruptive or provocative behavior on the ward, should alert the clinician that psychiatric factors must be investigated.

   Delusional beliefs can cause psychotic patients to seek surgery. Some psychotic patients appear quite normal superficially and may not spontaneously disclose their motivations. Postoperatively, ideas about the surgical procedure may be incorporated into their delusional system, with bizarre results. Open-ended questioning about the meaning of the illness is a good way to elicit motivation, once the clinician's suspicions are aroused.

5. *Prior adverse psychological reaction to surgery.* While obtaining the patient's past surgical history, ask if any emotional problems, "nervous breakdown," or psychiatric hospitalization occurred after surgery. A history of a prolonged psychotic episode or major depression postoperatively is an indication for psychiatric assessment prior to elective surgery. Repetition of either of these events would represent major morbidity for the individual.

6. *Organic brain syndrome.* Dementia places a patient at major risk for postoperative delirium. Old age, history of prior brain damage or substance abuse, and the impression of a "poor historian" suggests the possibility of underlying cognitive defects and should

prompt a careful mental status assessment. Formal testing by a psychologist can be very helpful in these cases. If dementia is present, several measures can be recommended (see Table 20.8).

Cognitive dysfunction has prognostic value in patients scheduled for cardiac surgery. Willner et al. (60, 61) screened patients preoperatively with a word analogy test. Extremely poor performance on this test of abstract reasoning was more predictive of long-term outcome (morbidity and mortality at 18 months and 5-year follow-up) than was age, pump time, medical diagnosis, surgical procedure, or New York Heart Association (NYHA) class. Patients with both preoperative psychiatric symptoms (determined by interview) and cognitive dysfunction had a 63% 5-year mortality rate, compared with 11% for the remaining patients. Depression was the most common psychiatric problem in this group, and deaths included one suicide. With the improved operative survival in heart surgery, psychological factors should be recognized as making an important contribution to overall outcome.

7. *Drug dependency states.* Habituation to a wide variety of legal and illegal substances may be encountered in surgical patients. When drug dependency is recognized, it can be dealt with safely either by preoperative detoxification or perioperative maintenance, depending on the urgency of the situation. It is the undetected habituation, often in the "unlikely" individual, that poses major risks. Substantial alcohol use is common both in elderly patients and in those who consider themselves moderate social drinkers. Specific inquiry (number and type of drinks per day) should be made of all patients who drink ethanol. Abrupt discontinuation of benzodiazepines can cause withdrawal symptoms, including seizures and hallucinations. Patients may be unaware that the "nerve pill" or pre-scription headache remedy that they chronically consume contains a barbiturate. Inordinate demands for parenteral pain medication upon hospitalization should raise a suspicion of narcotic addiction. A nonjudgmental attitude, combined with explanation, will elicit an accurate drug and alcohol history from the majority of patients.

PREOPERATIVE EVALUATION OF THE PATIENT WITH KNOWN PSYCHIATRIC ILLNESS

Most patients with psychiatric illnesses tolerate surgery normally and do not present special management problems. It is important to recognize the occasional instance when the pharmacologic treatment of psychiatric illnesses may increase surgical morbidity (Table 20.8). Frequent concerns in preoperative assessment of psychiatric patients include the risk of postoperative psychiatric problems, the management of acutely psychotic patients, and the interaction of psychotropic drugs with commonly used perioperative drugs.

ROLE OF THE PSYCHIATRIC ILLNESS

Patients with schizophrenia who are cooperative and functional do not comprise an excessively high risk group (62). Psychotic symptoms may even improve transiently during the time that the patient focuses energy on physical concerns. These patients are usually able to understand the necessity for surgery and to give informed consent. An exception is a patient whose perception of his illness is part of a delusional system. This patient, by definition, is unable to understand the nature of the problem or the give informed consent. Most patients with controlled psychosis can have uneventful operative courses, especially if the hospital staff does not display undue anxiety about the patient's psychiatric problems. Patients with manic-depressive illnesses or unipolar depressions are not at any increased risk when not experiencing affective problems.

In contrast to the above, the acutely manic or psychotic patient who is agitated or combative is a major management problem and should be stabilized with drugs, if possible, prior to surgical intervention. Around-the-clock nursing is required because of the danger of self-harm or patient elopement. The severely psychotic, hallucinating patient is frequently insensitive to physical stimuli and may fail to report pain or other significant physical symptoms. In cases of trauma or surgical emergencies, careful observation is required. These considerations also apply to patients in the midst of psychotic or agitated depressions, in whom the risk of suicide should always be kept in mind.

Patients who require long-term psychiatric hospitalization present special diagnostic and management problems (63). This population includes severely affected schizophrenics, mentally deficient individuals, and patients, often in the geriatric age group, with organic brain syndromes. Often, no history can be gleaned from these noncommunicative, mute or incoherent, paranoid, and perhaps actively hallucinating patients. These patients also are unlikely to report physical symptoms, including pain. For example, bowel perforation or other surgical catastrophes can occur without apparent distress. Therefore, reliance must be placed on physical examination and laboratory studies. Efforts at examination are often met with extreme physical resistance, as are therapeutic measures.

Preoperative evaluation in such patients should focus on practical management considerations. For example, no information will be gained and the omnipresent potential for patient injury enhanced if the consultant sends resistant patients for pulmonary function testing, computerized tomography, barium enemas, and other examinations requiring patient cooperation. If a test is deemed essential to patient care, it can usually be obtained with special planning: patient sedation, provision of extra attendants, and prior notification to radiology staff.

Patient resistance should also be considered when making recommendations for postoperative care. For example, in a patient with Chronic Obstructive Pulmonary Disease (COPD) needing abdominal surgery, the need for physical restraints combined with total lack of cooperation postoperatively creates a setup for pulmonary problems. Special nursing care will be required.

Superimposed postoperative delirium occurs with regularity in this group of patients, further complicating management. In general, although the presence of a severe, chronic psychiatric condition per se does not increase surgical risks, the potential for morbidity is high because of the patient's unpredictable behavior and lack of cooperation.

PSYCHOTROPIC DRUGS

The question of maintenance or discontinuation of psychotherapeutic drugs is frequently raised in the preoperative evaluation of psychiatric patients. Three separate issues need to be addressed when making recommendations:

1. Possible adverse drug interaction with anesthetic agents;
2. Drug withdrawal effects; and
3. Adverse psychiatric response to stopping medication.

MAO Inhibitors

Patients taking MAO inhibitors have the highest potential for life-threatening drug interactions. These agents have prolonged biologic action because their enzyme inhibition is irreversible. Serious hypertensive responses to pressors have been reported up to 2 weeks after discontinuation of MAO inhibitors. For elective surgery, these drugs should be stopped at least 2 weeks prior to the contemplated procedure. If emergency surgery is necessary in a patient taking MAO inhibitors, several points should be stressed:

1. Actions of many drugs and anesthetic agents will be prolonged and potentiated.
2. Fatal hyperpyrexic reactions have occurred with narcotics, especially meperidine.
3. Pressors should be avoided if possible. When absolutely necessary, use direct-acting agents and expect exaggerated responses (64).
4. Early notification of anesthesiology is advisable. During the procedure, blood pressure should be monitored via arterial line. The patient should be observed in an ICU until stable and not requiring introduction of additional drugs.

Abrupt discontinuation of MAO inhibitors will not cause withdrawal symptoms.

Tricyclic Antidepressants

The anticholinergic, cardiodepressant, and alpha-adrenergic blocking properties of the tricyclics have synergistic effects with anesthetic agents possessing similar properties. For this reason, it is often advantageous to withhold tricyclics for several days prior to operation, and restart them a few days postoperatively. Such brief discontinuation does not precipitate a return of depression. Mild abstinence symptoms (nausea, stomach pain, diarrhea, headache, and dizziness) can be seen with abrupt cessation and should not be mistaken for intercurrent illness or postoperative complications. Tricyclics should not be restarted in patients with postoperative ileus, urinary retention, or cardiac arrhythmias since they can worsen these problems. In the emergency situation, remember that tricyclics: *(a)* can potentiate the response to pressors (64) and *(b)* may cause paradoxical hypotension if epinephrine is used.

Antipsychotic Agents

Phenothiazines (prochlorperazine) and butyrophenones (droperidol) are frequently used as preoperative and anesthetic potentiating agents, so that interactions among these drugs are well known to anesthesiologists. Patients on chronic antipsychotic medication can undergo surgical procedures without special precautions. Due to the long biologic half-life of antipsychotics, exacerbation of the underlying condition is not usually a concern when drugs are stopped for short periods. If an acutely psychotic or manic patient requires surgery, parenteral drugs may be used postoperatively. Mild gastrointestinal and CNS abstinence symptoms, including dyskinesias, can occur postoperatively when antipsychotics are stopped abruptly before surgery (65). These respond to symptomatic management or to reinstitution of the drugs. Patients taking anticholinergics for antipsychotic-induced parkinsonism can develop rigidity or other symptoms when both drugs are stopped simultaneously, since anticholinergics have a much shorter half-life.

LITHIUM

Therapeutic lithium levels potentiate the effects of anesthetic agents (66). If this property is kept in mind, general anesthesia poses no special risk to the patient on lithium maintenance. For elective procedures, lithium can be stopped 1 or 2 days before operation. Withdrawal symptoms do not occur. Lithium should not be restarted postoperatively until the patient has fully stabilized and is at baseline for fluid intake, medication, and renal function. Some manic-depressive patients will relapse if off lithium for several weeks.

POSTOPERATIVE DELIRIUM: EVALUATION AND MANAGEMENT

Epidemiology

In prospective studies, a surprisingly high proportion of patients have been shown to develop temporary cognitive deficits after surgery. Because most patients try to conceal these symptoms, postoperative delirium is often not recognized clinically unless it causes florid behavioral changes. The incidence of postoperative delirium varies with the type of surgical procedure: Up to 10% of general surgery patients and 30% of cardiotomy patients will experience this complication.

Characteristically, delirium begins on the third day after surgery and persists for 24–36 hours. However, the patient may emerge from anesthesia in a delirious state, or the delirium may last for several weeks. Although postoperative delirium is, by definition, a reversible state, the potential for substantial morbidity exists during the time patients are agitated and uncooperative.

Differential Diagnosis of Altered Mental Status after Surgery

Postoperative neurologic disorders, psychiatric disturbances, and delirium are often confused with one another. **The majority of patients with postoperative changes in mental status are delirious.** Even the floridly hallucinating, paranoid patient is much more likely to have an organic syndrome than a primary psychiatric problem. Careful mental status and neurologic examination is the logical first step in evaluating patients with postoperative behavioral changes. On this basis, the patient's disorder can be assigned to one of the following groups, and evaluated accordingly:

1. *Neurologic deficit.* Abnormal neurologic findings such as papilledema, paresis, or sensory loss do not occur in delirium, and suggest the presence of a complication within the central nervous system. However, nonspecific signs such as tremor and asterixis are frequently seen in delirious patients. Multifocal myoclonus, the Babinski sign, and the suck, snout, or grasp reflexes occur occasionally. Patients with aphasias, often felt to be "confused," lack the alterations in consciousness found in delirium. Certain neurologic diseases, such as Wer-

nicke's encephalopathy, nonparetic stroke, subdural hematoma, and microembolization may present as confusion without focal findings, and are therefore included under the differential diagnosis of delirium.

2. *Postoperative psychiatric reaction.* Patients with postoperative psychiatric syndromes are usually distinguishable because of adequate cognitive function on mental status testing. Individuals with severe anxiety attacks, psychosis, mania, or marked depression occurring after surgery should be seen by a psychiatrist. Sometimes a psychiatric condition will affect the patient's cognitive function and raise the question of organicity (e.g., "delirious mania," depressive pseudodementia, acute psychotic reaction). In these cases, the internist and psychiatrist must jointly evaluate the condition.

3. *Organic hallucinosis.* Occasionally, a mentally clear patient will report vivid visual and/or auditory hallucinations. Usually, a drug reaction is the cause. The clear sensorium distinguishes this syndrome from delirium.

4. *Delirium.* Delirium is diagnosed by the presence of characteristic alterations in mental status (page 492) and diffuse slowing of the EEG. Patients with acute postoperative psychoses in whom a differentiation of delirium from "functional" psychosis is not possible should be investigated for causes of delirium, and evaluated by a psychiatrist. The EEG can be helpful in these cases.

Etiologic Factors in Postoperative Delirium

Delirium reflects a diffuse alteration in cerebral function due to changes in brain metabolism. Etiologic factors are usually *outside* the CNS. Delirium as a response to nonspecific conditions such as sensory deprivation or pain has been termed the "ICU psychosis." However, postoperative delirium is often the earliest indication that a significant complication has occurred. Patients should be thoroughly evaluated for serious problems, such as sepsis or heart failure. If major underlying disorders have been ruled out, the patient's delirium may be attributed to "ICU psychosis." Unfortunately, this term is often used to explain an alteration in mental status which should, in fact, be further investigated. Table 20.9 reviews etiologic factors in post-surgical delirium.

Specific surgical settings are associated with an increased risk of delirium. Disturbances of cerebral circulation during cardiopulmonary bypass probably contribute to the higher incidence of delirium after cardiac surgery. The patient's physical condition is the most significant preoperative predictor of postcardiotomy delirium. Risk of delirium increases with degree of cardiac impairment, presence of organic brain syndrome, and complexity of surgical procedure. Psychological factors are much less significant (68).

Eye surgery is also associated with a higher risk of postoperative delirium. Sensory deprivation is an important contributing factor.

Several circumstances predispose the multiple trauma patient to delirium. If there is a possibility of head trauma, cerebral concussion, contusion or subdural hematoma may be present. Meningitis can result from occult basilar skull fracture. Fat embolism may present with delirium and respiratory distress from 12–72 hours after trauma (69). The alcoholic trauma patient who receives a glucose infusion without thiamine supplementation may emerge from anesthesia with a severe confusional state due to Wernicke's encephalopathy. Delirium tremens may also begin immediately postoperatively, or may be delayed in onset up to a week by anesthetic agents and postoperative medications.

Drugs contribute to postoperative delirium. The potential for delirium is proportional to the number of drugs administered. Standing orders for sedatives or hypnotics often result in an intoxicated patient when metabolites accumulate over several days. Numerous drugs used in the postoperative period can cause delirium at therapeutic or higher blood levels.

Delirium resembles an atropinic psychosis. The finding that physostigmine reverses some postoperative deliria implicates anticholinergic drug toxicity in the etiology. Tune et al. followed the mental status of cardiotomy patients pre- and postoperatively (70). Serum anticholinergic activity was determined. There was a strong correlation between the occurrence of postoperative delirium and the level of cholinergic receptor blocking activity in the patient's blood. Drugs with anticholinergic properties should be stopped, if possible, when a patient becomes delirious, and such drugs should be avoided in therapy.

Table 20.9. Selected Etiologic Factors for Delirium in the Postsurgical Setting

Trauma patients
    Fat embolism
    Subdural hematoma
    CNS infection
    Wernicke-Korsakoff encephalopathy
    Drug withdrawal states
Postcardiotomy
    Cumulative anticholinergic toxicity
    Preexisting deficits
    Heart failure/fluid overload
All postanesthesia
    Acute porphyria
    Delirium tremens
    Seizure disorder: Postictal state
                "Psychomotor status"
General
    Fever/pain/sleep deprivation
    Sensory deprivation/isolation from personal
      contact
    Immobilization

Evaluation of the Patient with Postoperative Delirium

Steps in the evaluation of the delirious patient are presented in Table 20.10. General physical examination should be directed towards evidence of infection, cardiopulmonary problems, or drug reac-

Table 20.10. Evaluation of the Patient with Postoperative Delirium

1. Mental status and neurologic examination
     Distinguish delirium from psychiatric or neu-
       rologic complications
2. General physical examination
     Fever
     Papilledema
     Meningismus
     Cardiopulmonary dysfunction
     Stigmata of liver disease
3. Review preoperative course
     Did nurses note disorientation or "sundown-
       ing"?
     Possibility of head trauma
     Prolonged malnutrition, hyperalimentation
     Fever preoperatively
4. Review anesthesia record
     Intraoperative hypoxemia or hypotension
     Hypothermia
     Drugs
     Complications
5. Review current medications
6. Historical factors (obtain from friends, relatives)
     Preexisting dementia: forgetfulness, wander-
       ing, confusion, emotional lability
     Alcoholism
     Other substance abuse
     Prescription drugs
7. Laboratory studies

Electrolytes	Calcium
Glucose	Magnesium Blood gases
BUN	Phosphate Urinalysis
CBS and differential	
If clinically indicated: Drug screens	
	Serum NH_4

8. CXR, EKG
     Obtain EEG if required for confirmation of
       delirium
9. Lumbar puncture if no evidence of CNS mass
     lesion or raised intracranial pressure

tions. Chart review will often reveal contributory preoperative or operative factors. Inquiry among the patient's friends
or relatives can yield valuable information on pre-hospital mental status and
drug use. Laboratory data are essential.
An EEG is useful when the diagnosis of
delirium is in question. Lumbar puncture
should be performed in all patients with
unexplained delirium postoperatively, if
no contraindication exists.

Treatment

Four types of interventions are used, in
the order enumerated, to manage postoperative delirium.

1. *Treatment of precipitating conditions.*
   Hypoxemia, anemia, heart failure, and
   other contributors should be vigorously corrected. All nonessential drugs
   must be withdrawn. If a drug withdrawal syndrome such as delirium tremens is present, specific therapy should
   be instituted. Alcoholic patients should
   receive thiamine.
2. *Environmental manipulation.* Ideally,
   the patient should be placed in a quiet
   environment and provided with round-
   the-clock attendants. Extraneous
   stimulation is avoided. Clocks, calen-
   dars, signs, and verbal techniques are
   used to reassure and reorient the patient.
3. *Use of restraints.* Extremely agitated
   or combative patients require restraints to prevent self-harm. The patient's position must be changed frequently. This technique can be quite
   effective when combined with reassurance and reorientation.
4. *Use of antipsychotic agents.* Antipsychotic agents are indicated only when
   other measures have failed and the
   patient remains uncontrollable. Haloperidol is the drug of choice, at a dosage of 1–5 mg i.m. hourly until calm-
   ing occurs. Some clinicians prefer
   phenothiazines (such as chlorpromazine) because of their greater sedating
   effects; however, these drugs have more
   cholinergic activity and cardiovascular
   interactions. Antipsychotics are contraindicated if a sedative-hypnotic drug
   withdrawal syndrome is suspected (because of lowering of the seizure threshold). Although physostigmine can
   abruptly reverse the symptoms of delirium in some cases, its use is not
   generally recommended because of the

potential for serious cardiovascular side effects.

PSYCHOTROPIC DRUGS: AN OVERVIEW FOR THE INTERNIST

Among the most widely prescribed drugs in the United States are those that are used to alter mood, thinking processes, or other abnormal mental states. Many of these agents have far-reaching interactions outside the psychiatric sphere. The following overview of psychotropic drugs emphasizes their effects on organ systems and disease states, rather than their use in specific psychiatric conditions.

ANTIPSYCHOTIC AGENTS

PHARMACOLOGY

These drugs, also called "major tranquilizers" or "neuroleptics" are a structurally diverse group of compounds with antipsychotic activity. The central characteristic shared by all antipsychotic agents is the ability to block receptors for transmitter substances, such as dopamine, norepinephrine, serotonin, and ace-

tylcholine. Blockage of receptors occurs both within and outside the central nervous system, causing an unusually wide range of side effects, including movement disorders and neuroendocrine effects.

The antipsychotic agents now available are from five chemical classes. Each class of neuroleptic has a different profile of receptor interaction, producing various degrees of anticholinergic and antihistaminic action, alpha-adrenergic blockade, sedation, hypothalamic-pituitary derangement, and unwanted neurologic symptoms (Table 20.11). Consideration of which side effects are best avoided or produced in a particular patient can play a major role in drug selection. Generally, the low-potency, higher milligram dose agents cause more autonomic, cardiovascular, and idiosyncratic side effects. On the other end of the spectrum, high-potency drugs, which are relatively free of these problems, result in many more extrapyramidal reactions.

The pharmacology of antipsychotic agent metabolism is still not well understood. The drugs are erratically absorbed orally. They are metabolized in the liver and

Table 20.11. Side Effects of Antipsychotic Agents [a]

Class	Generic Name	Anticholinergic Effects	Extrapyramidal Effects	Orthostatic Hypotension	Special Problems
1. Phenothiazines	Chlorpromazine	H	M L	H	B, D, and E
Aliphatic	Promazine	H [b]	M L	H	B, D, and E
	Triflupromazine	H	M	M	B, D, and E
Piperadine	Thioridazine	H	L	M H	B, E, and F
	Prochlorperazine	M L	H	M	B, D, and E
Piperazine	Fluphenazine	M L	H	L	B, D, and E
	Trifluoperazine	M L	H	L	B, D, and E
2. Thioxanthenes	Thiothixene	M	H	M L	B
3. Butyrophenones	Haloperidol	L	H	L	B
4. Dibenzoxazepine	Loxapine	M	M H	M L	
5. Dihydroindoline	Molindone	M	M	L	

[a] A. *All can cause rashes and photosensitivity, and (rarely) cause blood dyscrasias.*
   B. *Cholestatic jaundice seen rarely. Hepatocellular enzyme elevations also can occur.*
   D. *Lenticular opacities may appear after long-term dosage.*
   E. *Can inhibit ejaculation.*
   F. *Pigmentary retiropathy at high doses.*
[b] *High = H; Moderate = M; Low = L.*

excreted in the urine. The phenothiazines have active metabolites that can be detected in the body up to 6 months after discontinuation. (Appendix B summarizes drug dosages.)

CARDIOVASCULAR INTERACTIONS

Cardiovascular effects of the antipsychotic agents are quite variable. Low-potency agents such as chlorpromazine are powerful vasodilators due to peripheral alpha-adrenergic blockade, effects on central vasoregulatory centers, and direct vessel wall dilatation. Orthostatic hypotension is common, and acute parenteral doses cause a predictable decrease in systolic blood pressure, even in the supine subject. Tolerance to the hypotensive effects usually occurs after several weeks. Mild tachycardia can occur with agents having a vagolytic action. All these effects are minimal with the high-potency agents such as the butyrophenones.

EKG changes are frequent with the use of low-potency antipsychotics. Electrophysiologic studies of thioridazine have demonstrated quinidine-like effects on conducting tissue and muscle, with a decrease in the rate of rise of phase zero of the action potential, lowering of the amplitude of phase 2, and prolongation of phase 3 (72). The effective refractory period is lengthened. Surface EKG tracings show lengthening of the QT_c with increasing dosage. About 50% of patients taking thioridazine will have fluctuating T wave changes (widening, notching, flattening, or frank inversion). These changes appear to be potassium dependent: i.e., they are reversible with potassium administration or after an overnight fast, and accentuated after a meal (73). They can be mistaken for the changes of progressive ischemia if the timing of the EKGs is not known. Similar changes have been reported in 20% of patients taking chlorpromazine, but in much lower frequency with piperazines and thioxanthenes. Haloperidol does not appear to cause T wave changes. Prolongation of PR and QRS intervals, AV block, and ST depression have also been reported with phenothiazines.

Like quinidine, the antipsychotic agents have both anti-arrhythmic properties and the capacity to induce dysrhythmias. Ectopic atrial and ventricular beats, supraventricular and ventricular tachycardias, and ventricular fibrillation have been reported. There have been a number of cases of sudden deaths in otherwise healthy patients taking phenothiazines. Thioridazine is most frequently implicated. Arrhythmias are much less common with the high-potency agents; however, serious rhythm disturbances and unexplained deaths have been reported in young patients taking high doses of haloperidol. The pathogenesis of these cardiac rhythm disturbances is still not well understood. Prolongation of repolarization with increased possibility for reentry may contribute to the serious ventricular arrhythmias.

Experimentally, low-potency antipsychotic agents cause mild myocardial depression at therapeutic doses. Cases of cardiomyopathy have been reported after prolonged treatment.

INTERACTIONS WITH OTHER ORGAN SYSTEMS

Neuroendocrine regulatory systems may be altered by treatment with neuroleptics. Body temperature control is impaired both at the hypothalamic level and through anticholinergic impairment of sweating. Patients are quite vulnerable to hyperpyrexia and heat stroke. Decreased prolactin inhibitory hormone can lead to elevated serum prolactin levels, causing galactorrhea and menstrual irregularities, or gynecomastia and decreased serum testosterone in men. Neuroleptics have been implicated in SIADH in a number of cases. High doses of chlorpromazine can impair glucose tolerance. The cause for the weight gain or the peripheral edema which can occur is unknown, but does not appear to be hormone-related.

The anticholinergic properties of the low-potency antipsychotic agents can lead to toxicity. Constipation is common, and functional bowel obstruction and perforation have been reported. A high index of suspicion is necessary to diagnose this complication in the acutely psychotic patient. Urologic problems include urinary retention or obstruction in the elderly, inhibition of ejaculation (especially with thioridazine), and priapism. Blurred vision is a frequent complaint. Patients with glaucoma can be treated with antipsychotics if followed by an ophthalmologist.

Long-term chlorpromazine treatment may cause lupus-like serologic changes, including a positive ANA, and serum antibodies to double-stranded DNA. Prolongation of the PTT by a circulating anticoagulant is also common, and splenomegaly can occur. Clinical lupus is quite rare (74).

Movement Disorders

All of the neuroleptic drugs have the capacity to produce a number of movement disorders, presumably as a result of pharmacologic action on dopamine receptors of the striato-nigral system and basal ganglia. Probably because dopaminergic blockade results in relative overactivity or disinhibition of cholinergic neurons in this system, most of the associated movement disorders respond well to anticholinergic drugs. Neuroleptics, which have greater milligram potency and less anticholinergic activity, are more likely to produce these syndromes. **Familiarity with these reactions is important, since they can occur in any patient treated with neuroleptics and can be confused with a number of other psychiatric/medical disorders.** There are four forms:

1. *Acute dystonic reaction.* These occur early in the course of treatment (first dose to 1 week). The patient develops muscle group spasm—torticollis, opisthotonos, oculogyric crisis, dysarthria, dysphagia, myoclonic twitching. Dystonic reactions occur most frequently in the young and can result from a single dose of phenothiazine used in a nonpsychiatric setting, such as for preanesthetic or antiemetic medication. Treatment is with oral or parenteral anticholinergics/antihistamines (Table 20.12), or with diazepam. Of these, benztropine is associated with the least amount of sedation and other adverse effects.

2. *Akathisia.* During the first weeks to months of therapy, patients may develop a syndrome of motor restlessness, which can take the form of twitching, rocking, agitation, pacing, or even running. This complication can easily be attributed to the patient's underlying illness and be mistakenly treated with increased dosage, whereas the treatment of choice is dose reduction and anticholinergics. Change to another class of drugs may be necessary.

3. *Extrapyramidal disorders.* During the first month of neuroleptic therapy, patients may complain of weakness and painful muscles, or they are noted to be akinetic, expressionless, and rigid. With longer treatment, patients can present with more classic parkinsonism: shuffling gait, drooling, and tremors. The incidence of the complication is much higher in the elderly, paralleling the age distribution for Parkinson's disease in the general population. Dosage should be reduced or medication changed when this complication appears. This drug-induced disorder also responds well to anticholinergic medications. Amantadine may be used in refractory cases, or where anticholinergics are not well tolerated, but levodopa is not effective.

With the use of large doses of neuroleptics, a more severe, life-threatening extrapyramidal syndrome has been reported, especially in young patients. The clinical state—rigidity and mutism—closely resembles catatonia, with

Table 20.12. Treatment of Drug-Induced Movement Disorders

I. Available Drugs:

Type	Generic Name	Trade Name	Daily Dose Range/mg
Anticholinergic	Benztropine	Cogentin	1–6
	Trihexyphenidyl	Artane, others	1–10
	Procyclidine	Kemadrin	6–20
	Biperiden	Akineton	2–6
Antihistaminic*	Diphenhydramine	Benadryl, others	100–200
	Orphenadrine	Disipal	50–250
Other	Amantadine	Symmetrel	100–300

*More sedating than anticholinergic

II. Disorders:

Side Effect	Onset after Starting Antipsychotic		Treatment
Acute dystonias	1–5 days	Initial	Cogentin 1–2 mg i.v. or i.m
			Benadryl 25–50 mg i.v. or i.m.
			Valium slow i.v., orally
		Follow-up	Continue agent orally for several days only
Akathisia	1–70 days	Initial	Dose reduction
			Oral anticholinergic or antihistaminics
			Benzodiazepines
		Follow-up	Change drug class if necessary
Parkinsonism	1–70 days		Dose reduction
			Oral antihistaminics or anticholinergics
			Amantadine
Catatonia	Early during high-dose therapy		Discontinuation
			Benzodiazepines
			Bromocriptine

which it may easily be confused (75). Pharyngeal muscle dysfunction can lead to dehydration, inanition, or aspiration. Pulmonary embolism can occur. Treatment includes drug discontinuation, aggressive supportive care, and therapy with anticholinergics or amantadine, which may be more effective in this situation. Psychotic thyrotoxic patients seem especially vulnerable to this complication.

4. *Malignant syndrome.* The "malignant neuroleptic syndrome" is a rare, serious, neuromuscular complication of antipsychotic therapy whose onset resembles drug-induced catatonia. After treatment with neuroleptic agents, the patient, often a young male, develops severe extrapyramidal signs such as dystonias, rigidity, or muscular hypertonia. This is followed shortly by pronounced hyperthermia, stupor, or coma, and evidence of autonomic dysfunction, such as tachycardia, pallor, fluctuations in blood pressure, and incontinence. In 40% of patients, leukocytosis and striking elevations of CPK may occur (76). Frank rhabdomyolysis and myoglobinuria may occur. The EEG may be normal. Rapid diagnosis is essential, since significant mortality has been reported in this disorder. Infections such as meningitis and encephalitis, as well as other causes of the catatonic syndrome (see page 493), must be ruled out. The primary treatment of the malignant syndrome is discontinuation of antipsychotic agents.

Symptoms persist for 5–10 days after stopping the neuroleptic (up to 1 month if a depot formulation was used). Dantrolene or high-dose benzodiazepine therapy has been used with some success in this disorder (77). It is not clear whether this syndrome represents a disturbance of central regulatory mechanisms, or is a muscular disorder similar to malignant hyperthermia.

5. *Tardive Dyskinesia.* This is a late, sometimes *irreversible,* complication of neuroleptic therapy, consisting of bizarre, involuntary, buccal-lingual-facial movements which can progress, in severe cases, to involve the extremities. Most cases occur after 6 months or more of therapy, frequently in the context of drug discontinuation or decreased dosage. Between 10–20% of patients treated for longer than 1 year will develop such symptoms. The syndrome is felt to be secondary to denervation supersensitivity of dopamine receptors in the basal ganglia. It is not responsive to anticholinergics. Increased dosage of neuroleptics will temporarily control the motor manifestations, but has the potential of leading to more severe problems. This syndrome is often socially devastating to those afflicted. Because of this serious complication of therapy, the indications for long-term neuroleptic use should be reviewed carefully in each patient and dosage kept to the minimum required. Chronic, prophylactic treatment with anticholinergic drugs is not recommended, since early symptoms of tardive dyskinesia could be masked. During neuroleptic drug withdrawal, "tardive" dyskinesia should not be diagnosed until 6–12 weeks have elapsed, since "withdrawal-emergence" dyskinesias may temporarily appear during this period.

ANTIPSYCHOTIC AGENT OVERDOSE

Although these drugs are used frequently for self-poisoning, they are rarely implicated in overdose fatalities because of their high therapeutic index. Deaths have been reported from doses as low as 500 mg/day of thioridazine.

Supportive care is the cornerstone of therapy. A few specific points should be remembered:

1. Most antipsychotics (except thioridazine) are potent antiemetics. Gastric lavage should be used to remove stomach contents since induced emesis will often fail and wastes time. Hemodialysis is not helpful.
2. A lag period of hours can occur before onset of severe symptoms in poisoning with high-potency agents such as haloperidol.
3. Body temperature should be monitored carefully. Hyperpyrexia can occur. Hypothermia, less likely to be recognized, can lead to cardiovascular collapse.
4. Hypotension is usually the result of vasodilatation and can be treated with fluid replacement under appropriate monitoring. Pressors with beta adrenergic activity (e.g., epinephrine, dopamine) should not be used since they can induce a paradoxical fall in blood pressure in the presence of intense alpha-adrenergic blockade. Hypertension may occur with high-potency agents, and can be managed with a vasodilator.
5. Fatalities from cardiovascular toxicity occur with low-potency agents. The clinical picture includes heart block (delayed conduction), ventricular irritability and ventricular tachycardia (prolonged repolarization facilitating reentry), and decreased cardiac output (direct myocardial toxicity with thioridazine and chlorpromazine). Any patient with a prolonged QT interval should be monitored. Anticholinergic symptoms may be prominent. Regarding management of such patients:

   • Symptomatic heart block is treated with temporary transvenous pacing.

- Physostigmine may be used *with great caution* for supraventricular tachyarrhythmias (SVT). SVT may be difficult to distinguish from VT in the presence of delayed conduction and wide QRS complexes. **Physostigmine can lead to increased block, hypotension, and other complications.**
- Lidocaine is the drug of choice for ventricular dysrhythmias. Quinidine, procainamide, and disopyramide are contraindicated since their effect on conduction is similar to the phenothiazines. If lidocaine fails, dilantin can be tried. Propranolol has also been effective. However, since beta-blockade can precipitate heart block in this situation, placement of a pacing wire is recommended before starting propranolol therapy. Marked prolongation of the QT and repetitive episodes of polymorphous VT of the "torsades de points" form, which have been reported with thioridazine and may occur with other low-potency agents (78,79), are often unresponsive to conventional antiarrhythmic therapy. The treatment of choice is overdrive ventricular pacing or rapid atrial pacing (80,81). Increasing the heart rate and shortening repolarization time with isoproterenol is also effective. However, isoproterenol can cause hypotension in this setting.
- Heart failure can occur. Digoxin and conventional measures are indicated.

6. Signs of CNS toxicity will vary depending on the agent ingested. Two extremes of the clinical spectrum are:

   - *Predominant anticholinergic toxicity.* Patients taking antipsychotics with potent anticholinergic properties can develop confusion, stupor, coma, and seizures. Supportive therapy is usually adequate. If manifestations are life-threatening, or if no cardiovascular complications exist, physostigmine can be used to reverse CNS toxicity.
   - *Predominant CNS excitation.* This can be seen with piperazine phenothiazines, thioxanthenes, and haloperidol. Agitation, delirium, hypertonia, extrapyramidal symptoms, and seizures can occur. Diphenhydramine, 25 mg i.v., can improve extrapyramidal symptoms and dystonic reactions.

TRICYCLIC AND RELATED ANTIDEPRESSANTS

Pharmacology

These widely prescribed drugs have recognized efficacy in the treatment of endogenous depression, and are also used to treat other depressive illnesses and pain syndromes. Tricyclics and related drugs block the re-uptake of amine neurotransmitters into presynaptic nerve endings, thus increasing their concentration at the synapse. However, these drugs vary widely in their specificity of receptor blockade as well as in their degree of anticholinergic and antihistaminic activity (Table 20.13). In usual clinical practice, most currently available drugs are felt to have equivalent antidepressant action, and **choice of an agent is usually based on consideration of side effects.**

The relationship of blood levels to therapeutic response is imperfectly understood. Drug levels are not routinely monitored; rather, initial dosage is low (Table 20.14) and is increased slowly over several weeks. However, plasma levels are helpful for monitoring therapy in elderly or medically ill patients, in individuals who develop side effects, and in those who do not respond to treatment. Underdosage or an inadequate trial are frequent reasons for treatment failure.

Central Nervous System Effects

Actions on the CNS are widespread. The drugs are not CNS "stimulants": nor-

Table 20.13. Pharmacologic Properties of Tricyclic Antidepressants

Agents	α-Adrenergic Blockade (82)	Anticholinergic Effects (83)	Antihistaminic Effects	Sedation (84)
Tertiary amines				
Amitriptyline	+ + +	+ + + + +	+ + +	+ + + +
Doxepin	+ + +	+ + +	+ + + +	+ + + +
Imipramine	+ +	+ + +	+ +	+ +
Trimipramine	+ + +	+ + +	+ + +	+ +
Secondary amines				
Nortriphyline	+ +	+ + + +	+ + +	+ +
Protriptyline	+ +	+ + + + +	+	Minimal
Desipramine	+ +	+ +	+	+
Dibenzoxazepine				
Amoxapine	+ +	+	+ +	+ +
Tetracyclic				
Maprotiline	+ +	+ + +	+ + +	+ + + +
Other				
Fluoxetine	0		0	+
Tradozone	+ + +	+/−	+/−	+ + +

mal subjects given tricyclics will experience sedation, difficulty concentrating, and mild dysphoria. Antidepressants can cause seizures in patients without a previous history of epilepsy. The effect is dose-related. Depressed patients with epilepsy can be treated with tricyclics, but blood levels should be monitored. Other neurologic effects of antidepressants are listed in Table 20.15.

Cardiovascular Interactions

The cardiovascular effects of antidepressant agents are complex (34,86). Orthostatic hypotension is frequent and occasionally may be severe (87). The incidence of orthostatic hypotension is similar in all age groups; however, the elderly are more likely to develop symptoms. Postural blood pressure changes

Table 20.14. Dosages of Tricyclic Antidepressants

Generic Name	Trade Name(s)	Initial Dose (mg)	Usual Daily Dose (mg) Average Adult	Elderly
Imipramine	Tofranil others	25–75	75–200	20–100
Amitriptyline	Elavil	25–75	75–150	20–100
Desipramine	Norpramin	25–75	150–200	20–100
Nortriptyline	Pamelor	40–75	50–100	10–75
Doxepin	Sinequan Adapin	25–75	75–150	30–200
Protriptyline	Vivactil	15	15–40	10–30
Amoxipine	Asendin	150	200–300	100–200
Maprotiline	Ludiomil	25–75	75–150	50–75
Trimipramine	Surmontil	75	50–150	50–100
Fluoxetine	Prozac	20	20–80	
Trazodone	Desyrel	150	150–400	

Table 20.15.   Side Effects of Tricyclic Antidepressants

Effect	Comment
Anticholinergic	
Dry mouth	
Blurred vision	
Urinary hesitancy	Older males
Delayed ejaculation	
Precipitation of glaucoma	Extremely rare: treated glaucoma is not contraindication
Constipation	Cases of ileus and intestinal perforation have been reported
Antihistaminic	Amitriptyline reported 20 times more potent than cimetidine at H_2 receptor
Endocrine	
Gynecomastia, galactorrhea	Uncommon
No known effect on thyroid function	
Priapism	Particularly with trazodone
Neurologic	
Agitation, disorientation: atropinic delirium	Elderly patient Reversible with physostigmine
Parkinsonism	Agents with little anticholinergic effect
Mania	Patients with manic/depressive illness
Uncontrollable rage reaction	Younger patient Not dose-related
Ataxia, dysarthria	Older patient
Seizures	With maprotiline
Stimulant effects	Fluoxetine

appear early in treatment at subtherapeutic plasma levels and are not dose-related. Tolerance often does not occur. In the individual patient, the magnitude of pretreatment orthostatic drop is the best predictor of the subsequent degree of drug-induced blood pressure change. These agents vary in their tendency to cause orthostatic hypotension. Imipramine treatment frequently results in marked standing blood pressure drops even in the healthy adult, while other drugs have lesser effects (Table 20.16).

Tricyclics and tetracyclics alter the

Table 20.16.   Cardiovascular Effects of Antidepressant Drugs at Therapeutic Blood Levels

Agent	Orthostatic Hypotension	Increase in Heart Rate, BPM	Prolongation of EKG Intervals		
			PR	QRS	QTC
Amitriptyline (88)	+ + +	16	±	±	±
Imipramine (86)	+ + + +	7	+ + +	+ + +	+ + +
Nortriptyline (89)	+	16	+	+	+
Desipramine (90,91)	+	15	+ +	+ +	+ +
Amoxapine (92)	+	Increases seen	±	±	±
Maprotiline (93)	+ + +	10	+	+	+
Fluoxetine (32)	minimal	Decreased, 3	0	0	0
Trazodone	transient	No	0	0	0
Doxepin (32)	+	Not significant	Not significant		

electrical properties of the heart through quinidine-like effects on conducting tissue. Electrophysiologic studies in animals reveal dose-related decrease in velocity of phase 0 depolarization, reduction in action potential amplitude, and slowed conduction velocities (94). Psychiatric dosages of tricyclics cause EKG changes in up to 40% of patients: increased PR interval, widening of the QRS complex, nonspecific ST and T wave changes, and increased QT_c. Intervals are usually not prolonged out of the normal range, and changes may revert toward pretreatment values with prolonged therapy or upon discontinuation. His bundle electrocardiography of patients taking amitriptyline or nortriptyline demonstrates normal AH conduction with plasma-level related prolongation of HV conduction times. While alterations in conduction are benign and asymptomatic in most patients, occasionally supraventricular tachyarrhythmias, bundle branch block, or complete heart block have been observed, especially in patients with underlying conduction system disease. Variable slowing of distal conduction in susceptible patients may facilitate reentrant ventricular arrhythmias and ventricular tachycardia. Sudden death has been reported in healthy young patients taking tricyclics. The nontricyclic fluoxetine has been reported not to cause conduction change (32).

Because tricyclic and tetracyclic antidepressants have been reported to cause myocardial depression in overdosage, there has been concern over their use in patients with heart failure. Recent studies have shown that, even in patients with preexisting myocardial dysfunction, **use of these agents does not usually result in demonstrable deterioration of cardiac function** (34,95).

Overdosage

Tricyclic antidepressant (TCA) overdosages account for approximately 10% of overdosages requiring hospital admission, but cause a higher percentage of serious or fatal cases. For example, in 1982, TCA overdose was the third most common drug-related cause of death in the United States (96). **When tricyclics are suspected, any but the most trivial ingestion must be considered serious.** The presence of seizures, coma, dysrhythmias or conduction defects suggests poisoning with these agents. Physostigmine reversal of coma occurs in tricyclic antidepressant overdosage, but is not completely specific as a diagnostic maneuver, since the drug can also lighten hypnosis caused by diazepam, other sedatives, and any anticholinergic drug. An ingestion history of 20 mg/kg (10 times the usual daily dose) or a plasma level greater than 1000 ng/ml constitutes a serious overdosage. Fatalities occur frequently with ingestion greater than 35 mg/kg. However, vagaries in absorption, metabolism, and distribution make blood levels more predictive of outcome. Some data suggest that findings on EKG may be the best predictor of the severity of overdosage. Prolongation of a previously narrow QRS complex to over 100 msec may identify patients who are at risk for serious complications such as arrhythmias or seizures. In one study, ventricular arrhythmias occurred only in patients with a QRS duration of 0.16 seconds or greater (97). It should be kept in mind that newer agents with different effects on cardiac conduction may not show the same profile with overdosage. Amoxapine overdose is characterized by seizures and status epilepticus. Prolongation of the QRS interval is not a guide to severity of overdosage with this drug. Similarly, fluoxetine and trazodone do not have marked effects on the EKG during overdose. Maprotiline has a long half-life: prolonged coma has been seen with this tetracyclic drug, along with the typical manifestations of tricyclic overdose.

Although good supportive care remains the mainstay of treatment, attention to specific aspects of therapy can be lifesaving in tricyclic overdosage. Gastrointestinal absorption is markedly delayed because of gastric atony and ileus. Emetics are often unsuccessful secondary to the antiemetic effects of these drugs and may result in aspirations. Lavage can recover a significant proportion of the total dose up to 12 hours after ingestion.

Activated charcoal binds these drugs and should also be administered. Cathartics can be given to offset decreased peristalsis. Because of avid protein binding and tissue concentration of tricyclics, dialysis and hemoperfusion are not effective. Any patient with a serious overdose should be monitored in an ICU. The duration of monitoring required is not clear. Major cardiac complications usually manifest themselves in the first 24 hours (98).

Management of Complications

Symptoms of anticholinergic poisoning, such as fever, tachycardia, and bowel or bladder paralysis, are best treated supportively if possible. CNS toxicity includes agitation, delirium, grand mal seizures, and coma. Generalized neuromuscular irritability may give rise to pseudoseizures, peculiar episodes of myoclonic jerking which occur with a normal EEG. Diazepam is recommended to treat seizures acutely, and phenytoin may also be used.

Most tricyclic overdose fatalities are due to cardiovascular toxicity. Serious overdoses manifest hypotension, supraventricular tachyarrhythmias, conduction disturbances with widened QRS complexes, and ventricular arrhythmias. The combination of slowed conduction and myocardial irritability makes treatment difficult. The following measures can be tried:

1. *Avoidance of acidosis.* Metabolic acidosis often accompanies significant poisoning. **Protein binding of the tricyclic antidepressants is highly pH-dependent, with an 8-fold <u>decrease</u> in free drug over a 0.8 rise of pH.** Also, animal studies suggest that elevated serum potassium levels may enhance tricyclic toxicity on membranes. Cardiac toxicity can sometimes be reversed dramatically by sodium bicarbonate therapy, or hyperventilation, ideally monitored by arterial blood gases to a pH of approximately 7.45. Reversal of acidosis, if present, is the initial treatment of choice for cardiovascular toxicity (99).

2. *Arrhythmias.* Lidocaine or dilantin can be used to treat ventricular arrhythmias. Quinidine, procainamide, or disopyramide are contraindicated because they may further compromise conduction. Supraventricular tachycardia with wide, aberrant complexes may easily be mistaken for ventricular tachycardia, but should be treated continuously with physostigmine, if necessary. Propranolol must also be used cautiously because of possible myocardial depression. Rhythms of the "torsades des pointes" type may be treated as previously outlined.

3. *Blocks.* Conduction defects may improve with alkalinization; however, ventricular pacing may be required. Prophylactic use of i.v. phenytoin for "early" conduction abnormalities (1° AV block or intraventricular conduction delay) has been reported (100).

4. *Blood pressure.* Hypotension is due to generalized vasodilation with low filling pressures, and/or to myocardial depression. Therefore, initial management includes fluid replacement, as well as correction of pH. If these measures fail, pressors can be tried. Norepinephrine or other alpha-adrenergic agents are the drugs of choice. Because of alpha-blockade, pressors with beta-agonist activity can lead to worsening of hypotension. Dobutamine may be used to counteract myocardial depression.

5. *Use of physostigmine.* This agent has been reported to reverse coma, stop seizures, slow sinus tachycardia and SVT, and improve ventricular irritability in tricyclic overdose. However,

use of the drug can lead to cholinergic crisis, seizures, hypotension or complete heart block. Therefore, physostigmine (1–3 mg slow i.v.) should be reserved for treating life-threatening complications where its use is pharmacologically plausible, such as uncontrollable hypertension or supraventricular tachycardia with circulatory compromise.

Recovery from tricyclic overdose is often prolonged, since drug half-life in this situation may be 45–80 hours, and many drugs have active metabolites. Plasma levels can remain above therapeutic for 4–5 days.

LITHIUM

Over 250,000 patients in the United States are now receiving lithium for psychiatric conditions. The drug is uniquely effective as prophylaxis for the profound mood variations of manic depression (bipolar affective disorder). Lithium also prevents recurrent attacks of mania in patients with unipolar affective disorder and may prevent recurrent depression in certain patient groups. Administration of lithium to an acutely manic patient will gradually restore a normal mood state over 10 days to several weeks.

PHARMACOLOGY

The drug's mechanism of action is unknown. Lithium can substitute for sodium and potassium intracellularly and thus alter membrane potential. It interacts with many cation-dependent enzyme and receptor systems. For example, hormone-mediated adenyl cyclase activity is reduced at several sites (101). The drug is not a sedative and does not cause noticeable CNS effects in normal volunteers.

Lithium is well absorbed orally with peak blood levels being achieved 2–4 hours after a dose. Redistribution into tissue is slower, and adverse effects can occur at "absorptive peaks" of blood levels. For this

reason, the drug is usually given in divided doses. The lithium ion is ultimately distributed throughout the total body water, achieving a steady state in 5–7 days. Ninety-five percent of lithium excretion is renal, with a serum half-life of 18 hours. Since about 80% of filtered lithium is reabsorbed in the proximal tubule and loop of Henle, lithium clearance is usually about one-fifth the patient's creatinine clearance. Increased proximal absorption of sodium will augment lithium reabsorption as well. Sodium depletion will cause increased lithium levels in a patient on chronic therapy. In contrast, salt loading has only a minor effect on lithium clearance.

Lithium has a very low therapeutic index, so that monitoring blood levels is essential. By convention, levels are obtained 12 hours after the last dose. Blood levels are only a guideline since certain patients, especially the elderly, can have symptoms of toxicity at "therapeutic" levels. Maintenance of the lowest level compatible with control of mood disturbance is the therapeutic goal (Table 20.17).

SIDE EFFECTS

Fatigue, gastrointestinal (GI) upset, and weakness are often transient problems during initiation of lithium therapy. A fine tremor, which may respond to beta-blockers, is quite common with chronic treatment. Polyuria is a frequent complaint (see below). The etiology of the weight gain sometimes seen with lithium therapy is obscure. Insulin requirements of diabetics may change. Other side effects and drug interactioins of lithium are summarized in Table 20.18.

CARDIOVASCULAR EFFECTS

Unlike many other psychoactive drugs, lithium has slight cardiovascular actions. Depression or flattening of T waves, resembling hypokalemia, is a frequent EKG finding during lithium therapy. With higher blood levels, T wave inversion and U waves can occur (103). The QT interval

Table 20.17. Lithium Therapy

	Lithium Dosage and Blood Levels	
Condition	Average Dose mg/day (300-mg tabs)	Therapeutic Blood Levels mEq/L (12 hr after oral dose)
Mania Chronic administration (no dose change for 5–7 days)	1200–3600	0.9–1.4
Adult	900–1500	0.4–1.2
Elderly		0.4–0.6
Toxic Levels		>1.6
Serious adult overdose		>3.0
Serious elderly overdose		>1.6
Frequently fatal overdose		>5.0

Monitoring lithium therapy	
Initial	Renal and thyroid history
	Urinalysis, electrolytes, 24-hr urinary volume and creatinine clearance, T4 and T3U, TSH
	Serum lithium and creatinine weekly for 1 month, then every 3 months for 1 year, then every 3 months
	TSH every 3 months for 1 year, then every year
	Yearly urinary volume and creatinine clearance
Maintenance	If TSH elevated, check thyroid function
(Check lithium level if intercurrent illness, dieting, diuretics, or fever occur)	

Drug interactions with lithium	
Indocin	Raises lithium level
Neuromuscular blockade	Potentiated
Dilantin, tegretol	↑ CNS toxicity
Iodide	Hypothyroidism
Antipsychotic agents	Enhance lithium neurotoxicity, higher incidence of neuroleptic malignant syndrome (109,110)
Diuretics	Increased lithium level

is not affected and ST segments do not change at rest or during exercise (104).

Lithium does occasionally affect atrial impulse generation. Reversible sinus node dysfunction (sinus bradycardia, sinus arrest, exit block) causing Stokes-Adams attacks has been precipitated with lithium therapy; however, premature atrial contractions may be suppressed. Conduction defects can also occur, including bundle branch block and complete heart block. The frequency of PVCs can increase during lithium treatment. All of these cardiac effects are uncommon. Short-term lithium therapy does not affect cardiovascular performance as assessed by exercise testing.

LITHIUM AND THE KIDNEY

Some controversy surrounds the effect of lithium on renal function. On initiation of lithium therapy, approximately 50% of patients will have transient polyuria. With chronic treatment, about 25% have somewhat increased urine volumes, and less than 10% have polyuria of greater than 3 L per day. Very rarely, this complication is irreversible when lithium is stopped (106). Lithium causes decreased renal sensitivity to ADH through inhibition of ADH-sensitive adenyl cyclase, and possibly through another mechanism distal to the formation of cyclic AMP (107). Plasma ADH levels rise in most patients taking

Table 20.18.   Side Effects of Lithium Therapy

I. At therapeutic levels

Initial	Nausea, abdominal pain, diarrhea, weakness, fatigue
Chronic	Tremor
	Polydipsia, polyuria
	Edema
	Weight gain
	Psoriasis exacerbation
	Leukocytosis (WBC 10–14,000—neutrophilia with lymphocytopenia) (+) ANA: clinical lupus rare
	Extrapyramidal signs

II. Symptoms of lithium overdose

	Disturbances of Consciousness	Cerebellar	Neuromuscular	Other
Spectrum of increasing severity	Drowsiness	Coarse tremor	Fasiculations	Extrapyramidal signs
	Confusion			
	Stupor	Ataxia	Twitching	
	Coma	Nystagmus	Myoclonus	Localizing sign
	Convulsions	Dysarthria	Reflex asymmetry	
			Hypertonia	

lithium, presumably in compensation. Nevertheless, many patients will be unable to maximally concentrate their urine in response to water deprivation. Exogenously administered vasopressin will not cause further urinary concentration. In addition to this nephrogenic diabetes insipidus, lithium can impair tubular secretion of acid. Other aspects of renal function, including glomerular filtration rate, diluting capacity, and renin levels, are not usually affected by lithium.

Persistent nephrogenic diabetes insipidus and also renal failure are reported sequelae of lithium poisoning. A few cases of nephrotic syndrome have been associated with lithium treatment (108).

Progressive impairment of urinary concentration occurs over years of lithium exposure. This defect improves slowly on discontinuation. Biopsies of polyuric patients and those who have had repeated episodes of lithium toxicity have shown interstitial fibrosis with tubular atrophy and some sclerotic glomeruli (109). These findings are obviously nonspecific and have also been reported in patients with affective disorders who have never

received lithium. The current consensus is that long-term lithium probably can cause structural renal damage, specifically interstitial nephropathy, in some patients. Renal changes are probably related to plasma lithium levels, and to duration of therapy. Impairment of concentrating ability is the most prominent sequela of lithium nephropathy. It has been difficult to document drug-related decreases in GFR in patients who have undergone long-term therapy (110, 111).

A baseline renal evaluation should be done whenever prolonged lithium therapy is contemplated. Patients with persistent polyuria may constitute a vulnerable subgroup and should have more frequent determination of creatinine clearance. Lithium levels should be kept as low as possible (112).

If symptomatic, the polyuria of lithium therapy may be diminished by several drugs. Thiazide diuretics decrease urine flow but may cause changes in lithium and potassium levels and in volume status. Amiloride also diminishes lithium-induced polyuria without affecting potassium or lithium levels (111, 113). The use of indomethacin has also been reported (114).

ENDOCRINE EFFECTS

Changes in thyroid function are the most frequent endocrine effects of lithium therapy. Lithium acts at many points of glandular activity: it blocks TSH-dependent adenyl cyclase, and decreases iodine uptake, iodination of tyrosine, and release of thyroxine. Approximately 30% of patients taking lithium will have increased TSH levels during the first year, 5% will have mild chemical hypothyroidism, and 3% will develop a goiter. An occasional patient, at any point during chronic lithium therapy, will evidence clinical hypothyroidism. **This may present in atypical forms (hallucinations, depression) and may be mistaken for a resurgence of the psychiatric illness.** This complication is higher in women and in those with preexisting thyroid disease. Treatment is via replacement therapy. A few cases of thyrotoxicosis related to lithium have been reported anecdotally. Hyperparathyroidism may be increasingly common in patients who have had long-term treatment (115).

OVERDOSAGE

Although lithium is sometimes ingested with suicidal intent, the majority of cases of lithium toxicity result from chronic therapy. Intercurrent illness, fever, diuretics, dieting, or other causes of volume depletion can precipitate toxicity in the previously well-maintained patient. Acute overdose frequently presents with GI symptoms. In contrast, when blood levels rise gradually toward and above 2 meq/liter, only such nonspecific problems as lethargy, confusion, and weakness may appear, delaying diagnosis. At higher blood levels, progressive neuromuscular irritability, cerebellar signs, and disturbances of consciousness are noted (Table 20.19). Oliguria, anuria, and irreversible renal failure can occur, as well as ST changes, QT_c prolongation, and arrhythmias; how-

Table 20.19. MAO Inhibitors

Agent	Initial Dose mg	Daily Dose Range, mg
Phenelzine (Nardil)	15	60–90
Tranylcypromine (Parnate)	10	20–60
Isocarboxazide (Marplan)	30	10–20

Side effects of MAO inhibitors:

System	Effects
Cardiovascular	Orthostatic hypotension
	Decreased cardiac output (sympatholytic)
Central nervous system	Mild euphoria—tranylcypromine
	Stimulation
	Tremor
Autonomic nervous system	Mild anticholinergic effects
GI tract	Constipation
Peripheral nervous system	Phenelzine-neuropathy (pyridoxine-deficient)
General	Peripheral edema
	Loss of appetite
	Hyperphagia

ever, CNS toxicity causes most morbidity. The fatality rate of serious lithium overdose is estimated at 10–15% (116).

Initial treatment of lithium overdose includes removal of gastric contents, followed by continuous nasogastric (NG) suction, since the ion is secreted into the stomach. Clinical estimation of the patient's condition may be deceptive: deterioration can occur many hours after ingestion and progress, despite falling lithium levels. Lithium blood levels should always be determined and followed. Toxicity appears to be in proportion to the duration of exposure to high lithium levels, as well as to the absolute level. Normally, levels of 3 meq/liter are indicative of serious overdose, and more than 5 meq/liter has a high fatality rate; however, individual variations are great. It is difficult to increase renal lithium excretion significantly, although various methods (osmotic diuresis, aminophylline, acetazolamide) have been recommended. A practical measure, if cardiac and renal function permit, is to ensure a good urine output via saline diuresis, since decreased urine flow will lead to lithium retention. Dialysis is the method of choice for lowering serum lithium levels. Indications for dialysis include a lithium level greater than 4 meq/liter, or severe toxicity. Dialysis should be continued until the level is less than 1 meq/liter. Because of reequilibration from tissue, blood levels will rebound after cessation of dialysis.

Most patients with serious overdose will present with some degree of renal insufficiency, accompanied by decreased renal concentrating ability. Frank nephrogenic DI may ensue, with voluminous output of dilute urine. This syndrome is not responsive to vasopressin. Treatment includes careful attention to electrolyte balance and fluid replacement. Polyuria can persist for weeks to months after an iintoxication.

MONOAMINE OXIDASE (MAO) INHIBITORS

Because of their potential for serious adverse reactions, MAO inhibitors are not widely used for the treatment of depression. However, they have been demonstrated to be effective in many types of depression, and are possibly superior in patients with "atypical" depression (117). Three drugs are currently available (Table 20.19).

Pharmacology

The MAO inhibitors irreversibly inactivate monoamine oxidase (MAO), an intracellular enzyme which degrades epinephrine, norepinephrine, dopamine and 5-HT. Catecholamine-o-methyl transferase (COMT), which matabolizes circulating amines, is not affected. After a dose of an MAO inhibitor, elevated levels of the above amines can be measured in body tissues, such as heart, and in the blood. MAO inhibitors also affect enzyme systems in gut, liver, and other areas.

MAO inhibitors are well absorbed orally. Effects of the drugs last for up to 2 weeks after discontinuation. As with tri-

cyclics, several weeks are required for an antidepressant effect to occur. Orthostatic hypotension, a major side effect, also progresses over weeks and can be so severe as to require discontinuation. Other side effects are listed in Table 20.19.

Drug Interactions

Although the direct effects of the MAO inhibitors are relatively benign, multiple drug interactions may occur. As a result of inhibition of various enzyme systems, MAO inhibitors potentiate and prolong the action of other drugs, including barbiturates, alcohol, antihypertensives, and tricyclic antidepressants (Table 20.20). After discontinuation of an MAO inhibitor, there should be a delay of 2 weeks before starting a tricyclic or another MAO inhibitor to avoid serious interaction. Meperidine (Demerol) can cause severe hyperpyrexia when administered to a patient on an MAO inhibitor.

Hypertensive crisis, the "tyramine reaction," is the best-known serious complication of the use of these drugs. Tyramine escapes its normal gut and hepatic degradation and acts on nerve endings to release the increased amounts of norepinephrine present. Patients develop severe headache, nausea, vomiting, fever, and signs of increased adrenergic activity, including pronounced hypertension. Of importance is the fact that many sympathomimetic drugs, especially indirect acting agents, can cause this response (Table 20.20). Direct adrenergic agents are less likely to cause hypertension since they are metabolized by COMT. Reduction of blood pressure with i.v. phentolamine is the treatment of choice for this reaction. Intramuscular (i.m.) chlorpromazine (for alpha-blockade) has also been used successfully.

Overdose

MAO inhibitors are lethal drugs in overdose: The estimated fatal dose of tranylcypromine is 250 mg (25 pills). If

Table 20.20. Drugs Interacting with MAO Inhibitors

Drug Class	Drug	Effect
Antihypertensives	Reserpine	↑ BP
	Alpha-methyldopa	↑ BP
	Propranolol	↑ BP
	Guanethidine	↓ BP
Sympathomimetics	Pseudoephedrine	Hypertensive crisis
Cold remedies	Ephedrine	Indirect-acting agents worse
Diet pills	Phenylephrine	
Decongestants	Epinephrine	
	Isoproterenol	
	Norepinephrine	
	Dopamine	
	Amphetamines	
	Metaraminal	
Anesthetic agents	Succinylocholine	Potentiated
	Barbiturates, alcohol, analgesics	
Antiparkinson agent	L-Dopa	Hypertensive crisis
Oral hypoglycemics		Potentiated
Tricyclics		Agitation, ↑ BP, seizures, hyperpyrexia
Narcotics[a]	Meperidine	Hyperpyrexia, coma, BP fluctuation

[a] Narcan may reverse or improve.

seen early, patients will present a deceptively benign picture since there is a lag period of up to 12 hours until effects begin. Overdosed patients will develop signs of CNS, autonomic, and neuromuscular irritability, hypertension, seizures, coma, and malignant hyperpyrexia. The following points are important:

1. Gastric lavage is indicated. Acidification of the urine hastens excretion. If a suspected lethal dose has been ingested, consider dialysis.
2. Treat hypertension with phentolamine, and with a vasodilator if necessary. Beta-blockade may also be helpful, but should not be started until after the patient is on an alpha- or ganglionic blocker to avoid worsening of hypertension.
3. Hypotension can occur. If pressors are necessary, use a direct-acting agent such as norepinephrine, and use with great caution.
4. Monitor blood glucose since hypoglycemia may develop.
5. Monitor body temperature. A clinical response to dantrolene has been reported in a case of hyperpyrexia and coma resulting from phenylzine overdose (118).

Appendix A

Medical Illnesses That Can Present with Psychiatric Symptoms

Endocrine Disorder	Comments
Hyperthyroidism	Anxiety, agitation, hyperactivity, paranoia, rarely psychosis
Hypothyroidism	Affective changes, esp. depression, anxiety, slowed mentation, hallucinations
Hyperparathyroidism, hypercalcemia	Personality changes, anxiety, hyperactivity, delusions, paranoia
Hypoparathyroidism, primary or surgical	Anxiety, paresthesias, dissociative changes
Hypercortisolism	Depression most common. Also agitation, paranoia, mania
Adrenal insufficiency	Depression. Occasionally, paranoia or organic brain syndrome
Insulinoma	Episodic personality changes, dementia
Pheochromocytoma	Episodic anxiety Psychoses reported
Hypopituitarism	Anxiety, depression, thought disorder
Acromegaly	Personality changes
Diabetes mellitus	Depression, fatigue, impotence
Abrupt decrease in gonadal function	Vasomotor changes, sweating, flushing, anxiety

Nervous System	

Cerebral hypoxia
  Low cardiac output
  CO poisoning
  Hypoxemia
	Irritability, poor memory, concentration defects, personality changes

Huntington's chorea	Personality changes and subtle dementia seen early
Multiple sclerosis	Protean manifestation
Psychomotor epilepsy	Episodic behavioral abnormalities, episodic dizziness, may have hallucinations during attack
Parkinson's disease	Resembles depression
Dementia Alzheimer's disease	Personality changes, anxiety, depression
Space-occupying lesions Chronic subdural hematomas, tumors, esp. frontal lobe or midline	Personality change: cases presenting as psychosis have been reported

Meningeal infiltration
  CNS sarcoid
  Carcinomatous meningitis
  Infections: TB
       Cryptococcal
       Other fungi
	Neuropsychiatric complaints, headache, fatigue

Neurosyphilis	Personality changes; dementia
Encephalitis Herpes	Because of frontal/temporal lobe predominance, may present with hallucinations, psychosis, personality changes
Others	Severe postencephalitic fatigue syndromes may occur in elderly people

Nervous System	**Comments**
Postconcussive syndrome	Irritability, trouble concentrating, fatigue; may be mistaken for endogenous depression or hypochondriasis
Normal pressure hydrocephalus	Dementia, ataxia, and incontinence are classic triad: personality changes may be prominent

Neuromuscular disease
  Myasthenia gravis
  ALS
  Muscular dystrophies
  Myopathies
	Patient may appear to be "hysterical," have anxiety, or hypochondriasis. Patients with weakness may appear depressed.

Cerebrovascular disorders
  Embolic: Subacute bacterial endocarditis
         Atrial myxoma
         Transient ischemic attack
         Fat emboli
	Fatigue, episodic dizziness or visual loss without objective signs. Frank delirium and hallucinations may occur.

Hemorrhagic: Subarachnoid Intracerebral	Can present as acute confusional state with combative or agitated patient
Migraine	Hemiplegic migraine may be confused with conversion reaction in young person; other unusual manifestations resemble anxiety attacks; careful history usually diagnostic
Stroke	Aphasias may resemble psychotic episode
Sleep apnea	Accompanying hypersomnolence, history of snoring

Metabolic

Acute intermittent porphyria (varigate porphyria)	Anxiety most common; "neurotic" complaints: psychosis can occur in acute episodes.
Wilson's Disease	May present as any psychiatric illness: adolescent turmoil, anxiety, psychosis
Uremia	Fatigue, lassitude, irritability
Electrolyte, calcium, phosphorus imbalance	Delirium, hallucinations, paranoia
Hepatic failure	Apathy, fatigue may resemble depression

Pulmonary

Asthma	Attacks of dyspnea may resemble episodic anxiety
Chronic obstructive pulmonary disease	Irritability, severe fatigue, dyspnea

Other causes of air hunger:
  Salicylate overdose
  Pulmonary embolism
  Chronic pulmonary hypertension
	Absence of objective signs may lead to diagnosis of hyperventilation syndrome

CO_2 narcosis	Delirium, somnolence

Toxic

Manganese	"Manganese madness": psychosis, parkinsonism, organic brain syndrome. Psychosis may be presenting syndrome (ore workers, miners).
Lead: Chronic	Irritability, fatigue, organic brain syndrome combined with abdominal complaints, peripheral neuropathy, extrapyramidal signs.
Subacute	Headache, dizziness, irritability, mood change, weakness, abdominal complaints.

Toxic	**Comments**
	Wide variety of occupational/avocational exposure.
Mercury	
Elemental (chronic)	"Erethism": easy blushing, anxiety, depression, irritability, emotional instability
	Intention tremor
	Occupational exposure (inhalant)
Organomercurials	Erethism, dementia, tunnel vision, paresthesias, cerebellar signs
	"Minimata disease"
	Environmental pollution, occupational exposure
Thallium	Psychosis, hallucinations, irritability; also gastrointestinal irritation and neurologic signs. All variable. Alopecia 1–3 weeks after exposure.
Insecticides	Vague inability to concentrate, dizziness,
Polyhalogenated polyaromatics; chronic poisoning	headache, weakness, occupational or environmental pollution

Deficiency Diseases

Zinc	Apathy, confusional state, depression. May have dermatitis. Clinical setting for nutritional deficiency.
Vitamin B_1	Hallucinations, depression, or dementia can accompany hematologic or neurologic manifestations.
Pyridoxine	Hallucinations, confusion, peripheral neuropathy
Magnesium	Delirium, hallucinations, illusions, or psychosis in clinical setting of alcoholism or nutritional deficiency
Thiamine (Werneke's encephalopathy)	May present as acute confusional state
Tryptophan (Pellagra)	"Diarrhea, dermatitis, dementia" but earliest signs may be neuropsychiatric

Rheumatologic

Polymyalgia rheumatica, temporal arteritis	May present as depression in elderly
Lupus cerebritis	Neuropsychiatric symptoms may be prominent in lupus

Cardiovascular

Valvular heart disease	Case history and physical exam can usually
Heart block, arrhythmias	differentiate from anxiety attack or
Congestive heart failure	depression

Systemic Infections

Pneumonia	In elderly, may present with hallucinations, confusional state
Mononucleosis	Extreme fatigue and malaise may resemble depression
Brucellosis	Prolonged debility associated with infection: can present with anxiety attacks
Malaria	Schizophreniform psychosis, delirium
HIV	"AIDS dementia complex": depression, dementia, organic psychosis

Appendix B

Dosage of Antipsychotic Agents

Drug	Trade Name	Initial Dose mg	Daily Dose Range mg	Approximate Equipotent Dose to 100 mg Chlorpromazine
1. Phenothiazines				
Aliphatics				
Chlorpromazine	Thorazine, Chlor-Pz Others	25–100 orally 25–50 i.m.	100–1000	100
Promazine	Sparine and others	25–50	25–1000	100
Triflupromazine	Vesprin	20–50	20–150	25
Piperidines				
Thioridazine	Mellaril	25–100	30–800	100
Mesoridazine	Serentil	30–50		50
Piperacetazine	Quide	20–50	20–160	10
Piperzines				
Prochlorperazine[a]	Compazine,[a] others	5–10	15–125	15
Acetophenazine	Tindal	20–40	40–80	20
Carphenazine	Proketazine	25–50	25–400	25
Fluphenazine	Prolixin, permitil	2.5–5.0	.5–20	3
Perphenazine	Trilafon	5–10	2–64	10
Trifluoperazine	Stelazine	2–4	2–30	5
2. Thioxanthenes				
Chlorprothixene	Taractan	orally 25–50 i.m. 125–25[b]	75–600	50
Thiothixene	Navane	2–5	6–60	5
3. Butyrophenones				
Haloperidol	Haldol	2.5–5.0	3–30	2
Droperidol	Inapsine	2.5–10		
4. Dihydroindolones				
Molindone	Moban	5–10		20
5. Dibenzoxazepines				
Loxapine	Loxitane	10–20		

[a] No antipsychotic efficacy.
[b] Every 1–3 weeks as depot form.

READINGS

Epidemiology

1. Chandler JD, Gerndt JE: The role of the medical evaluation in psychiatric inpatients. *Psychosomatics* 29:410–416, 1988.
2. Koranyi EK: Undiagnosed physical illness in psychiatric patients. *Ann Rev Med* 33:309–316, 1982.
3. Davies DW: Physical illness in psychiatric outpatients. *Br J Psych* 3:27–33, 1965.
4. Hall RCW, Popkin MK, Devaul RA, et al.: Physical illness presenting as psychiatric disease. *Arch Gen Psychiatr* 35:1315–1320, 1978.
5. Hall RCW, Gardner ER, Stickrey SK, et al: Physical illness manifesting as psychiatric disease: II. Analysis of a state hospital inpatient population. *Arch Gen Psychiatry* 37:989–995, 1980.

Mental Status Examination

6. Strain JJ, Fulop G, Lebovits A, et al: Screening devices for diminished cognitive capacity. *Gen Hosp Psychiatr* 10:16–23, 1988.
7. Chandler JD, Gerndt J: Cognitive screening tests for organic mental disorders in psychiatric inpatients. A hopeless task? *J Nerv Ment Dis* 176:675–681, 1988.

Delirium

8. Lipowski ZJ: Delirium updated. *Compr Psychiatry:* 21:190–196, 1980.
9. American Psychiatric Association: *Diagnostic and Statistical Manual of Mental Disorders,* ed 3, revised. Washington, D.C., American Psychiatric Association, 1987.

Catatonia

10. Abrams R, Taylor MA: Catatonia. A prospective clinical study. *Arch Gen Psychiatry* 33:579–581, 1976.
11. Gelenberg AJ: The catatonic syndrome. *Lancet* 1:1339–1341, 1976.
12. Gelenberg AJ, Mandel MR: Catatonic reactions to high-potency neuroleptic drugs. *Arch Gen Psychiatry* 34:947–950, 1977.

Organic Mental Syndromes

13. Cummings JL: Organic psychosis. *Psychosomatics* 29:16–26, 1988.
14. Manschreck TC, Petri M: The paranoid syndrome. *Lancet* 2:251–253, 1978.
15. Stondemire A, Riethr AM: Evaluation and treatment of paranoid syndromes in the elderly: a review. *Gen Hosp Psychiatry* 9:267–274, 1987.
16. Krauthammer C, Klerman GL: Secondary mania. Manic syndromes associated with antecedent physical illness or drugs. *Arch Gen Psychiatry* 35:1333–1339, 1978.
17. Cummings JL: Organic Psychoses, Delusioinal disorders and secondary mania. *Psychiatr Clin North Am* 9:293–311, 1986.

Medical Illnesses Causing Psychiatric Syndromes

18. MacCrimmon DJ, Wallace JE, Goldberg WM, et al: Emotional disturbance and cognitive deficits in hyperthyroidism. *Psychosom Med* 41:331–340, 1979.
19. Whybrow PC, Prange AJ, Treadway CR: Mental changes accompanying thyroid gland dysfunction. *Arch Gen Psychiatry* 20:48–63, 1969.
20. Smith KC, Barish J, Correa J, et al: Psychiatric disturbance in endocrinologic disease. *Psychosom Med* 34:69–86, 1972.
21. Gabuzda DH, Hirsh MS: Neurologic manifestations of infection with human immundodeficiency virus. *Ann Intern Med* 107:383–391, 1987.
22. Navia BA, Prich RW: The acquired immunodeficiency dementia complex as the presenting or sole manifestation of human immunodeficiency virus infection. *Arch Neurol* 44:65–69, 1987.
23. Bach MC, Boothy JA: Dementia associated with human immunodeficiency virus with a negative ELISA. *N Engl J Med* 315:891–892, 1986.

Approach to the Psychiatric Patient

24. Larson EB, Mack LA, Watts B, et al: Computed tomography in patients with psychiatric illnesses: Advantage of a "rule-in" approach. *Ann Intern Med* 95:360–364, 1981.
25. Goodstein RK: Guide to CAT scanning in hospital psychiatry: *Gen Hosp Psychiatry* 7:367–376, 1985.

26. Beresford TP, Blow FC, Hall RCW, et al: CT scanning in psychiatric inpatients: II. Clinical data predicting scan results. *Psychosomatics* 29:321–327, 1988.

The Hypertensive Patient

27. Raisfeld IH: Cardiovascular complication of antidepressant therapy. Interactions at the adrenergic neuron. *Amer Heart J* 83:129–133, 1972.
28. Croog SH, Levin S, Tevta MA et al: The effects of antihypertensive therapy on the quality of life. *N Engl J Med* 314:1657–1664, 1986.
29. Hansten PD, Horn JR (eds): *Drug Interaction* Philadelphia, Lea & Febiger, 1989.

The Cardiac Patient

30. Glassman AH, Johnson LL, Giardina EV, et al: The use of imipramine in depressed patients with congestive heart failure. *JAMA* 250:1997–2001, 1983.
31. Stoudemire A, Adkinson P: Use of cyclic antidepressants in patients with cardiac conduction disturbances. *Gen Hosp Psychiatry* 10:389–397, 1988.
32. Fisch C: Effect of fluoxetine on the electrocardiogram. *J Clin Psychiatry* 46:42–44, 1985.
33. Smith RC, Chojnacki ML, Hu R, et al: Cardiovascular effects of therapeutic doses of tricyclic antidepressants: Importance of blood level monitoring. *J Clin Psychiatry* 41:57–63, 1980.
34. Veith RC, Raskind MA, Caldwell JH, et al: Cardiovascular effects of tricyclic antidepressants in depressed patients with chronic heart disease. *N Engl J Med* 306:954–959, 1982.

The Patient with Renal Disease

35. Viederman M, Rusk GH: Psychotherapeutic agents in renal failure. *Am J Med* 62:529–532, 1977.
36. Port FK, Kroll PD, Rosenzweig J: Lithium therapy during maintenance hemodialysis. *Psychosomatics* 20:130–131, 1979.
37. McAllister CJ, Soowden EB, Stone WJ: Toxic psychosis induced by phenothiazine administration in patients with chronic renal failure. *Clin Nephrol* 10:191–195, 1978.

Endocrine Disturbances in the Psychiatric Patient

38. Carney MWP, Macleod S, Sheffield BF: Thyroid function screening in psychiatric in-patients. *Br J Psychiatry* 138:154–156, 1981.
39. Cohen KL, Swigar ME: Thyroid function screening in psychiatric patients. *JAMA* 242:254–257, 1979.
40. Gruen PH: Endocrine changes in psychiatric diseases. *Med Clin North Amer* 62:285–295, 1978.
41. Prange AJ, Loosen PT: Some endocrine aspects of affective disorders. *J Clin Psychiatry* 41:29–34, 1980.
42. Carroll BJ, Feinberg M, Greden JF, A specific laboratory test for the diagnosis of melancholia. *Arch Gen Psychiatry* 38:15–22, 1981.

Anorexia Nervosa

43. Schwabe AD, moderator. Anorexia nervosa. *Ann Intern Med* 94:371–381, 1981.
44. Boyar RM: Endocrine changes in anorexia nervosa. *Med Clin North Am* 62:297–303, 1978.
45. Warren SE, Steinberg SM: Acid-base and electrolyte disturbances in anorexia nervosa. *Amer J Psychiatry* 136:415–418, 1979.
46. Mart MS, Faragher BS: The hematology of anorexia nervosa. *Br J Hematology* 23:737–749, 1972.
47. Bowers TK, Eckert E: Leukopenia in anorexia nervosa. Lack of increased risk of infection. *Arch Intern Med* 138:1520–1523, 1978.
48. Gottdiener JS, Gross HA, Henry WL: Effects of self-induced starvation on cardiac size and function in anorexia nervosa. *Circulation* 58:425–433, 1978.
49. Drossman DA: Anorexia nervosa: a comprehensive approach. *Adv Intern Med* 28:339–361, 1983.
50. Cuellar RE, Van Thiel DH: Gastrointestinal consequences of the eating disorders: anorexia nervosa and bulimia. *Am J Gastroenterol* 81:1113–1124, 1986.
51. Saleh JW, Lebwohl P: Metacloplamide induced gastric emptying in patients with anorexia nervosa. *Am J Gastroenterol* 74:127–132, 1980.
52. Heymsfield SB, Bethel RA, Ansley VD, et al: Cardiac abnormalities in cachectic repletion. *Am Heart J* 95:584–594, 1978.

Electroconvulsive Therapy

53. Consensus conference. Electroconvulsive therapy. *JAMA* 254:2104–2108, 1985.
54. Bidder TG: Electroconvulsive therapy in the medically ill patient. *Psychiatric Clin North Amer* 4:391–405, 1981.
55. Troup PJ, Small JG, Milstein V, et al: Effect of electroconvulsive therapy on cardiac rhythm, conduction, and repolarization. *PACE* 1:172–177, 1978.
56. Abiuso P, Dunkelman R, Proper M: Electroconvulsive therapy in patients with pacemakers. *JAMA* 240:2459–2460, 1978.
57. Gerring JP, Shields HM: The identification and management of patients with a high risk for cardiac arrhythmias during modified ECT. *J Clin Psychiatry* 43:140–143, 1982.
58. Dec OW, Stern TA, Welch C: The effects of electroconvulsive therapy on serial electrocardiograms and serum cardiac enzyme values. *JAMA* 2540:2525–2529, 1985.

General Psychological Risk Factors for Surgery

59. Rockwell DA, and Pepitone Rockwell R: The emotional impact of surgery and the value of informed consent. *Med Clin North Am* 63:1341–1350, 1979.
60. Willner AE, Rabiner CJ, Wisoff BG, et al: Analogy tests and psychopathology at follow-up after open-heart surgery. *Biol Psychiatry* 11:687–696, 1976.
61. Willner AE, Rabiner CJ: Psychopathology and cognitive dysfunction five years after open-heart surgery. *Compr Psychiatry* 20:409–418, 1979.

Preoperative Evaluation of the Patient with Known Psychiatric Illness

62. Solomon S, McCartney JR, Saravay SM, et al: Postoperative hospital course of patients with history of severe psychiatric illness. *Gen Hosp Psychiatry* 9:376–382, 1987.
63. Kampmeier RH: Diagnosis and treatment of physical disease in the mentally ill. *Ann Intern Med* 86:637–645, 1977.
64. Boakes AJ, Laurence DR, Tech PC, et al: Interactions between sympathomimetic amines and antidepressant agents in man. *Br Med J* 1:311–315, 1973.
65. Dilsaver SC, Coffman JA: Antipsychotic withdrawal phenomena in the medical-surgical setting. *Gen Hosp Psychiatry* 10:438–446, 1988.
66. Havdala HS, Borison RL, Diamond BI: Potential hazards and applications of lithium in anesthesiology. *Anesthesiology* 50:534–537, 1979.

Postoperative Delirium

67. Wever RJ, Oszko MA, Bolender BJ, et al: The intensive care unit syndrome: causes, treatment and prevention. *Drug Intell Clin Pharm* 19:13–20, 1985.
68. Dubin WR, Field HZ, Gastfriend DR: Postcardiotomy delirium. A critical review. *J Thorac Caradiovasc Surg* 77:586–594, 1979.
69. Dines DE, Burgher IW, Okazaki H: The clinical and pathological correlation of the fat embolism syndrome. *Mayo Clin Proc* 50:407–411, 1975.
70. Tune LE, Holland A, Folstein MF, et al: Association of postoperative delirium with raised serum levels of anticholinergic drugs. *Lancet* 2:651–653, 1981.
71. Moore DP: Rapid treatment of delirium in critically ill patients. *Am J Psychiatry* 134:1431–1432, 1977.

Psychotropic Drugs

72. Elkayam U, Frishman W: Cardiovascular effects of phenothiazines. *Am Heart J* 100:397–401, 1980.
73. Chouinard G, Annable L: Phenothiazine-induced ECG abnormalities. Effect of a glucose load. *Arch Gen Psychiatry* 34:951–954, 1977.
74. Zarrabi MH, Zucker S, Miller F, et al: Immunologic and coagulation disorders in chlorpromazine-treated patients. *Ann Intern Med* 91:194–199, 1979.
75. Gelenberg AJ, Mandel MR. Catatonic reactions to high potency neuroleptic drugs. *Arch Gen Psychiatry* 34:947–950, 1977.
76. Carnoff SN: The neuroleptic malignant syndrome. *J Clin Psychiatry* 41:79–83, 1980.
77. Fricciore GL, Cassem NH, Hooberman D, et al: Intravenous lorazepam in neuroleptic-induced catatonia. *J Clin Psychopharmacol* 3:338–342, 1983.

78. Sclarovsky S, Strasberg B, Lewin RF, et al: Polymorphous ventricular tachycardia: Clinical features and treatment. *Am J Cardiol* 44:339–344, 1979.

79. Fowler NO, McCall D, Chon T, et al: Electrocardiographic changes and cardiac arrhythmias in patients receiving psychotropic drugs. *Am J Cardiol* 37:223–230, 1980.

80. Smith W, Gallagher JJ: Les torsades de pointes: An unusual ventricular arrhythmia. *Ann Intern Med* 93:578–584, 1980.

81. Khan MM, Logan KR, McComb JM, et al: Management of recurrent ventricular tachyarrhythmias associated with Q-T prolongation. *Am J Cardiol* 47:1301–1308, 1981.

82. Richardson JW, Richelson E: Antidepressants: A clinical update for medical practitioners. *Mayo Clin Proc* 59:330–337, 1984.

83. Blackwell B, Stefopoulos A, Enders P, et al: Anticholinergic activity of two tricyclic antidepressants. *Am J Psychiatry* 135:722–724, 1978.

84. Hollister LE: Tricyclic antidepressants. *N Engl J Med* 299:1106–1109, 1978.

85. Glassman AH, Bigger T: Cardiovascular effects of therapeutic doses of tricyclic antidepressants. *Arch Gen Psychiatry* 38:815–820, 1981.

86. Glassman AH, Rouse SP, Giardina EV, et al: Cardiovascular effects of tricyclic antidepressants. Meltzer HY (ed): *Psychopharmacology: The third generation of progress.* New York, Raven Press, 1987.

87. Hayes JR, Born GF, Rosenbaum AH: Incidence of orthostatic hypotension in patients with primary affective disorders treated with tricyclic antidepressants. *Mayo Clin Proc* 52:509–512, 1977.

88. Ziegler VE, Co BT, Biggs JT: Electrocardiographic findings in patients undergoing amitriptyline treatment. *Diseases of the Nervous System* 38:697–699, 1977.

89. Freyschuss U, Sjogvist F, Tuck D, et al: Circulatory effects in man of nortriptyline, a tricyclic antidepressant drug. *Pharmacol Clin* 2:68–71, 1970.

90. Veith RC, Friedel RO, Bloom V, et al: Electrocardiogram changes and plasma desipramine levels during treatment of depression. *Clin Pharmacol Ther* 27:796–802, 1980.

91. Rudorfer MY, Young RC: Desipramine: Cardiovascular effects and plasma levels. *Am J Psychiatry* 137:984–986, 1980.

92. Smith RS, Ayd FJ: A critical appraisal of amoxapine. *J Clin Psychiatry* 42:238–242, 1981.

93. Burckhardt D, Roeder E, Muller V, et al: Cardiovascular effects of tricyclic and tetracyclic antidepressants. *JAMA* 239:213–216, 1978.

94. Brennan FJ: Electrophysiologic effects of imipramine and doxepin on normal and depressed cardiac purkinje fibers. *Am J Card* 46:599–606, 1980.

95. Roose SP, Glassman AH, Giardina EV, et al: Nortryptyline in depressed patients with left ventricular impairment. *JAMA* 256:3253–3257, 1986.

96. Callahan M, Kassel D: Epidemiology of fatal tricyclic antidepressant ingestion: implications for management. *Ann Emerg Med* 14:1–9, 1985.

97. Boehnert MT, Lovejoy FH: Value of the QRS duration versus the serum drug level in predicting seizures and ventricular arrhythmias after an acute overdose of tricyclic antidepressants. *N Engl J Med* 313:474–479, 1985.

98. Goldberg RJ, Capore RJ, Hunt JD: Cardiac complications following tricyclic antidepressant overdose. *JAMA* 254:1772–1775, 1985.

99. Frommer BA, Kulig KW, Marx JA, et al: Tricyclic antidepressant overdose. A review. *JAMA* 257:521–526, 1987.

100. Hagarman GA, Hanasiro PK: Reversal of tricyclic-antidepressant-induced cardiac conduction abnormalities by phenytoin. *Ann Emerg Med* 10:82–86, 1981.

101. Singer I, Rotenberg D: Mechanisms of lithium action. *N Engl J Med* 289:254–260, 1973.

102. Reisberg B, Gershon S: Side effects associated with lithium therapy. *Arch Gen Psychiatry* 36:879–887, 1979.

103. Demers RG, Heninger GR: Electrocardiographic T-wave changes during lithium carbonate treatment. *JAMA* 218:381–386, 1971.

104. Tilkian AG, Schroeder JS, Kao JJ, et al: Effect of lithium on cardiovascular performance: Report on extended ambulatory monitoring and exercise testing before and during lithium therapy. *Am J Card* 38:701–708, 1976.

105. Tilkian AG, Schroeder JS, Kao JJ, et al: The cardiovascular effects of lithium in man. *Am J Med* 61:665–670, 1976.

106. Simon NM, Garber E, Arieff AJ: Persistent nephrogenic diabetes insipidus after lithium carbonate. *Ann Intern Med* 86:446–447, 1977.

107. Forrest JN, Cohen AD, Torretti J, et al: On the mechanism of lithium-induced diabetes insipidus in man and rat. *J Clin Invest* 53:1115–1123, 1974.

108. Richman AV, Masco HL, Rifkin SI, et al: Minimal-change disease and the nephrotic syndrome associated with lithium therapy. *Ann Intern Med* 92:70–71, 1980.

109. Hansen HE, Hestbech J, Sorensen JL, et al: Chronic interstitial nephropathy in patients on long-term lithium treatment. *Q J Med* 48:577–591, 1979.

110. Hullin RP, Coley VP, Birch NJ, et al: Renal function after long-term treatment with lithium. *Br Med J* 1:1457–1459, 1979.

111. Boton R, Graviria M, Batlle DC: Prevalence, pathogenesis and treatment of renal dysfunction associated with chronic lithium therapy. *Am J Kidney Dis* 10:329–345, 1987.

112. Amdisen A, Grof P: Lithium and the kidney. *International Drug Therapy Newsletter* 16:9–16, 1981.

113. Batlle DC, Riotte AB, Graviria M, et al: Amelioration of polyuria by amiloride in patients receiving long-term lithium therapy. *N Engl J Med* 312:408–414, 1985.

114. Allen HO, Jackson RL, Winchester MD, et al: Indomethacin in the treatment of lithium-in-

duced nephrogenic diabetes insipidus. *Arch Intern Med* 149:1123–1126, 1989.

115. Stancer HC, Forbath N: Hyperparathyroidism, hypothyroidism, and impaired renal function after 10 to 20 of lithium treatment. *Arch Intern Med* 149:1042–1045, 1989.

116. Hansen HE, Amdisen A: Lithium intoxication. *Q J Med* 186:123–144, 1978.

117. Murphy DL, Aulakh CS, Garrick NA, et al: Monoamine oxidase inhibitors as antidepressants. Meltzer HY (ed): *Psychopharmacology: The Third Generation of Progress.* New York, Raven Press, 1987.

118. Kaplan RF, Feinglass NG, Webster W, et al: Phenelzine overdose treated with dantrolene sodium. *JAMA* 255:642–644, 1986.

21
Special Topics

Richard J. Gross and William S. Kammerer

The preceding chapters have examined the effect of a single medical problem on the overall risk for anesthesia and surgical procedures. The opposite approach is used in this chapter, which discusses how the risks of selected operations are affected by common medical problems.

Since it is not possible to discuss all surgical procedures, the procedures were selected based on the prevalence of significant medical problems unrelated to the primary surgical disease and the availability of literature relating medical risk to the specific surgical procedure. Emphasis is given to selecting preoperative problems that are not discussed in standard textbooks. In addition, a number of special problems are included in this section which do not fit elsewhere in the book, including surgery in the elderly patient (over age 65) and consultation on the burn patient.

SURGICAL PROBLEMS IN THE ELDERLY

The evaluation of elderly patients for surgery has become increasingly important as the proportion of people over age 65 increases. Improvements in surgical and anesthesiological techniques have greatly reduced surgical risk, even for the very old (over 80 years) (1, 2), although some authorities have questioned a decrease in risk (6, 18, 35).

Mortality is increased for elderly patients for certain operations. However, in most cases, age itself is a relative, and not a prohibitive, risk factor. The effect of age on operative risk varies widely between different procedures, ranging from a very small increase in cataract extraction to a major increase for partial gastrectomy (Table 21.1).

Many physicians have not yet become accustomed to the changes in the effect of age on operative risk over the past 20 years. Most of this section will be devoted to outlining the effect of age on the risk of different operative procedures, the proportion of increased risk due to age itself versus that from concomitant disease, the interaction of age with other risk factors, and the degree to which the increased risk can be reduced (see also Chapter 3).

A consistent theme throughout this section will be that *a patient should neither be rushed into nor denied surgery solely because of age.*

Epidemiology

The risk of many operations is increased in the older age groups. The increased risk is due both to age itself and other accompanying disease found in older patients.

The age above which the risk of surgery is markedly increased has been moved back from 50–60 in the 1940s to 65–80 currently. Major surgery is now performed with acceptable risk in the healthy over 80 age group (27–34). It is not likely that the age contraindicating major surgery can be moved back much further because of the small proportion of patients above age 90. A more likely occurrence will be the use of age as a relative rather than absolute risk.

The risk of surgery is still increased in

Table 21.1. Representative Mortality for Selected Common Surgical Procedures in the Elderly[a,b]

Operation	Mortality (%)[b] All Adult Patients (age 20–up)	Elderly (age 65+)
All procedures	2 (.9% excluding age 65+)	5–10%
Non-body cavity		
Amputation	2–4	3–17
Cataracts	0.01–0.05	0.01–0.2
Hernia		
Elective	0.01	0.3
Emergency	0.1	1–3
All	0.05	1
Mastectomy (modified radical)	0.1	0.6
Radical neck dissection	0.1–1	11
Transurethral resection prostate	<0.4	0.2–2
Total hip replacement		5
Abdominal		
Appendectomy		
Without perforation	0.01	0.6
Perforated	0.1	6
Cholecystectomy (elective)	0.3–7	3–7
Colon resection (cancer)	5	10
Gastric		
Vagotomy-pyloroplasty	0.6	3–18
Partial gastrectomy	1–3	3–18
Thoracic and Cardiac		
Pneumonectomy	3–6	10–20
Aortic valve	5–10	15–20
Mitral valve	10	15–20
Coronary artery bypass graft	7	3–5
Vascular		
Aortic aneurysm (elective)	5	5–10%
Major bypass for peripheral vascular disease	5	15

[a] Derived in part from Refs. 3–6, 8, 11, 17–26.
[b] The mortality figures cited above are from representative series in the literature. The relative differences can be taken as accurate. The absolute mortality should NOT be considered definitive because of wide variation in series in the literature, recent improvements in mortality that have not appeared in the literature, and differences in patient population, severity of disease, and expertise between different centers.

elderly patients compared with other age groups. The overall risk for all operations in adults less than age 65 is 0.9% compared to 5–10% for patients over age 65 (Table 21.1). Table 21.1 should be interpreted as showing only relative differences, since there is wide variation in mortality depending on the year of the study and the center at which it was done.

In the very old (over age 80), surgical risk is elevated (about 10%) (Table 21.2), compared with patients less than age 65 (0.9%), and 65–80 (about 5%), but the risk

Table 21.2. Surgical Mortality in the Very Old

Study	Control Group (<age)	Age >80	>90
Denney (1972)			29%
Djokovic (1979)			6.2%
Adkins (1984)			13.4%
Michael (1984)			7.5%
Pollock (1987)	5%	20%	
Hosking (1989)			8.4%
Median	—	—	8.4%

Table 21.3. Anesthesia—Surgical Mortality in the Elderly

Study	≤65	65–70	70–80	80–90	90+
Djokovic, 1979				5%	9%
Marx, 1973	1–3%	4.3%	6.6%	7.8%	
Burnett, 1972				7–13%	
Kohn, 1973 (all ages)[a]	≈5%[b]	5%		12%	
Marshall, 1964				20%	13.5%
Lassen, 1962	2.5%	10.9%	14%	25%	
Coghill, 1967					
Elective surgery	8%		18%		
Emergency surgery	10%		23%		

[a] Age 70–75, 5%; age 75–90+, 12%.
[b] Age 60–70.

is not prohibitive. Reports on small numbers of patients age 100 or more (31, 34) show acceptable risks, but most of the procedures were minor.

The risk of anesthesia increases with age, with the largest difference being between the under and over 60–65-year age group (Table 21.3) (Fig. 21.1). Current series indicate overall mortality due to anesthesia and surgery is 1–2% below age 60 and increases to 5–15% above age 65. Within the group defined as elderly above age 65, there seems to be similar mortality between age 65–80 (Table 21.3). The risk then increases from about 5–10% to 10–20% in the 80 and above age group. However, more recent data suggest that surgery can be done above age 80–90 with a 5–10% mortality (28, 30–32). Thus, current evidence suggests there

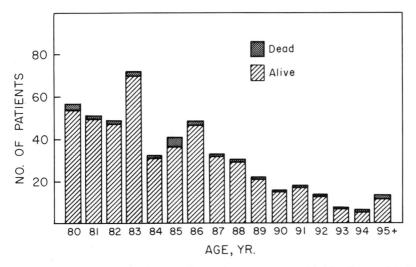

Figure 21.1. Perioperative mortality by age for patients over age 80 (the "very elderly"). There is no increase in mortality with increasing age *over* age 80. Note the "surprisingly" low mortality for such an elderly group of patients. (From Djokovic JL, Hedley-Whyte J: Prediction of outcome of surgery and anesthesia in patients over 80. *JAMA* 242:2302, 1979, with permission, copyright 1979, American Medical Association.)

is not or is only slightly increased in patients over age 65 (Table 21.1), with the exception of radical neck dissection.

The increased surgical risk in the elderly is related to the type of surgery. The risk of surgery not involving body cavities is not or is only slightly increased in patients over age 65 (Table 21.1), with the exception of radical neck dissection.

Major abdominal and thoracic surgery have significantly increased risk in the elderly. An important factor in this increased risk is the higher incidence of emergency procedures and the marked increased risk of emergency procedures in elderly patients.

A number of other factors beside age contribute to the increased operative risk in the elderly (see Table 21.7, p. 550). An understanding of these factors is crucial because they determine the very wide variation in operative risk between patients of the same age. The most important factors are sex, type of anesthesia and surgery, overall medical condition, certain specific diseases (such as heart or lung disease), and general physical and psychological status.

SEX

Perioperative mortality was 6.6% for females and 5.6% for males in a study of patients over 80. There are suggestive data that risk may be lower for females under certain circumstances. Females may have a lower anesthetic mortality (14); pulmonary disease may represent a lower risk in females (16); and females undergoing cholecystectomy may have a lower mortality than males (17). Adequate controls have not been examined to determine whether these are real associations or are due to confounding variables.

TYPES OF ANESTHESIA

Spinal anesthesia does not necessarily offer a lower risk than general anesthesia (12, 27) (see p. 24). Local anesthesia or regional block carries a very low risk. The anesthesia literature indicates a higher mortality for procedures under local compared with other types of anesthesia, but this is due to selection of the worst cases for local procedures. There has generally been a very small increment in operative mortality with age for elective procedures that are done under local anesthesia, such as cataract extraction.

SURGICAL PROCEDURE

Major determinants of surgical risks in the elderly are the urgency of the procedure and need to enter the peritoneal or pleural cavities. Emergency or urgent surgery consistently has had a much higher (three times) mortality than the same surgery done electively (18, 35). The increment in risk for emergency surgery is proportionately much higher for elderly than young patients. The higher risk for emergency surgery has been supported by mortality in general surgical series (Table 21.1) (Fig. 21.2) and series for specific operations (Tables 21.4 and 21.5).

Abdominal or thoracic surgery has had a much greater increment in risk (as well as an absolutely high risk) than surgery not involving body cavities (Table 21.1).

There is only slightly increased risk to non-body cavity surgery, especially if done under local or regional anesthesia (such as cataract extraction or elective hernia repair). Notable exceptions are neurosurgery and radical neck dissection (1, 10, 11). Pneumonectomy is also done with increased risk in the elderly, although the effect of age on less extensive resection is not as well documented. The risk of major vascular surgery in the elderly has fallen greatly to where it approaches that of younger patients if proper patient selection and appropriate procedures are utilized.

Thus, elective surgery not involving body cavities can be done at a relatively low risk in the elderly. A major decrement in risk can also be obtained by doing body cavity surgery electively rather than urgently.

The finding of surgically uncorrectable

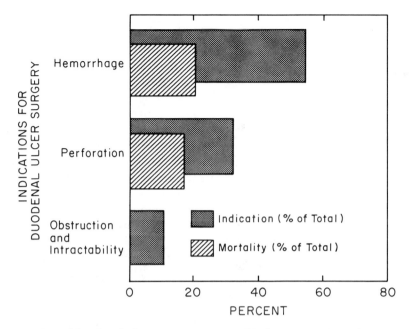

Figure 21.2.   Mortality of duodenal ulcer surgery among elderly patients by indication for surgery. Emergency indications for surgery carried a higher mortality. (From Ferris P: Surgical management of the elderly. *Hosp Prac* 11:68, 1976, with permission (chart by A. Miller).)

Table 21.4.   Elective versus Emergency Surgery in the Elderly

	Elective Operations	Emergency Operations	Age Group
Cole			
Three series prior to 1960	6.5%	18.5%	>60
Two series— 1957, 1965	5.0	24%	>70
Marshall, 1964	10%	20%	>80

Table 21.5.   Mortality for Elective versus Emergency Surgery in the Elderly—Selected Procedures

	Mortality	
	All Patients	Elderly (age 65+)
Appendectomy		
Elective	0.01%	0.2–0.8%
Emergency	0.03%	4–20%
Cholecystectomy		
Elective	0.2%	3%
Emergency	2%	5–10%

disease at the time of surgery (e.g., extensive mesenteric infarction or disseminated cancer) greatly increases surgical risk and accounts for a significant proportion of perioperative mortality in the elderly (1, 43). Surgery for malignancy in the elderly has a higher risk than for other conditions. These factors cannot usually be modified, but do affect surgical risk.

GENERAL HEALTH

Important measures of operative risk have been overall scales of severity of illness, which are independent of specific organ system disease. The scales have graded severity of an illness in a spectrum from healthy to terminally ill. The best known general measure is the American Society of Anesthesiologists (ASA) scale (see p. 22). Operative mortality increases as ASA status declines from healthy (class I) to moribund (class V). There is some evidence supporting ASA status as a risk factor independent of age

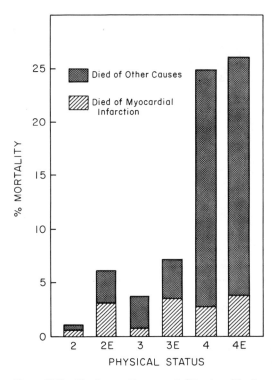

(Fig. 21.3) (1, 17). The healthy elderly patient is at less risk than the patient rated moderately to severely ill overall, without making specific reference to the organ system involved.

GENERAL CONDITION

The patients' general condition refers to their overall physical and psychological status as assessed by such factors as nutrition, debility, and daily activities, as compared with "general health" above, which refers to overall severity of illness. The physician's overall general opinion of the status is still important. Some au-

thors have contrasted the term physiological age with chronological age to describe the differences in physical conditioning and activity of older patients of the same age. It is important that the physician's overall assessment is factual, objective, and accurate. Too often, physicians make a quick, poorly thought-out statement about the patient's general condition on which life and death decisions are made. In our experience and from our review of the literature, most physicians base their assessment of the patient's general condition on three factors: nutrition, activity, and psychological status. The more commonly used negative terms are malnutrition, debility (or inanition), and will to live.

The objective measures of *nutritional status* previously given (see p. 38) are applicable to older patients. Many of these measures were validated on elderly, hospitalized populations. It is important that multiple objective measures be used and then combined with the physician's own assessment, since no single measure now available is accurate.

Activity level (36, 38) is best described by contrasting the example of the 70-year-old patient active in family life, gardening, and tennis, with the bedridden, demented nursing home patient of the same age. Assessment of activity should include the patient's daily activities, whether the patient lives or can live alone, independence for activities of daily living, and muscle mass. The term *debility* is used to describe a patient with loss of muscle mass and ability to perform activities. The term *inanition* refers to the loss of interest in doing daily activity, as well as the ability to do them.

Several factors contribute to the patient's *psychological status* before surgery. The patient's attitude toward surgery and his feelings about its outcome are important. Although no study has proven that the patient's predictions of surgical outcome correlate with actual results, most clinicians dealing with elderly patients have found a correlation. The patient's overall will to live is important, his living (social) situation previously and the situation to which he will return postoperatively is important to "quality of life."

SPECIFIC ORGAN SYSTEM DISEASE

Dysfunction of several organ systems is responsible for much of the perioperative mortality in the elderly. Unrelated organ system disease contributes substantially to the increased surgical risk in the elderly (21, 35, 37, 38, 43, 50).

Preexisting *cardiac disease* increases operative risk, especially coronary artery disease or congestive heart failure (3, 13, 28, 40, 76). Age over 70 has been shown to be a risk factor independent of preexisting heart disease for postoperative cardiac complications (76). Weaker associations have been made between preoperative pulmonary disease, age over 70, and postoperative morbidity (3, 5, 14, 17).

"Causes" of postoperative mortality in the elderly are given in Table 21.6. Cardiac disease is the most frequent cause of mortality. Infection and sepsis are the second most common cause of perioperative mortality. Renal failure is a significant contributing factor to mortality in the elderly. Inadequate data are available on whether preoperative renal disease or intraoperative acute renal failure is the more important determinant of postoperative morbidity.

Diagnostic Activities and Approaches

Extensive preoperative evaluation is necessary because of the wide variety of concomitant medical conditions and the need for general health information in this age group (see Chapter 23).

The information from initial evaluation should be reviewed for specific risk factors in the elderly when the data base is complete. It has been our experience that risks are commonly misjudged in the elderly unless clinicians review the patient record with specific risk factors in mind.

The record should be examined for two

Table 21.6. "Causes" of Mortality Postoperatively in Elderly Patients[a]

Cause	Djokovic (1979)	Cole (1950– 1952)[b]	Randall (1968)	Kohn (1973)	Miller (1977)	Palmberg (1979)
Heart disease (all)	32%	24%	12%	12%	17%	13%
Myocardial infarction	29%				17%	2%
Congestive heart failure	3%					
Pulmonary emboli	3%	11.6%	5.5%	12%	6%	33%
Chronic obstructive lung disease	3%	—[c]	—[c]			
Infection (total)	26%	33%	56%	16%		
Pneumonia (± sepsis, atelectases)	26%	18%	28%	16%	56%	26%
Sepsis (includes peritonitis)		15%	28%		22%	
Gastrointestinal				4%		
Liver disease						
Bleeding					6%	6%
Renal failure	3%	7.5%	0%	8%		
Miscellaneous (total)	34%	23%	18%	38%		10%
Carcinoma	6%	12%	18%	16%		
Subarachnoid hemorrhage	6%					
Mesenteric infarction	19%					
Ruptured aortic aneurysm	3%					

[a] Compiled from series in the bibliography.
[b] Average of three series.
[c] Pulmonary deaths included in pneumonia mortality.

Table 21.7. Known Factors Increasing Operative Risk in the Elderly (in addition to age)

A. **Patient**
1. ? Sex
2. General health (ASA status; healthy vs. chronic disease)
3. General condition
   Nutrition (malnutrition)
   Activity (debility, inanition)
   Psychological status (attitude toward surgery, will to live, social situation)

B. **Specific organ disease**
1. Cardiac (coronary artery disease, congestive heart failure)
2. Infection or sepsis (especially pneumonia)
3. Renal disease
4. Less important or common: COPD, liver disease, congestive failure, dementia

C. **Type of surgery**
1. Body cavity vs. non-body cavity
2. Elective vs. emergency
3. Type of anesthesia
4. Finding of surgically uncorrectable disease or malignancy

sets of risk factors (Table 21.7). First, does the patient have diseases of organ systems which place the elderly at particularly high risk: cardiac disease (especially coronary artery disease), infection or sepsis (especially pneumonia), chronic obstructive lung disease, or chronic renal failure?

Secondly, general risk factors characteristic of the patient and the type of surgery should be assessed (Table 21.7). Finally, the assessment of the benefit to the patient in terms of quality of life and, if applicable, longevity is even more crucial in the elderly than in other age groups. Assessment of cardiac status is discussed on p. 107.

Patients over age 60–65 undergoing major surgery should have spirometry done routinely because of the increased severity and frequency of pulmonary complications in this age group.

Routine tests of renal function using the serum creatinine and blood urea nitrogen may be misleading. Serum creatinine may be falsely low due to reduced muscle mass. The urea nitrogen may be falsely low due to poor intake or falsely high due to volume depletion. Glomerular filtration rate falls with increasing age. A normal serum creatinine of 1.0 mg/dl in an 80-year-old may represent loss of the 50% of renal function which is lost before the creatinine rises. A creatinine clearance can resolve questions of renal function.

Infection or sepsis may be clinically subtle in sick elderly patients. In very old patients, a careful and often repeated search for infection should be made in the presence of even nonspecific signs of infection such as unexplained low-grade fever, unexplained leukocytosis, or "downhill" course (see p. 394).

A notoriously inaccurate way to assess mental status is the physician's impression of the patient based on conversation or history taking. A baseline formal mental status examination should be done as part of the neurological examination on elderly surgical patients.

Preliminary studies have indicated that surgical risk in the elderly may be more precisely measured by invasive assessments of cardiac and pulmonary function (44, 45). Very high mortality was confined to patients with poor ventricular function and large A-V oxygen differences. We do not recommend routine catheterization to define surgical risk because of the lack of data on validity of these measurements. However, determination of cardiac output and A-V oxygen differences may be worthwhile *additional* pieces of data to obtain in patients in whom the decision for major surgery is borderline. Until further information is available on the validity of these measurements, they should not be the *sole* reason for a decision for or against surgery.

Management Principles

PREOPERATIVE MANAGEMENT

The decision to operate on an elderly patient remains a difficult clinical problem (47). There is an increased surgical risk, but less tolerance of the effects of surgically uncorrected disease and of emergency surgery.

In judging the effect of surgery on longevity, most clinicians do not recognize that the average 70–80-year-old has a *mean* life expectancy of 8 years (46). Elderly patients are too often refused surgery because "they only have 1 or 2 years to live." The other major consideration in the elderly is that the end point is often not a major increase in longevity as in younger age groups, but improvement in the quality of life.

. . The balance of benefit versus risk of surgery in the elderly can usually be determined with the general guidelines previously given (see p. 18). In using this schema, the benefits considered must include *accurate* assessment of longevity and quality of life, including the *patient's* feelings about his future and the surgery. The assessment must focus on those general factors and specific organ diseases (Table 21.7) that most affect mortality in the elderly, in addition to specific medical risk factors applicable to all patient groups (43).

The age at which surgical risk increases has changed over the past 30 years. The degree of risk has also changed from a prohibitive 25+% to 5–10%. The 5–10% still indicates a significantly higher risk than the 0.9% for young patients. Another perspective can be obtained by realizing that while a 5–10% risk is regarded as large by today's standards, it was a quite acceptable risk only 20–30 years ago. The data above show that this major increase of risk *may not* occur until age 65–70 rather than age 55–65.

Deciding on surgery on the basis of the factors listed above (Table 21.7) seems complex because the set of risk factors listed are not familiar to most nongeriatric physicians. Once the list is mastered, they are no more complex than other medical decisions. Although these risk factors provide a more precise estimate of surgical risk, they should complement, not supplant, the clinician's overall judgment.

Nutritional supplementation by oral, nasogastric, or intravenous hyperalimention should improve surgical risk due to malnutrition in the elderly. In using these modalities, the risks of nutritional interventions, particuarly aspiration pneumonia and sepsis, should be recognized (see p. 38).

Preoperative management of specific organ system problems in the elderly is covered in the preceding chapters on each system (e.g., cardiovascular disease).

POSTOPERATIVE MANAGEMENT

Several considerations are important in the postoperative management in the elderly. Elderly patients are more often confused postoperatively due to residual effect of anesthetics, analgesics, fever, and electrolyte disturbances. The stress of surgery and unfamiliar surroundings are also frequent precipitating causes. Changes in mental status postoperatively are often missed until they are severe, unless they are specifically looked for. Simple measures to prevent confusion include returning the patient to the same room occupied preoperatively, allowing the presence of familiar objects and relatives, avoiding the use of unnecessary instrumentation, and using smaller doses of analgesics and hypnotics.

After prolonged bed rest, mobilization is more difficult for elderly than younger patients. The elderly should be gotten out of bed and ambulated as quickly as possible. Judgment should be used in not ambulating patients who have inadequate relief of pain or who are too weak. Blood pressure should be taken lying, sitting, and standing before ambulating elderly patients who have been at bed rest for more than 2–3 days because of the frequent occurrence of orthostatic hypotension. In the absence of volume depletion, patients suffering from mild orthostatic hypotension with no or minimal symptoms may be helped out of bed more slowly with elastic leg stockings. Severe orthostatic hypotension with marked symptoms may require use of tilt tables and physical therapy.

More meticulous attention than usual should be paid to maintaining fluid and electrolyte balance and oxygenation. Major complications may result from small errors in management in elderly patients which would not affect younger patients.

Postoperative infections often present subtly in the elderly. The elderly also tolerate untreated infections and undrained abscesses poorly. The lack of tolerance is for both acute development of septic shock and for development of a chronic downhill course. Elderly patients may not recover from subacute infection even with vigorous therapy and nutritional support if discovered late in the course. Subtle signs that should lead to a careful search for infection may be low-grade fever, leukocytosis, or unexplained downhill course. One should not expect to find all the unusual signs of infection in any given elderly patient (see also p. 394).

Special Considerations

Several operations are done frequently in the elderly and have special considerations besides those listed above.

HERNIA (ELECTIVE)

Elective hernia repair has a slightly increased risk in the elderly. Many surgeons are repairing hernias under local anesthesia. While the risk with local anesthesia is very small in the absence of unstable coronary artery disease, the benefit of performing elective surgery on asymptomatic hernias in the elderly is still controversial (17, 49).

TRANSURETHRAL PROSTATE RESECTION

See page 576.

PARTIAL COLECTOMY

Colon resection for cancer carries an increased risk in the elderly because of the major intra-abdominal nature of the procedure and the risk of infection (50–52). The increased risk is also due to more frequent emergency operations and complicated presentations (obstruction, perforation). Operation is usually undertaken in all but very poor risk patients because of the ultimate fatal nature of the disease and lack of alternative procedures. Possible alternative procedures for low-lying rectal carcinoma are fulgeration and laser, although it should be realized that these often require multiple general anesthesias and are not curative.

ULCER OPERATIONS

There is a markedly increased mortality for ulcer operations in the elderly. The increased risk is in part due to more elderly patients being operated on for complications and having emergency surgery (Fig. 21.2) (55). Other contributing factors to increased mortality are the major, intra-abdominal nature of the procedure and the closeness to the diaphragm with resulting pulmonary compromise. Medical treatment should be used for peptic ulcer disease in elderly patients, unless complications supervene. In elderly patients requiring operation, most surgeons will perform the simplest definitive procedure for the complication rather than extensive "curative" surgery. The most common complications are cardiac and pulmonary.

APPENDICITIS

Appendicitis retains its classical reputation as an operation with greatly increased mortality in the elderly, whether uncomplicated or for perforation (Table 21.1). Although British studies indicate medical therapy may be an alternative in *some* patients, operation remains the treatment in the United States for all patients. Early diagnosis and operation is essential, since the risk is much higher if perforation occurs (0.6% versus 6–10%).

AORTIC ANEURYSM

See p. 558.

Gynecologic procedures have been performed with a low mortality in elderly women (6, 58), although many of the procedures reported have been through a vaginal rather than abdominal approach.

Age over 70 years has been felt to be a relative contraindication to lung resection in many centers. One recent study (59) reported an operative mortality of 4% among patients with lung resection over age 70, although about one-half of patients had conservative amounts of lung resected (e.g., segmental or wedge resection) rather than pneumonectomy. Twenty percent of patients had major complications. This compares to a 17% operative mortality in prior studies (59). Risk factors for perioperative morbidity were congestive heart failure, previous pulmonary resection, and extent of lung resected. This study would indicate lung resection can be performed in selected patients over age 70 with an acceptable mortality, if proper patient selection, certain lung-sparing operative techniques, and good supportive care are used. Confirmation with studies at other institutions should be done.

ABDOMINAL AORTIC ANEURYSM

Epidemiology

The prevalence of abdominal aortic aneurysms at autopsy ranges from 0.6–1.0% in modern series (60). The frequency of abdominal aneurysms in clinical populations has not been accurately determined because of difficulty in diagnosing small or asymptomatic aneurysms; however, abdominal aneurysms are not a common disease. The only known risk factors for arteriosclerotic abdominal aneurysms are hypertension, arteriosclerosis in other vessels, and, rarely, previous dissection.

The mortality of untreated abdominal aneurysms is high. The only unselected series of non-operative patients found a 33% mortality at 1 year and an 81% mortality at 5 years after the diagnosis of an aneurysm (61). A 5-year mortality of 64–90% was found in a larger number of series of patients who did not undergo operation because of too high risk or patient refusal (Fig. 21.4) (66, 77, 82, 85–89).

In comparison, the 5-year mortality for patients undergoing elective aneurysm repair was 40–63% (Fig. 21.4). The survival curves for operated patients are consistently better than and do not overlap with non-operated or autopsy series. The survival of patients in operated series falls about midway between unoperated patients and an aged adjusted normal population (Fig. 21.4). The primary cause of late death was coronary artery disease. Late complications of aneurysm repair, such as infection and graft failure, are rare and represent only about 1% of late mortality.

A converse approach can be taken by examining autopsy series for the percentage of unoperated patients dying *of their aneurysm* rather than of another cause. Of patients dying and coming to autopsy, the major cause of death is the aneurysm itself (25–50%), rather than another cause with the aneurysm remaining intact. Other causes of death in patients with an intact aneurysm at autopsy are cardiac, renal, respiratory failure, stroke, and cancer (62, 90).

Although there is no randomized series, improved survival for *elective* resection of known aneurysms is strongly supported by the consistently improved survival of electively operated patients in all series (Fig. 21.4) and by retrospective data indicating that the aneurysm is the most common cause of death.

The lack of a reliable parameter that will predict aneurysm rupture with a high degree of accuracy is a major deterrent to deferring operation and following these patients. No clinical or laboratory finding

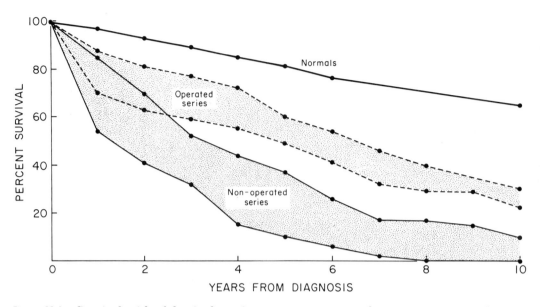

Figure 21.4. Survival with abdominal aortic aneurysms: operated versus non-operated series (data from Refs. 60–62, 64, 66, 71, 77, 79, 82, 83, 85, 87–89, 90).

can either predict the chances of aneurysm rupture or signify an impending rupture that will occur within a short period of time with enough certainty to be clinically useful.

The factor found to be consistently predictive of rupture is aneurysm size. Aneurysms over 7 cm have a 50% or more risk of rupture, with about one-quarter occurring during the first year after diagnosis (63). Aneurysms between 4–7 cm have about a 25% risk of rupture (62, 63).

In one study performing ultrasound every 3 months, small aneurysms (less than 6 cm) grew an average of 0.4 cm per year. There was considerable individual patient variation from 0–0.6 centimeters, and sudden asymptomatic large increases in size did occur in nine (19%) patients. Fourteen (29%) patients required resection for development of symptoms or sudden increase in aneurysm size after being followed from 3 months to 5 years. Thus, when followed by serial ultrasound for a short period of time, only a small number of patients unexpectedly ruptured aneurysms. However, many patients had to undergo operation for increased aneu-

rysm size or symptoms, and a significant number of patients developed unexpected asymptomatic changes in size between ultrasound examinations.

The risk of aneurysm rupture must be compared with the risk of surgery. The risk of elective aneurysm surgery decreased from 11% in 1952–1960 to 5% in a current series (Table 21.8). More dramatic than the average figures in Table 21.8 is the fact that many series in the decade 1952–1960 had 25–50% mortality, whereas the range of mortality after 1970 was no greater than 2.5–6%. Operative mortality is lower for patients without heart disease (Fig. 21.5).

The "cause" of perioperative death in elective aneurysm surgery provides the best insight to risk factors, despite the difficulty in assessing causes of deaths in patients with multiple problems (Table 21.9).

The major cause of postoperative mortality is cardiac disease. Most series label the majority of cardiac deaths as due to myocardial infarction, without providing sufficient data to separate these from other cardiac causes of death. Both pulmonary

Table 21.8.   Operative Mortality for Elective Abdominal Aneurysm Repair

Study Period[a]	Operative Mortality			No. of Studies	Reference
	Median	Mean	Range		
1952–60	11%	13%	0–50%	21	60
1960–70	12%	11%	0–20%	14	60, 66
1970–	5%	5%	2.5–6%	3	68, 70, 75, 91, 92, 93

[a] Dates refer to when the series was collected and not date of publication. Series spanning more than one decade were placed in the decade in which most patients were operated on or, if evenly divided, into the later decade.

and renal deaths have decreased greatly since 1970 (70, 75–76, 79, 127). Pulmonary causes of death have included pneumonia, respiratory failure, and pulmonary embolism. Preoperative renal failure and surgical complications greatly increase the chances of postoperative renal failure (127–129).

Postoperative stroke accounted for about 12% of deaths, although several recent series (72, 75, 76) report no death due to stroke.

As illustrated in Table 21.9, the majority of deaths were due to medical causes of cardiac, cerebrovascular, pulmonary, or renal complications and not to surgical technique.

The frequency of postoperative medical complications (Table 21.10) is less certain because many series do not state whether only non-fatal or all complications are reported. There is a similar relative ranking of problems as with mortality with two exceptions. Pulmonary complications are relatively more common than pulmonary deaths, primarily due to the occurrence of atelectasis. Gastrointestinal (GI) bleeding was a frequent complication, but infrequently listed as the major or contributing cause of death. Certain

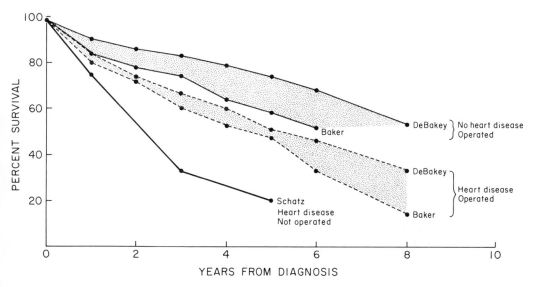

Figure 21.5   Effect of heart disease on survival of operated patients with abdominal aneurysms (data from Refs. 60, 71, 89, 98).

Table 21.9. Medical Causes of Postoperative Mortality in Elective Aneurysm Repair: Literature Review 1955–1980[a]

Cause	Percentage of Deaths[b]	
	Range	Median
Cardiac (all)	20–100	40
Arrhythmia/arrest	3–25	—[c]
MI	12–100	34
CHF	3–50	—[c]
Cerebrovascular (stroke)	0–25	12
Pulmonary (including pneumonia)	6–41	12
PE and phlebitis	2–18	8
Renal	10–50	25
Surgical and miscellaneous	?	?

[a] Derived from Refs. 65–83, 90.
[b] Total exceeds 100% because of multiple causes of death.
[c] Too few studies for accurate median.

gastrointestinal complications, including pancreatitis, jaundice, mesenteric infarction, and gastric dilatation, are rare.

A similar perspective on risk factors is provided by examining the concomitant

Table 21.10. Postoperative Complications in Elective Abdominal Aneurysm Repair: Literature Review 1955–1980[a]

	Percentage of Patients	
	Range	Median
Cardiac (all)	2–47	9
Arrhythmia/arrest	1–14	4
MI	1–15	4
CHF	2–37	—[b]
Cerebrovascular (stroke)	0–11	1
GI bleeding[c]	1–5	2
Pulmonary	2–56	9
PE and phlebitis	1–11	1
Renal	1–13	6

[a] Derived from Refs. 65–83, 92.
[b] Too few studies and widely varying results to give meaningful estimates of median.
[c] Less frequent GI complications were jaundice, pancreatitis, mesenteric infarction and gastric dilatation.

Table 21.11. Preexisting Medical Problems in Patients Undergoing Elective Abdominal Aneurysm Repair: Literature Review 1955–1980[a]

	Percentage of Patients	
	Range	Median
Cardiac (all)	23–56	40
Angina	14–21	15
MI (± angina)	18–47	22
CHF	3–16	—[b]
Valvular heart disease	1–3	2
Hypertension	28–54	43
Cerebrovascular (all)	3–25	8
Stroke	3–7	5
Diabetes	7–22	9
Pulmonary	18–50	—[b]
Renal	3–22	7

[a] Derived from Refs. 63–76.
[b] Too few studies and too widely scattered results to estimate a meaningful average.

medical problems in patients presenting for elective abdominal aneurysm repair (Table 21.11).

The information on causes of mortality or morbidity after operation must be interpreted with caution because of widely varying criteria for diagnosis, retrospective assessment of cause of death, and combining elective and ruptured aneurysm statistics in many series.

The role of coronary artery disease as the major risk factor of operation is consistently shown by its high prevalence in aneurysm patients, and its frequency as a cause of mortality and morbidity. Preexisting clinical heart disease increases the risk of cardiac complications during aneurysm repair (64, 75, 140). The severity of the heart disease by the New York Heart Association classification increases operative risk (66, 140).

The evaluation of patients for elective aneurysm repair below will emphasize cardiac evaluation because of the predominant role of heart disease in determining operative risk. Other important risk factors are pulmonary, renal, and cerebrovascular disease.

Diagnostic Activities and Approaches

A complete history, physical examination, and admission laboratory data base are necessary in aneurysm patients because of the common occurrence of multisystem disease and the risk to multiple organ systems during surgery (120). Spirometry should be performed on all patients because of the risk of pulmonary complications. A creatinine clearance is helpful to document baseline renal function.

During the workup, attention should be paid for any signs indicating concomitant undiscovered malignancy since this occurs in a significant number of patients (133).

The preoperative evaluation should focus on cardiovascular disease, which is the major risk factor for aneurysm surgery.

Non-invasive tests are useful in patients in whom the existence or severity of cardiac heart disease is uncertain clinically. Recent data (111) indicate dipyridamole thallium stress tests are predictive of cardiac complications postoperatively in aneurysm patients (see also p. 113). However, there are insufficient data for a positive test to be the *sole* basis for decision making. Stress tests should not be performed on patients without cardiac symptoms to detect asymptomatic cardiac disease in most instances because of its false-positive and false-negative rates in asymptomatic patients and lack of data relating stress test performance to surgical risk.

Non-invasive evaluation of left ventricular function (e.g., MUGA scan) is useful in evaluating operative risk, with an ejection fraction (EF) below 35% being high risk in preliminary studies (110, 116). However, aortic surgery has been performed on such patients with an acceptable mortality (110).

Until more definitive studies are available, non-invasive studies (including MUGA scans, dipyridamole thallium stress tests) should serve as additional valid information in assessing risk, but should not be the sole basis for deciding on surgery or cardiac catheterization.

The role of coronary angiography and coronary artery bypass grafts in symptomatic patients is uncertain because of lack of controlled data showing that prior bypass surgery decreases operative mortality (see p. 128). Uncontrolled studies are conflicting, concluding that *routine* coronary angiography is indicated in all patients (113), some patients (112, 115, 117), or not indicated (108). Most high-risk patients as determined by coronary angiography have symptomatic coronary disease clinically (108, 117). The operative risk in the patient who has had a prior coronary artery bypass is low at 2–4% (112, 113, 115, 117). Until randomized, controlled trials yield a definitive answer, coronary angiography is not routinely indicated before aortic aneurysm repair or in the asymptomatic patient. The decision in the symptomatic patient should be based on clinical and laboratory data on the severity of the coronary disease, as well as local experience.

Catheterization is indicated in some moderate and all severe cases of congestive failure due to potentially correctable causes, especially valvular heart disease. The more precise assessment of the degree of failure and left ventricular function by catheterization will allow more precise estimation of how the patient's cardiac function will tolerate aneurysm surgery, although only qualitative guidelines can be given (see p. 155) for first doing valvular surgery.

The management of patients with cerebrovascular disease during aneurysm surgery is controversial. Most of the controversy about prophylactic carotid endarterectomy has centered on surgery for aneurysms and peripheral vascular disease. This subject is reviewed in detail in Chapter 19 (see p. 470).

Consideration of endarterectomy should be limited to patients at high risk of stroke due to symptomatic transient ischemic attacks or high-grade stenoses. Endarterectomy *may* be indicated in *some* patients whose bruits represent high-grade stenosis by non-invasive testing and whom the surgeon feels will be difficult operative cases with high likelihood of hypotension.

The decision for patients with transient ischemic attacks is the priority of two necessary surgical procedures, rather than preoperative prophylaxis. In most cases, it would be desirable to do the endarterectomy first, since the aneurysm repair can be done after a relatively brief wait and an asymptomatic aneurysm does not complicate carotid surgery.

Patients with chronic renal failure have undergone aortic aneurysm surgery, but the risk is increased, especially for creatinines over 4 mg/dl (128, 129). Baseline assessment of renal function, and possible use of a Swan-Ganz catheter to tightly control intravascular volume should be considered. Planning should be done for possible perioperative hemodialysis in patients with creatinine over 4 mg/dl (129).

Postoperative Management

The major treatable problems postoperatively are cardiac, pulmonary, and renal complications. The only preventable postoperative problem precipitating stroke is hypotension.

Patients undergoing aneurysm surgery are usually placed in an ICU postoperatively, with intensive monitoring of rhythm and blood pressure. Patients with significant preoperative coronary artery disease should probably be monitored for at least 4–5 days, based on the risk of postoperative myocardial infarction and cardiac death extending to this time.

Indications for Swan-Ganz pulmonary artery catheterization in aortic aneurysm surgery are not firmly established, despite growing experience (121–126) (see also p. 92). A Swan-Ganz catheter is indicated in the less common aneurysms extending above the renal arteries, because of the larger hemodynamic changes with cross-clamping the suprarenal aorta. The hemodynamic response to infrarenal cross-clamping during surgery is larger in patients with coronary disease (122, 124). The indications for and use of Swan-Ganz catheterization in all patients with coronary disease vary widely between centers, and no general recommendation can be given. Most centers tend to use Swan-Ganz catheters in high-risk cardiac patients.

Special Considerations

THE AGED PATIENT (see also p. 543)

The effect of age on mortality from aortic aneurysm surgery is important because aneurysm is a disease of the elderly. Ten to 20% of aneurysm surgery is done in patients over age 70.

Patients 70–80 years old generally have been considered very high risks for aneurysm repair because of their age and the major extent of surgery. Earlier experience suggested that patients had a very high incidence of complications and mortality (77, 97).

DeBakey's series showed patients age 60–69 had an 11% and patients 70–90 years old had a similar 12% operative mortality (64). Several recent series showed that elective resection could be done in selected good-risk patients older than 75–80 years with a 5% mortality quite comparable to other age groups (96–100). The incidence of cardiac, renal, and respiratory postoperative complications was comparable to those in younger patients. Survival curves for operated patients were close to those of the general population. Patients not having surgery had a 50% mortality in 1 year, which was about equally split between ruptured aneurysm and cardiac disease.

Current results would suggest that age greater than 70–80 years alone does not markedly raise operative risk and is not a contraindication. Most authors note that it is important to consider the "physiologic" rather than chronologic age of the patient. If the conditions of surgical expertise, patient condition, and lack of major organ disease are met, it is reasonable to offer elective surgery to patients older than 80, because of the risk of rupture within a short period of time and the reasonable 6–10-year life expectancy of this age group.

RUPTURED ABDOMINAL AORTIC ANEURYSMS

Rupture of an abdominal aneurysm is an acute emergency leaving no time for preoperative medical evaluation. Postoperatively, the most common cause of death is a progressive decline manifest by hypotension and multiple organ failure. Although different series (101–106) may classify this as due to surgery, hypotension, arrhythmia, myocardial infarction, or renal failure, the course is similar in its characteristics. The major approach to the patient is surgical repair of the aneurysm and postoperative maintenance of blood pressure. Cardiac and renal complications should be anticipated in management. Daily routine monitoring of renal function (creatinine, urine output), electrocardiograms, and cardiac isoenzymes should be performed. Complications with ruptured aneurysms are more closely related to preoperative shock and operative course, rather than to preexisting disease in contrast to elective cases.

The most important consideration regarding ruptured aneurysm is prevention, since marked improvement in operative technique in the past 20 years has had little effect on mortality for ruptured aneurysm.

MESENTERIC ISCHEMIA AND INFARCTION

Ischemia of the bowel is a rare complication of aneurysm surgery (130–132). The colon is more frequently involved than the small bowel in ischemia after aneurysm resection.

The typical presentation of ischemia bowel post-aneurysm surgery is the onset of bloody diarrhea, abdominal pain, and hypotension. The ischemic bowel may also present as hypotension without other signs or apparent causes. Other atypical presenting problems are gastric dilation, vomiting with or without coffee grounds, abdominal distention and ileus, diarrhea without blood, and fever. The most frequently made incorrect diagnoses are myocardial infarction (hence the reason for medical consultation) and diarrhea. Diarrhea has often been attributed mistakenly to antibiotic colitis, postoperative bowel dysfunction, and tube feedings.

The workup when this complication is suspected depends upon what tests the patient's condition permits. Sigmoidoscopy is helpful, as rectum and sigmoid are often but not always involved (130). The diagnosis can also be made by barium enema; often repeat laparotomy is necessary.

COINCIDENTAL MALIGNANCY AND AORTIC ANEURYSM

An unsuspected malignant lesion is found in 3–5% of patients presenting for elective aneurysm replacement due to the age of the population (133–135a). The occurrence of both unsuspected carcinoma and an aneurysm raises the question of which lesion has surgical priority.

No absolute rule can be made on which lesion should be repaired first, but general guidelines are available (133–135a). The risk of aneurysm rupture should be considered based on aneurysm size and symptomatology. The extent of the malignancy should be assessed in terms of risk of spread over an interval period and whether there are metastases precluding cure and shortening longevity. Surgical considerations are which surgery will allow more rapid recovery and a shorter period to the second operation. The surgeon will often want to remove an abdominal malignancy (usually carcinoma of the colon) first so that he is not working with potentially infective material near a newly placed graft.

GASTROINTESTINAL BLEEDING

Gastrointestinal bleeding occurs in 0–3% of aneurysm replacements. The most usual cause of lower GI bleeding or melena is intestinal ischemia. Upper gastrointestinal bleeding is usually related to stress gastritis.

JAUNDICE AFTER ANEURYSM REPAIR

Jaundice occurs infrequently after elective aneurysm repair (75). The literature and our experience have found that jaundice usually occurs in patients with multiple possible etiologies, and it is not possible to specify a single cause. The causes of jaundice are similar to those for other operations (see p. 258). Severe, sustained hypotension and multiple transfusions commonly occur and may be more frequent causes of jaundice in aneurysm surgery.

Profound jaundice can occur after surgery for ruptured aortic aneurysms. The most likely cause is hypotension and shock. These patients have a high mortality because of severe ischemic damage to the other organs (137).

Liver dysfunction and jaundice may be a manifestation of sepsis in either elective or ruptured aneurysm repair. Infection should be sought in any patient with unexplained hepatic abnormalities.

GRAFT INFECTION

Early postoperative infection of aortic replacement grafts occurs in 1–3% of patients (138). Presenting symptoms include fever, distal embolization, and GI bleeding from aortoenteric fistulae.

Infection is documented by obtaining positive blood cultures. Blood cultures obtained from venous samples are usually adequate to discover graft sepsis. Occasionally, arterial blood will produce positive cultures when venous cultures are negative.

Cultures obtained at the time of oper-ation from the aneurysm or abdominal cavity may be positive in up to 20% of patients; only a few of these will develop early or late infection (138). No specific factor is predictive of which patients with positive operative cultures will develop sepsis. Prophylactic antibiotics are usually administered (see p. 378).

CATARACT SURGERY

Epidemiology

Consultation is often requested on patients undergoing cataract surgery because of their advanced age and multiple concomitant diseases. Cataract surgery can be performed under either local or general anesthesia. The only absolute requirements for general anesthesia are poor patient cooperation, coughing, inability to lie still due to discomfort, and certain more complicated procedures.

The overall mortality from cataract surgery has been reported as 0.005–0.05%, depending on the center and type of anesthesia used. If only patients over age 65 are considered, mortality has been reported to be 0.01–0.2% (141–143) (Table 21.1). There was one death in 20,000 cataract extractions under local anesthesia (0.005%) in one series (141). The risk is similar for local and general anesthesia (141–143, 149).

Operative manipulation and several adrenergic drugs administered intraocularly can affect blood pressure and pulse during cataract surgery (Table 21.12) (146–153). Manipulation or pressure on the eye may produce bradycardia (oculocardic reflex). The bradycardia is potentiated by underlying conduction system disease or hypoxia (146). The reflex is not fully prevented by preoperative atropine, but can be abolished by retrobulbar block with lidocaine.

The pupil is dilated during surgery with topical administration of adrenergic agents such as epinephrine and phenylephrine. Agents that produce miosis such as acetylcholine may also be administered post-

Table 21.12. Selected Reported Side Effects of Ophthalmologic Drops[a]

Type (Drug)	Reaction
1. Adrenergic	
(Phenylephrine)	HTN[b] (severe)
	Coronary spasm; MI
	Cardiac arrest
	Subarachnoid hemor-
	rhage and HTN
(Epinephrine)	PVCs
2. Beta-Blocker	Bradycardia
(Timolol)	Hypotension
	Syncope
	CHF
	Bronchospasm
3. Cholinergic	Cholinergic symptoms
(Pilocarpine)	
4. Anticholinergic	CNS (confusion, halluci-
(Atropine)	nation)
	SVT
5. Anticholinesterase	Anticholinesterase
(Echothiopate)	toxicity
	Cardiac arrest

[a]Table includes examples of side effects selected from case reports; numerous other possible reactions exist based on pharmacology of these agents. From references 146–153, 242.
[b]Abbreviations: HTN, hypertension; MI, myocardial infarction; CHF, congestive heart failure; CNS, central nervous system; SVT, supraventricular tachycardia.

operatively. It has been our experience that these rarely produce significant changes in blood pressure, pulse, or systemic complications. However, sympathetic agents have been shown to produce marked hypertension and tachycardia in occasional patients. Similarly, acetylcholine and timolol have produced bradycardia, hypotension, or bronchospasm in an occasional patient (Table 21.12) (146–153, 242).

Diagnostic Activities and Approaches

Most patients tolerate this surgery well, even in the presence of moderately severe chronic cardiac or pulmonary disease. We do not feel that moderately severe coronary disease is a contraindication to this operation as long as the patient's disease is stable and they are more than 6 months postmyocardial infarction.

The operation should be done under local anesthesia in high-risk patients because this poses no additional problems to the surgeon in most cases and probably lowers operative risk. General anesthesia should be considered for the patient who is very anxious about undergoing this surgery under local anesthesia. The small risk of general anesthesia may be preferable to the stress of anxiety. Increases in blood pressure and pulse due to topical drugs usually produce no symptoms and can be managed by withholding additional amounts of adrenergic agents. Short-acting antihypertensives such as Arfonad or nitroprusside can be used when marked hypertension, accompanied by symptoms, develops. Propranolol can be used for tachycardia and atropine for bradycardia hypotension. Short-acting agents are preferable since the duration of action of most of the interocular agents is brief. Use of drugs to reverse side effects from topical anticholinergics or β-blocking agents is rarely required, if careful monitoring of the patient's vital signs is performed and as small a dose as necessary of mydriatrics is used.

CHOLECYSTECTOMY

Epidemiology

The problem of managing gallbladder disease in cardiac patients has long been a subject of controversy. No adequate recent study is available on the incidence of coronary artery disease among patients undergoing cholecystectomy. A 1955 report found 100 patients with coronary artery disease among 5891 patients undergoing cholecystectomy (2%) (154).

Most studies of medical complications of cholecystectomy were done in the 1950s–1960s and are not necessarily applicable to current techniques. Studies from that era reported a mortality of 3–10% in patients with ischemic heart disease. Cardiac problems were implicated in 33–70% of perioperative deaths (154–155).

The increased risk of cholecystectomy in cardiac patients has been comparable to that of other major intra-abdominal procedures. An increased risk for cholecystectomy above that of other major abdominal procedures has not been shown in modern studies.

The performance of a cholecystectomy carries a significantly increased morbidity and mortality in patients with chronic obstructive lung disease. Cholecystectomy shares this risk with other upper abdominal procedures. The increased risk is due to the closeness of the procedure to the diaphragm with resulting atelectasis and hypoventilation. The risk of significant pulmonary complications or death was 20% in patients undergoing upper abdominal procedures compared with 9% for lower abdominal procedures. Total pulmonary morbidity was 5% in patients undergoing upper abdominal procedures compared with 2.5% in patients undergoing other types of operations (156).

Diagnostic Activities and Approaches

Patients with ischemic heart disease requiring surgery have a significantly increased risk for cholecystectomy. The increase in risk is less well documented for other types of heart disease.

In addition, spirometry should be performed on patients for cholecystectomy with any history of smoking, lung, or cardiac disease because of the high incidence of atelectasis and hypoventilation due to the upper abdominal incision.

Management Principles

PREOPERATIVE MANAGEMENT

Most patients should receive pulmonary therapy to prevent atelectasis; this is especially important in patients with both cardiac and pulmonary disease.

A common clinical dilemma is the need for cholecystectomy in patients with mod-erate to severe cardiac or pulmonary disease. The occurrence of symptomatic cholelithiasis and cholecystitis present a significant risk of developing recurrent episodes and complications, such as Gram-negative sepsis, that may exceed 20–50% over a short period of time. Patients with cardiopulmonary disease tolerate these complications of gallbladder disease and emergency surgery poorly. The clinical dilemma posed is that the high risk of surgery is often equal to or exceeded by the high risk of not operating.

Moderate to severe ischemic heart disease should be optimally controlled with β-blockers and nitrates. Patients remaining at high risk due to recent myocardial infarction or unstable angina may warrant cardiac catheterization, bypass surgery, or use of the intra-aortic balloon pump.

Cholecystotomy is an acceptable alternative procedure for the high-risk cardiac patient. Cholecystotomy can be done under local anesthesia, with lower operative risk. Some surgeons do not favor cholecystotomy since 20% of patients will require cholecystectomy because of recurrent symptoms due to obstruction of the common bile duct. The operation does work well for the majority of patients, and many of those requiring reoperation will have their medical condition improve or will die of other causes in the interval.

Treatment with oral chenodeoxycholic acids is not helpful in the acutely symptomatic patient because of the delay until stones dissolve; its effectiveness in preventing symptomatic attacks is uncertain. Gallstone lithotripsy remains experimental.

In summary, gallstones that are clearly symptomatic have a high risk of complications over a relatively short period of time, and these complications are poorly tolerated by patients with severe cardiac disease. Some patients with moderate to severe cardiac disease can be optimally managed medically to prepare them for surgery. Some are candidates for cardiac catheterization, and the remainder should be considered for the alternative procedure of cholecystotomy. Only the few patients with end-stage heart disease should not be considered for any treatment.

Patients with mild to moderate pulmonary disease usually can undergo cholecystectomy. Pre- and postoperative pulmonary therapy is important. Patients with severe pulmonary disease present a difficult clinical problem. Cholecystotomy may not lower the risk as much as in cardiac patients, since the same subcostal incision is used.

Special Considerations

The problems posed by cholecystectomy in patients over age 65 are discussed on page 543.

DENTAL PROCEDURES AND SURGERY

Epidemiology

The major considerations in cardiac patients undergoing dental procedures are those of anesthesia. The most common concern is arrhythmias, but other possible complications include angina, myocardial infarction, congestive failure, and sudden death. Local anesthesia presents the problems of the use of small quantities of epinephrine with the local anesthetic and the effect of anxiety and pain on the cardiac problem. Patients with valvular and septal lesions require prophylaxis for subacute bacterial endocarditis.

The causes of death during dental procedures will be considered first, followed by effects of dental anesthesia on myocardial function, and arrhythmias.

Death has occurred during dental anesthesia in both young, healthy patients and in patients with cardiac disease. Mortality risks from general dental anesthesia are estimated at 1:250,000 to 1:850,000 (157–158, 161). The risk with local anesthesia for dental work is not known, but is felt to be lower than general anesthesia (157). The cause of most den-

tal anesthetic deaths remains speculative (157, 158).

Deaths during general dental anesthesia presented in two ways in one study (158). Respiratory symptoms often associated with airway problems tended to occur "early" in anesthesia. Sudden cardiovascular collapse occurred most often during recovery from anesthesia without any symptoms; the cause of these deaths remains obscure. "Early" respiratory arrest accounted for 60% of the deaths; "later" cardiovascular collapse of unknown cause accounted for 40%. Deaths during dental anesthesia have been attributed to fainting in the sitting position, arrhythmia, halothane, local injection of adrenalin, aspiration, medication errors, hypotension, and cardiac arrest (159–161). The first manifestation noticed by the dentist is most often hypotension, but evidence is lacking on whether the initiating cause is a primary hypotensive event, arrhythmias, or respiratory arrest (159–161).

Numerous reviews have discussed the management of dental procedures in patients with cardiovascular disease (162, 181).

Very limited experience (240) indicate minor dental procedures can be done under local anesthesia with monitoring in the perimyocardial infarction period without high risk, but more patients need to be studied to define the risk.

Arrhythmias are common in both healthy and cardiac patients undergoing dental procedures. The incidence of arrhythmia is similar for local (mean = 22%) and general (mean = 25%) anesthesia (Tables 21.13 and 21.14).

Under general anesthesia, the most common arrhythmias are nodal rhythm and premature ventricular contractions (PVC) (Table 21.15). Complex PVCs are more common than simple PVCs. Supraventricular arrhythmias and premature atrial contractions are less frequent. High-grade arrhythmias such as transient ventricular tachycardia and heart block were seen in only a small percentage of pa-

Table 21.13. Arrhythmias with Dental Procedures: General Anesthesia

Study	Number	Number of Patients with Arrhythmias (%)
Ryder, 1970	243	71 (29%)
Christenson, 1959		(18%)
Christenson, 1961[a]	417	(9%)
Kaufman, 1966	40	20 (50%)
Meyer, 1966	23	3 (13%)
Tolas, 1967	52	8 (15%)
Tuohy, 1968		(27%)
Rollmon, 1968		(18%)
Fisch, 1969[a]	103	44 (43%)
Alexander, 1971	203	84 (41%)
Miller, 1970	102	76 (75%)[a,b]
Ryder, 1971	544	129 (39%)
Forbes, 1960	100	13 (13%)
Rafel, 1972	55	0 (0%)
Gotta, 1976	109	46 (42%)
Ostroff, 1977	21	12 (50%)
Auscoll, 1954	109	20 (18%)
Hanna, 1983	30	13 (43%)
Mean		25%[c]
Median		18%[c]
Range		0–50%

[a] Reporting number of procedures rather than patients and/or numbers of arrhythmias rather than number of patients with arrhythmias.
[b] Includes sinus tachycardia.
[c] Excluding sinus tachycardia.
[d] Derived in part from Refs. 169–180.

tients. No reported patient had sustained high-grade arrhythmias or died during monitoring in the combined series of over 2000 patients.

The types of arrhythmias seen under local anesthesia differ from those arrhythmias seen with general anesthesia (Table 21.15). First, simple PVCs were more common than complex PVCs. Second, premature atrial contractions were more frequent than nodel rhythm. Transient second- and third-degree heart block was observed. No instances were observed of ventricular tachycardia, cardiac arrest, or death.

The effect of general dental anesthesia on blood pressure has not been well documented. Sinus tachycardia occurs frequently with general dental anesthesia, with pulse rates exceeding 100 in 10–40% of patients.

A large number of experimental studies have examined the effect of local anesthesia, with or without epinephrine, on blood pressure and pulse under well-controlled circumstances (163–166). Local anesthesia with epinephrine produces a small rise in blood pressure (systolic $1 - 6 \pm 7$ mm Hg, diastolic $0.5–3 \pm 4$ mm Hg) and pulse ($1 - 5 \pm 5$ beats/min) (163–166). A spectrum of changes occurs in individual patients, including a significant number of patients with no alteration in vital signs.

The use of small amounts of epinephrine with the local anesthetic does not seem to cause a major additional increase in blood pressure or pulse (169) in most patients. The evidence suggests that use

Table 21.14. Arrhythmias with Dental Procedures: Local Anesthesia[a]

Study	Number	Epinephrine	Patients with Arrhythmia (%)	Comment
Ryder, 1970	97	Yes	9 (9%)	Fainting 3 (30%)
Rafel, 1972	49	Some	0 (0%)	
Williams, 1963	63	Yes	15 (29%)	Cardiovascular collapse
Barkin, 1978	225	Yes	36 (16%)	Oscilloscope without printout
Hughes, 1966	77	Yes	25 (32%)	
Hughes, 1966	31	Yes	15 (48%)	
Mean			22%	
Median			16%	
Range			0–48%	

[a] Derived in part from Refs. 169, 171.

Table 21.15.   Type of Arrhythmias with Dental Anesthesia[a]

	Number of Series	PAC	SVT	Simple PVC	Complex PVC	V-Tach	V-Fib	Nodal	2–3° Heart Block	Sinus Brady-cardia and Other Brady-arrhythmias	Com-pli-cations
Local anes-thesia	5	21% (0–40%)	0% (0%)	47% (47–48%)	13% (7–20%)	0% (0%)	0% (0%)	6% (0–20%)	5% (0–13%)	22% (11–13%)	Syncope Collapse, 3 pa-tients
General anes-thesia	11	3% (8–13%)	4% (0–25%)	14% (0–96%)	38% (0–58%)	9% (0–66%)	0% (0%)	24% (0–78%)	0.3% 0–3%	16% 12–23%	?

[a] Partially derived from Refs. 168–179.

of epinephrine results in lower blood pressure and pulse due to better anesthesia and pain control. Use of mild sedation may block the systolic blood pressure rise in hypertensive, but possibly not normotensive patients.

In summary, the literature would suggest, on the average, that epinephrine causes little change in vital signs during dental procedures. Similar changes in blood pressure and pulse result from anxiety and pain. The mean figures, however, do not reflect a small number of patients who may have large increases in blood pressure and pulse rates.

Preoperative Management

A frequent question is which cardiac patients should be hospitalized for dental work. Hospitalization has the advantage of better blood pressure and EKG monitoring, the availability of an anesthesiologist for monitoring while the dentist is doing the procedure, and the availability of medical personnel should complications arise.

Indications for hospitalization include moderate to severe angina, recent myocardial infarction, or significant arrhythmias. Patients with mild angina or myocardial infarction greater than 6 months previously with no major residual compromise usually can be done in the office

under local anesthesia in most instances. Patients with ischemic heart disease requiring general anesthesia should be done on an inpatient basis, although we recognize this is a very conservative approach. Very anxious patients requiring extensive, painful procedures should also be hospitalized, because anxiety-induced stress alters blood pressure and pulse as much as anesthesia. Patients with valvular heart disease or congestive failure can be treated under local anesthesia as outpatients, except for those with severe disease. Bacterial endocarditis prophylaxis should be given to patients with valvular heart disease (see p. 387) and may require hospitalization, since parenteral prophylactic regimens are difficult to provide on an outpatient basis.

The recent advent of same-day surgery units raises the question of whether dental procedures in cardiac patients can be done in these units with resultant cost savings. Although reported experience with dental patients is lacking, experience with other types of surgery in patients with ischemic heart disease demonstrates that risk extends beyond the period when the patient is under anesthesia. Until further experience is documented, we feel patients with significant ischemic heart disease, arrhythmias, and severe congestive failure should be hospitalized for at least 24 hours after dental procedures.

When extensive dental work requiring large doses of local anesthetic are planned, either multiple, staged procedures on different days should be done or general anesthesia considered. Mild sedation with a benzodiazepine or short-acting barbiturate may be helpful, especially in very anxious patients. Preliminary studies indicate beta-blockers *may* reduce the incidence of arrhythmias during dental general anesthesia, but further study is needed (180). Elective dental surgery should be deferred after myocardial infarction. Similar to other minor elective surgery, very limited experience indicates minor procedures can be done for emergencies if the patient is in marked pain, but the patient should be monitored, and epinephrine avoided or minimized.

Intra- and Postoperative Management

Patients manifesting arrhythmias under general anesthesia should be checked to make sure they are not hypoxic by obtaining arterial blood gases. In general, arrhythmias under anesthesia do not require long-term drug therapy. Patients manifesting serious arrhythmias should be treated acutely and reevaluated when stable for chronic anti-arrhythmic agents.

Most physicians are willing to discharge dental patients with cardiac disease 24 hours after their procedure if no complications occur.

Special Considerations

BACTERIAL ENDOCARDITIS PROPHYLAXIS

Dental procedures are a classic cause of subacute bacterial endocarditis. Prophylaxis should be provided for all dental work, except routine examination. Prophylaxis should be provided even for minor procedures such as teeth cleaning, extraction of loose teeth, and gum work.

The current recommended parenteral prophylactic regimens are difficult to give on an outpatient basis. Until definitive data are available, the use of more con-

venient oral regimens versus more intensive parenteral regimens must be based on considerations in the individual patient, as outlined in Chapter 16.

ANTICOAGULANT THERAPY

Anticoagulant therapy reAuires special management for dental extractions. Bleeding may not occur immediately during the procedure and may be delayed for hours to several days. A number of small series have reported dental extraction on anticoagulated patients without complications (Table 21.16). These series have attributed the lack of bleeding to maintaining the anticoagulation in a low therapeutic range (1.5–2 times control) and have noted that most bleeding has been reported in patients with prothrombin times in the high therapeutic to excessive range (2.5 or more times control).

The risk of stopping anticoagulants for several days is small in patients with artificial heart valves (see p. 158); extensive series have not been reported for briefly discontinuing anticoagulation for other indications.

Dental extraction presents the risk of excessive, significant bleeding, at least in some patients on anticoagulation. Therefore, we prefer to stop coumadin 24–48 hours before planned dental procedures and to administer aquamephyton if nec-

Table 21.16.   Dental Procedures in Patients on Anticoagulant Therapy

Study	Number	Prothrombin Time (control = 14 sec)	Complications
Askey (182)	11	14–51%	None
Frank (183)	25	15–40%	None
Ziffer (184)	2	39 sec	? excessive bleeding
Behrman (185, 187)	45	18–37 sec	None
Shira (186)	18	17–51 sec	3 excessive bleeding
Scopp (188)	2	31–39 sec	2 excessive bleeding

essary to normalize the prothrombin time (within 2 seconds of control). Coumadin may be restarted from immediately to 48 hours after the procedure, depending on the extent of the procedure and perioperative bleeding. In patients at high risk for thromboembolic phenomenon, heparin may be started within 12–24 hours if bleeding is minimal and continued until the prothrombin time is therapeutic from coumadin. Discontinuing anticoagulation for the short period of time represents a very low risk of thromboembolism and avoids bleeding.

Patients with dental and facial trauma should be managed according to the extent of their injury and trauma. The major risk is subcutaneous bleeding into the planes of the face and neck with resulting hematoma and possibly airway obstruction. All anticoagulated patients with a history of significant orofacial trauma should be hospitalized for observation, whether or not bleeding is apparent. When forceful blunt trauma or bleeding occurs, the anticoagulant should be withheld and vitamin K_1 administered. Fresh frozen plasma may need to be administered in the presence of significant acute bleeding, major fractures, or soft-tissue trauma. A major mistake is to assume that the absence of bleeding in the emergency room is reassuring. Delayed bleeding from hours to several days after trauma represents a major risk.

PULMONARY DISEASE

There is no reported experience with dental extractions in patients with pulmonary disease. Most patients with mild to moderate chronic obstructive lung disease tolerate dental procedures under local anesthesia well in the outpatient setting.

Patients with severe lung disease may have trouble with maintaining an adequate tidal volume resulting in hypoxia, during manipulation of the mouth, although this sequence of events has not been well documented. Dental work on these patients should be performed in an inpatient setting. General anesthesia should be avoided.

Patients with asthma pose the increased risk of bronchospasm during induction or awaking from anesthesia. The inpatient operating room should be considered for patients with moderate to severe asthma undergoing general anesthesia, and some with severe asthma undergoing local procedures. Hospitalization should also be considered for patients with poorly compensated asthma. The major risk of bronchospasm is in the immediate postoperative period so that these patients are good candidates for same-day surgery units and do not necessarily require 24 hours of observation.

Asthmatics should be on a theophylline bronchodilator before procedures are performed, even if they are normally in a stable state without bronchodilators. The bronchodilator should be taken orally the morning of surgery for local procedures and a dose administered at midnight for patients who will be NPO for general anesthesia the following morning.

DENTAL INFECTIONS

The bacteriology of the oropharynx, gums, and teeth are complex (189, 190). Most aerobic and anaerobic organisms can be found in the mouth. In addition, certain unusual organisms, such as actinomyces and nonpathogenic aerobic and anaerobic organisms, can be found in the mouth. In addition, certain unusual organisms, such as actinomyces, and nonpathogenic bacteria, such as fusobacterium, may cause infection. The most common aerobic organism isolated is *Streptococcus*. The most common anaerobic organisms are *Peptostreptococcus* and *Bacteroides*. Most of the organisms commonly isolated are sensitive to penicillin, including most *Bacteroides* (Table 21.17).

It is important to differentiate the location of infection, since the natural history and treatment vary. Infection may occur in the dental pulp, periodental area,

Table 21.17. Microbiology of Dental Infections[a]

Organism	% of Infections Isolated (N = 31)
Aerobic	
Streptococcus	14 (45%)
Anaerobic	
Bacteroides	21 (68%)
Fusobacterium	7 (23%)
Peptostreptococcus	16 (52%)
Peptococcus	7 (23%)
Actinomyces	4 (13%)

[a] Organisms isolated from more than 10% of patients. Data from Ref. 189.

pericoronal area, mandible, maxilla, and retropharyngeal facial spaces (189). The major, life-threatening complications are bacteremia and extension to retropharyngeal spaces, cavernous sinus, sinuses, and Ludwig's angina.

The most important general principle is to carefully evaluate patients with dental infections for spread to the jaw (osteomyelitis), nearby structures (cellulitis, sinusitis), and facial plains of the head and neck. A careful examination of the head, neck, and throat should be performed. In questionable cases or seriously ill patients, an otolaryngology consultation should be suggested. X-rays of the jaw, sinuses, and soft-tissue neck films are often helpful.

It is important to recognize two rare, life-threatening syndromes. Ludwig's angina presents with board-like edema below the mandible, the inability to close the mouth, and elevation of the tongue. Obstruction may produce difficulties in swallowing and respiration. Infection of the retropharyngeal space may be manifested by high fever, rigors, pain, and trismus of the mandible, dysphasia, and difficult breathing. The importance of recognizing these syndromes is the necessity for rapid and radical surgical drainage.

Minor infections limited to the area of teeth and gums may usually be treated with oral penicillin. Routine culturing is not necessary unless there is a failure to respond. Culture should be obtained on infections that are anatomically more extensive or in severely ill patients. It is important to obtain both aerobic and anaerobic cultures since both types of organisms are usually involved. In seriously ill patients, high-dose intravenous penicillin is the drug of choice (10–20 million units/day in divided doses). Acceptable alternatives are clindamycin or a second/third-generation cephalosporin with anaerobic activity.

Prompt, adequate drainage is a cornerstone of therapy for dental infections, since most involve localized pus. Institution of antibiotic therapy should not produce complacency toward adequate drainage. The duration of antibiotic therapy depends on the severity of infection. In most cases, 10–14 days of therapy is sufficient. Longer durations of therapy (from 2–6 weeks) is necessary in osteomyelitis and extensive facial infections.

BURNS

Burn injury and its treatment may involve complications of every organ system (Table 21.18). Most of the complications are managed by routine burn care protocols by the surgeon. This section will further discuss in detail the three complications which most commonly lead to medical consultation in pulmonary injury, infection, and stress-induced gastrointestinal bleeding. Other complications for which consultation may be occasionally requested will be briefly summarized with reference to appropriate literature.

Pulmonary Complications

EPIDEMIOLOGY

Pulmonary complications occur in one-quarter to over one-half of patients with extensive burns and contribute to over one-half of burn deaths (198–207). The multiple causes of pulmonary complications in burn patients can be divided into early and late problems. *Early problems*

Table 21.18. Complications of Burns Contributing to Mortality[a]

Complications	No. of Cases
Nonbacterial	
Early shock or cardiac failure	12
Glottic burns and/or inhalation of smoke	7
Carbon monoxide poisoning	2
Pulmonary edema and/or atelectasis	11
Aspiration of vomit	2
Acute renal failure	24
Pulmonary embolism	5
Hypokalemia	4
Cardiac arrest	4
Hepatic jaundice	2
Hemorrhage from duodenal ulcer	1
Acute encephalopathy	1
Acute dilation of the stomach	3
Agranulocytosis and thrombocytopenia	1
Others	12
Total	91
Bacterial	
Septicemia (including pyemia)	60
Bronchopneumonia	56
Acute pyelonephritis	16
Meningitis	2
Enterocolitis	3
Gas gangrene	1
Others	3
Total	141

[a] From Sevitt S: Death after burning. *Med Sci Law* 6:36–44, 1966, with permission.

are caused by direct thermal injury and carbon monoxide poisoning, mainly at the time of presentation or within several days of injury. *Late complications* occurring after 24 hours include chemical injury to the lung from combustion-product pneumonia, adult respiratory distress syndrome, atelectasis, pulmonary emboli, and complications of mechanical ventilation (pneumothorax).

DIAGNOSTIC ACTIVITIES AND APPROACHES

Findings suggestive of direct inhalation injury are burns due to fires in enclosed spaces, facial burns, wheezing, carbonaceous sputum, and lung findings by auscultation. None of these findings are specific, and a significant number of patients may lack such findings. Indirect laryngoscopy should be performed as soon as possible when upper airway damage is suspected.

Carbon monoxide levels should be obtained in all patients involved in fires in closed spaces. Arterial oxygen saturation is helpful only if measured directly.

The diagnosis of inhalation injury to the lower respiratory tract and lung may be clinically difficult. A number of tests have been proposed for diagnosis including xenon ventilation scans, bronchoscopy, and pulmonary function testing. None of these studies has been definitely established as a procedure of choice, and they may be difficult to obtain in severely injured patients. Many patients have to be followed clinically, with symptomatic treatment without a firmly established diagnosis.

MANAGEMENT PRINCIPLES

Burned patients with upper airway injuries need to be followed closely for airway obstruction. An endotracheal tube should be used, since tracheostomy is accompanied by a significant mortality in burn patients. Carbon monoxide poisoning should be treated with 100% oxygen and hyperventilation.

Inhalation injury to the lower respiratory tract should be treated by bronchodilators, and pulmonary toilet. The use of steroids is controversial (191, 204). Patients requiring mechanical ventilation should receive positive end expiratory pressure (PEEP). PEEP may shorten the duration of symptomatic lung injury, especially if initiated early.

Infectious Complications

EPIDEMIOLOGY

Infections remain the primary cause of burn mortality. Infections are a significant factor in 60–75% of burn deaths (191–192). The most common sites of infection are pneumonia and the burn wound itself. Sites of intravenous and urinary tract catheterization are the next most likely sites of infection.

The organisms involved in infection of burned patients are similar regardless of the burn site because of common environmental exposure and bacteremic seeding from the burn wound (191). The types of organisms involved have changed greatly over the past 30 years. Infection with group A *Streptococcus* occurred early in the course of the burn wound. These infections are now prevented by prophylactic low-dose penicillin and topical antibiotics.

Infection now tends to occur after the first week. Predominant bacteria are Gram-negative bacteria (especially pseudomonas); *Staphylococcus,* and fungi, especially *Candida,* are also commonly involved.

DIAGNOSTIC ACTIVITIES AND APPROACHES

Early in the treatment of the burn, a mild leukocytosis may be found secondary to the burn injury itself (190, 191); leukocytosis over 20,000 favors infection. Localizing symptoms and signs are frequently absent.

Atypical presentation of infections in burn patients are frequent as are isolated hypothermia, hypotension, hypoxia, worsening of the burn wound, or sloughing of skin grafts. In patients with possible infection, a careful examination of the chest, urine, and sites of instrumentation (urinary tract, intravenous) is important in localizing a site of infection. The burn wound should be cultured by quantitative biopsy, since swab cultures cannot differentiate between colonization and infection. A colony count of greater than 10^5 bacteria/g of tissue is indicative of infection of the burn wound (190).

MANAGEMENT PRINCIPLES

Prevention of infection is crucial, since burned patients are immunosuppressed and do not always respond to antibiotic treatment. Prophylactic treatment involves application of topical antibiotics and, in many centers, prophylactic low-dose (1.2–2.4 million units per day) penicillin for the first 1–3 days. Limiting the number of and meticulous attention in inserting intravenous and urinary tract catheters are important. Proper attention to asepsis in caring for the burned patient and prevention of cross-infection in burn units are also important. A passive vaccine shows promise in decreasing the incidence and mortality of pseudomonas infections (191).

Infections in burned patients must be treated early, since these immunosuppressed patients may rapidly succumb to infection.

In general, suspected infection should be treated early and should not wait for positive cultures. In the common situation where a site cannot be positively identified, appropriate coverage includes an aminoglycide antibiotic active against pseudomonas, and a semi-synthetic penicillin active against *Staphylococcus.*

Proper local care should include removal and culturing of catheters suspected of infection, debridement of the burn wound, surgical removal of infected veins, and pulmonary toilet. Careful attention should be paid to other complications, especially hypoxia and hypotension.

Gastrointestinal Bleeding

EPIDEMIOLOGY

Clinical studies have found evidence for upper gastrointestinal bleeding and gastritis in about one-half of patients with large burn injuries. Less common is frank gastroduodenal ulceration occurring in 12–25% of patients and life-threatening hemorrhage occurring in 5%. Serial endoscopy have shown gastric erosions are present in most large burns and occur early within 72 hours after injury (191, 194–197). Additional risk factors for more severe gastroduodenal injury are sepsis, hypoxia, and hypotension (197). Both intensive prophylactic antacid therapy and, possibly, cimetidine have been shown to prevent major gastrointestinal hemorrhage after burn injury.

DIAGNOSTIC ACTIVITIES AND APPROACHES

There is no consensus on which patients ought to be endoscoped. Patients with sufficient bleeding to require consideration of surgery ought to be endoscoped. Endoscopy should also be performed in patients whose past history or the time course of bleeding suggest preexisting lesions not related to burns, such as esophageal variances in the alcoholic. A search for occult sepsis and disseminated intravascular coagulation should be made in the absence of known infection or respiratory insufficiency, since one of these is frequently present in patients with bleeding.

MANAGEMENT PRINCIPLES

Both occult and major bleeding after burns can be prevented by the administration of an intensive antacid regimen, sucralfate, or, possibly, cimetidine. Hourly antacids sufficient to maintain a gastric pH > 3.5 should be administered prophylactically to patients with burns covering more than 20–50% of the body surface or with the additional risk factors of sepsis and respiratory insufficiency.

Abnormalities of Liver Function

Liver enzymes are elevated after extensive burn injury in as many as one-half of patients. The pattern is one of a hepatocellular injury with the greatest elevation of transaminases. Liver function tests may become elevated within 24 hours of injury and may take 2–3 weeks to return to normal. Abnormal liver function tests occurring late after the initial burn injury should suggest the possibility of sepsis or hypotension. Important differential diagnoses include sepsis, acalculous, cholecystitis, and pancreatitis.

Cardiovascular Complications

EPIDEMIOLOGY

Myocardial depression occurs after second–third-degree burns over 40–60% of body surface, depending on the burn depth. Cardiac output may drop to one-third of previous levels (191, 192, 193). Myocardial depression is due to both volume depletion and a plasma factor causing myocardial depression (191–193). Myocardial depression can lead to clinical congestive heart failure with the massive fluid replacement routinely given as therapy.

Myocardial infarction occurs in a few percent of burns, usually in elderly patients with extensive injuries (191).

Hypertension has been reported as a complication of burns in children but not in adults. Hypertension after burns in adult patients can usually be explained by prior hypertension or fluid overload.

DIAGNOSTIC ACTIVITIES AND APPROACHES

Congestive heart failure may be extremely difficult to diagnose in burn patients. The major differential diagnosis is pulmonary burn injury and acute respiratory distress syndrome. Swan-Ganz catheterization is useful in resolving difficult cases. Patients with severe heart disease may benefit from pulmonary artery pressure monitoring, but the risk of infection should be recognized.

Myocardial infarction may be difficult to diagnose, as the presenting symptoms are often congestive heart failure, arrhythmias, or shock, which may have many other explanations in these patients.

Neuropsychiatric Disorders

Patients with large burns may present a spectrum of psychiatric complications ranging from mild grief to psychosis. These must be differentiated from an acute organic brain syndrome which can follow burn injury. The organic syndrome may range from mild lethargy to delirium or coma. There are no localizing neurological signs, but pupillary abnormalities, abnormalities of extraocular muscles, cerebellar signs, and seizures have been reported.

The organic delirium is usually seen in extensive burns exceeding 50% of body surface. The neurological syndrome may not begin until 2–3 weeks after injury. The onset may be related to sepsis. Management focuses on adequate treatment of the burn injury, sepsis, and any potentiating metabolic abnormalities.

Mild lethargy and confusion in the burned patient may be the presenting symptom of metabolic abnormalities or sepsis, especially occurring early in the course. The diagnosis of delirium secondary to burn injury should not be made until other abnormalities have been excluded, especially if the features or timing of onset is atypical.

Renal and Electrolyte Complications

Acute renal failure may be caused by hypovolemia early in the course of burns and by septicemia later during hospitalization. Both oliguric and non-oliguric renal failure have been reported. Multiple electrolyte and acid-base abnormalities occur both due to the burn and its treatment (see ref. 191). Mild to moderate hyponatremia occurs 3–7 days after injury. The mechanism of the hyponatremia is not firmly established, but is probably related to fluid therapy and mobilization of burn fluid. Treatment is restriction of free water.

Electrical Injury

EPIDEMIOLOGY

Little quantitative literature exists on medical complications of electrical injury. Complications can be divided into those occurring during the hospital course and chronically weeks to years after injuries. The most frequent acute complications are cardiac arrhythmias, respiratory arrest, renal failure, and central nervous system damage (191, 208–210).

The most immediate, generalized effect of electrical injury is cardiac arrhythmias (usually ventricular fibrillation) and respiratory arrest.

After the initial resuscitation, many electrocardiographic changes have been reported, including bundle-branch block, A-V dissociation, premature atrial and ventricular beats, and sustained supraventricular and ventricular arrhythmias. Ischemic changes on the electrocardiogram have included nonspecific ST-T wave changes in most patients and changes typical of myocardial infarction in an occasional patient (208–209). Most studies have been done without utilizing cardiac scans or myocardial isoenzymes to establish whether myocardial infarction has occurred.

Patients with these ischemic changes have been reported to tolerate required surgical procedures without cardiac complications (208–209).

Although respiratory arrest is a contributing cause to hypoxia and cardiac arrhythmias, other pulmonary injuries are uncommon. Occasional patients will suffer a localized pneumonitis and pleural effusion related to the entrance wound. As with burns, pneumonia is a frequent and important complication.

A large number of patients have renal damage or failure due to multiple causes. Factors implicated in renal failure have included direct electrical damage to the kidneys, the initial hypotension, tissue breakdown products, and myoglobinuria.

Damage to the nervous system includes initial coma and spinal cord injury due to current or vertebral fractures. The course of these changes is quite variable, but permanent damage is frequent, especially with spinal cord lesions (208).

Submucosal hemorrhages throughout the gastrointestinal tract occur with electrical injuries. An occasional death is due to hemorrhagic necrosis of the bowel, especially the colon. Stress-induced gastric bleeding is a frequent problem as with burns. The most frequent cause of death in electrical injuries is infection (208). In addition to the common sites for the other types of burns, infection of necrotic muscle is an important source of sepsis, and prompt debridement is important.

DIAGNOSTIC ACTIVITIES AND APPROACHES

Serial electrocardiograms and continuous monitoring for arrhythmias are important. Although there is a lack of reported experience, cardiac isoenzymes (CPK-MB) should be of diagnostic help. In questionable cases of cardiac injury, [99]technetium or thallium scans should be obtained. Renal function, urine output, electrolytes, and acid-base status should be measured frequently during the first several days, as severe acidosis is common. During the recovery period from the acidosis, profound hypokalemia may suddenly occur.

MANAGEMENT PRINCIPLES

Patients with electrical injuries usually present with cardiac and respiratory arrest. Resuscitation attempts should be prolonged, as complete cardiac and neurological recovery have been reported, even in patients requiring several hours of resuscitation. There are no data to establish how long monitoring should be continued, but it should be for a minimum of 3 days or until the acute stage of injury has resolved. Surgery for debridement should not usually be delayed because of possible cardiac damage, as it is required for the patient to survive, and seems to have acceptable risk, even in the presence of EKG abnormalities (209, 210).

All patients should have sufficient amounts of intravenous fluids to maintain blood pressure and urine flow. The amount of fluid required to maintain blood pressure and urine output is highly variable and no set regimen is established, in contrast to burn injuries (208). Most authors recommend that mannitol be given soon after injury to reduce myoglobin-induced renal damage. Severe acidosis is common and should be treated vigorously with sodium bicarbonate. The acidosis will plateau after the first several days, and is then followed by a period during which severe potassium depletion may occur. It is therefore important to monitor the serum potassium very frequently, not only during bicarbonate replacement but for several days thereafter.

PELVIC EXENTERATION

Epidemiology

Pelvic exenteration is an uncommon radical surgical procedure indicated for recurrent cancer of the cervix and for certain cases of rectal cancer involving the genital tract. Even on large gynecologic oncology services, the frequency averages only one per month. The frequency of pelvic exenterations will further decrease with current radiation therapy techniques and with earlier diagnosis by routine Pap smears. Because of the extensive nature of this procedure, most gynecologic oncologists recommend that it be performed only by teams experienced in the technique and in the management of the postoperative complications most frequently seen. The 2-year survival for recurrent cancer of the cervix treated conservatively approaches zero. With current surgical techniques and supportive care, the 2-year survival for those patients treated with pelvic exenteration approximates 50%, with a 2–13% surgical mortality.

Preoperative Evaluation

Proper patient selection is a keystone in minimizing surgical morbidity and mortality. Tumor spread beyond the pelvis, positive peritoneal cytology, or para-aortic and pelvic node involvement make the possibility of a successful outcome remote. Nutritional status, circulating volume, electrolyte, and acid-base balance must be as close to normal as possible before surgery is undertaken.

Unrelated conditions substantially increasing morbidity and mortality are impaired renal function, cardiac failure, and poorly controlled diabetes mellitus (212–213). Many gynecologists consider these disorders to be relative contraindications to the procedure.

Preoperative evaluation should focus on assessment of cardiac and renal function. Time should be allowed to achieve good control of diabetes mellitus.

In addition, psychosocial abnormalities (mental retardation, psychosis) profoundly alter the necessary patient cooperation needed for successful rehabilitation and make proper postoperative stoma care improbable.

The use of central hyperalimentation pre- and postoperatively has had a major impact on optimizing the patient's condition and preventing infection, debility, and postoperative fistulae, and on improving wound healing (211). In addition, the routine use of preoperative prophylactic antibiotics (usually an aminoglycoside plus clindamycin) has also contributed to the prevention of postoperative wound infections. Patient support groups and stomal therapists contribute crucial emotional comfort and essential practical advice.

Postoperative Care

In a review of 296 patients at the M. D. Anderson Hospital, Rutledge et al. (212) grouped postoperative complications into early (day 1–7), intermediate (day 7–90), and late (greater than 90 days) phases (Table 21.19).

In the first 7 days postoperatively, complications could generally be categorized as primarily medical, whereas those occurring later were more likely to be surgical.

The most common medical complications are cardiac, thromboembolic, renal failure, pneumonia, sepsis, and gastrointestinal bleeding (Table 21.20). Particular management problems during the first postoperative week are replacement of blood and fluids and nutritional support. For example, the operative field has been

Table 21.19. Complications of Pelvic Exenteration in 296 Patients[a]

	Number	% of Total
Early (day 1–7)		
(1) Cardiac failure, MI, pulmonary emboli, DVT, CVAs, DIC	31	33
(2) Uremia	17	20
(3) Pneumonia	18	20
(4) Sepsis (pyelonephritis, pelvic infections, peritonitis)	21	23
(5) GI bleeding	2	2
Intermediate (day 7–90)		
(1) Sepsis, pneumonia, wound infection	41	35
(2) Intestinal obstruction and fistulas	41	35
(3) Uremia, urinary fistulae, leakage, pyelonephritis	34	29
(4) Cardiovascular	2	1
Late (>90 days)		
(1) Chronic UTI	31	38
(2) Uropathy (stones, renal failure)	15	18
(3) Intestinal obstruction	13	16
(4) Stoma retraction, herniation	12	16
(5) Perineal herniation	10	12

[a] From Rutledge et al: *Am J Obstet Gynecol* 129:881, 1977. Used with permission.

compared to a 10% third-degree burn, with maintenance and replacement crystalloids and colloids calculated accordingly (213a).

Table 21.20. Complications of Pelvic Exenteration in 37 Patients at the Milton S. Hershey Medical Center, 1972–1979[a]

	N	%
Sepsis	7	20
Wound infection	5	15
Phlebitis	4	12
Pneumonia	2	6
Hepatitis	1	3
Small bowel obstruction	5	15
Urinary and GI conduit fistulae	6	17

[a] From Curry et al.: *Gynecol Oncol* 11:119, 1981. Used with permission.

RADICAL NECK SURGERY

Epidemiology

Most internists conceive of radical neck dissection as a mutilating procedure with high surgical morbidity and mortality. However, radical neck dissection (i.e., the unilateral, *en bloc* removal of the lymph nodes and drainage of the neck) gives a cosmetically good result, except when combined with extensive oral facial resections or with total laryngectomy. Aggressive plastic and reconstructive techniques can often restore patients with resections of the face and mandible to good physiologic function and fair cosmetic results. Average blood loss is 1–3 units, and the average duration of surgery is from 1–3 hours. However, operating time of up to 10 hours may be required in complicated cases, e.g., in those with previous uncoordinated radiation therapy or "redo" operations.

Overall surgical mortality is 1–3% with unilateral radical neck dissection and 2–5% for bilateral radical neck dissection. Except for the very old (over age 70), radical neck dissection is a well-tolerated procedure by the aged, with surgical morbidity and mortality in appropriately prepared patients approximately that of other *major* surgical procedures in this age group (Tables 21.21 and 21.22). The major causes of increased mortality in the very old are aspiration pneumonia, malnutrition, and cardiovascular disease.

Table 21.21.   Operative Mortality for Radical Neck Dissection [a]

Age	Number	
All ages	2.8%	2.8%
≤49	0/83	0%
50–59	5/211	2.4%
60–69	3/258	1.2%
70–79	6/131	4.6%
80+	6/31	19.4%

[a] From McGuirt et al.: *Laryngoscope* 87:1378, 1977. Used with permission.

Table 21.22.   Type of Surgical Procedure Related to Cause of Death [a]

	Pulmonary	Cardiovascular	Multiple Stress
Jaw-neck	1	4	1
Laryngectomy-pharyngectomy	3		1
Radical neck dissection		2	1

[a] From McGuirt et al.: *Laryngoscope* 87:1378, 1977. Used with permission.

Older and ill patients are often advised against surgery and referred for extensive radiation therapy because of the bias of many physicians that many of these patients will not outlive their primary disease. However, many patients survive long enough to present for complex surgery at an even older age. Primary radiation therapy uncoordinated with surgery often compromises the ideal surgical approach and increases surgical morbidity (by 30–40% in many series) by leading to extensive fibrosis, edema, disruption of tissue planes, and altered perfusion.

Diagnostic Activities and Management

Preoperative preparation and attention to detail play a major role in decreasing surgical morbidity and mortality. Nutritional status should be restored as closely to normal as possible via either enteral or parenteral approaches. If the oral-pharyngeal space is to be penetrated, prior treatment of periodontal disease should be vigorously pursued and appropriate antibiotic coverage planned. Most studies report a significant decrease in postoperative infections with the use of cephalosporin (1 g preoperatively, 500 mg every 6 hr for four doses postoperatively). Alternative antibiotic regimens are clindamycin, cephalosporin (or penicillin or clindamycin) plus tobramycin. A single dose of antibiotic preoperatively followed by administration for 1–3 days postoperatively has been recommended, as has continuing prophylactic antibiotics for 5–7 days. No data prove the superiority of a two-drug regimen or prolonged administration. In addition, patients should be fully prepared emotionally for the recovery period and for any further planned plastic and reconstructive surgery.

Postoperative Management

Camnitz et al. (215) have conveniently divided surgical complications into intraoperative, early, and late postoperative phases. Intraoperative complications are primarily mechanical and treated by immediate surgical correction (e.g., jugular vein bleeding, air embolism, carotid sinus syndrome, carotid thrombosis, cranial and phrenic nerve injuries, pneumothorax, and thoracic duct injury). The internist is rarely involved in their diagnosis or management.

Early (1–7 days) postoperative complications vary according to the type of surgery. With radical neck dissection alone, most complications are usually of cardiovascular origin; whereas with pharyngectomies or laryngectomies, pulmonary complications predominate (Table 21.22). With radical neck dissection alone, cough is not impaired.

When a tracheostomy is required, drying of the airway and a poor cough with retention of secretions, atelectasis, and pneumonia are of constant concern. Tracheostomy cuffs must be fully inflated when using positive pressure breathing to avoid forcing oral-pharyngeal contents into the wound. Fistula formation and wound infections are more common when the oral-pharyngeal space has been surgically entered. With the use of closed-suction drainage catheters placed in the wound at surgery, the incidence of these complications has been substantially reduced but is still frequent, occurring in 20% or more of patients.

Agitation and irrational behavior postoperatively may be due to hypoxia. Arterial blood gases should be obtained. Tra-

cheal obstruction due to hematomas or seromas should always be considered. Other causes of agitation, such as urinary retention, delirium tremens, and ICU psychosis, should also be considered.

Late complications (>30 days) are often related to tumor recurrence or surgical mishaps (jugular vein ligation, loss of skin flaps, carotid erosion, etc.). In total laryngectomy patients treated with radiation therapy, hypothyroidism may occur late.

In summary, with careful preoperative preparation, avoidance of preoperative radiation therapy uncoordinated with surgery, and the use of prophylactic antibiotics, radical neck dissection, laryngectomies, and pharyngectomies can be safely performed even in the aged, with good functional and cosmetic results.

TRANSURETHRAL PROSTATE RESECTION

Transurethral prostate resection (TURP) is among the most common operation in elderly males. The risk of such surgery is very small (about 1%), even when done in patients with severe chronic disease.

Epidemiology

Several operations are performed for benign prostatic hypertrophy, including transurethral, suprapubic, and, less commonly, retropubic prostatectomy. Radical prostatectomy is performed for carcinoma of the prostate. Only transurethral prostate resection for benign disease will be discussed, since it is the most common operation and has a lower risk than other procedures. Suprapubic and radical prostatectomy constitute major surgery with comparable cardiopulmonary risk to major lower intraperitoneal procedures. These more extensive procedures have an increased risk compared with transurethral resection of sepsis from urinary tract infection and thromboembolism.

Current series indicate that TURP can be performed with a 1% overall mortality. The major consideration is the existence

Table 21.23.   Risk of Prostate Surgery[a]

| | Mortality | | | |
	All Patients	Patients with Cardiac Disease	Total Number (Cardiac)	Cause of Mortality
Erlik, 1968	0.93%	0.96%	539 (104)	3 pulmonary emboli 1 CVA 1 pulmonary emboli and MI
−Additional cases	0%	0%	135 (27)	
Thompson, 1962		5%	192 (192)	7 MI 1 CHF 1 SBE
Skinner, 1964		2%	124 (124)	

[a] Derived in part from Refs. 218 and 219.

of cardiac disease. Perioperative mortality was not increased in patients with (0.76%) compared to those without (0.74%) cardiac disease in Erlik's combined series of 674 patients (218) (Table 21.23).

A 5% mortality was reported for patients undergoing TURP after myocardial infarction (219). TURP has been performed within 6 months of a myocardial infarction without a major increase in mortality, but experience is limited, and prudence dictates waiting for 6 or more months post-infarction, if possible.

The major causes of postoperative mortality after TURP are infection, pulmonary emboli, and cardiac complications (241). Most of the small number of myocardial infarctions occurred late after surgery (5 or more days) in the two reported series.

The risk of thrombophlebitis has been variously estimated from 7 to 80% in patients undergoing all types of prostate surgery (225). Studies of only transurethral resection found an incidence of deep vein thrombosis (DVT) of 7–10% by ^{125}I fibrinogen scanning, and 5% by phleborography (Table 21.24).

The incidences of *fatal* pulmonary emboli after *all* types of prostatectomy was 1% in the international low-dose heparin trial (222). The available data suggest thrombophlebitis is not as frequent a complication with TURP as many clinicians feel or as with other methods of prostate surgery.

The incidence of Gram-negative sepsis after transurethral prostatectomy is also lower in current series (average 1–8%) than with other types of prostatectomy in earlier studies (see p. 381) (232).

Thus, TURP represents a relatively safe operation from the viewpoint of medical problems. The feared complications of thromboembolic events, sepsis, and myocardial infarction are much lower than in older series or when prostatectomy is done by other methods, but still accounts for most of the small current mortality.

Table 21.24.   Risk of Thrombophlebitis with Transurethral Prostate Resection[a]

Study	Diagnostic Study	No. with TURP	Thrombophlebitis (%)
Mays, 1971	^{131}I fibrinogen	20	2 (10%)
Nicolardes, 1972	^{131}I fibrinogen	29	2 (7%)
Crawford, 1978	Phleborheography	150	7 (5%)
Van Arsdalen	Venography	29	2 (7%)

[a] From Refs. 220, 225, and 230–231.

Diagnostic Activities and Approaches

The initial data base should emphasize the cardiac and pulmonary systems. Pulmonary function tests do not need to be routinely performed in the absence of any history of physical findings of *clinically* significant pulmonary disease, because of the low incidence of pulmonary complications. Assessment of renal function, urine culture, and often IVP are routinely performed by the urologist. Abnormalities of renal function need to be further investigated prior to surgery.

Management Principles

PREOPERATIVE MANAGEMENT

Transurethral prostate resection can be performed on most patients, including those with stable, severe chronic disease. The most important concomitant disease is coronary artery disease.

Patients with recent myocardial infarction (1–6 months) should have their TURP deferred. In patients who do not tolerate Foley catheter drainage or with repeated complications, surgery earlier than 6 months can be considered because of the small increase in risk (waiting a *minimum* of 6–12 weeks is recommended, depending on individual circumstances).

Prophylaxis for prevention of thromboembolic events is controversial because there are inadequate data specifically for prostatectomy. Elastic stockings and early ambulation should be used for all patients as general measures. Various drug regimens that are used include low-dose heparin and aspirin, but no regimen has proven efficacious.

POSTOPERATIVE MANAGEMENT

Any new signs suggestive to deep venous thrombosis warrant obtaining a venogram because of the inaccuracy of clinical diagnosis. Postoperative fevers are a frequent occurrence; a close search should be made for infection, especially of the urinary tract. Prompt therapy should be instituted for suspected urinary tract infection because of the risk of Gram-negative sepsis.

Special Considerations

CEREBROVASCULAR DISEASE

Cerebrovascular accidents extended or recurred in two of 22 (10%) patients undergoing TURP who had a prior stroke in one study (234). No information was given on the patients' condition or the elapsed time since the previous cerebrovascular accident (CVA). In our experience, the recurrence of CVA has not been as high, perhaps due to patient selection, allowing an adequate time of (6–12 weeks) post-stroke, and good perioperative maintenance of blood pressure. Preoperative evaluation of patients for TURP after a stroke should include an evaluation to exclude neurological problems as a major contributing cause to difficulty with micturition.

HYPONATREMIA

Rarely, marked drop in serum sodium occurs shortly after transurethral prostatectomy. (235–237). The hyponatremia may be marked, with sodium falling from normal to below 120 mEq/L. The fall in serum sodium results from absorption of irrigating fluid. This problem occurred more frequently when sterile water was used as an irrigating solution than with current solutions which contain mannitol or sodium chloride.

The drop in serum sodium is acute and therefore often accompanied by severe symptoms, including confusion, coma, and seizures. Rarely, the major manifestation will be focal neurological signs. A syndrome of cortical blindness due to hyponatremia after prostatectomy has been labeled the "TURP reaction." This is not specific for prostatectomy, as focal signs have been reported with hyponatremia in other circumstances.

Electrolytes should be obtained immediately if a patient develops new central nervous symptoms or other symptoms suggestive of hyponatremia after TURP. Treatment depends on the patient's intravascular volume. Since most patients will be *fluid-overloaded,* furosemide and hypertonic saline are the usual treatment (see p. 197).

READINGS

1. Djokovic JL, Hedley-Whyte J: Prediction of outcome of surgery and anesthesia in patients over 80. *JAMA* 242:2301–2306, 1979.
2. Ferris P: Surgical management of the elderly. *Hosp Pract* 11:65–71, 1976.
3. Miller R, Marlar K, Silvay G: Anesthesia for patients aged over ninety years. *NY St J Med* 77:1421–1425, 1977.
4. Kohn P, Zekert F, Vormittag E, et al: Risks of operation in patients over 80. *Geriatrics* 28:100–105, 1973.
5. Marshall WH, Fahey PJ: Operative complications and mortality in patients over 80. *Arch Surg* 88:896–904, 1964.
6. Ziffren SE: Comparison of mortality rates for various surgical operations according to age groups, 1951–1977. *J Am Geriatr Soc* 10:433–438, 1979.
7. Burnett W, McCaffrey J: Surgical procedures in the elderly. *Surg Gynecol Obstet* 134:221–226, 1972.
8. Denney JL, Denson JS: Risk of surgery in patients over 90. *Geriatrics* 27:115–118, 1972.
9. Cogbill CL: Operation in the aged: mortality related to concurrent disease, duration of anesthesia, and elective or emergency operation. *Arch Surg* 94:202–205, 1967.
10. Glenn F: Surgical principles for the aged patient, in Reichel W (ed): *Clinical Aspects of Aging.* Baltimore, Williams & Wilkins, 1978, pp 367–382.
11. McGuirt WF, Loevy S, McCabe BF, et al: The risk of major head and neck surgery in the aged population. *Laryngoscope* 87:1378–1382, 1977.
12. Marx GF, Mateo CV, Orkin LR: Computer analysis of postanesthetic deaths. *Anesthesiology* 39:54–58, 1973.
13. Cole WH: Medical differences between the young and the aged. *J Am Geriatr Soc* 18:589–614, 1970.
14. Rashad KF, Goldman EJ, Graff TD, et al.: Baltimore Anesthesia Study Committee: Factors in geriatric anesthesia mortality. *Anesth Analg* 44:462–648, 1965.
15. Lassen HK: Geriatric problems in surgery. A clinical review with a statistical survey of mortality rates as related to age. *J Gerontol* 17:167–179, 1962.
16. Tarhan S, Moffitt EA, Sessler AD, et al: Risk of anesthesia and surgery in patients with chronic bronchitis and chronic obstructive pulmonary disease. *Surgery* 74:720–726, 1973.
17. Bunkey JP, Barnes BA, Mosteller F (eds): *Risks and Benefits of Surgery.* New York, Oxford, 1977, pp 223–245.

18. Linn BS, Linn MW: Evaluation of results of surgical procedures in the elderly. *Ann Surg* 195:90–96, 1982.
19. Greenburg AG, Salk RP, Farris JM, et al: Operative mortality in general surgery. *Am J Surg* 144:22–28, 1982.
20. Santos AL, Gelperin A: Surgical mortality in the elderly. *J Am Geriatr Soc* 23:42–46, 1975.
21. Palmberg S, Hirsjarvi E: Mortality in geriatric surgery. *Gerontology* 25:103–112, 1979.
22. Cogbill TH, Landerscasper J, Strutt P, et al: Late results of peripheral vascular surgery in patients 80 years of age and older. *Arch Surg* 122:581–586, 1987.
23. Reiss R, Deutsch AA: Emergency abdominal procedures in patients above age 70. *J Gerontol* 40:154–158, 1985.
24. Loop FD, Lytle BW, Cosgrove DM, et al: Coronary artery bypass graft surgery in the elderly. *Cleve Clin J Med* 55:23–34, 1988.
25. Hochberg MS, Derkac WM, Conkle DM, et al: Mitral valve replacement in elderly patients: Encouraging postoperative clinical and hemodynamic results. *J Thoracic Cardiovasc Surg* 77:422–426, 1979.
26. De Bono AHB, English TAH, Milstein BB: Heart valve replacement in the elderly. *Br Med J* 2:917–919, 1978.
27. Dripps RD, Lamont A, Eckenhoff JE: The role of anesthesia in surgical mortality. *JAMA* 178:261–266, 1961.
28. Goldman L: Supraventricular tachyarrhythmias in hospitalized adults after surgery. Clinical correlates in patients over 40 years of age after major noncardiac surgery. *Chest* 73:450–454, 1978.
29. Pollock AV, Evans M: Major abdominal operations on patients aged 80 and over: an audit. *Brit Med J* 295:1522, 1987.
30. Michel SL, Stevens L, Amodeo P, et al: Surgical procedures in nonagenarians. *West J Med* 141:61–63, 1984.
31. Hosking MP, Warner MA, Lobdell CM, Offord KP, et al: Outcomes of surgery in patients 90 years of age and older. *JAMA* 261:1909–1915, 1989.
31A. Warner MA, Hosking, MP, Lobdell, CM, Offord, KP, et al: Surgical procedures among those ≥ 90 years of age. *Ann Surg* 207: 380–386, 1988.
32. Adkins RB, Scott HW: Surgical procedures in patients aged 90 years and older. *South Med J* 77:1357–1364, 1984.
33. Denny JL, Denson JS: Risk of surgery in patients over 90. *Geriatrics* 27:115–118, 1972.
34. Katlic MR: Surgery in centenarians. *JAMA* 253:3139–3141, 1985.
35. Rosenthal RA, Andersen DA: Surgery in the elderly. In Andres R, et al. (eds): *Principles of Geriatric Medicine.* New York, McGraw-Hill, 1985, pp 909–932.
36. Seymour DG, Pringle R: Post-operative complications in the elderly surgical patient. *Gerontology* 29:262–270, 1983.
37. Wilder RJ, Fishbein RH: Operative experience

with patients over 80 years of age. *Surg Gynecol Obstet* 113:205–212, 1961.

38. Keating HJ: Preoperative considerations in the geriatric patient. *Med Clin North Am* 71:569–583, 1987.

39. Cogbill CL: Operation in the aged. *Arch Surg* 94:202–205, 1967.

40. Gerson MC, Hurst JM, Hertzberg VS, et al: Cardiac prognosis in noncardiac geriatric surgery. *Ann Intern Med* 103:832–837, 1985.

41. Bistrian BR, Blackburn GL, Hallowell E, et al: Protein status of general surgical patients. *JAMA* 230:858–860, 1974.

42. Organ CH, Finn MP: The importance of nutritional support for the geriatric surgical patient. *Geriatrics* 32:77–84, 1977.

43. Reiss R, Haddad M, Deutsch A, et al: Prognostic index: prediction of operative mortality in geriatric patients by use of stepwise logistic regression analysis. *World J Surg* 11:248–251, 1987.

44. Del Guercio LRM, Cohn JD: Monitoring operative risk in the elderly. *JAMA* 243:1350–1355, 1980.

45. Lewin I, Lerner AG, Green SH, et al: Physical class and physiologic status in the prediction of operative mortality in the aged sick. *Ann Surg* 174:217–231, 1971.

46. Andersen B, Ostberg J, et al: Long-term prognosis in geriatric surgery. *J Amer Geriatr Soc* 20:255–258, 1972.

47. Seymour DG, Vaz, FG: Aspects of surgery in the elderly: preoperative medical assessment. *Brit J Hosp Med* 37:102–112, 1987.

48. Gerson MC, Hurst JM, Hertzberg VS, et al: Cardiac prognosis in noncardiac geriatric surgery. *Ann Int Med* 103:832–837, 1985.

49. Guillen J, Aldrete JA: Anesthetic factors influencing morbidity and mortality of elderly patients undergoing inguinal herniorrhaphy. *Amer J Surg* 120:760–763, 1970.

50. Boyd JB, Bradford B, Watne A: Operative risk factors of colon resection in the elderly. *Ann Surg* 192:743–746, 1980.

51. Greenburg AG, Salk RP, Peskin GW: Mortality and gastrointestinal surgery in the aged. *Arch Surg* 116:788–791, 1981.

52. Greenburg AG, Salk, RP, Pridham D: Influence of age on mortality of colon surgery. *Amer J Surg* 150:65–70, 1985.

53. Blake R, Lynn J: Emergency abdominal surgery in the aged. *Br J Surg* 63:956–960, 1976.

54. Steiger E, Seltzer MH, Rosato FE, et al: Cholecystectomy in the aged. *Ann Surg* 174:142–144, 1971.

55. Mitty WF: *Surgery in the Aged: Seventy-five Years of Age and Over.* Springfield, Illinois, Charles C Thomas, 1966.

56. Randall HT: The treatment of cancer in the older patient, in Powers JH (ed): *Surgery of the Aged and Debilitated Patient.* Philadelphia, WB Saunders, 1968. Quoted in Cole WH: Medical differences between the young and the aged. *J Am Geriatr Soc* 8:589–614, 1970.

57. Schein CJ: A selective approach to surgical problems in the aged. in *Clinical Geriatrics.* Philadelphia, JB Lippincott, 410–427, 1971.

58. Panayiotis G, Ellenbogen A, Grunstein S: Major gynecologic surgical procedures in the aged. *J Amer Geriatr Soc* 26:459–462, 1978.

59. Breyer RH, Zippe C, Pharr WF: Thoracotomy in patients over age seventy years. *J Thorac Cardiovasc Surg* 81:187–193, 1981.

60. Gore I, Hirst AE Jr: Arteriosclerotic aneurysms of the abdominal aorta: A review. *Prog Cardiovasc Dis* 16:113–150, 1973.

61. Estes JE Jr: Abdominal aortic aneurysm: A study of one hundred and two cases. *Circulation* II:258–264, 1950.

62. Darling RC, Messina CR, Brewster DC, et al: Autopsy study of unoperated abdominal aortic aneurysms: the case for early resection. *Cardiovasc Surg* 56:II-161-II-164, 1976.

63. Bernstein EF, Fisher JC, Varco RL: Is excision the optimum treatment for all abdominal aortic aneurysms? *Surgery* 61:83–93, 1967.

64. DeBakey ME, Crawford ES, Cooley DA, et al: Aneurysm of abdominal aorta: analysis of results of graft replacement therapy one to eleven years after operation. *Ann Surg* 160:622–638, 1964.

65. Friedman SA, Hufnagel CA, Conrad PW, et al: Abdominal aortic aneurysms: Clinical status and results of surgery in 100 consecutive cases. *JAMA* 200:1147–1151, 1967.

66. Szilagyi DE, Smith RF, DeRusso FJ, et al: Contribution of abdominal aortic aneurysmectomy to prolongation of life. *Ann Surg* 164:678–697, 1966.

67. Couch NP, Lane FC, Crane C: Management and mortality in resection of abdominal aortic aneurysms. A study of 114 cases. *Am J Surg* 119:408–415, 1970.

68. Stokes J, Butcher HR Jr: Abdominal aortic aneurysms. Factors influencing operative mortality and criteria of operability. *Arch Surg* 107:297–301, 1973.

69. Gardner RJ, Lancaster JR, Tarnay TJ, et al: Five-year history of surgically treated abdominal aortic aneurysms. *Surgery Gynecol Obstet* 130:981–987, 1970.

70. Thompson JE, Hollier LH, Patman RD, et al: Surgical management of abdominal aortic aneurysms: Factors influencing mortality and morbidity—A 20-year experience. *Ann Surg* 181:654–660, 1975.

71. Baker AG Jr, Roberts B, Berkowitz HD, et al: Risk of excision of abdominal aortic aneurysms. *Surgery* 68:1129–1134, 1970.

72. Levy JF, Kouchoukos NT, Walker WB, et al: Abdominal aortic aneurysmectomy: a study of 100 cases. *Arch Surg* 92:498, 1966.

73. Cannon JA, Van De Water J, Barker WF: Experience with the surgical management of 100 consecutive cases of abdominal aortic aneurysm. *Am J Surg* 106:128–141, 1963.

74. Hall AD, Zubrin JR, Moore WS, et al: Surgical treatment of aortic aneurysm in the aged: A review of 100 patients. *Arch Surg* 100:455–459, 1970.

75. Young AE, Sandberg GW, Couch NP: The reduction of mortality of abdominal aortic aneurysm resection. *Am J Surg* 134:585–590, 1977.

76. Gardner RJ, Gardner NL, Tarnay TJ, et al: The surgical experience and a one to sixteen year follow-up of 277 abdominal aortic aneurysms. *Am J Surg* 135:226–230, 1978.

77. Esselstyn CB Jr, Humphries AW, Young JR, et al: Aneurysmectomy in the aged? *Surgery* 67:34–39, 1970.

78. May AG, DeWeese JA, Frank I, et al: Surgical treatment of abdominal aortic aneurysms. *Surgery* 63:711–721, 1968.

79. Hicks GL, Eastland MW, DeWeese JA, et al: Survival improvement following aortic aneurysm resection. *Ann Surg* 181:863–869, 1975.

80. Interhospital Cardiovascular Study Group of the University of Toronto: Surgical treatment of abdominal aortic aneurysms in Toronto: A study of 1013 patients. *Can Med Assoc J* 107:1091–1094, 1972.

81. Vasko JS, Spencer FC, Bahnson HT: Aneurysm of the aorta treated by excision: Review of 237 cases followed up to seven years. *Am J Surg* 105:793, 1963.

82. MacVaugh H III, Roberts B: Results of resection of abdominal aortic aneurysm. *Surg Gynecol Obstet* 113:17–23, 1961.

83. Voorhees AB Jr, McAllister FF: Long term results following resection of arteriosclerotic abdominal aortic aneurysms. *Surg Gynecol Obstet* 117:355–358, 1963.

84. Baker AG Jr, Roberts B: Long-term survival following abdominal aortic aneurysmectomy. *JAMA* 212:445–450, 1970.

85. Foster JH, Bolasny BL, Gobbel WG Jr, et al: Comparative study of elective resection and expectant treatment of abdominal aortic aneurysm. *Surg Gynecol Obstet* 129:1–9, 1969.

86. Gliedman ML, Ayers WB, Vestal BL: Aneurysms of the abdominal aorta and its branches. A study of untreated patients. *Ann Surg* 146:207–214, 1957.

87. Klippel AP, Butcher HR Jr: The unoperated abdominal aortic aneurysm. *Am J Surg* 111:629–631, 1966.

88. Szilagyi DE, Elliott JP, Smith RF: Clinical fate of the patient with asymptomatic abdominal aortic aneurysm and unfit for surgical treatment. *Arch Surg* 104:600–606, 1972.

89. Schatz IJ, Fairbairn JF II, Juergens JL: Abdominal aortic aneurysm. A reappraisal. *Circulation* 26:200–205, 1962.

90. Crawford ES, Saleh, SA, Babb, JW, et al: Infrarenal abdominal aortic aneurysm. *Ann Surg* 193:699–709, 1981.

91. McCabe CJ, Coleman WS, Brewster DC: The advantage of early operation for abdominal aortic aneurysm. *Arch Surg* 116:1025–1029, 1981.

92. Diehl JT, Cali RF, Hertzer NR, et al: Complications of abdominal aortic reconstruction. *Ann Surg* 197:49–56, 1983.

93. Soreide O, Lillestol J, Christense O, et al: Abdominal aortic aneurysms: survival analysis of four hundred thirty-four patients. *Surgery* 91:188–193, 1982.

94. Wolffe JB, Colcher RE: Diagnosis and conservative management of atherosclerotic aneurysms of the abdominal aorta. *Vasc Dis* 3:49–57, 1966.

95. Bernstein EF, Dilley RB, Goldberger LE, et al: Growth rates of small abdominal aortic aneurysms. *Surgery* 80:765–773, 1976.

96. O'Donnell TF Jr, Darling RC, Linton RR: Is 80 years too old for aneurysmectomy? *Arch Surg* 111:1250–1257, 1976.

97. Edmunds LH Jr: Resection of abdominal aortic aneurysms in octogenarians. *Ann Surg* 165:453–457, 1967.

98. Roger VL, Ballard DJ, Hallett JW, et al: Influence of coronary artery disease on morbidity and mortality after abdominal aortic aneurysmectomy: a population-based study 1971–1987. *J Am Coll Cardiol* 14:1245–1252, 1989.

99. Sterpetti AV, Schultz RD, Feldhaus RJ, et al: Abdominal aortic aneurysm in elderly patients. *Amer J Surg* 150:772–776, 1985.

100. Cogbill TH, Landercasper J, Strutt PH, et al: Late results of peripheral vascular surgery in patients 80 years of age and older. *Arch Surg* 122:581–586, 1987.

101. Stallworth JM, Price RG Jr, Hughes JC III, et al: Surgical treatment of ruptured abdominal aortic aneurysms. *Ann Surg* 155:711–720, 1962.

102. Ottinger LW: Ruptured arteriosclerotic aneurysms of the abdominal aorta. Reducing mortality. *JAMA* 233:147–150, 1975.

103. Alpert J, Brief DK, Parsonnet V: Surgery for the ruptured abdominal aortic aneurysm. *JAMA* 212:1355–1359, 1970.

104. Darling RC: Ruptured arteriosclerotic abdominal aortic aneurysms. A pathologic and clinical study. *Am J Surg* 119:397–401, 1970.

105. Van Heeckeren DW: Ruptured abdominal aortic aneurysms. *Am J Surg* 119:402–407, 1970.

106. Hiatt JCG, Barker WF, Machleder HI, et al: Determinants of failure in the treatment of ruptured abdominal aortic aneurysm. *Arch Surg* 119:1264–1268, 1984.

107. Cooperman M, Pflug B, Martin EW Jr, et al: Cardiovascular risk factors in patients with peripheral vascular disease. *Surgery* 84:505–509, 1978.

108. Yeager RA, Weigel RM, Murphy ES, et al: Application of clinically valid cardiac risk factors to aortic aneurysm surgery. *Arch Surg* 121:278–281, 1986.

109. White GH, Advani SM, Williams RA, et al: Cardiac risk index as a predictor of long-term survival after repair of abdominal aortic aneurysm. *Amer J Surg* 156:103–107, 1988.

110. Kazmers A, Cerqueira MD, Zierler RE: Perioperative and late outcome in patients with left ventricular ejection fraction of 35% or less who require major vascular surgery. *J Vasc Surg* 8:307–315, 1988.

111. Cutler BS, Leppo JA: Dipyridamole thallium 201 scintigraphy to detect coronary artery disease before abdominal aortic surgery. *J Vasc Surg* 5:91–100, 1987.

112. Blombery PA, Ferguson, IA, Rosengarten DS, et al: The role of coronary artery disease in complications of abdominal aortic aneurysm surgery. *Surgery* 101:150–155, 1987.

113. Hertzer NR, Beven EG, Young JR, et al: Cor-

onary artery disease in peripheral vascular patients. *Ann Surg* 199:223–232, 1984.

114. Toal KW, Jacocks MA, Elkins RC: Preoperative coronary artery bypass grafting in patients undergoing abdominal aortic reconstruction. *Amer J Surg* 148:825–829, 1984.

115. Reul GJ, Cooley DA, Duncan JM, et al: The effect of coronary bypass on the outcome of peripheral vascular operations in 1093 patients. *J Vasc Surg* 3:788–798, 1986.

116. Pasternack PF, Imparato AM, Bear G, et al: The value of radionuclide angiography as a predictor of perioperative myocardial infarction in patients undergoing abdominal aortic aneurysm resection. *J Vasc Surg* 1:320–325, 1984.

117. Ruby ST, Whittemore, Couch NP, et al: Coronary artery disease in patients requiring abdominal aortic aneurysm repair. *Ann Surg* 201:758–764, 1985.

118. Acinapura AJ, Rose DM, Kramer MD, et al: Role of coronary angiography and coronary artery bypass surgery prior to abdominal aortic aneurysmectomy. *J Cardiovasc Surg:* 28:552–557, 1987.

119. Beven EG: Routine coronary angiography in patients undergoing surgery for abdominal aortic aneurysm and lower extremity occlusive disease. *J Vasc Surg* 3:682–684, 1986.

120. Hollier LH: Surgical management of abdominal aortic aneurysm in the high risk patient. *Surg Clin North Am* 66:269–279, 1986.

121. Pasternack PF, Imparato AM, Baumann FG, et al: The hemodynamics of β-blockade in patients undergoing abdominal aortic aneurysm repair. *Circ* 76(suppl III):III-1–III-7, 1987.

122. Attia RR, Murphy JD, Snider M, et al: Myocardial ischemia due to infrarenal aortic cross-clamping during aortic surgery in patients with severe coronary artery disease. *Circ* 53:961–965, 1976.

123. Bush HL Jr, LoGerfo FW, Weisel RD, et al: Assessment of myocardial performance and optimal volume loading during elective abdominal aortic aneurysm resection. *Arch Surg* 112:1301–1305, 1977.

124. Cohen JL, Wender R, Maginot A, et al: Hemodynamic monitoring of patients undergoing abdominal aortic surgery. *Amer J Surg* 146:174–177, 1983.

125. Kalman PG, Wellwood MR, Weisel RD, et al: Cardiac dysfunction during abdominal aortic operation: the limitations of pulmonary wedge pressures. *J Vasc Surg* 3:773–781, 1986.

126. Huval WV, Lelcuk S, Allen PD, et al: Determinants of cardiovascular stability during abdominal aortic aneurysmectomy. *Ann Surg* 199:216–222, 1983.

127. Porter JM, McGregor F Jr, Acinapura AJ, et al: Renal function following abdominal aortic aneurysmectomy. *Surg Gynecol Obstet* 123:819–825, 1966.

128. Bush JL: Renal failure following abdominal aortic reconstruction. *Surgery* 93:107–109, 1983.

129. Cohen JR, Mannick JA, Couch NP, et al: Abdominal aortic aneurysm repair in patients with preoperative renal failure. *J Vasc Surg* 3:867–870, 1986.

130. Johnson WC, Nabseth DC: Visceral infarction following aortic surgery. *Ann Surg* 180:312–318, 1974.

131. Smith RF, Szilagyi DE: Ischemia of the colon as a complication in the surgery of the abdominal aorta. *AMA Arch Surg* 80:806–821, 1960.

132. Welling RE, Roedersheimer R, Arbaugh JJ, et al: Ischemic colitis following repair of ruptured abdominal aortic aneurysm. *Arch Surg* 120:1368–1370, 1985.

133. Szilagyi DE, Elliott JP, Berguer R: Coincidental malignancy and abdominal aortic aneurysm problems of management. *Arch Surg* 95:402–411, 1967.

134. Tilson MD, Fief EL, Harvey M: Malignant neoplasia in patients with abdominal aortic aneurysms. *Arch Surg* 119:792–794, 1984.

135. Lobbatok VJ, Rothenberg RE, LaRaja RD, et al: Coexistence of abdominal aortic aneurysm and carcinoma of the colon: a dilemma. *J Vasc Surg* 2:724–726, 1985.

135a. Nora JD, Pairolero PC, Nivatvongs S, et al: Concomitant abdominal aortic aneurysm and colorectal carcinoma: priority of resection. *J Vasc Surg* 9:630–636, 1989.

136. Ouriel K, Ricotta JJ, Adams JT, et al: Management of cholelithiasis in patients with abdominal aortic aneurysm. *Ann Surg* 198:717–719, 1983.

137. Hermreck AS, Proberts KS, Thomas JH: Severe jaundice after rupture of abdominal aortic aneurysm. *Am J Surg* 134:745–748, 1977.

138. Ernst CB, Campbell HC Jr, Daugherty ME, et al: Incidence and significance of intra-operative bacterial cultures during abdominal aortic aneurysmectomy. *Ann Surg* 185:626–633, 1977.

139. Fisher DF, Yawn DH, Crawford ES: Preoperative disseminated intravascular coagulation associated with aortic aneurysms. *Arch Surg* 118:1252–1255, 1983.

140. Goldman L, Caldera DC, Southwick FS, et al: Cardiac risk factors and complications in noncardiac surgery. *Medicine (Baltimore)* 57:357–370, 1978.

141. Snow JC, Sensel S: A review of cataract extraction under local and general anesthesia at the Massachusetts eye and ear infirmary. *Anesth Analg* 45:742–747, 1966.

142. Duncalf D, Gartner S, Carol B: Mortality in association with ophthalmic surgery. *Amer J Ophthalmol* 69:610–615, 1970.

143. Lynch S, Wolf GL, Berlin I: General anesthesia for cataract surgery: A comparative review of 2217 consecutive cases. *Anesth Analg* 53:909–913, 1974.

144. Petruscak J, Smith RB, Breslin P: Mortality related to ophthalmological surgery. *Arch Ophthalmol* 89:106–109, 1973.

145. Jedeikin RJ, Hoffman S: The oculocardiac reflex in eye surgery anesthesia. *Anesth Analg* 56:333–334, 1977.

146. Rongey KA, Weisman H: Hypotension following intraocular acetylcholine. *Anesthesiology* 36:412, 1972.

147. Solosko D, Smith RB: Hypertension following 10 per cent phenylephrine ophthalmic. *Anesthesiology* 36:187–189, 1972.
148. McReynolds WU, Havener WH, Henderson JW: Hazards of the use of sympathomimetic drugs in ophthalmology. *Arch Ophthalmol* 56:176–179, 1956.
149. Adler AG: Perioperative management of the ophthalmology patient. *Med Clin North Am* 71:561–567, 1987.
150. Adler AG, McElwain GE, Merli GJ, et al: Systemic effects of eye drops. *Arch Intern Med* 142:2293–2294, 1982.
151. Merli GJ, Weitz H, Martin JH, et al: Cardiac dysrhythmias associated with ophthalmic atropine. *Arch Intern Med* 146:45–47, 1986.
152. Adler AG, McElwain, Martin JH: Coronary artery spasm induced by phenylephrine eyedrops. *Arch Intern Med* 141:1384–1385, 1981.
153. Heath P, Geiter CW: Use of phenylephrine hydrochloride in ophthalmology. *Arch Ophthal* 41:172–177, 1949.
154. Alexander S, McAlpine FS: Cholecystectomy in the cardiac patient. *Med Clin North Am* 50:495–500, 1966.
155. Mendelsohn D Jr, Monheit R: Electrocardiographic and blood-pressure changes during and after biliary-tract surgery. *N Engl J Med* 254:307–313, 1956.
156. Tarhan S, Moffitt EA, Sessler AD, et al: Risk of anesthesia and surgery in patients with chronic bronchitis and chronic obstructive pulmonary disease. *Surgery* 74:720–726, 1973.
157. Consensus Conference: Anesthesia and sedation in the dental office. *JAMA* 254:1073–1076, 1985.
158. Coplans MP, Carson, I: Deaths associated with dentistry. *Brit Dent J* 153:357–362, 1982.
159. Cardiac irregularities during dental anaesthesia. *Lancet* 1:754, 1966.
160. Bourne JG: Deaths with dental anaesthetics. *Anaesthesia* 25:473–481, 1970.
161. Brierley JB, Miller AA: Fatal brain damage after dental anaesthesia. Its nature, etiology, and prevention. *Lancet* 2:869–873, 1966.
162. Chamberlain FL: Management of medical-dental problems in patients with cardiovascular diseases. *Mod Concepts Cardiovasc Dis* 30:697–700, 1961.
163. Cheraskin E, Prasertsuntarasai T: Use of epinephrine with local anesthesia in hypertensive patients. III. Effect of epinephrine on blood pressure and pulse rate. *JADA* 57:507–519, 1958.
164. Salman, I, Schwartz SP: Effects of vasoconstrictors used in local anesthetics in patients with diseases of the heart. *J Oral Surg* 13:209–213, 1955.
165. Cheraskin E, Prasertsuntarasai T: Use of epinephrine with local anesthesia in hypertensive patients. IV. Effect of tooth extraction on blood pressure and pulse rate. *JADA* 58:61–68, 1959.
166. McCarthy FM: A clinical study of blood pressure responses to epinephrine-containing local anesthetic solutions. *J Dental Res* 36:132–141, 1957.
167. Forbes AM: Halothane, adrenaline and cardiac arrest. *Anaesthesia* 21:22–27, 1966.
168. Tolas AG, Allen GD, Ward RJ: Comparison of effects of methods of induction of anesthesia on cardiac rhythm. *J Oral Surg* 25:54–59, 1967.
169. Williams RM, Keyes M, Becker DJ, et al: Electrocardiographic changes during oral surgical procedures under local anesthesia. *Oral Surg Oral Med Oral Pathol* 16:1270–1275, 1963.
170. Ryder W: Hazards during anesthesia or sedation for dental procedures. *Proc R Soc Med* 64:82–83, 1971.
171. Rafel SS: Electrocardiographic changes during outpatient oral surgery. *J Oral Surg* 30:898–899, 1972.
172. Christenson GR, Hebert CL, Driscoll EJ: Intravenous barbiturate anesthesia for dental outpatients. *Anesth Analg* 40:77–86, 1961.
173. Ryder W: The electrocardiogram in dental anaesthesia. *Anaesthesia* 25:46–62, 1970.
174. Fisch C, Ochler RC, Miller JR: Cardiac arrhythmias during oral surgery with halothane-nitrous-oxide-oxygen anesthesia. *JAMA* 208:1839–1842, 1969.
175. Ostroff LH, Goldstein BH, Pennock RS: Cardiac dysrhythmias during outpatient general anesthesia—a comparison study. *J Oral Surg* 35:793–797, 1977.
176. Driscoll EJ, Christenson GR, White CL: Physiologic studies in general anesthesia for ambulatory dental patients. *Oral Surg Oral Med Oral Pathol* 12:1496–1514, 1959.
177. Alexander JP: Dysrhythmia and oral surgery. *Br J Anaesth* 43:773–777, 1971.
178. Kaufman L: Unforeseen complications encountered during dental anaesthesia. *Proc R Soc Med* 59:731–734, 1966.
179. Miller JR, Redish CH, Fisch C: Factors in arrhythmia during dental outpatient general anesthesia. *Anesth Analg* 49:701–706, 1970.
180. Hanna MH, Heap, DG, Kimberlyey, PS: Cardiac dysrhythmia associated with general anaesthesia for oral surgery. *Anaesthesia* 38:1192–1194, 1983.
181. Cintron A, Medina R, Reyes AA,: Cardiovascular effects and safety of dental anesthesia and dental interventions in patients with recent uncomplicated myocardial infarction. *Arch Intern Med* 146:2203–2204, 1986.
182. Askey JM, Cherry CB: Dental extraction during dicumarol therapy. *California Med* 84:16–17, 1956.
183. Frank BW, Dichhaus DW, Claus EV: Dental extractions in the presence of continual anticoagulant therapy. *Ann Intern Med* 59:911–913, 1963.
184. Ziffer AM, Scopp IA, Beck J: Profound bleeding after dental extractions during dicumarol therapy. *N Engl J Med* 256:351–354, 1957.
185. Behrman SJ: Dental surgery during continuous anticoagulant therapy. *J Am Dent Assoc* 62:172–180, 1961.
186. Shira RB, Hall RJ, Guernsey LH: Minor oral surgery during prolonged anticoagulant therapy. *J Oral Surg Anesth Hosp D Serv* 20:93–99, 1962.

187. Behrman SJ, Wright IS: Dental surgery during continuous anticoagulant therapy. *JAMA* 175:483–488, 1961.
188. Scopp IW, Fredrics H: Dental extractions in patients undergoing anticoagulant therapy. *Oral Surg Oral Med Oral Pathol* 11:470–474, 1958.
189. Chow AW, Roser SM, Brady FA,: Orofacial odontogenic infections. *Ann Intern Med* 88:392–402, 1978.
190. Burke JF: Burns, in Mandell GL, Douglas RG, Bennett JE (eds): *Principles of Infectious Diseases*. New York, John Wiley, 1979.
191. Pruitt BA Jr: Other complications of burn injury in Artz CP, Moncrief JA, Pruitt BA (eds): *Burns: A Team Approach*. Philadelphia, WB Saunders, 1979, pp 523–552.
192. Sevitt S: A review of the complications of burns, their origin and importance for illness and death. *J Trauma* 19:358–369, 1979.
193. Aikawa N, Martyn JAJ, Burke JF: Pulmonary artery catheterization in thermodilution cardiac output determination in the management of critically burned patients. *Am J Surg* 135:811–817, 1978.
194. Czaja AJ, McAlhany JC, Pruitt BA Jr.: Acute gastroduodenal disease after thermal injury. An endoscopic evaluation of incidence and natural history. *N Engl J Med* 291:925–929, 1974.
195. McAlhany JC, Czaja AJ, Pruitt BA Jr: Antacid control of complications from acute gastroduodenal disease after burns. *J Trauma* 16:645–657, 1976.
196. McElwee HP, Sirinek KR, Levine BA: Cimetidine affords protection equal to antacids in prevention of stress ulceration following thermal injury. *Surgery* 86:620–624, 1979.
197. Czaja AJ, McAlhany JC, Pruitt BA Jr: Acute duodenitis and duodental ulceration after burns. Clinical and pathological characteristics. *JAMA* 232:621–624, 1975.
198. Markley K: Burn care: Infection and smoke inhalation. *Ann Intern Med* 90:269–270, 1979.
199. DiVincenti FC Pruitt BA Jr, Reckler JM: Inhalation injuries. *J Trauma* 11:109–117, 1971.
200. Bartlett RH, Nicole M, Travis MJ: Acute management of the upper airway in facial burns and smoke inhalation. *Arch Surg* 111:744–749, 1976.
201. Zikria BA, Weston CC, Chodoff M: Smoke and carbon monoxide poisoning in fire victims. *J Trauma* 12:641–645, 1972.
202. Petroff PA, Mander EW, Clayton WH: Pulmonary function studies after smoke inhalation. *Am J Surg* 132:346–351, 1976.
203. Zawacki BE, Jung RC, Joyce J: Smoke, burns, and the natural history of inhalation injury in fire victims: A correlation of experimental and clinical data. *Ann Surg* 185:100–110, 1977.
204. Mellins RB, Park S: Respiratory complications of smoke inhalation in victims of fires. *J Pediatr* 87:1–7, 1975.
205. Pruitt BA Jr, Erickson DR, Morris A: Progressive pulmonary insufficiency and other pulmonary complications of thermal injury. *J Trauma* 15:369–379, 1975.
206. Schall GL, McDonald HD, Carr LB: Xenon ventilation-perfusion lung scans. The early diagnosis of inhalation injury. *JAMA* 240:2441–2445, 1978.
207. Moylan JA: Smoke inhalation and burn injury. *Surg Clin North Am* 60:1533–1540, 1980.
208. Apfelberg DB, Masters FW, Robinson DW: Pathophysiology and treatment of lightning injuries. *J Trauma* 14:453–460, 1974.
209. Burda CD: Electrocardiographic changes in lightning stroke. *Am Heart J* 72:521–524, 1966.
210. Rouse RG, Dimick AR: The treatment of electrical injury compared to burn injury: A review of pathophysiology and comparison of patient management protocols. *J Trauma* 18:43–46, 1978.
211. Ford JH Jr, RC Dudan, JS Bennett: Parenteral hyperalimentation in gynecologic oncology patients. *Gynecol Oncol* 1:70–75, 1972.
212. Rutledge FN, JP Smith, JT Wharton: Pelvic exenteration: Analysis of 296 patients. *Am J Obstet Gynecol* 129(8):881–892, 1977.
213. Curry LC, Nahhas WA, AE Jahshan: Pelvic exenteration: A 7-year experience. *Gynecol Oncol* 11:119–123, 1981.
213A. Shepherd JH, Chamber MG: Complications of gynecological cancer surgery: a review. *J Royal Soc Med* 79:289–293, 1986.
214. McGuirt WF, Loery S, McCabe BJ: The risks of major head and neck surgery in the aged population. *Laryngoscope* 87:1378–1382, 1977.
215. Camnitz PS, Biggers WP, Fischer ND: Avoidance of early complications following radical neck dissection. *Laryngoscope* 89:1553–1562, 1979.
216. Becker GD, CJ Parell: Cefazolin prophylaxis in head and neck cancer surgery. *Ann Otol Rhinol Laryngol* 88:183–186, 1979.
217. Dornfeld L, Kelin LA. (eds): Symposium on medical aspects of genitourinary surgery. *Urol Clin North Am* 3:197–449, 1976.
218. Erlik D, Valero A, Birkhan J: Prostatic surgery and the cardiovascular patient. *Br J Urol* 40:53–61, 1968.
219. Thompson GJ, Kelalis PP, Connolly DC: Transurethral prostatic resection after myocardial infarction. *JAMA* 182:908, 1962.
220. Crawford ED, Dumbadge I, Ratledge HW: Deep venous thrombosis following transurethral resection of the prostate: Diagnosis by phleborheography. *J Urol* 120:438–441, 1978.
221. Allen NH, Jenkins JD, Smart CJ: Surgical haemorrhage in patients given subcutaneous heparin as prophylaxis against thromboembolism. *Br Med J* 1:1326, 1978.
222. An international multicentre trial prevention of fatal postoperative pulmonary embolism by low doses of heparin. *Lancet* 2:45–51, 1975.
223. Coe NP, Collins REC, Klein LA: Prevention of deep vein thrombosis in urological patients: A controlled, randomized trial of low-dose heparin and external pneumatic compression boots. *Surgery* 83:230–234, 1978.
224. Kakkar VV, Spindler J, Flute PT: Efficacy of low doses of heparin in prevention of deep-vein

thrombosis after major surgery—a double-blind, randomized trial. *Lancet* 2:101–106, 1972.

225. Nicolides AN, Field ES, Kakkar VV: Prostatectomy and deep-vein thrombosis. *Br J Surg* 59:487–488, 1972.

226. Williams HT: Prevention of postoperative deep-vein thrombosis with perioperative subcutaneous heparin. *Lancet* 2:950–952, 1971.

227. Nicolaides AN, Desai S, Douglas JN: Small doses of subcutaneous sodium heparin in preventing deep venous thrombosis after major surgery. *Lancet* 2:890–893, 1972.

228. Becker J, Bergström S, Saltzman GP: Occurrence and course of thrombosis following prostatectomy—a phlebographic investigation. *Acta Radiol Diagn* 10:513–533, 1970 (New Series).

229. Rosenberg IL, Evans M, Pollock AV: Prophylaxis of postoperative leg vein thrombosis by low dose subcutaneous heparin or peroperative calf muscle stimulation: A controlled clinical trial. *Br Med J* 1:649–651, 1975.

230. Mayo ME, Halil T, Browse NL: The incidence of deep vein thrombosis after prostatectomy. *Br J Urol* 43:738–742, 1971.

231. VanArsdalen KN, Barnes RW, Clark G: Deep vein thrombosis and prostatectomy. *Urology* 21:461–463, 1983.

232. Murphy DM, Flakiner FR, Carr M: Septicemia after transurethral prostatectomy. *Urology* 22:133–135, 1983.

233. Wan RL, Irvine AH, Jendale ST: Nonoliguric renal failure after transurethral prostatic resection. *Urology* 8:114–117, 1976.

234. Moisey CU, Rees RWM: Results of transurethral resection of prostate in patients with cerebrovascular disease. *Br J Urol* 50:539–541, 1978.

235. Henderson DJ, Middleton RG: Coma from hyponatremia following transurethral resection of prostate. *Urology* 15:267–271, 1980.

236. Sunderrajan S, Bauer JH, Vopat RL: Postransurethral prostatic resection hyponatremic syndrome. *Amer J Kid Dis* 4:80–84, 1984.

237. Campbell HT, Fincher ME, Sklar AH: Severe hyponatremia without severe hypoosmolality following transurethral resection of the prostate (TURP) in end-stage renal disease. *Amer J Kid Dis* 12:152–155, 1988.

238. Clayman RV, Ortlip SA, Eckfeldt JH: Diagnostic specificity of creatine kinase isoenzymes after transurethral operations. *J Urol* 130:279–282, 1983.

239. Antila LE, Markkula, Iisalo H: Ten years' experience of geriatric aspects in surgery of patients with benign prostatic hyperplasia. *Acta Chir Scand Suppl* 357:95–96, 1966.

240. Cintron G, Medina R, Reyes AA: Cardiovascular effects and safety of dental anesthesia and dental interventions in patients with recent uncomplicated myocardial infarction. *Arch Intern Med* 146:2203–2204, 1986.

241. Sheldon CA: Perioperative care of the urologic patient. *Urol Clin North Am* 10:1–199, 1983.

242. Everitt DE, Avorn J: Systemic effects of medications used to treat glaucoma. *Ann Intern Med* 112:120–125, 1990.

22

Medical Illness During Pregnancy

William S. Kammerer

The intensive growth phase of high-risk obstetrics continues. Both internists and obstetricians show an increasing interest in collaborating in the care of pregnant patients with active medical problems as part of a high-risk team.

Our purpose is not to review every medical problem that can occur in pregnancy but, rather, to highlight new information and management techniques of common maternal medical problems pertinent to the internist involved in high-risk obstetrics.

DIABETES MELLITUS

Strict physiologic control of maternal blood sugar, along with improved methods for determining fetal distress before and at term, have revolutionized expectations in diabetic pregnancies. A decrease in fetal loss and in perinatal morbidity and mortality from a rate of 25–75% (Table 22.1) to <4–5% (Table 22.2)

has been demonstrated in juvenile-onset diabetics. **It has become clear that the more physiologic the control, the better the perinatal outcome.** These observations have encouraged obstetricians to use aggressive measures to maintain the mean maternal blood sugar below 100 mg/100 ml throughout pregnancy. The development of simple, accurate, and portable outpatient methods (Glucochek, Glucometer II, Chemstrips bG, etc.) with which to measure blood sugar has made it possible to achieve this goal in essentially any setting.

In general, as pregnancy advances, the need for dietary modifications and for multiple meal-related injections of short- and intermediate-acting insulins become mandatory in order to achieve this degree of control (Fig. 22.1). While the risks of hypoglycemic episodes would appear to be slightly increased, they are usually mild and easily recognized and controlled. In addition, brief maternal hypoglycemia does

Table 22.1. Diabetes in Pregnancy: Correlations with Outcome[a]

Class	Onset	Duration	Complication	Fetal Loss (%)[b]
A	Pregnancy	Gestation		4.4
B	Over 19 years of age	Less than 10 years		6.8
C	10–19 years of age	10–19 years		23
D	Under 10 years of age	More than 20 years	Calcified leg vessels, retinopathy	23
E	Under 10 years of age	More than 20 years	Pelvic vascular calcification	75
F	Under 10 years of age	More than 20 years	Renovascular disease, albuminuria	75
H	Usually <10 years	Usually >20 years	Arteriosclerotic cardiovascular disease	95
R	Under 10 years of age	More than 20 years	Retinitis proliferans	?

[a] Adapted from Pedersen J, et al: *Diabetes* 23:302–305, 1974. Used with permission.
[b] Without strict physiologic control of blood sugar and with delivery between 36th and 38th weeks of gestation.

Table 22.2.   Fetal Loss in Diabetic Pregnancy: Correlation with Blood Sugar Control[a]

Mean Blood Sugar	Fetal Loss (%)
Less than 100 mg/100 ml	4
100–150 mg/100 ml	16
More than 150 mg/100 ml	24
(Nondiabetic)	(2–4)

[a] After Karlson K, et al: *Am J Obstet Gynecol* 112:213–220, 1972. Used with permission.

not substantially increase the risk for abnormalities in fetal development or well-being, and is much less of a risk to the fetus than intermittent hyperglycemia or ketoacidosis.

It should be stressed that **efforts to control maternal blood sugar should not be relaxed during labor and delivery.** The practice of giving only a fraction of the usual daily dose of insulin at the onset of labor increases the risk of ketoacidosis, which is associated with an increased incidence of the fetal respiratory distress syndrome. More accurate control can be obtained with constant infusion, low-dose (1–2 units per hour) regular insulin intravenously with hourly blood sugar determinations done in the labor and delivery suite.

Ketoacidosis occurring during pregnancy ($HCO_3 < 10–17$ meq/L) is associated with alarmingly high rates of fetal loss (30–50%) and with congenital abnormalities of the central nervous system and impaired intellectual function in surviving fetuses. As with all diabetics, but especially during pregnancy when severe ketoacidosis can develop within 8–12 hours, constant vigil and effort should be practiced to avoid this complication.

Blood sugars should be monitored regularly, as many of the symptoms of ketoacidosis during pregnancy mimic those of normal pregnancy. In addition, other poor prognostic signs of pregnancy (preeclampsia and pyelonephritis) should be sought for and controlled. While the course of diabetic vascular complications affecting the eye and kidney is unpredictable during pregnancy, rarely do they actually improve. Even with optimal control of blood sugar, renal function and vision may deteriorate to the point where therapeutic abortion must be considered (5).

While the obstetrician will usually assume the major responsibility for the care of the pregnant diabetic, the internist can also have a major impact on the outcome. Despite achieving optimal blood sugar control in the latter two-thirds of gesta-

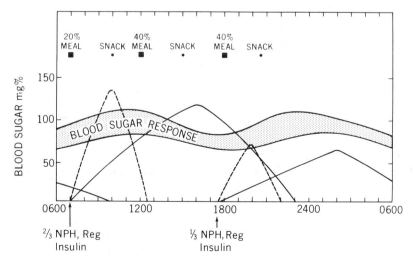

Figure 22.1. Split-dose intermediate- (NPH, Lente, Monotard) and rapid-acting (regular, Semilente, Actrapid) insulins for the control of blood sugar during pregnancy.

tion, the incidence of congenital abnormalities in diabetic pregnancies has not consistently decreased. **Congenital abnormalities remain 3–5 times more frequent in diabetics** than in nondiabetics (12% vs. 3%, respectively), and lethal congenital abnormalities are seven times more common (2.3% vs. 0.3%). This may be explained by the fact that most antenatal care does not begin until 8–10 weeks after conception. During this critical period of fetal development, diabetic control is often being maintained at traditional prepregnancy levels. The internist may be the individual best placed, then, to improve on this situation. With appropriate control for 2–3 months or more prior to conception and during the first trimester, an optimum environment for pregnancy might be provided, with a concomitant decrease in congenital abnormalities. Miller et al. (6) found that HbA_{1c} levels below 7–8.5% in the first trimester were associated with a significant decrease in major congenital abnormalities (0–5% vs. 23%). In the poorly controlled diabetic, proteins critical for early fetal development may become glycosylated (as with Hb → HbA_{1c}) and be unable to function properly (7–9).

In addition, the sensitive and challenging task of family counseling often falls to the internist. While with modern methods of care, maternal mortality due to diabetes mellitus during pregnancy should approach zero, long-term maternal complications must be addressed. Fifty percent of juvenile-onset diabetics not treated with laser beam therapy will be legally blind (visual acuity less than 20/200) by 20 years from the date of onset. Similarly, in juvenile diabetics who develop diabetic nephropathy, the average duration until the onset of severe renal failure and death is 17–22 years. Overall, the average survival for the pregnant juvenile-onset diabetic is reported to be 8 years for those with vascular disease and 20–30 years for those without. The internist must carefully weigh these long-term risks and realities against what it will mean to the young diabetic to have a child.

HEART DISEASE IN PREGNANCY

Epidemiology

Until recently, cardiac disease has been reported in 2–4% of all pregnancies, with the great majority (75–90%) being rheumatic valvular disease, especially mitral stenosis (over 75% of the total). In the past 25 years, the prevalence of rheumatic heart disease in the U.S. has steadily decreased. Fewer patients with significant acquired cardiac disease are being seen now during pregnancy, and of these, rheumatic valvular disease is no longer quite as common. Of the congenital cardiac disorders, ventricular septal defect, atrial septal defect, pulmonary stenosis, patent ductus arteriosus, and coarctation of the aorta account for 75% or more of the total.

Pathophysiology

The physiologic changes of pregnancy result in a substantial increase in cardiac work. This is most notable in patients with pulmonary hypertension and cyanotic heart disease. Oxygen consumption increases 15–20%, reflecting the hypermetabolic state of pregnancy; blood, plasma, and total body water volumes increase by some 20–30%; and the pulse rate increases by an average of 10–12 per minute. In addition, the effect of adding 20–30 pounds of weight must be considered. Cardiac output increases steadily from the 12th week to a peak of 30–50% over baseline by the 24th week.

In general, the increased cardiac work caused by these various changes become maximal between the 27–32nd week of pregnancy, giving rise to the **clinical maxim that if heart failure develops before the 24th week of pregnancy, medical management will be unsuccessful, and conversely, heart failure developing after the 32nd week will**

respond to medical management and that the stress of normal labor and vaginal delivery can be tolerated. During labor and delivery, a sudden increase in cardiac output related to pain, anxiety, and uterine contractions should be anticipated. Adequate pain relief (conduction anesthesia without epinephrine) and positioning the mother on her side can help maintain cardiovascular stability during labor.

Rheumatic Valvular Heart Disease

Pregnancy is generally well tolerated in women with mitral stenosis accurately classified according to the New York Heart Association (Table 22.3) as Class I or II and without significant pulmonary hypertension. **However, acute pulmonary edema may occur even in Class I or II patients,** most often in association with the development of atrial fibrillation. In addition to arrhythmias and the physiologic changes of pregnancy, other factors, such as pulmonary emboli, infective endocarditis, recurrent rheumatic carditis, and other associated valve lesions must also be considered when a patient with previously stable Class I or II mitral stenosis develops heart failure.

The incidence of both maternal and fetal morbidity becomes substantial in New York Heart Association Class III and IV patients and makes surgical repair during pregnancy an important consideration (Table 22.4). This is especially so for women who develop refractory congestive heart failure or pulmonary edema early in pregnancy, whatever the prepregnancy

Table 22.3. New York Heart Association Classification of Heart Disease

Functional Class	Therapeutic
I. No symptoms on normal exertion.	A. No restriction
II. + symptoms on normal exertion	B. No competitive exercise
III. + + symptoms on normal exertion. VC[a] 30% below normal	C. Slight restriction
IV. Symptoms at rest. VC 35–50% below normal.	E. Complete bed rest

[a]VC, vital capacity.

New York Heart Association classification. With current surgical techniques and postoperative care, necessary surgical correction of rheumatic mitral stenosis, especially with closed valvotomy, can offer both the mother and the fetus a better chance for survival than medical therapy alone.

Patients with rheumatic valvular disease should be maintained on antibiotic prophylaxis against recurrent acute rheumatic fever and rheumatic carditis throughout pregnancy. In addition, they should receive penicillin and streptomycin prophylactically for any invasive procedures (see SBE prophylaxis below).

Congenital Heart Disease

The reported experience with congenital heart defects during pregnancy is less extensive than with rheumatic valvular heart disease. Patients with atrial or ventricular septal defects or patent ductus

Table 22.4. Maternal and Fetal Mortality Rates for Patients with Rheumatic Mitral Stenosis

| | Normal Pregnancy | Medical Therapy Alone | | | Mitral Valvotomy and Valvuloplasty | Mitral Valve Replacement |
		NYHA Class I and II	Class III	Class IV		
Maternal mortality (%)	0.03	0.05	4–6	25–40	2–10	5
Fetal mortality (%)	2–4	4–6	30	50	5–25	30–40

arteriosus without significant pulmonary hypertension can generally tolerate pregnancy and vaginal delivery without undue difficulty. As in patients with acquired heart disease, the development of congestive heart failure before the 24th week of gestation bodes ill for successful medical management. If surgery is required for these defects during pregnancy, both maternal and fetal mortality have been well within those reported with closed mitral valvotomies for rheumatic mitral stenosis (Table 22.4). However, with prolonged extracorporeal circulation, hypothermia and difficulties in maintaining maternal pressure above 80 mm Hg may lead to decreased uteroplacental blood flow, placing the fetus at very high risk.

Women with right-to-left shunts and hypoxia (such as tetralogy of Fallot and Eisenmenger's syndrome), and with primary pulmonary hypertension, **especially those with hematocrits greater than 60%,** tolerate pregnancy extremely poorly, with spontaneous abortions in the first trimester occurring almost 100% of the time. Those with lesser degrees of cyanosis with hematocrits between 45–55% tolerate pregnancy somewhat better (approximately 50–60% fetal loss). Women with obstructive lesions (such as aortic stenosis, pulmonary stenosis, coarctation of the aorta, and idiopathic hypertrophic subaortic stenosis) are somewhat more likely to tolerate a full-term pregnancy, with a fetal loss between 25–50%. At delivery, excessive, rapid blood loss can quickly precipitate shock and must be avoided.

In general, children born to women with congenital heart disease are frequently found to be dysmature and small for age and have an incidence of associated congenital abnormalities of 20% overall, and of 3–10% of congenital heart defects.

Women with well-functioning prosthetic valve replacements and good left ventricular function before conception and who are closely followed from the time of conception will usually tolerate pregnancy without serious difficulty as far as cardiac symptoms are concerned. However, difficulties with anticoagulant control during pregnancy, labor and delivery, and in the postpartum period lead to frequent, serious peripheral embolic complications (12).

A high rate of fetal loss (up to 33%) has been reported in these patients. This may be related, in part, to the use of warfarin anticoagulants with their associated problems of fetal hemorrhage and embryopathy. With the more frequent use of porcine valves or the use of heparin throughout pregnancy, this high rate of fetal loss may decrease.

Congenital mitral valve prolapse has been reported in up to 6% of the general population. Some have associated it with an increased incidence of malignant arrhythmias and embolic strokes in patients younger than 40 years old. Rayburn and Fontana's (20) recent report of 42 pregnancies in 25 patients with mitral valve prolapse constitutes the only systematic study of this condition during pregnancy to date. As intravascular volume increases during pregnancy, the click and murmur associated with congenital mitral valve prolapse decreased in intensity. They found no associated pathology in their patients. Compared with controls, there was no increase in maternal or fetal complications. There would appear to be no need to use antiarrhythmics or anticoagulants, nor concern regarding the development of congestive heart failure during normal pregnancy and vaginal delivery. While definitive data are lacking, there is no apparent increased risk for SBE developing during normal vaginal delivery, and we do not recommend prophylactic antibiotics under these circumstances.

Peripartum Cardiomyopathy

A peculiar form of heart failure may occur in the last 2 weeks of gestation or within 2–5 months of delivery. It is most often found in women age 30 or above and with two or more previous pregnancies. The etiology is unknown, with most authors speculating on a hypersensitivity reaction to the products of conception or diffuse coronary artery spasm. Generally, peripartum cardiomyopathy is a diagnosis of exclusion, to be differentiated from heart failure associated with toxemia, nephritis, nutritional or infectious cardiomyopathies, or idiopathic hypertrophic subaortic stenosis. Pathologically, the condition is characterized by cardiac dilatation and hypertrophy with extensive mural thrombi, and by diffuse subendocardial fibrosis and degeneration. Clinically, patients develop the rapid onset of congestive heart failure with persistent tachycardia and supraventricular arrhythmias, and frequent arterial embolization. In 50% of patients, heart size returns to normal within 6–12 months of delivery. Symptomatic improvement with prolonged bed rest, diuretics, and digitalis is the rule in this group. Mortality in this group approximates 14%. In the other half, cardiomegaly and failure persist and are resistant to all therapy. Mortality is reported to be 85% within 5 years. Subsequent pregnancies will almost always be associated with recurrence and worsening of heart failure in the latter group, while in the former, recurrences are less predictable. **Because emboli are so common in both groups, all of these patients should be anticoagulated** (21).

Marfan's Syndrome

Marfan's syndrome is inherited as an autosomal dominant trait with a high degree of penetrance. Pregnancy greatly increases the risk of aortic aneurysm and dissection, especially in the third trimester. All women with this syndrome should receive effective contraceptive treatment. If pregnant, therapeutic abortion should be seriously considered. If the pregnancy has progressed to term with no evidence of cardiac or aortic disease, vaginal delivery is not thought to impose an undue stress and should be allowed, with cesarean section reserved for obstetrical indications.

Cardiac Arrhythmias

An increased frequency of paroxysmal atrial tachycardia (PAT) has been reported in pregnancy, especially in the third trimester and during labor. Those with PAT before conception usually experience an increase in frequency, duration, and severity of attacks. When cardiac function is otherwise normal, these constitute no real increase in maternal or fetal risk with appropriate therapy. For those with underlying heart disease (rheumatic heart disease, coronary, or hypertensive heart disease), the increase in rate may quickly precipitate congestive heart failure. In these patients, prompt control is required. There are no contraindications to digitalis and quinidine during pregnancy (24). Similarly, electrical cardioversion has been safely performed on multiple occasions during pregnancy (25, 26) and verapamil has also been effectively employed with apparent safety for the fetus (27).

Atrial fibrillation and flutter occur only rarely during pregnancy in patients with normal hearts and are seen primarily in patients with advanced rheumatic heart disease. Hyperthyroid patients are an obvious exception to this generalization. When associated with rheumatic heart disease, both maternal and fetal risks are greatly increased, especially for congestive heart failure and as related to complications of anticoagulation.

Premature ventricular contractions, while possibly of increased incidence in pregnancy, are of no risk to patients with otherwise normal hearts. Avoidance of caffeine, nicotine, and alcohol may decrease the frequency. Propranolol can be considered for symptomatic patients, but depressed respiration, bradycardia, and hypoglycemia may occur in the newborns of patients taking this medication.

Complete Heart Block

In current practice, most women with complete heart block already have permanent pacemakers implanted at the time of conception. For those who do not, the majority with congenital complete heart block tolerate pregnancy and labor and delivery surprisingly well. Nor is there any increase in fetal wastage. The development of congestive heart failure or Stokes-Adams attacks, however, would necessitate the prompt insertion of a permanent pacemaker.

Whether the pacer rate should be increased 5–10 beats per minute during pregnancy has not been studied, but could be considered for those with early signs and symptoms of congestive heart failure.

SBE Prophylaxis at Delivery

While the documented incidence of significant bacteremia associated with normal vaginal delivery is less than 1% (Table 22.5), SBE prophylaxis remains common practice in the USA for patients with valvular heart disease. Several obstetrical factors which increase the likelihood of SBE have been identified (Table 22.6) and prophylaxis in these situations should be undertaken. In addition, pa-

Table 22.6. Obstetrical Risk Factors in Subacute Bacterial Endocarditis (SBE)

Documented
  Manual removal of placenta
  Prolonged (? > 12 hr) rupture of membranes
  Abortion, induced
  Cesarean section
Possible
  Forceps
  Amniocentesis

tients with prosthetic valves and those with prior episodes of SBE (as well as patients with ventricular-atrial shunts for hydrocephalus) are felt to be at very high risk and should be given prophylaxis even with normal vaginal deliveries. Given the very low incidence of significant bacteremia with normal vaginal deliveries, SBE prophylaxis for patients at low risk (IHSS, mitral valve prolapse, permanent pacemakers) is not recommended. From the data available, it would not appear that patients with rheumatic or congenital valvular disease routinely need SBE prophylaxis for normal vaginal delivery.

HYPERTENSION AND PREGNANCY

While it is primarily the obstetrician who detects and manages hypertension

Table 22.5. Incidence of Puerperal Bacteremia in 1121 Patients[a]

			Blood Cultures			
Authors	Year	No. of Patients	Total No.	Time	Percent Positive	Organisms Isolated
Burwell and Metcalfe	1948	17	74	Not stated	0	
Readleaf and Fadell	1959	101	202	At delivery; within 24 hr	7.2	Micrococcus and haemolytic streptococcus
Baker et al.	1966	396	1779	At delivery; 12, 24, 48 hr	0.39	E. coli, Aerobacter pseudomonas
Baker and Hubbell	1967	519	2583	Delivery of placenta; 15 min, 30 min, 12 hr, 24 hr	0.77	E. coli, S. viridans, bacteroides, pseudomonas
Sugrue et al.	1979	83	299	Within 30 min of delivery	0.1	Anaerobic gram-negative bacilli, mixed growth

[a]From Sugrue, et al. (29).

during pregnancy, the internist will often be consulted for assistance in the management of maternal complications. In addition, the remote prognosis for the mother needs to be understood in order to arrange appropriate long-term follow-up. The internist, therefore, needs to be familiar with current concepts of etiology, risks, and management of toxemia of pregnancy (pregnancy-induced hypertension).

While defined as the presentation of hypertension (greater than 140/90 mm Hg), proteinuria (greater than 250 mg/L), and edema after the second trimester, these women may not always have true preeclampsia. Only 4% of over 4000 patients referred by obstetricians for evaluation of toxemia in Finnerty's (30) experience were eventually diagnosed as true preeclamptics. The great majority of these patients were found to have preexisting hypertension, glomerulonephritis, pyelonephritis, or asymptomatic bacteriuria. Medical risk factors for the development of toxemia include diabetes mellitus, chronic hypertension, labile hypertension in early pregnancy, previous severe preeclampsia or frank eclampsia, and obesity.

While the exact etiology of toxemia remains to be determined, it is characterized pathophysiologically by arteriolar spasm and decreased intravascular volume. Finnerty emphasizes the importance of finding retinal arteriolar spasm and generalized retinal edema in differentiating patients with true toxemia from those with preexisting hypertension. Preexisting hypertension, however, is associated with an increase in the incidence and severity of toxemia, with a resultant increase in both maternal and fetal morbidity and mortality. While treatment of preexisting hypertension does not necessarily decrease the incidence of preeclampsia, it will decrease both maternal and fetal complications. While there is no place for the use of thiazides in the treatment of the usual edema of pregnancy,

their addition to the treatment of preexisting hypertension unresponsive to methyldopa or hydralazine may be appropriate. In true preeclampsia, on the other hand, thiazides are not used in that they will further decrease intravascular volume and uteroplacental blood flow. Methyldopa and hydralazine, because they do not significantly decrease blood flow to the placenta, are currently the drugs most commonly employed by obstetricians. Under experimental conditions, methyldopa has been reported to slightly decrease uterine-placental blood flow, while hydralazine increases it. Neither has been associated with an increase in fetal anomalies, and there is some evidence to suggest that treatment of hypertension with Aldomet may improve overall fetal mortality and morbidity. Propranolol and atenolol would appear to be safe for use throughout pregnancy and probably also decrease the incidence of fetal wastage in patients with chronic hypertension (32–34).

For patients in hypertensive crisis (blood pressure greater than 180/120), intravenous hydralazine every 2–4 hours or by constant infusion is the usual drug of first choice. Both diazoxide and nitroprusside have been used to successfully control maternal blood pressure, but have not improved the high frequency of fetal loss (33–50%) in this condition (35).

Even among obstetricians sensitive to the many potential manifestations of eclampsia, **consultations to internists occur for complications of unrecognized toxemia.** Goodlin (36) reports 28 such incidents, including three referred for retinal abnormalities or visual complaints, six for renal abnormalities, four for hepatitis or cholelithiasis, one each for upper GI bleeding, pancreatitis, and appendicitis, seven for epilepsy or brain tumor, two for heart failure, and three with thrombocytopenia for idiopathic thrombocytopenic purpura or disseminated intravascular coagulation. The "HELLP Syndrome" (Hemolysis, Elevated Liver enzymes, and Low Platelets) is also being increasingly recognized in toxemia patients (37). Clearly, the internist, no less than the obstetrician, must think of toxemia even in the absence of its more common signs and symptoms for almost any pregnant patient ill in the last trimester.

The treatment of severe preeclampsia is complex and varies in detail from institution to institution. The internist should be prepared to assist in the treatment of the more common complications, i.e., congestive heart failure, hypertensive crisis, renal failure, disseminated intravascular coagulation, and seizures. At this stage, the definitive therapy is most always the delivery of the fetus. The treatment of maternal complications should not be compromised for the sake of fetus. Patients with severe hypertension are usually able to be controlled with parenteral hydralazine or methyldopa. Diazoxide and nitroprusside should be avoided initially, if possible, due to unpredictable profound lowering of blood pressure with the former and the theoretical danger of cyanide accumulation in the fetus with the latter.

Postpartum, it is important to bear in mind the remote effects of toxemia in recommending appropriate follow-up. In general, nulliparous eclamptics experience no increase in the occurrence of chronic hypertension, but for women who develop eclampsia as multiparas, the incidence of chronic hypertension is increased. The late development of adult-onset diabetes mellitus is increased by 2.5 for nulliparas and by 4 for multiparas. In a 20–40 year follow-up of 267 eclamptic patients, Chesley (38) reports no increase in mortality for white nulliparas, but an increase of 2–5 times expected in white multiparas and all black eclamptics. How much of this increase is related to previous occasionally cavalier attitudes towards the treatment of chronic hypertension and of adult-onset diabetes mellitus remains to be seen.

CARDIOVASCULAR DRUGS IN PREGNANCY

In addition to the maternal indications for use of vasoactive and cardiac drugs, it is important to take into consideration their effects on myometrial tone and excitability and uterine-placental blood flow, as well as the possible physiologic and teratogenic effects on the fetus.

For the most part, it appears as though uterine-placental blood flow lacks substantial autoregulatory capacity and varies pari passu with maternal cardiac output, volume, and peripheral vascular resistance. The general characteristics of the drugs considered are outlined in Table 22.7, although some variability between compounds within the same class is to be expected.

Selected β-agonists (terbutaline and ritodrine), currently used experimentally as tocoleptics (often in combination with betamethasone) may present a special problem. Several individual case reports of congestive heart failure or acute pulmonary edema have recently been re-

Table 22.7. Effect of Cardiovascular Drugs on Uterine-Placental Blood Flow (UPF) and Myometrial Tone and Contractility (MC)

	Adrenergic Agonists			Adrenergic Blockers		Aldomet	Hydrala-zine	Diazoxide	Digitalis
	α	β	$\alpha+\beta$	α	β				
UPF	↓	No Δ	Low dose primarily β	No Δ	?	± ↓	↑	↓	?– ↑
MC	↑	↓	High dose primarily α	↓	No Δ–? ↑	No Δ	No Δ	No Δ	↑

ported in previously healthy women with this combination when given with rapidly infused large volumes of i.v. fluids. The etiology, frequency, and overall significance are not yet known, although some investigators report a frequency as high as 5 per 100. Fluid overloading also seems to be a common feature in these patients. Also, insulin requirements have been reported to double when ritodrine is used in insulin-requiring diabetics with premature labor. Diabetic ketoacidosis may develop in these patients unless carefully monitored. In addition, it has been suggested that subclinical idiopathic hypertrophic subaortic stenosis (IHSS) could be worsened by β-agonists and predispose to the development of acute pulmonary edema. It is important, therefore, that all patients receiving β-agonists as tocoleptics have hourly measurements of intake and output and receive a careful clinical examination for evidence of IHSS.

The dilutional effect of increasing maternal blood and total body water volumes and the increase in creatinine clearance during pregnancy can be of clinical significance. Digitalis and quinidine blood levels, for example, may be decreased by 40%, and dose adjustments throughout pregnancy may be required to maintain a stable clinical effect.

Because of fetal shunting through the foramen ovale and the ductus arteriosus, placental pooling of blood, and perhaps placental detoxifying enzymes, it is uncommon to see physiologic effects of most drugs in the fetus. It is estimated that increases in the usual maternal dose of 2–10 times would be needed to achieve drug effects in the fetus comparable to those seen in the mother at usual therapeutic doses.

THYROID DISORDERS

Hyperthyroidism, hypothyroidism, and solitary thyroid nodules developing during pregnancy present major diagnostic challenges and frustrations, and often give rise to strongly held and widely differing opinions regarding optimal therapy.

Hyperthyroidism

Hyperthyroidism is reported to occur at a rate of 1 per 1500 to 2000 pregnancies. Clinical diagnosis is frequently confused by and delayed due to the similarity of symptoms caused by the hypermetabolic state of pregnancy. The presence of persistent resting tachycardia (pulse greater than 100), onycholysis, weight loss, muscle wasting, and exophthalmos are helpful clinical clues in this situation. While an exact incidence is not available, fetal wastage, stillbirths, and spontaneous abortions associated with untreated moderate to severe maternal hyperthyroidism are increased (74% prematurity and 26% perinatal mortality, as reported by Montoro and Mestman (49).

DIAGNOSIS

Radionuclide thyroid uptake studies and scans are contraindicated in pregnancy. Wide fluctuations in plasma iodine and thyroxine-binding globulin make interpretation of triiodothyronine resin uptake (T_3RU) and iodine-linked thyroid hormone assays difficult. Total T_4 iodine increases by a factor of 1.5, and T_3RU decreases by 1.9 during pregnancy. However, the free T_4 index (Total $T_4 \times T_3RU$) remains fairly constant throughout normal pregnancy. Maternal free-thyroxine levels correlate fairly closely with cord blood levels. However, a normal maternal free-thyroxine does not preclude fetal hypothyroidism (51). Serial measurements of the free-T_4 index, free-thyroxine and total T_3 levels are the most accurate and convenient laboratory means by which to confirm clinical observations and to monitor therapy.

THERAPY

The major emphasis in the therapy of hyperthyroidism during pregnancy should be to avoid overtreatment. Most young, previously healthy pregnant women will tolerate the symptoms of mild to moderate hyperthyroidism without difficulty, making overly vigorous and rapid therapeutic maneuvers unnecessary. With the development of rapid and highly accurate radioimmunoassays for T_3, free-thyroxine (T_4), and the free-T_4 index, the medical therapy of hyperthyroidism with thioamides has become much easier to monitor and control. Both propylthiouracil (PTU) and methimazole rapidly cross the placenta and can lead to fetal goiter and cretinism. Marchant et al.'s studies (52) in patients undergoing therapeutic abortions suggest that only ⅓ as much PTU as methimazole crosses the placenta; however, this has not been confirmed in term pregnancies. T_3 and T_4 cross the placenta poorly, if at all, and should not be relied upon to protect the fetus from the effects of the thioamides. In addition, their use leads to increased amounts of thioamides needed to control maternal hyperthyroidism. Dosages of less than 100–150 mg of PTU per day or 10–15 mg of methimazole per day generally will not result in fetal hypothyroidism, although a transient (3–5 days) decrease at birth in the T_4 has been reported. Once maternal signs and symptoms are corrected, daily doses of PTU or methimazole can usually be reduced to less than 100 or 10 mg, respectively, and can often be discontinued entirely in the second or third trimester without exacerbations.

Both PTU and methimazole have been infrequently associated with an increase in congenital malformations (ectodermal dysplasia and aortic atresia most commonly), and fetal loss associated with PTU therapy is reported to be approximately 9%. Methimazole has certain theoretical advantages over PTU. Its long half-life (12 hours vs. 2–4 hours for PTU) makes its use for convenient once per day dosage more rational. In addition, it does not interfere with peripheral conversion of T_4 to T_3. As the fetus' mechanism for this transformation is immature and inefficient, it could be argued that it would be less deleterious to the fetus.

Subtotal thyroidectomy has been an important alternative to medical therapy, and in certain situations remains so. In experienced centers, surgical maternal mortality approaches zero, and fetal loss in large series is reported to be 5–6%. Recurrent laryngeal nerve palsies and postoperative hypoparathyroidism are extremely rare (53).

However, the inherent risk of surgery and general anesthesia to both the mother and, especially in the first trimester, to the fetus must be considered. In addition, more than 50% of hyperthyroid patients treated medically will attain lasting remissions and will need no further therapy. In most instances, with accurate and rapid laboratory monitoring of the medical therapy of hyperthyroidism, and with surgical experience decreasing in many centers, surgery is usually reserved for several specific situations. Patients with drug sensitivity to or toxicity from the thioamides are one such group. Also, patients requiring more than 300 mg per day of PTU or 30 mg per day of methimazole for control should be considered for surgery, as these larger amounts are associated with an increasing incidence of fetal hypothyroidism and developmental anomalies. Women with toxic nodular goiters should also be considered for surgery, as they often require large doses of thioamides for control. Also, women wishing to have more children and who fail to remain euthyroid off of medical therapy should be considered for surgery in that there is an increased incidence of congenital anomalies in the offspring of patients who have been maintained for long periods of time on thioamides and who are taking them at the time of conception. In addition, paradoxically, pregnancy will occasionally ameliorate hyperthyroidism in the first trimester in patients on stable doses of thioamides. These patients may then become hypothyroid, with potential major detrimental effects to the newly conceived fetus.

The role of β-adrenergic blockers in the therapy of hyperthyroidism in pregnancy is unsettled. While rapidly relieving many of the maternal signs and symptoms, an increasing number of adverse effects on the fetus are being reported. These include: depressed respiration at birth, postnatal bradycardia, and hypoglycemia. Their current role should probably be limited to short-term use to control maternal signs and symptoms while establishing euthyroidism with PTU or methimazole, or in preparation for surgery. While combining iodine with propranolol in the nonpregnant preoperative patient has resulted in rapid clinical and laboratory control and an improved surgical field, the use of iodine in pregnancy is contraindicated in that even very small amounts of iodine (12 mg per day) can cause fetal goiter.

Finally, postpartum exacerbations of hyperthyroidism, often to the point of thyroid storm, while infrequent in properly treated patients, should be anticipated.

Hypothyroidism

Traditionally, maternal hypothyroidism has been associated with an increased frequency of fetal wastage and congenital anomalies. The outcome (10% perinatal death, 10% congenital anomalies) as reported by Montoro et al. (50) of 11 pregnancies in 9 hypothyroid patients suggests that previous estimates may have been too high. Nonetheless, **maternal hypothyroidism should be treated with full replacement doses of thyroid hormone.** A common clinical situation is that of a young woman being treated with small doses of thyroid hormone for symptoms suggestive of hypothyroidism antepartum, who then becomes pregnant. Regardless of the degree of antepartum hypofunction, these patients should be given full replacement

doses during pregnancy. A recent report (54) demonstrated hypothyroidism-associated lymphocytic thyroiditis in 17% of clinically normal women examined 6–12 weeks postpartum. Theoretically, it has been suggested that a compound containing both T_3 and T_4 (such as Thyrolar or Euthroid) be used, as T_3 is thought to cross the placenta in small amounts. Even though it is not clear that maternal thyroid hormone is necessary for normal fetal development, it does appear necessary for normal uteroplacental function. Every effort should be made to ensure adequate maternal thyroid hormone replacement in order to minimize the increased incidence of stillbirths associated with maternal hypothyroidism. The total T_3 and the T_4 index (and TSH in primary hypothyroidism) should be monitored throughout pregnancy to assure adequate replacement.

Solitary Thyroid Nodules

The evaluation of the solitary thyroid nodule that appears during pregnancy is complicated by the prohibition against the use of radionuclide scans to determine if, in fact, the nodule is solitary, or "hot" or "cold." Ultrasound and CAT scans are helpful alternatives in visualizing multiple nodules. They might also help to determine whether a nodule is cystic or solid, although a cystic lesion is not necessarily benign. Spickled calcifications within the nodule suggest neoplasia. Elevations of serum calcitonin levels are associated with medullary carcinoma. Aspiration biopsy, if positive, will help to determine appropriate therapy. However, a negative biopsy is no guarantee of benignity. The usefulness of needle aspiration biopsies depends almost entirely upon the experience and expertise of the cytologist. Even groups with an extensive experience report a false-negative rate of up to 10% and a false-positive rate of 5%.

Diagnostic suppression of simple colloid nodules or cysts may not occur in pregnancy due to control factors other than TSH operative during gestation. Therefore, a lack of responsiveness of ≥50% does not necessarily indicate malignancy.

Cunningham and Slaughter (47), in their series of 26 solitary thyroid nodules discovered and removed during pregnancy found that nine (35%) were true adenomas and eight (30%) papillary carcinomas, five of which had already metastasized to local nodes at the time of surgery. There was no evidence for an increased frequency of either adenomas or carcinomas in pregnancy. Because of the high frequency of carcinomas in solitary thyroid nodules in young women, they recommended that suspicious nodules found during the first and second trimester be removed at that time; while for those discovered late in pregnancy, delaying removal until delivery did not constitute an unduly high risk to the mother.

Conversely, it has been argued that follicular and papillary adenocarcinomas, even when locally metastatic, are generally indolent tumors with excellent long-term survival expectations and that the risks of surgery and anesthesia during pregnancy to the mother and fetus are greater than waiting until after delivery for definitive surgery. In addition, for malignant carcinoma of the thyroid, surgery does not improve outcome and should not be attempted during pregnancy.

ASTHMA

Many of the normal physiologic changes of pregnancy are relevant to the clinical course of asthma. Tidal volume and oxygen consumption increase. The increase in progesterone in the second and third trimesters stimulates respiration and reduces airway resistance. Maternal cortisol levels increase. Cell-mediated immunity is decreased. IgE is normally reduced during pregnancy. In asthmatics, a stable or increasing IgE level is said to be helpful in detecting those whose asthma may become worse during pregnancy.

The incidence of asthma in pregnancy is reported to be between 0.4 and 1.3%. The concensus of published reports on the general clinical course of asthma during pregnancy is that one-third get better, one-third remain unchanged, and one-third get worse. When looked at more in terms of the severity of asthma prior to conception, more specific conclusions are possible. Sixty-seven to ninety percent of women with mild to moderate asthma will be either unchanged or better, and 10–33% will be worse. **Of those with severe asthma (requiring steroids or with weekly symptoms), only 15–50% will remain unchanged or do better, and 45–85% will be worse.** In addition, the response of asthma in earlier pregnancies tends to be the same in subsequent pregnancies. In general, then, women with mild to moderate asthma can be expected to remain stable or do better and those with severe asthma to become worse during pregnancy.

There is a slight increase in prematurity (14.0 vs. 9.3%) among asthmatics. Perinatal mortality is also reported to be increased, most often in the poor with severe asthma.

Therapy for asthma during pregnancy is similar, for the most part, to that of nonpregnant patients. Aminophylline preparations cross the placenta, but at usual therapeutic doses have no major ill effects on the fetus. Terbutaline has not been associated with any untoward effects in pregnant asthmatics, but when used in a high-dose continuous i.v. drip in combination with steroids as a tocoleptic, it has been associated with acute pulmonary edema in patients with previously normal hearts. Prednisone, 8 mg/day (or equivalent), does not result in any increased fetal morbidity or mortality. Betamethasone and dexamethasone are not inactivated by placental enzymes, whereas prednisone (and most other corticosteroids) is. Thus, the former cross the placenta intact in a significantly higher amount than prednisone and should not be used for the treatment of asthma during pregnancy (59, 60). However, the usual medical complications of corticosteroids, such as gastrointestinal bleeding and diabetes mellitus, must be remembered and sought for. In addition, "stress steroid coverage," as discussed in Chapter 13, should be provided during labor to steroid-dependent asthmatics. Prophylactic cromalyn therapy is safe for use during pregnancy and seems appropriate prior to labor and delivery in those women with exertionally induced asthma.

Tetracycline, iodine, and morphine, as well as aspirin in those asthmatics sensitive to it, should be avoided during pregnancy. Immunotherapy (desensitization) has not been associated with adverse fetal effects and may be safely continued during pregnancy.

NEUROLOGIC DISORDERS IN PREGNANCY

Epilepsy

With an estimated prevalence of 4.4 per 1000 in pregnancy, internists need to be familiar with the implications of epilepsy in pregnancy. A small percentage of patients will improve during gestation, perhaps related to more faithful adherence to their treatment program. **Even with only one seizure in the 9 months before conception, 25% of patients will experience more frequent seizures during pregnancy.** If greater than one seizure has occurred in that time frame, 60% will worsen. Seizures occurring for the first time during pregnancy, especially if focal, may be associated with arteriovenous malformations or brain tumor.

Medical control of epilepsy during pregnancy is complicated by a much increased plasma clearance of diphenylhydantoin and phenobarbital, beginning early in the first trimester. Monthly blood levels and appropriate adjustments are necessary in order to maintain therapeutic levels. Congenital malformations (primarily cleft lip and palate and the fetal hydantoin syndrome) are 2–3 times more common in women taking regular daily doses of diphenylhydantoin at the time of conception and during the first trimester. If possible, antenatal control should be established with one drug, preferably phenobarbital, and adjusted monthly as indicated to maintain control. While tegretol and sodium valproate have not, as yet, been associated with human congenital malformations, they have been in animals and should not be considered safe until so proven.

Other Disorders

Mononeuropathies, particularly carpal tunnel syndrome, meralgia paresthetica, and Bell's palsy occur more frequently in pregnancy, presumably related to rapid weight gain and increased total body fluid volumes. They regularly improve postpartum. While the activity and exacerbations of multiple sclerosis decrease or are unaffected during pregnancy, they do increase by 20–40% over controls in the 9-month postpartum period (65).

The course of myasthenia gravis is unpredictable during pregnancy. Postpartum exacerbations are common, though, and should be anticipated. Also, significant fatigue may complicate labor, necessitating frequent parenteral anticholinesterase for control. In particularly difficult cases, thymectomy during pregnancy could be considered. Approximately 40% of patients so treated will improve.

INFECTIONS IN PREGNANCY

General Considerations

Influenza A, rubeola, rubella, mumps, bacterial sepsis, and toxoplasmosis pose special problems during pregnancy due to the increased incidence of fetal wastage associated with these conditions. Obviously, appropriate vaccination against viral illnesses should be assured before conception. Poliomyelitis and yellow fever vaccination can be given during pregnancy if required (67). Weekly chloroquine prophylaxis against malaria, while not absolutely without risk, is much less likely to cause fetal damage than acute malaria in a non-immune and should be used when the mother is at high risk for contracting malaria.

Overwhelming bacterial sepsis, especially with group B streptococcus, increases the risk of spontaneous abortion due to hypoxia, hypotension, and infection of the amnion or the fetus itself.

Standard doses of antibiotics may fail to provide adequate serum levels due to increased maternal blood volume, increased creatinine clearance, and placental and fetal pooling. Antibiotic dosage should be increased if serum levels are subtherapeutic and the patient is not clinically responding. Penicillins, cephalosporins, chloramphenicol, and erythromycin pose no particular risks for the fetus, although the estolate form of erythromycin should be avoided due to an increased risk of cholestatic jaundice of pregnancy in the mother. Aminoglycosides may cause fetal ototoxicity. Tetracycline should be avoided due to fetal bone and dental enamel toxicity. Trimethoprim may be teratogenic due to its anti-folic acid activity. Sulfas, at term, are associated with an increased risk of kernicterus (68). The isoquinolone antibiotics (ciprofloxacin, norfloxacin) are contraindicated due to fetal bone and cartilage toxicity.

Specific Infections

Localized bacterial infections during pregnancy generally pose no increased risk to the mother or fetus if treated promptly and appropriately. With current antibiotic and supportive therapy, bacterial and mycoplasma pneumonias pose no special risks for the fetus. However, in mothers at high risk for complications (ethanol abuse, asthmatics, diabetics, sickle-cell disease, valvular heart disease), an increase in both maternal and fetal morbidity and mortality can be anticipated.

When appropriately treated with isoniazid and ethambutol, active pulmonary tuberculosis has not been associated with increased risk of fetal loss or malformation. When indicated, pulmonary resections for tuberculosis have been accomplished during pregnancy with only a slight increase in risk of fetal loss.

Women who have acquired toxoplasmosis before pregnancy are not at risk for increased fetal wastage or congenital infections of the newborn. However, when contracted during pregnancy (approximately 1 per 1000 pregnancies in U.S.), about one-third of these fetuses will become infected. In 90% of these cases, a positive serology is the only manifestation of infection at birth. This is especially so when the maternal infection was contracted in the third trimester. However, in long-term follow-up of these asymptomatic cases, a possible increase in central nervous system and eye damage has been noted. In the other 10%, severe or fatal central nervous system infections are found in the fetus. There is a higher likelihood of this outcome when maternal infections were contracted during the first trimester. Treatment of the mother with spectinomycin or pyrimethamine-sulfadizine, while perhaps decreasing the frequency of fetal infection, has not been shown to decrease the severity of fetal infection, and therapeutic abortion may be indicated, especially for those mothers in whom the infection was documented to have developed in the first trimester.

Rising titers of IgM antibodies detected by ELISA testing are highly supportive of recent toxoplasma infection.

HEMATOLOGY

Anemia of Pregnancy

The anemia of pregnancy is usually mild to moderate, with hemoglobin concentrations rarely below 10 grams/dl. Anemia becomes manifest at about the 8th week of pregnancy and slowly progresses until the 32nd to 34th week, at which time it becomes stable and then improves just before delivery. The anemia is dilutional since the red cell volume actually increases during pregnancy by about 20%, but the increase in plasma volume is approximately 30–40%. Although the hemoglobin concentration is decreased, the hypervolemic state ensures the mother and fetus of excellent blood perfusion and oxygen supply. The anemia of pregnancy is often worsened by concomitant iron and/ or folic acid deficiency. There is an increased utilization of iron and folic acid by the fetus during its maturation. The mother will lose approximately 700 mg of iron during a single pregnancy. It is appropriate to give every pregnant woman preventive iron and folic acid supplements. After pregnancy, iron should be given for several months to replete marrow iron stores.

Thrombocytopenia

The etiology of thrombocytopenia in pregnancy (Table 22.8) can often be quickly surmised from the associated clinical and laboratory findings. Several of these causes are of a self-limited obstetric nature and the internist would not generally be expected to be involved. In the others, the assistance of the internist will often be requested in managing the overall clinical problem. The management of most of these disorders is the same in pregnancy as at other times. However, idiopathic thrombocytopenic purpura (ITP) requires further mention.

Table 22.8. Thrombocytopenia in Pregnancy

Abruptio placentae
Retained placental parts
Hydatidiform mole
Pregnancy-induced hypertension (toxemia) with DIC
Malignant nephrosclerosis of pregnancy
Folic acid deficiency
Drugs (thiazides, oral hypoglycemics, etc.)
Lymphoma (leukemia)
Systemic lupus erythematosus
Thrombotic thrombocytopenic purpura
Idiopathic thrombocytopenic purpura

The majority of cases of ITP occur in young women but the frequency of ITP is not increased with pregnancy nor does the severity of the condition appear to be aggravated by pregnancy. **Asymptomatic patients with ITP need not be treated during pregnancy just to correct a low platelet count** (77). Before labor and delivery, no special therapy is required unless the mother is bleeding or at very high risk (platelets less than $20,000/mm^3$). Prednisone, 60–100 mg per day, is employed initially, with splenectomy reserved for unresponsive cases. An increase in both maternal and fetal morbidity and mortality can be expected when splenectomy is required.

The circulating maternal IgG antibody to platelet-associated antigen in ITP readily crosses the placenta and may cause thrombocytopenia in the fetus. There is an increased risk of spontaneous abortion (7–30%) in women with ITP compared to normals (10–15%). The fetus with less than $50,000–100,000$ platelets/mm^3 is at high risk for clinically significant bleeding (often intracranial) due to the trauma of even a normal vaginal delivery. However, not all offspring from mothers with ITP are significantly thrombocytopenic, but current methodology for predicting which infant will be at risk is imperfect. Fetal scalp blood sampling during labor can provide helpful information but at the risk of excessive bleeding in the thrombocytopenic (less than 50,000 platelets/mm^3) fetus. Retrospective surveys suggest that when maternal platelets are greater than $100,000/mm^3$, fetal thrombocytopenia is less likely to be clinically significant (25%) compared to when maternal platelets are less than $100,000/mm^3$ (80%). In one recent report (79) the level of maternal circulating antiplatelet antibody correlated with both the presence and the extent of neonatal thrombocytopenia. In general, elective caesarean section is the preferred mode of delivery unless the maternal and fetal platelet counts are $>100,000/mm^3$. As the IgG antibody persists after splenectomy in women with ITP, cesarean section is always recommended in these cases as it is impossible to estimate fetal platelet counts under these circumstances.

Infusing high doses (300–400 mg/kg/day) of gamma-globulin intravenously for 4–5 days has resulted in transient increases in platelet counts to near normal levels and normalization of the bleeding time (80). While this approach has not been prospectively studied in pregnancy, several case reports suggest that it will be successful in the management of ITP during labor and delivery. Since it may take up to 3 weeks for IgG to effectively cross the placenta, it has been suggested that intermittent high-dose gamma-globulin be started 3–4 weeks before the estimated delivery date (77b, 81).

Sickle Cell Disease

Pregnancy and the postpartum period are potentially hazardous times for a mother with sickle cell (SC) disease. Women with sickle cell trait have no higher incidence of complications during pregnancy than a woman with normal hemoglobin. Hemoglobin SC disease is a relatively mild disorder, but during pregnancy, manifestations similar to those encountered with homozygous (SS) sickle cell anemia, as well as a peculiar, often fatal syndrome of bone marrow infarction and fat embolization may occur.

The pregnant sickle cell patient at risk should be closely supervised during pregnancy and a difficult, lengthy labor should be avoided. However, routine cesarean section is not recommended. Although there are increased dangers for the pregnant woman, they are usually not so overwhelming as to interrupt pregnancy or prevent a desired pregnancy. Spontaneous abortion is more common in such women, babies tend to be small, and perinatal mortality is high. Most normal women have a decrease in the hematocrit during pregnancy due to hemodilution.

This also occurs in women with sickle cell anemia, and their hematocrit values may be less than 20% without significant symptoms. Transfusion is not required for an asymptomatic woman. It is not clear whether a decreased oxygen-carrying capacity is harmful to the fetus.

The value of exchange transfusion in the management of infarctive crisis in pregnancy is now well established (82, 83). Partial exchange transfusion should be performed if a serious crisis occurs, and the patient should be maintained with blood containing less than 50% sickle cells. Blood should always be cross-matched as the patient enters labor because of the increased danger of hemorrhage in an anemic patient. If transfusion is required, a hematocrit of 25% appears to be the level at which sickle cell blood is closest to normal viscosity. During labor, the patient should be kept warm and watched for signs of circulatory overload. Regional or spinal anesthesia should be used for delivery and supplemental oxygen should be used throughout the delivery process. Many such women have no crisis at all during pregnancy and are not hospitalized until the time of delivery.

COLLAGEN VASCULAR DISEASES

While often categorized as a group of diseases of similar pathogenesis and of overlapping clinical findings and laboratory abnormalities, the collagen vascular diseases are characterized by major differences in their response to pregnancy. A familiarity with these differences is critical for the internist for counseling regarding pregnancy and for monitoring and managing these patients during gestation. The three most common of these disorders occurring during pregnancy are rheumatoid arthritis, systemic lupus erythematosus, and scleroderma.

Rheumatoid Arthritis

The prevalence of rheumatoid arthritis (RA) in the general female population is approximately 0.5%, but would be somewhat less overall in the child-bearing age group. A cascade of case reports and retrospective series over the past 40 years attests to the general impression that **RA improves during pregnancy but has a tendency to be exacerbated postpartum.** For example, Persellin (84) points out that in 75% of 274 pregnancies complicated by RA, the mothers improved: 74% within the first trimester, 20% more in the second, and 6% more in the third. Improvement was not related to age, severity of disease, rheumatoid factor titers, or duration of disease. Unfortunately, 95% of patients experience an exacerbation postpartum, two-thirds within the first 2 months, the remainder by 6 months. Exacerbations are not related to lactation or return of menses. However, there is no cumulative progression of disease compared with nonpregnant patients.

No consistently adverse effects of maternal RA on the fetus have been documented. Rheumatoid factor is not transmitted to the fetus. However, small-for-age infants are common in patients with an active, generalized vasculitis complicating their RA.

The ameliorating effect of pregnancy on RA has stimulated a continuing search for a therapeutic principle that could be applied in the nonpregnant state. A number of anecdotal reports of improvement with maternal blood products, cord serum, and placental extracts exist, but no consistent benefit has been shown in controlled trials. While cortisols are increased in pregnancy, the beneficial effect of pregnancy seems independent of this increase. RA titers are generally unchanged in pregnancy. T lymphpocyte function has been shown to be decreased in pregnancy and it has been suggested that this is responsible for the improvement seen, but specific details and analyses are lacking. Circulating "pregnancy proteins," more specifically the pregnancy zone protein, an α_2 globulin which stabilizes lysosomal membranes, and preg-

nancy α glycoprotein which suppresses monocyte activity are also said to play a major role. A remission in one pregnancy is generally predictive of similar results in subsequent pregnancies and vice-versa.

While administering steroids prophylactically postpartum will diminish the likelihood and severity of an exacerbation, pharmacologic doses could be required for up to 2–6 months. Due to the likelihood of severe side effects and dependency, they are better employed only when other less toxic drugs (aspirin, nonsteroidal anti-inflammatories) are unsuccessful.

Scleroderma

In the absence of renal involvement, the effect of pregnancy on scleroderma and vice-versa is unpredictable. In a review of the literature, Karlen and Cook (85) report that 40% of patients showed no change, 12–22% improved, and 39–42% worsened. **When renal involvement complicates scleroderma, either before or during pregnancy, the experience for both mother and fetus has been disastrous,** with a maternal mortality approaching 100%. Most authorities recommend therapeutic abortion if any decrease in renal function develops.

The effect of scleroderma on fetal outcome is not entirely settled. By and large, if the mother's condition remains stable, no consistent increase in fetal complications or loss has been noted. When otherwise, there is an increase in prematurity and perinatal death of up to 30% (87, 88, 88a).

Systemic Lupus Erythematosus

Systemic lupus erythematosus (SLE) has been estimated to occur with a frequency of 1 in 1660 pregnancies. **Unlike RA, however, rarely is the patient's clinical condition improved during pregnancy.** For patients in remission at the time of conception, the likelihood of an exacerbation approximates 25%. For pa-

Table 22.9. Systemic Lupus Erythematosus (SLE) in Pregnancy

SLE	Exacerbation
In remission when conceived	25%
Active SLE when conceived	70%
SLE with active nephritis when conceived	75–85%
(Exacerbations most common in 3rd trimester or 1st 2 weeks postpartum)	

tients with active SLE, 70% will worsen and of those with active lupus nephritis, 75–85% will worsen (Table 22.9). Most exacerbations occur in the third trimester or in the first 2 weeks postpartum. (92)

In addition to deteriorating renal function, other major medical problems frequently encountered are thrombocytopenia, pulmonary vasculitis, and a generalized flare with polyserositis and fever. In addition, "preeclampsia" has been reported in 18–25% of SLE pregnancies, compared to an average rate of 3%. The great majority of these appear to be manifestations of lupus nephritis, as many will improve or stabilize with steroids, whereas the tendency in preeclampsia would be to deteriorate further with steroid therapy. In addition, SLE patients with "circulating anticoagulant" are at high risk for bleeding complications at delivery.

Rarely will patients with active SLE improve with pregnancy. However, the exacerbations associated with pregnancy do not appear to ultimately change the long-term course of the disease as far as overall morbidity and mortality are concerned.

Increasing attention is being focused on the *"obstetric-lupus syndrome."* These patients are usually identified by having had multiple recurrent fetal losses, usually in the second or third trimester. When nonpregnant, they are usually healthy but when pregnant, they may develop hypertension, arthropathies, thrombocytopenia,

a prolonged partial thromboplastin time and a positive test for the "lupus anticoagulant." However, tests for antinuclear antibodies are characteristically negative. The "lupus anticoagulant" is in fact an anticardiolipin antibody, and these patients represent a subset of a larger group of patients with the "anticardiolipin syndrome" (93). There is some evidence to suggest that treatment with prednisone and low-dose aspirin may improve fetal outcome and will improve the mother's clinical state (94).

The effect of SLE on the fetus varies with the activity of the disease at the time of conception. For patients in remission or who develop SLE postpartum, a frequency of 25–30% of stillbirths or prematurity is to be expected, compared to an average rate of 10%. For patients with active SLE at the time of conception, the frequency is 45%, and for those with active lupus nephritis, the rate is over 50% (Table 22.10). It has been suggested that patients with persistently high levels of lymphocytotoxic antibodies during pregnancy are more likely to experience stillbirths and prematurity. The proposed pathogenesis involves a placental immune complex vasculitis due to absorption of these antibodies by trophoblastic antigens. Whether immunosuppressive therapy could reduce the percentage of fetal loss in these patients has not been determined in prospective studies. While steroids and immunosuppressive drugs will improve the maternal course, they have not been shown to directly reduce

Table 22.10. Effect of SLE on Fetus

Mother	Fetus
In remission or SLE developed postpartum	25–30% stillbirths or prematurity
Active SLE, without nephritis	45% prematurity, stillbirth
Active SLE, with nephritis	≥50% prematurity, stillbirth

the high incidence of fetal wastage in patients with active SLE.

Congenital abnormalities in the fetus have generally been few and well tolerated and include a transient discoid lupus rash, thrombocytopenia, and circulating antinuclear antibodies. Recently, however, a number of reports have appeared describing an often fatal complete heart block and endocardial fibrosis in the fetuses of patients with collagen vascular disorders, most frequently with SLE (95).

Blood levels of C'_3 are increased in normal pregnancies. **In patients with SLE, a stable or decreasing level of C'_3 heralds a worsening course in 75–85% of cases.** Increasing titers of antinuclear antibodies are predictive of an exacerbation in 40%. In patients with a decreasing C'_3 and increasing ANA titers, steroid therapy should begin or be increased, even if the patient appears clinically stable at the time. Also, because of the high frequency of postpartum exacerbations, especially in patients with active SLE, steroids should be instituted or increased prophylactically 1 week before delivery and continued for at least 1 week postpartum. If the clinical course is unstable, or if the titer of C'_3 is worsening, increased steroids should be continued for 6–8 weeks.

The average life expectancy postpartum of the patient with active proliferative lupus nephritis is 2 years without dialysis. Five-year survival with membranous or proliferative lupus glomerulonephritis is 20%, and 40% in patients with CNS lupus. The internist must carefully consider these realities, as well as the morbidity associated with this disease, when counseling a patient with SLE regarding pregnancy.

Dermatomyositis/Polymyositis

A recent report by Gutierrez et al. (96) documents a high rate of fetal loss (>50%) in patients with dermatomyositis/polymyositis, especially in those whose disease began during pregnancy. Treatment with prednisone, while improving maternal symptoms, did not appear to decrease the high rate of fetal loss.

Drug Therapy of Collagen Vascular Diseases During Pregnancy

GENERAL PRINCIPLES

As the severity of rheumatoid arthritis is almost always decreased during pregnancy, it is frequently possible to decrease or eliminate drugs that were required for control of signs or symptoms antepartum. Systemic lupus erythematosus, on the other hand, not infrequently exacerbates during pregnancy and requires a decision to increase or begin new drug therapy. Therapy is often mandatory to protect the mother. In this situation, maternal considerations should outweigh fetal risks. As yet, no consistently effective therapy exists for scleroderma. Therapeutic abortion is often recommended when scleroderma renal disease begins or worsens during pregnancy.

DRUGS

Aspirin

The major maternal concern with aspirin is gastrointestinal bleeding, especially in the presence of gastric stasis or hyperemesis gravidarum.

Questionable teratogenicity has been reported in animal studies but not in humans. A possible increased incidence of fetal bleeding caused by aspirin effects on platelets has been reported. Also, aspirin tends to prolong labor and is associated with an increased frequency of postmaturity.

Nonsteroidal Anti-inflammatories

While teratogenicity studies in rodents at doses similar to those used in man have not demonstrated an increased risk, no human studies are available and these drugs are not recommended for use in pregnancy. Phenylbutazone is probably embryotoxic and should be specifically avoided in pregnancy.

Gold

Gold is highly protein-bound and crosses the placenta poorly, if at all. It has been safely used throughout pregnancy, but due to limited observations, it should probably be discontinued whenever possible in pregnancy.

Hydroxychloroquine

This drug intercolates with the DNA molecule and is capable of causing chromosomal damage. In addition, it accumulates in the fetal uveal tract and should be avoided in pregnancy.

Corticosteroids

Relatively little fetal toxicity has been directly associated with high-dose steroid therapy in pregnancy. Possibilities of adrenal gland suppression, masculinization of the female fetus, and intrauterine growth retardation have been mentioned. An increased frequency of cleft palate in animal studies has been reported but no increase in human fetal malformations have been demonstrated. Intra-articular steroids provide a safer alternative to oral or parenteral steroids where appropriate.

Immunosuppressives

Imuran and cytoxan have been used safely throughout pregnancy but overall experience has been limited. In general, they are to be avoided when possible.

RENAL DISEASE DURING PREGNANCY

Urinary Tract Infections

Over the past 20 years, a considerable amount of data has been accumulated on the frequency of bacteriuria during pregnancy, and of its effect on maternal and fetal health. Bacteriuria, most often asymptomatic, occurs in 4–6% of pregnancies and is stable at that figure from the second month of gestation on. While it is often speculated that anatomic changes in the urinary tract occurring during pregnancy are responsible, bacter-iuria usually occurs before these changes are present.

Untreated bacteriuria during pregnancy will progress in 25–40% to acute pyelonephritis, usually in the third trimester. Successful therapy of bacteriuria will reduce this incidence to near zero. Up to 10% of pregnant bacteriuric patients will have abnormal IVPs, although the changes often seem inconsequential. Whether women with bacteriuria or pyelonephritis during pregnancy with a normal IVP will subsequently develop significant renal disease has not been established.

Methodologic difficulties and concomitant factors, such as smoking, nutritional status, and differing socioeconomic profiles, have contributed to confusion regarding the effect of bacteriuria on fetal well-being. Naeye (101) has clarified part of this issue. In a large series of patients with concomitant perinatal disorders (amniotic fluid infections, congenitally malformed infants, umbilical cord compression, large placental infarcts, abruptio placenta, growth-retarded placenta, Rh disease, and placental previa), those with bacteriuria had twice the fetal mortality as those without (42/1000 vs. 21/1000). This difference is even more pronounced in mothers with associated acetonuria or hypertension. In addition, hypertension was 85% more frequent in those women with bacteriuria and pyuria than those without.

Nephrolithiasis

Somewhere between 25–30 g of calcium are mobilized from the maternal skeleton to the fetus during the second half of gestation. 1,25-dihydroxy-vitamin D levels are substantially increased in pregnancy, probably through the action of estrogens, progesterones, and human placental lactogen, as parathyroid hormone remains normal throughout pregnancy. This results in increased intestinal absorption of calcium to balance the large fetal needs.

Nephrolithiasis occurs in approximately 1 per 1400 pregnancies, being found with equal frequency in each trimester. In nonselective series of patients, the great majority are idiopathic. Most will have associated urinary tract infections. Coe and colleagues, on the other hand, found that, among recurrent stone formers, 41% had idiopathic hypercalcinuria, 13% infected struvite stones, 13% hyperuricosuria, 10% primary hyperparathyroidism, 3% cystinuria, and 19% were idiopathic (103). In their patients with recurrent renal calculi, the frequency of stone formation did not increase with pregnancy, but urinary tract infections did, with an average incidence of 40%.

Surgical removal of stones is indicated for recurrent or persistent infections or a high degree of obstruction. Internal ureteral stents with antibiotic prophylaxis has also been successfully employed intrapartum for relief of pain and obstruction (105). The high incidence of associated acute urinary tract infections and the occasional patient with primary hyperparathyroidism account for the increased incidence of fetal loss (approximately 6%) reported in the literature.

Effect of Pregnancy on Underlying Renal Disease

Recent reviews (106–109) of this subject conclude that for women with inactive renal disease with a serum creatinine of less than 1.5 mg/100 ml, pregnancy poses little increase in risk for either the mother or the child. A probable exception is for women with active lupus nephritis, as discussed earlier. There appears to be a slight trend for small-for-date babies and prematurity, but there is no significant difference from normal in live births. On the other hand, for women with active renal disease and a serum creatinine of greater than 1.5 mg/100 ml, deterioration

of renal function, increased diastolic blood pressure, increased proteinuria, and increased urinary tract infections are to be expected. In addition, postpartum follow-up reveals a high frequency (50%) of rapid continuing deterioration in renal function in this group. Fetal loss and premature, complicated deliveries are similarly greatly increased in this group.

Renal Failure During Pregnancy and Postpartum

By far the most common causes of renal disease during pregnancy are infections and toxemia. Finnerty (31) emphasizes the importance of carefully evaluating patients with a diagnosis of toxemia for urinary tract infections, in that eradication of such infections will often eliminate the clinical features of "toxemia." He stresses the presence of retinal sheen in patients with true toxemia in helping to differentiate them from patients with urinary tract infections.

Also specific to pregnancy is the entity of "idiopathic postpartum renal failure" (112). While only 50 cases have been reported to date, a wider spectrum of this disorder is now being recognized. Characterized by the rapid onset of renal failure, microangiopathic hemolytic anemia, and thrombocytopenia following a normal gestation and delivery, it was initially thought to be uniformly fatal. Recently, milder cases have been recognized with complete recovery within 1 month of onset. Clinically, the disorder is characterized by oliguria, bleeding, and variable hypertension and cardiac failure. Pathologic changes include fibrin deposition in the glomeruli and a fibrinoid necrosis of arteries in the kidney, lung, brain, and spleen. Many clinical and pathologic features are shared with the hemolytic uremic syndrome in children, disseminated intravascular coagulation, thrombotic thrombocytopenic purpura, and the generalized Schwartzman reaction. Heparin, antiplatelet drugs, corticosteroids, and fibrinolytic therapy with streptokinase have all been tried, but are infrequently successful.

GASTROINTESTINAL AND HEPATOBILIARY DISORDERS IN PREGNANCY

Jaundice

Some degree of jaundice is reported in approximately 1 per 1500–3000 pregnancies. The majority are caused by viral hepatitis (20–40%), recurrent cholestasis of pregnancy (25–75%), toxemia (10%), and cholelithiasis (5%).

Viral Hepatitis

The majority of cases are due to hepatitis B, and most (90%) appear in the third trimester. Most cases are clinically benign. In the U.S. and Europe, there is no increase in incidence or severity during pregnancy but in developing countries, there may be an increase in both, especially in the third trimester. Cases occurring in the first or second trimester appear to present little risk to the mother or fetus, with very few cases of congenital transmission under these circumstances. Viral hepatitis B occurring in the third trimester, however, is frequently (75%) associated with transmission to the newborn, with transmission via the fecal-oral route at birth, or transplacentally of approximately equal incidence. A large percentage of these infants have become chronic HB$_S$Ag carriers, with many progressing to chronic hepatitis and cirrhosis. Therefore, infants born to mothers with hepatitis B in the third trimester should all receive high-titer hepatitis B γ-globulin whether sero-positive or not (67b). If seropositivity returns after initial therapy, they should be retreated. With the advent of a hepatitis B vaccine, all infants from seropositive mothers should be actively immunized. The fetal risk of developing chronic active hepatitis

or of becoming a chronic carrier from mothers who are chronic carriers of HB$_S$Ag is not clear. Studies in the United States suggest a 10% incidence, but in Taiwan and Bougainville (Solomon Islands), up to one-third of such infants become chronic carriers, with many developing chronic hepatitis and cirrhosis. If the mother is HB$_e$Ag-positive transmission occurs 80–90% of the time, with 85% of infected infants becoming chronic carriers (115).

Cirrhosis

Cirrhosis with portal hypertension due to chronic active hepatitis or to extrahepatic portal vein obstruction carries unacceptable risks of both maternal mortality (25–45%) from esophageal bleeding or hepatic failure and of fetal death (50%). Even with successful shunt surgery for extrahepatic portal vein obstruction, the risk of major, and often fatal, gastrointestinal bleeding is intolerable. In addition, immunosuppressive therapy used in chronic active hepatitis may be teratogenic. Even with a successful pregnancy, maternal life expectancy is much reduced, leaving the family with a motherless child. Women with these disorders should be fully informed of the risks involved with pregnancy and should be advised of appropriate birth control.

Acute Yellow Atrophy of Pregnancy

While the incidence of this disorder is low (1 per 13,328 deliveries) (121), it is a devastating disease with extremely high fetal (85%) and maternal (75%) mortality. Clinically, it occurs late in the third trimester, with headaches, nausea, vomiting, abdominal pain, jaundice, hematemesis, and stupor. It is characterized by rapidly developing hepatic and renal failure, disseminated intravascular coagulation, and coma. Pathologically, there is little hepatic necrosis but a diffuse, panlobular microvacuolar fatty infiltration, with the liver being characteristically small and not palpable. The pathologic changes are very similar to those seen in Reye's syndrome. Thus, it has been speculated that a partial deficiency of ornithine transcarbamylase may be the basic biochemical etiology. Based on this analogy, it has been suggested that intravenous infusion of ornithine or citrelline may be therapeutic, but no such case reports are available. Emergency cesarean section or vaginal delivery, when possible, may improve fetal salvage and perhaps maternal survival as well (122). Anti-thrombin III levels may be very low and specific replacement is of value in controlling clinical manifestations of disseminated intravascular coagulation. While subsequent pregnancies have been few, they all proceeded normally with no liver abnormalities (123).

Recurrent Cholestasis of Pregnancy

Twenty-five to 75% of cases of jaundice during pregnancy are the result of "recurrent cholestasis of pregnancy." While often described as benign, several studies report an incidence of up to 30% prematurity and fetal distress. In addition, there is a considerable amount of maternal morbidity due to persistent pruritis and, occasionally, troublesome nausea and vomiting.

This disorder occurs late in pregnancy and is thought to be due to a genetically determined increase in the usual impaired biliary secretory ability seen in late pregnancy. This change is mediated by an interaction of estrogens and progestins, which causes biliary stasis due to both an increase in reabsorption of bile into the plasma and a decreased secretion of bile into the biliary collection system. The predominant clinical feature is pruritis, along with a variable amount of anorexia, nausea and vomiting, and, usually, a mild degree of jaundice. The condition clears at delivery, but usually will recur in subsequent pregnancies or with the use of birth control pills.

Cholelithiasis

Cholecystectomies are performed at a rate of 1–2 per 5000 pregnancies, most commonly (85%) in the first or second trimester. A large percentage of these represent "acute biliary colic," as stones are found only 50% of the time. In retrospect, half have had similar symptoms before pregnancy. Despite alterations in bile salt composition and secretion during gestation, pregnancy itself probably does not increase the frequency of cholelithiasis. With the availability of improved ultrasound methodology, "skinny needle" cholangiography, and endoscopic retrograde cholangiopancreatography, the frequency of cholecystectomies during pregnancy will, in all probability, decrease.

When surgery is required, most authorities prefer to wait until the second trimester if at all possible, as the peak incidence of spontaneous abortions has then passed, the major fetal organ systems have formed, and the uterus has not yet become so large as to interfere with the surgical field. Fetal mortality with surgery for uncomplicated cholecystitis and cholelithiasis is approximately 5%, and there is no increased maternal mortality. However, when complicated by pancreatitis, fetal mortality rises to 60% and maternal mortality to 15%.

Crohn's Disease

In two recent reviews (125, 126) totaling 100 pregnancies, a slight increase in spontaneous abortions was noted, but otherwise there appeared to be no major effect of the disease on pregnancy or vice-versa, especially if the disease was quiescent at the time of conception (127). There has been noted, though, a tendency for the disease to flare in the immediate postpartum period in 5–25% of patients. Therefore, prophylactic corticosteroids should be considered for 1–3 months postpartum. In addition, many of these women are chronically ill and poorly nourished, and optimum nutritional support throughout pregnancy may present a major problem. The demonstration of the practicality and success of home total parenteral nutrition will make the care and outcome for these patients more optimistic (128). Medical management with corticosteroids is almost always the preferred therapy for exacerbations of chronic illness during pregnancy.

Ulcerative Colitis

The probability of exacerbations of ulcerative colitis during pregnancy (45%) does not differ from nonpregnant controls. However, for those women who do suffer a major relapse, the incidence of spontaneous abortions, particularly in the first trimester, is increased. Relapses are most likely to occur in the first trimester or postpartum. During these periods, endogenous maternal corticosteroids are relatively low or are falling, which, it has been speculated, accounts for the increased frequency of disease activity at these times. Surgical emergencies, such as toxic megacolon, are rare but devastating during pregnancy. Both maternal and fetal mortality approach 100% with this complication. Azulfidine will decrease the likelihood of recurrence of ulcerative colitis by up to 4-fold and should be continued throughout pregnancy. However, because it is potentially teratogenic, it is advisable to consider corticosteroids instead during the first trimester. Also, because of the increased likelihood of severe relapses during the first 3 months postpartum, corticosteroids should also be considered during this time.

READINGS

Diabetes Mellitus

1. White P: Pregnancy and diabetes, medical aspects. *Med Clin North Am* 49:1015–1024, 1965.
2. Mintz DH, Skyler JS, Chez RA: Diabetes mellitus and pregnancy. *Diabetes Care* 1:49–65, 1978.
3. Adashi EY, Pinto H, Tyson JE, et al.: Impact of maternal euglycemia on fetal outcome in diabetic pregnancy. *Am J Obstet Gynecol* 133:268–274, 1979.
4. Karlson K, Kjellmer I, et al.: The outcome of

diabetic pregnancies in relation to the mother's blood sugar level. *Am J Obstet Gynecol* 112:213–220, 1972.
5. Sinclair SH, Nesler CL, Schwartz SS, et al.: Retinopathy in the pregnant diabetic. *Clin Obstet Gynecol* 28:536–552, 1985.
6. Miller E, Hare JW, Cloherty JR, et al.: Elevated maternal hemoglobin A_{1c} in early pregnancy and major congenital anomalies in infants of diabetic mothers. *N Engl J Med* 304:1331–1334, 1981.
7. Goldman JA, Dicker D, Feldberg D, et al.: Pregnancy outcome in patients with insulin-dependent diabetes mellitus with preconceptional diabetic control: A comparative study. *Am J Obstet Gynecol* 155:293–297, 1986.
8. Fuhrmann K, Reiher H, Semmler K, et al.: Prevention of congenital malformations in infants of insulin-dependent diabetic mothers. *Diabetes Care* 6:219–223, 1983.
9. Freinkel N, Dooley SL, Metzger BE, et al.: Care of the pregnant woman with insulin-dependent diabetes mellitus. *N Engl J Med* 313:96–100, 1985.
10. Pedersen J, Molsted-Pedersen L, et al.: Congenital malformations: The possible role of diabetes care outside pregnancy, in *Pregnancy Metabolism, Diabetes and the Fetus*. London, Ciba Foundation Symposium #63, 1979, pp 265–271.

Heart Disease

11. Sullivan JM, Ramanathan KB: Management of medical problems in pregnancy—severe cardiac disease. *N Engl J Med* 313:304–309, 1985.
12. Iturbe-Alessio I, Fonseca MDC, Mutchinik O, et al.: Risks of anticoagulant therapy in pregnant women with artificial heart valves. *N Engl J Med* 315:1390–1393, 1986.
13. Harken DE, Taylor WJ: Cardiac surgery during pregnancy. *Clin Obstet Gynecol* 4:697–709, 1961.
14. Szekely P, Turner P, Snaith L: Pregnancy and the changing pattern of rheumatic heart disease. *Br Heart J* 35:1293–1303, 1973.
15. Zitnik RS, Brandenburg RO, Sheldon R, et al.: Pregnancy and open heart surgery. *Circulation* 39:Suppl. I, 257–262, 1969.
16. Ibarra-Perez C, Arevalo-Toledo N, Alvarez de la Cadena O, et al.: The course of pregnancy in patients with artificial heart valves. *Am J Med* 61:504–512, 1976.
17. Whittemore R, Hobbins JC: Pregnancy in women who have congenital heart defects. *Prim Cardiol* 3:26–31, 1977.
18. Sugrue D, Blake S, MacDonald D: Pregnancy complicated by maternal heart disease at the National Maternity Hospital, Dublin, Ireland, 1969 to 1978. *Am J Obstet Gynecol* 139:1–6, 1981.
19. Stevenson RE, Burton OM, Ferlauto GJ, et al.: Hazards of oral anticoagulants during pregnancy. *JAMA* 243:1549–1551, 1980.
20. Rayburn WF, Fontana M: Mitral valve prolapse and pregnancy. *Am J Obstet Gynecol* 141:9–11, 1981.
21. Homans D: Peripartum cardiomyopathy. *N Engl J Med* 312:1432–1437, 1985.

22. Demakis JG, Rahimtoola SH: Peripartum cardiomyopathy. *Circulation* 44:964–968, 1971.
23. Elias S, Berkovitz RL: The Marfan syndrome and pregnancy. *Obstet Gynecol* 47:358–361, 1976.
24. Rotmensch HH, Elkayam U, Frishman W: Antiarrhythmic drug therapy during pregnancy. *Ann Intern Med* 98:487–497, 1983.
25. Schroeder JS, et al.: Repeated cardioversion during pregnancy. Treatment of refractory paroxysmal atrial tachycardia during three successive pregnancies. *Am J Cardiol* 27:445–446, 1971.
26. Cullhed I: Cardioversion during pregnancy—case report. *Acta Med Scand* 214:169–172, 1983.
27. Klein V, Repke JT: Supraventricular tachycardia in pregnancy: Cardioversion with verapamil. *Obstet Gynecol* 63:16S–18S, 1984.
28. Mendelson CL: Disorders of the heartbeat during pregnancy. *Am J Obstet Gynecol* 72:1208–1301, 1956.
29. Sugrue D, Blake S, Troy P, et al.: Antibiotic prophylaxis against infective endocarditis after normal delivery: Is it necessary? *Br Heart J* 44:499–502, 1980.

Hypertension

30. Finnerty FA Jr: Toxemia of pregnancy as seen by an internist: An analysis of 1081 patients. *Ann Intern Med* 44:358–375, 1956.
31. Finnerty FA Jr: Hypertension and pregnancy. *Cardiovasc Med* 5:559–568, 1980.
32. Rubin PC: Beta-blockers in pregnancy (Current Concepts). *N Engl J Med* 305:1323–1326, 1981.
33. Rubin PC, Clark DM, Sumner DJ, et al.: Placebo-controlled trial of atenolol in treatment of pregnancy-associated hypertension. *Lancet* 431–434, 1983.
34. Redman CWG: Therapy of non-preeclamptic hypertension in pregnancy. *Am J Kidney Dis* IX:324–327, 1987.
35. Lindheimer MD, Katz AI: Hypertension in pregnancy. *N Engl J Med* 313:675–680, 1985.
36. Goodlin RC: Severe preeclampsia: Another great imitator. *Am J Obstet Gynecol* 125:747–753, 1976.
37. MacKenna J, Dover NL, Brame RG: Preeclampsia associated with hemolysis, elevated liver enzymes, and low platelets—an obstetric emergency? *Obstet Gynecol* 62:751–754, 1983.
38. Chesley LC: Eclampsia: The remote prognosis. *Semin Perinatol* 2:99–111, 1978.
39. Roberts JM: When the hypertensive patient becomes pregnant. *Contemporary Obstet Gynecol* 13:47–55, 1979.
40. Brinkman CR, Woods JR: Effects of cardiovascular drugs during pregnancy. *Cardiovasc Med* 1:231–251, 1976.
41. Tinga DJ, Ardnoose JG, Rudge P, et al.: Postpartum pulmonary edema associated with preventive therapy for premature labor. *Lancet* 1:1026–1027, 1979.
42. Wagner JM, Morton MJ, Johnson KA, et al.: Terbutaline and maternal cardiac function. *JAMA* 246:2697–2701, 1981.
43. Mordes D, Kreutner K, Metzger W, et al.: Dangers of intravenous ritodrine in diabetic patients. *JAMA* 248:973–975, 1982.

Thyroid Diseases in Pregnancy

44. Selenkow HA: Therapeutic considerations for thyrotoxicosis during pregnancy, in DA Fisher, GN Burrow (eds): *Perinatal Thyroid Physiology and Disease.* New York, Raven Press, 1975, pp 145–161.
45. Burrow GN: The thyroid in pregnancy. *Med Clin North Am* 59:1089–1097, 1975.
46. Burrow GN: Hyperthyroidism during pregnancy. *N Engl J Med* 298:150–153, 1978.
47. Cunningham MT, Slaughter DT: Surgical treatment of disease of the thyroid gland in pregnancy. *Surg Gynecol Obstet* 131:486–488, 1970.
48. Becker WF: Hyperthyroidism: An experience with 245 patients treated by thyroidectomy. *J Louisiana State Med Soc* 128:221–224, 1976.
49. Montoro M, Mestman J., et al.: Graves' disease and pregnancy (letter). *N Engl J Med* 305:48, 1981.
50. Montoro M, Collea JV, Frasier SO, et al.: Successful outcome of pregnancy in women with hypothyroidism. *Ann Intern Med* 94:31–34, 1981.
51. Momotani N, Noh J, Oyanagi H, et al.: Antithyroid drug therapy for Graves' disease during pregnancy—optimal regimen for fetal thyroid status. *N Engl J Med* 315:24–28, 1986.
52. Marchant B, Brownlie BEW, Hart DM, et al.: The placental transfer of propylthiouracil, methimazole and carbimazole. *J Clin Endocrinol Metab* 45:1187–1193, 1977.
53. Becker DV: Choice of therapy for Graves' hyperthyroidism. *N Engl J Med* 311:464–466, 1984.
54. Nikolai TF, Turney SL, Roberts RG: Postpartum lymphocytic thyroiditis—prevalence, clinical course, and long-term follow-up. *Arch Intern Med* 147:221–224, 1987.

Asthma in Pregnancy

55. Schatz M, Patterson R, Zeitz S, et al.: Corticosteroid therapy for the pregnant asthmatic patient. *JAMA* 233:804–807, 1975.
56. Greenberger P, Patterson R: Safety of therapy for allergic symptoms during pregnancy. *Ann Intern Med* 89:234–237, 1978.
57. Weinstein AM, Dubin BD, Podleski WK, et al.: Asthma and pregnancy. *JAMA* 241:1161–1165, 1979.
58. Turner ES, Greenberger PA, Patterson R, et al.: Management of the pregnant asthmatic patient. *Ann Intern Med* 93:905–918, 1980.
59. Greenberger PA, Patterson R: Management of asthma during pregnancy. *N Engl J Med* 312:897–902, 1985.
60. Ziment I, Au JP: Managing asthma in the pregnant patient. *J Respir Dis* 9:66–74, 1988.

Neurologic Disorders in Pregnancy

61. Hopkins A: Neurologic disorders. *Clin Obstet Gynecol* 4:419–433, 1977.
62. Montouris GD, Fenichel GM, McLain LW: The pregnant epileptic. *Arch Neurol* 36:601–603, 1979.
63. Donaldson JO: *Neurology of Pregnancy, Major Problems in Neurology,* vol 7. Philadelphia, WB Saunders, 1978.

Neurologic Diseases in Pregnancy

64. Dalessio DJ: Seizure disorders and pregnancy. *N Engl J Med* 312:559–563, 1985.
65. Nelson LM, Franklin GM, Jones MC: Risk of multiple sclerosis exacerbation during pregnancy and breast feeding. *JAMA* 259:3441–3443, 1988.
66. Nazir M: When myotonic dystrophy complicates pregnancy. *Medical Aspects of Human Sexuality* 72–83, 1987.

Infectious Diseases in Pregnancy

67. Levine MM, Edsall G, Bruce Chwatt LJ: Live-virus vaccines in pregnancy-risks and recommendations. *Lancet* 34–38, 1974.
68. Safety of antimicrobial drugs in pregnancy. In Abramowicz A (ed): *The Medical Letter* 27:93–95, 1985.
69. Kean BH: Clinical toxoplasmosis: 50 years. *Trans R Soc Trop Med Hygiene* 66:549–571, 1972.
70. Desmonts G, Couvreur J: Congenital toxoplasmosis: A prospective study of 378 pregnancies. *N Engl J Med* 290:1110–1116, 1974.
71. Frenkel JK: Congenital toxoplasmosis: prevention or palliation? *Am J Obstet Gynecol* 141:359–361, 1981.
72. Schwarz RH, Crombleholme WR: Antibiotics in pregnancy. *South Med J* 72:1315–1318, 1979.
73. Weinstein AJ: Treatment of bacterial infections in pregnancy. *Drugs* 17:56–65, 1979.
74. Flanagan, P, Hensler NM: The course of active tuberculosis complicated by pregnancy. *JAMA* 109:783–787, 1959.
75. Schwartz RH: Considerations of antibiotic therapy during pregnancy. *Obstet Gynecol* 58:95S–99S, 1981.

Hematology

76. Perkins RP: Thrombocytopenia in obstetric syndromes: A review. *Obstet Gynecol Surv* 34:101–114, 1979.
77. Burrows RF, Kelton JG: Incidentally detected thrombocytopenia in healthy mothers and their infants. *N Engl J Med* 319:142–145, 1988.
77a. Newland AC, Boots MA, Patterson KG: Intravenous IgG for autoimmune thrombocytopenia in pregnancy. *N Engl J Med* 310:261–262, 1984.
78. Carloss HW, McMillan R, Crosby WH: Management of pregnancy in women with immune thrombocytopenic purpura. *JAMA* 244:2756–2758, 1980.
79. Cines DB, Dusak B, Tomaski A, et al.: Immune thrombocytopenic purpura and pregnancy. *N Engl J Med* 306:826–831, 1982.
80. Fehr J, Hofmann V, Kappeler U: Transient reversal of thrombocytopenia in idiopathic thrombocytopenic purpura by high-dose intravenous gamma globulin. *N Engl J Med* 306:1254–1258, 1982.
81. Hoffman PC: Idiopathic thrombocytopenic purpura in pregnancy. *Clin Perinatol* 12:599–607, 1985.
82. Morris J, Wiser W: The use of prophylactic partial exchange transfusion in pregnancies associated with sickle cell hemoglobinopathies. *Obstet Gynecol* 48:516–520, 1976.
83. Koshy M, Burd L, Wallace D, et al.: Prophylactic red-cell transfusions in pregnant patients with sickle cell disease—a randomized cooperative study. *N Engl J Med* 319:1447–1452, 1988.

Collagen Vascular Diseases

84. Persellin RH: The effect of pregnancy on rheumatoid arthritis. *Bull Rheum Dis* 27:922–927, 1976–77 series.
85. Karlen JR, Cook WA: Renal scleroderma and pregnancy. *Obstet Gynecol* 44:349–354, 1974.
86. Cook WA: Raynaud phenomenon in pregnancy (letter). *JAMA* 235:145–146, 1976.
87. Ballou SP, Morley JJ, Kushner I: Pregnancy and systemic sclerosis. *Arthritis Rheum* 27:295–298, 1984.
88. Scarpinato L, Mackenzie AH: Pregnancy and progressive systemic sclerosis. Case report and review of the literature. *Cleve Clin Q* 52:207–211, 1985.
88a. Steen VD, et al.: Pregnancy in women with systemic sclerosis. *Arthritis Rheum* 32:151–157, 1989.
89. Scott JS: Systemic lupus erythematosus and allied disorders in pregnancy. *Clin Obstet Gynecol* 6:461–471, 1979.
90. Zulman JI, Tali N, Hoffman GS, et al.: Problems associated with the management of pregnancies in patients with systemic lupus erythematosus. *J Rheumatol* 7:37–49, 1980.
91. Fine LG, Barnett EV, Gabriel M, et al.: Systemic lupus erythematosus in pregnancy. *Ann Intern Med* 94:667–677, 1981.
92. Bobrie G, Liote F, Houillier P, et al.: Pregnancy in lupus nephritis and related disorders. *Am J Kidney Dis* IX:339–343, 1987.
93. Hughes GRV, Harris NN, Gharavi, AE: The anticardiolipin syndrome. *J Rheum* 13:486–488, 1986.
94. Branch DW, Scott JR, Kochenour NK, et al.: Obstetric complications associated with the lupus anticoagulant. *N Engl J Med* 313:1322–1326, 1985.
95. Litsey SE, Noonan JA, O'Connor WN, et al.: Maternal connective tissue disease and congenital heart block. Demonstration of immunoglobulin in cardiac tissue. *N Engl J Med* 312:98–100, 1985.
96. Gutierrez G, Dagnino R, Mintz G: Polymyositis/dermatomyositis and pregnancy. *Arthritis Rheum* 27:291–294, 1984.
97. Berkowitz RL, Coustan DR, Mochizuki TK: *Handbook for Prescribing Medications during Pregnancy*. Boston, Little, Brown & Co, 1981.

Renal Disease

98. Kass EH: Bacteriuria and pyelonephritis of pregnancy. *Arch Intern Med* 105:194–198, 1960.
99. Brumfitt W: The effects of bacteriuria in pregnancy on maternal and fetal health. *Kidney Int* 8:S113–S119, 1975.
100. Little PJ: Incidence of urinary infection in 5000 pregnant women. *Lancet* 2:925–928, 1966.

101. Naeye RL: Causes of the excessive rates of perinatal mortality and prematurity in pregnancies complicated by maternal urinary-tract infections. *N Engl J Med* 300:819–823, 1979.
102. Strong DW, Murchison RW, Lynch DF: Management of ureteral calculi during pregnancy. *Gynecol Obstet* 146:604–608, 1978.
103. Coe FL, Parks JH, Lindheimer MD: Nephrolithiasis during pregnancy. *N Engl J Med* 298:324–326, 1978.
104. Kumar R, Cohen WR, Epstein FH: Vitamin D and calcium hormones in pregnancy. *N Engl J Med* 302:1143–1144, 1980.
105. Loughlin KR, Bailey RB: Internal ureteral stents for conservative management of ureteral calculi during pregnancy. *N Engl J Med* 315:1647–1649, 1986.
106. Bear RA: Pregnancy in patients with renal diseases. A study of 44 cases. *Obstet/Gynecol* 48:13–18, 1976.
107. Leppert P, Tisher C, Cheng S, et al.: Antecedent renal disease and the outcome of pregnancy. *Ann Intern Med* 90:747–751, 1979.
108. Hou S: Pregnancy in women with chronic renal disease. *N Engl J Med* 312:836–839, 1985.
109. Ferris TF: Pregnancy and chronic renal diseases. *Kidney* 19:1–3, 1986.
110. Finkelstein FO, Kashgarian M, Hayslett JP: Clinical spectrum of postpartum renal failure. *Am J Med* 57:649–654, 1974.
111. Sun NC, Johnson WJ, Sung DT, et al.: Idiopathic postpartum renal failure: Review and case report of a successful renal transplantation. *Mayo Clin Proc* 50:394–401, 1975.
112. Hayslett JP: Postpartum renal failure. *N Engl J Med* 312:1556–1559, 1985.

Gastrointestinal and Hepatobiliary Disorders in Pregnancy

113. Schweitzer IL, Dunn A, Peters R, et al.: Viral hepatitis B in neonates and infants. *Am J Med* 55:762–771, 1973.
114. Beasley RP, Lin C-C, Wang KY, et al.: Hepatitis B immune globulin (HBIG) efficacy in the interruption of perinatal transmission of hepatitis B virus carrier state—initial report of a randomised doubled-blind placebo-controlled trial. *Lancet* 2:388–393, 1981.
115. Snydman DR: Hepatitis in pregnancy. *N Engl J Med* 313:1398–1401, 1985.
116. Holzbach RT: Jaundice in pregnancy—1976. *Am J Med* 61:367–376, 1976.
117. Rencoret R, Aste II: Jaundice during pregnancy. *Med J Aust* 1:167–169, 1973.
118. Varma RR, Michelsohn NH, Borkowk HI, et al.: Pregnancy in cirrhotic and non-cirrhotic portal hypertension. *Obstet/Gynecol* 50:217–222, 1977.
119. Cheng Y-S: Pregnancy in liver cirrhosis and/or portal hypertension. *Am J Obstet Gynecol* 128:812–822, 1977.
120. Varner M, Rinderknecht NK: Acute fatty metamorphosis in pregnancy: Maternal mortality and literature review. *J Reprod Med* 24:177–180, 1980.
121. Kaplan MM: Acute fatty liver of pregnancy. *N Engl J Med* 313:367–370, 1985.
122. Riely CA, et al.: Acute fatty liver of pregnancy. *Ann Intern Med* 106:703–706, 1987.
123. Rolfes DB, Ishak KG: Acute fatty liver of pregnancy: A clinicopathologic study of 35 cases. *Hepatology* 5:1149–1158, 1985.
124. Kammerer W: Non-obstetric surgery during pregnancy. *Med Clin North Am* 63:1157–1164, 1979.
125. Homan WP, Thorbjarnarson B: Crohn's disease and pregnancy. *Arch Surg* 111:545–547, 1976.
126. Donaldson LB: Crohn's disease: "Its gynecologic aspect." *Am J Obstet Gynecol* 131:196–202, 1978.
127. Donaldson RM: Management of medical problems in pregnancy—inflammatory bowel disease. *N Engl J Med* 312:1616–1618, 1985.
128. Tresadern JC, Falconer GF, Turnberg LA, et al.: Maintenance of pregnancy in a home parenteral nutrition patient. *JEPN* 8:199–202, 1984.
129. DeDombal FT, Watts JM, Watkinson G, et al.: Ulcerative colitis and pregnancy. *Lancet* 2:559–601, 1965.
130. Webb MJ, Sedlack RE: Ulcerative colitis and pregnancy. *Med Clin North Am* 58:823–827, 1974.

23

Evaluation of the Healthy Patient and the Ambulatory Surgery Patient

Richard J. Gross

A consensus has not been reached currently on the appropriate extent of the routine medical evaluation of the preoperative patient. This is due to the lack of data and clinical agreement. Other important factors are marked changes in clinical practice recently, the large number of patients (now over 50% of surgical patients) having outpatient surgery or same-day admission for surgery, general opinion that traditional, routine laboratory work has a low yield, and cost-cutting efforts.

Traditionally, the medical evaluation of the surgical patient by the internist has included the basic components of a comprehensive history and physical, admission laboratory work, chest x-ray, and EKG. Recently, more limited laboratory work has been recommended by expert consensus (1, 3); little information is available on more limited approaches to the history and physical examination.

The approach to the medical evaluation of the preoperative patient in this chapter will be based on the *limited* available data, expert consensus, clinical practices, and the author's experience (in the absence of definitive studies or expert consensus). Some of the recommendations are based on very limited data and the absence of expert consensus, but we felt that a practical approach to this type of evaluation is needed by internists, even in the absence of complete information.

This chapter will first discuss the basic evaluation of the "healthy" patient, fol-lowed by special aspects in the evaluation of the patient for ambulatory surgery or same-day surgical admission. There will also be a general discussion of cost-benefit (yield) studies in the preoperative patient, and then a summary of the literature on yield of preoperative diagnostic testing, so the reader can review the basis for our recommendations.

EVALUATION OF THE HEALTHY PATIENT

The basic medical evaluation preoperatively of the surgical patient, includes the core evaluation common to the patient who is presumably healthy other than his primary surgical disease and to the patient with multiple other illnesses. In the patient with multiple nonsurgical illnesses, additional clinical examination and laboratory testing will need to be added to further evaluate other diseases, but the core evaluation serves as a basic minimum for all other systems. This chapter will discuss this core evaluation; evaluation of other nonsurgical diseases is discussed in the appropriate organ system chapters. Decision making is discussed in Chapter 3 (p. 18).

History and Physical

Almost no objective studies are available, and there is no agreement among experts (see p. 628), to guide recommendations for the extent of the history and physical examination preoperatively. The numerous factors influencing the extent of examination make general rules difficult to apply to the individual patient. *Important factors that affect the extent of examination needed include the patient's age, interval since last comprehensive physical examination, type of anesthesia planned (general vs. spinal vs. regional/local), and nature of the surgery (minor, major).* Other considerations are discussed on p. 626, such as establishing a baseline for anticipated postoperative changes or complications.

The traditional consultation has included a comprehensive history and physical examination, EKG, chest x-ray urinalysis, and blood work (complete blood count, tests of hemostasis, blood urea nitrogen, creatinine, glucose, electrolytes, liver function tests; possibly 20 chemistry screens, serologic test for syphilis [STS]). This approach has been criticized for having low yield and high cost (1–3). At the other extreme, some analysis of the cost-benefits of preoperative testing have indicated that only a very limited examination or testing is worthwhile (this approach has *not* been proven) (3).

A practical approach we have used is *to select one of two general types of preoperative evaluation (Table 23.1): either a limited or comprehensive workup.* Guidelines for choosing between these alternative workups (Table 23.2) can be outlined generally, but the multiple factors in an individual patient listed above preclude rigid rules for choosing the type of workup. Generally, limited workups are appropriate for patients under age 40, with a recent (less than 1 year) complete physical examination, who are generally healthy without major organ system disease, and having local or regional anesthesia for a minor procedure. The comprehensive examination is more appropriate for inpatient consultations or patients previously unknown to the internist; the limited examination for patients previously seen by the internist undergoing minor outpatient surgery. In borderline situations, we would continue to err on the side of more

Table 23.1. General Preoperative History and Physical: Comprehensive vs. Limited Examination

Component of Workup	Limited Workup[a]	Comprehensive Workup[a]
History	HPI[b], past med. hx, allergies, medications; heart, lungs, hemostasis, endocrine, family hx of surgical/anesthesia problems, and new symptoms (especially upper respiratory infection)	HPI[b], past med hx, social hx, family, hx, allergies, medications, brief review of all systems
Physical examination	Vital signs, oral cavity, chest, heart, and abdomen	Complete physical examination
Laboratory[a]	Hematocrit, urinalysis, EKG (some cases >age 35), serum potassium (some cases), pregnancy test[c]	Chest x-ray, EKG (>age 35), complete blood count, blood urea nitrogen or serum creatinine, serum glucose, serum electrolytes, urinalysis, pregnancy test[c]

[a] Basic evaluation for screening and baseline data. Other tests may be added to evaluate known disease in a patient or to follow up findings in the preoperative history and physical examination see also Table 23.3.
[b] Abbreviations: HPI = history of present illness; hx = history.
[c] Women in childbearing age group.
(From Gross RJ: Preoperative planning for the ambulatory patient. In RL Barker, et al. (eds): *Principles of Ambulatory Medicine.* Baltimore, Williams & Wilkins, 1990, (in press) with permission.)

Table 23.2. Guidelines for Selecting the Type of General Preoperative Evaluation

Limited Workup	Comprehensive Workup
Age < 40	Age > 40 (especially > 60)
Established patient, previously examined by physician	New patient, unknown to physician
Recent comprehensive physical exam	No, old, or inadequate data base
Well patient	Patient with moderate-severe major organ disease
Local, regional, or spinal anesthesia	General anesthesia
Minor procedure	Major procedure (especially thoracic, abdominal, neurosurgical)

(From: Gross RJ: Preoperative planning for the ambulatory patient. In RL Barker, et al. (eds): *Principles of Ambulatory Medicine.* Baltimore, Williams & Wilkins, 1990 (in press) with permission.)

extensive workups, until more data are available on the adequacy of limited workups. Limited workups are not usually appropriate for patients with major organ system disease (cardiopulmonary, renal, liver, CNS), chronically ill patients, old patients without recent physical examinations, for very major procedures, and for patients who have major undiagnosed symptoms (e.g., chest pain).

The comprehensive workup is basically the traditional complete physical examination, with the omission of a few items of clinically low yield (i.e., the neurologic examination, except for mental status in the elderly). The limited examination includes more items than most "bare bones" analysis based on clinical experience. Obviously, other items should be added to either examination to further evaluate the patient's surgical disease or other known medical problems.

Additional questions need to be asked as part of the history in the preoperative patient that are not routinely asked or emphasized in routine medical patients (Table 23.4). Specific questions should include bleeding history from the patient, especially if clotting studies are not routinely obtained (see below and p. 325). A history of prior anesthesia should be obtained with inquiry about any anesthetic problems, particularly high unexplained fever or jaundice postoperatively (malignant hyperthermia, halogenated hydrocarbon anesthesia hepatitis). A history of

Table 23.3. Additional Preoperative Screening Tests for Common High-Risk Situations

High-Risk Situation	Screening Tests
Patient undergoing neurosurgical, cardiac, or vascular, or major abdominal procedure	Tests of hemostasis: platelet count, prothrombin time, partial thromboplastin time
Patient on diuretics, with vomiting/diarrhea, other abnormal fluid loss, cardiac disease, renal disease	Electrolytes
Patient with increased risk of active liver disease (e.g., alcoholism, drug addiction, homosexuality, dialysis patient, high-risk medications) who is undergoing general or spinal anesthesia	Liver function tests: serum aminotransferases, alkaline phosphatase, bilirubin hepatitis-associated antigen
Patient with increased risk of chronic pulmonary disease (e.g., smoker with ≥ 10 pack years) who is undergoing general anesthesia	Pulmonary function tests (see p. 60)
Patient with increased risk of tuberculosis (e.g., known exposure, underprivileged population, HIV-positive)	Chest x-ray, purified protein derivative skin test
Patient with increased risk of coronary artery disease (i.e., smoker, hypertensive, strong family history, diabetic, hyperlipidemia)	EKG
Malnourished patient or prolonged inability to eat.	Nutritional assessment (see p. 38)
Patient with cancer	Liver function tests, calcium

From: Gross RJ: Preoperative planning for the ambulatory patient. In RL Barker, et al. (eds): *Principles of Ambulatory Medicine.* Baltimore, Williams & Wilkins, 1990 (in press) with permission.

Table 23.4. Supplemental Screening History-Taking in the Surgical Patient (Medical Preoperative Evaluation)

1. Have you ever had abnormal bleeding, or been told you are a bleeder? (See also Tables 23.5 and 23.6).
2. Have you ever had a blood transfusion? If yes, any reaction *including* fever?
3. Have you ever had any problem with anesthesia, including fever?
4. Is anyone in your family a bleeder; or had problems (including fever) with anesthesia? or a blood transfusion?
5. What medications do you take? Do you take any nonprescribed (over-the-counter) drugs, including pills patients often don't consider medication (such as birth control pills/hormones, vitamin pills, or aspirin)?
6. Any history of alcohol or illicit-drug use?

Table 23.5. Brief, Screening Bleeding History[a,b]

1. Do you develop large bruises without a good reason? Have you bled a long time after minor cuts or trauma to your tongue, cheek, or lip? If so, how old were you when this began?
2. Have you had teeth extracted? If so, which ones? How long did you bleed after extraction? Did bleeding start up again a day or so later?
3. What operations have you had? Was bleeding after surgery or childbirth hard to stop? Were transfusions necessary? Did your wounds heal well?
4. Have you had general medical problems? What are these and how are they being treated? Have you had kidney, liver, or arthritic diseases?
5. What medicines do you take? Do you use over-the-counter drugs for colds, allergy, headaches, arthritis, menstrual cramps, backaches, or other pains? Have you taken any medicines, including antibiotics within the last 7–10 days?
6. Do you have any blood relatives who have experienced prolonged or excessive bleeding?

[a] Reproduced from Table 14.7; see p. 325 for discussion.
[b] Modified from Rappaport SI: Preoperative hemostatic evaluation: Which tests, if any? *Blood* 61:229–231, 1983.

prior transfusion and any reactions, especially fever (leukocyte sensitization) should be obtained. Family history should specifically ask for bleeding problems, anesthesia problems, as described above, and transfusion reactions. Although these questions ask about relatively rare problems, the problems are potentially catastrophic, and are not or cannot be screened for by other means. A few well-worded screening questions (Table 23.4) can cover these items quickly; an extensive question list is not needed unless something abnormal is present.

History of medication use should emphasize recent aspirin and aspirin-containing compound use, over-the-counter and nonprescribed compounds (again looking for aspirin), diuretics/hormones, and drugs patients often don't consider "medication" (aspirin and birth control pills are often omitted by patients). Alcohol and illicit drug use pose special problems for the anesthesiologist as well as the internist postoperatively and should be specifically inquired for.

Bleeding histories can vary from a single question to a prolonged, time-consuming review. Relatively brief lists of screening questions have been developed (see refs. 34, 35), but not well validated. A reasonable, brief screening bleeding history is described on p. 325 (reproduced in Table 23.5). Similar questions have been incorporated into patient self-completed questionnaires, which are widely used but not well validated. An extensive bleeding history is described in Table 23.6. We feel that at least the abbreviated bleeding history (Table 23.5), ought to be reviewed for patients with all but very minor surgery either by the physician or questionnaire.

Laboratory Tests

More studies (see pp. 628–635) are available on the yield and benefit of preoperative laboratory tests than the clinical examination, but many more confounding factors influence the selection of tests. Most studies only look at one factor (positive tests that change therapy) and not the many factors that influence the clinician's decision. Thus, while the available literature provides general guidelines, absolute rules cannot be given. The

Table 23.6.   Extensive Bleeding History and Physical Examination

A. **History**
1. Bleeding during childhood (circumcision, tonsillectomy and adenoidectomy, epistaxis, joints, soft tissues, lacerations)
2. Extent of bruising from minor trauma; any spontaneous bruising (including minor lacerations, and biting mouth) (ask specifically about bruises on trunk or abdomen, quantitate size)
3. Any delayed or delayed recurrent (more than 12–24 hours) postoperative bleeding; prolonged bleeding after surgery or procedures (more than 24 hours)
4. Menses
5. Dental extractions or work
6. Procedures (cardiac catheterization, etc.).
7. Prior surgery (abnormal or late bleeding)
8. Predisposing diseases (uremia, liver disease, malabsorption, malnutrition, autoimmune disease)
9. Medications (ASA, ASA-compounds, some NSAID, coumadin, heparin, medications high risk for thrombocytopenia, radiation therapy, chemotherapy)
10. Transfusions
11. Alcohol use
12. Family history of bleeding disorder

B. **Physical examination**
1. Signs of bleeding on skin and mucous membranes
2. Telangectasia, skin signs of liver or renal disease
3. Hepatosplenomegaly
4. Lymphadenopathy

approach we have used is to select one of two types of general preoperative testing: either a limited or comprehensive workup (Tables 23.1, 23.2, and 23.3), compatible with the approach used for the history/physical examination in the previous section. *General guidelines for choosing between limited and comprehensive laboratory testing are given (Table 23.2), but the many factors influencing an individual case need to be considered by the physician.*

The comprehensive workup includes most of the admission laboratory tests traditionally used by internists, with the deletion of routine liver enzymes, SMA-20 multichannel chemistry tests, clotting tests, and differential white count, which have not been shown to be of high yield. The limited laboratory workup includes a bare minimum on which there is consensus by most experts. It is appropriate for young, healthy patients, undergoing local or regional anesthesia, for minor procedures. Some additional laboratory tests, such as electrolytes, will be indicated by the history or clinical examination in most other circumstances.

Additional laboratory screening tests need to be added when the history-physical examination identifies certain high-risk groups (Table 23.3). Laboratory tests also need to be added to these basic panels to evaluate known or newly discovered medical problems (e.g., heart disease), the primary surgical problem, and as a baseline for potential postoperative problems in major surgery.

Non-invasive cardiac tests are covered in Chapter 10 (pp. 113–114).

A discussion of management appears on p. 622.

EVALUATION OF THE AMBULATORY SURGERY PATIENT

The number of surgical patients having their medical preoperative evaluation as outpatients has increased dramatically from almost none 15 years ago. Currently, in many hospitals, 50% or more of surgical cases are done as outpatients (Fig. 23.1); this does not include the many patients who are admitted the same morning as inpatient major surgery and, hence, have an outpatient medical consultation. More surgeons are requesting outpatient medical consultation, to avoid cancelling inpatient cases the night before, with the resultant utilization denials and a loss of operating room time (Table 23.8). A wide variety of surgical procedures are done on an outpatient basis, including those requiring general anesthesia (Tables 23.7a, 23.7b).

The medical preoperative evaluation of

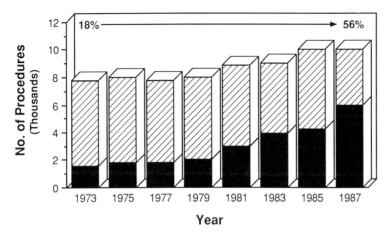

Figure 23.1. Numbers of ambulatory procedures (black bars) and surgical procedures (hatched bars) by year at Norwalk (Conn.) community hospital. Slightly modified from Laffaye HA: The impact of an ambulatory surgical service in a community hospital. *Arch Surg* 124:601, 1989, with permission. Copyright 1989, the American Medical Association.

surgical patients as outpatients in the office poses a number of unique problems not found or common in hospital settings. The two types of clinical and laboratory evaluation in the preceding section still apply to the outpatient setting; the differences in factors influencing the extent of the evaluation in the outpatient setting will be discussed below. There are also several management issues unique to the outpatient setting.

This section will include as "ambulatory" surgical patients both the patient for totally outpatient surgery and the patient admitted the morning of major, inpatient surgery. While this is not the usual definition of this term (which is usually applied to totally ambulatory surgery), both types of patients raise many similar

Table 23.7a.   Most Common Outpatient Surgical Procedures at One Connecticut Community Hospital[a]

1. Intraocular lens
2. Breast biopsy
3. Dilation and curettage
4. Myringotomy
5. Knee procedure
6. Hernia repair

[a]Data from ref. 6.

Table 23.7b.   Selected Procedures Not Routinely Reimbursed for Inpatient Stay in Maryland by Medicare (Proposed)

1. *Cardiovascular*
   Varicose vein ligation
2. *ENT*
   Myringotomy
   Many nasal and sinus operations
3. *Gastrointestinal*
   Endoscope
   Incision of perianal abscess
   Hemorrhoid procedures
   Unilateral inguinal hernia repair
4. *Gynecologic*
   D&C
   Laparoscope
   Local excision vaginal tumor
   Pelvic exam under anesthesia
5. *Ophthalmological*
   Cataract
6. *Orthopedic*
   Carpal tunnel release
   Bunionectomy
   Arthroscopy
   Trigger finger release
7. *Radiology*
   Arteriogram
   Myelogram
8. *Urology*
   Prostate biopsy
   Cystoscope
   Bladder biopsy
   Orchiectomy
9. *Other*
   Breast biopsy

Table 23.8.   Outpatient Preoperative Assessment—Why?

1. Same-day surgical centers (insurance)
2. Inpatient surgery—no preoperative days
3. Eliminates inefficiency of last-minute surgical cancellation for patient, surgeon, hospital/operating room/anesthesiologist, insurance company (cost).
4. Better care
5. Better patient satisfaction

Table 23.9.   Current Guidelines on Patient Eligibility for Ambulatory Surgery Based on Medical Condition (*Not* Considering Type of Surgery)

1. ASA Class I–II (some Class III for minor procedures)
2. Stable, compensated chronic medical problems; absence of acute medical problems.
3. No recent MI, unstable cardiac disease, or decompensated lung disease
4. If diabetic, not on insulin; if on insulin, stable, not brittle; patient capable of and able postoperatively to do self-monitoring (insulin-dependent diabetics should be done *early* in the morning)

issues for the internist (i.e., both have their preoperative medical evaluation on an outpatient basis).

This section assumes the prior section on evaluation of the healthy patient has been read.

Organizational Issues

The organization or rules for preoperative medical evaluation for ambulatory surgery vary widely between hospitals and recommendations by authors. Several policy issues ought to be firmly established in hospital policy (but often are not), and in the consulting internist's practice, because of the fragmentation of outpatient workups. These will also be useful to internists on hospital committees setting local hospital policy. Only an outline of recommendations can be given, because of the absence of a solid research base or even of a good description of current practices.

The first issue is: which patients are candidates for ambulatory surgery without admission, based on medical considerations (Table 23.9) (surgical considerations will not be discussed). However, these *medical* guidelines must be adjusted in light of the type of surgery and the individual situation. Even some excluded types of patients may undergo outpatient surgery under certain conditions, such as if the surgery is very minor (e.g., minor abscess drainage). Criteria for allowing outpatient surgery have continued to be liberalized over the past several years. Although initially, elderly patients were

excluded from outpatient surgery, there is currently no accepted maximum age limit. Most centers will not allow ambulatory surgery on many ASA (American Society of Anesthesiologists) Class III and any ASA Class IV or V patients. Some *stable* ASA Class III patients can have outpatient minor surgery, based on individual circumstances. Patients with unstable major organ medical disease generally need overnight observation. Recent acute myocardial infarction, unstable cardiovascular disease, or other types are generally considered contraindications to outpatient surgery. Juvenile-type, brittle diabetics usually require hospital admission for intravenous fluids and observation of glucoses.

Secondly, policies need to be established regarding *responsibility* for coordinating outpatient evaluation, management, and follow-up of medical problems (Table 23.10). A single person or at least clear lines of responsibility need to be delineated, since the internist may do the preoperative physical, the surgeon may obtain the laboratory results, and the anesthesiologist may be the one to interview the patient about changes in condition from the time of the physical to surgery. Clearly, there is a large possibility of loss of information (lab results), or errors in judgment based on poor coordination (e.g., the internist didn't know the patient's angina got worse). The various issues that need to be considered are given

Table 23.10. Recommended Hospital Policy Issues Regarding Administrative Aspects of Preoperative Evaluation

1. When should evaluation be done before surgery (? 24 hrs. to 7–10 days)?
2. Who does the evaluation (internist, surgeon, anesthesiologist, hospital nurse practitioner)?
3. What laboratory, EKG, and x-rays are routinely required by simple categories (age, presence/absence chronic disease). Where will lab work be done (? required at hospital)?
4. Who receives the laboratory, EKG, and x-ray results. (If sent to the surgeon, need to establish mechanism for internist to be routinely notified of abnormal results, **as well as surgeon**.)
5. Who is responsible for compiling data on history/physical, lab, EKG, and x-ray—making sure it was all completed, and making decisions regarding surgery based on results (surgeon, internist, anesthesiologist)?
6. What is the mechanism or who is responsible person to notify internist **routinely** if all abnormal results (#4) or changes in surgical plans (#5), if these are done by surgeon.
7. Who sends a copy of laboratory, EKG, and x-ray results to consulting internist even if normal (may go through normal channels or mail, as long as mechanism of notification of abnormal results)?
8. Who is responsible for interviewing patient on day of surgery, to see if an interval illness or worsened chronic disease has developed since medical evaluation days before; how is this to be documented? (This **cannot** be the internist.)
9. Who is responsible for instructing patient on preoperative orders (e.g., NPO after midnight)? Does this person know he should instruct about medical considerations—a.m. medications, ASA, patient to call if interval illness, etc.; see Table 23.12)?
10. Who is responsbile for postoperative patient instructions? Does this person know to give medical instructions (e.g., resumption of preoperative medications, call internist if worsened chest pain, etc.) (see Table 23.12).

in Table 23.10). From the internist's point of view, it is crucial he/she either obtain, personally review, or make certain an iron-clad system exists at the hospital to notify him/her of abnormal lab results. The person responsible for notification of changes in condition by the patient, and for instructing the patient on taking medications the morning of surgery and resumption postoperatively, should be clearly identified to all physicians *and to the patient.*

One person should really be responsible for coordinating this multifaceted effort. We believe that has to be the *surgeon,* since he/she is the only physician who has contact with all parties, and through the entire time span from preoperative evaluation through postoperative visit. In some hospitals, nurse practitioners are responsible for coordinating results and communication; this is acceptable as long as the practitioner relays abnormalities to *all* three physicians involved (not just the surgeon), and adequate physician backup is provided by the hospital for problem situations. This does not relieve the internist of the responsibility of reviewing laboratory data, instructing the patient, and assuring medical return appointment postoperatively, if needed.

A policy must be established regarding the appropriate interval before surgery for performance of the preoperative examination. Hospital policies vary between a maximum of 2 days to 2 weeks between examination and surgery. The longer interval makes administration of preoperative testing easier at the hospital since results are obtained well before surgery; it increases the chance of interval illnesses. Although no data are available, we feel that more than a 1 week interval between examination and surgery is too long for most chronically ill or elderly patients; a slightly longer interval of 10 days *may be* acceptable in an otherwise well, young, reliable patient. The shorter end of the interval usually depends on administrative convenience, rather than on medical considerations.

Other issues include where the laboratory, EKG, and x-ray are obtained (community laboratory versus hospital), and how the workup gets from the internist's office to the hospital (patient- versus physician-carried; the mails are too slow).

The routine preoperative medical evaluation is performed by different types of practitioners in different hospitals, including the primary physician (family practitioner or internist), surgeon, anesthesiologist, or hospital-based nurse practitioner or physician assistant (this is separate from preoperative medical consultation for a specific problem). No data and insufficient experience exist to show one practitioner is preferable. The allied health practitioners need physician supervision; we also feel they should be trained specifically in preoperative assessment, which is infrequently done. However, regardless of who does the *routine* preoperative evaluation, the internist should be involved on either a primary or consultative basis for chronically ill patients, patients with major organ disease, abnormal laboratory studies, and other high-risk patients.

Diagnostic Activities and Approaches

The selection of the extent of evaluation (see pp. 614) (Tables 23.1, 23.2; pp. 615) in the outpatient setting is influenced by the fact that the internist often knows the patient well (and has referred him to the surgeon); most surgical procedures done on an outpatient basis are minor; and only local or regional anesthesia will be required. Thus, for many similar ambulatory surgical patients, a limited workup will suffice.

However, a compelling reason for a comprehensive work-up exists at the other end of the spectrum, when an outpatient is seen for the first time by the internist for preoperative consultation. The internist will not have an opportunity to observe the patient even briefly for 12 hours overnight and will not see the patient postoperatively with the opportunity to make quick adjustments for preoperative oversights. Thus, the elderly, multiply chronically ill patient seen for the first time in consultation for outpatient surgery needs more attention than the same patient for an inpatient procedure.

We have identified several aspects of

clinical history-physical examination and management that are frequently forgotten in the outpatient setting (Tables 23.11, 23.12). The patient's problem list should be reviewed specifically with diseases increasing operative risk in mind. The patient who appears generally ill from multiple diseases or malnutrition should not be underestimated because no one disease is severe. Medication history is important, including over-the-counter medications, recent corticosteroid use (within 1 year), aspirin, and anticoagulant use. Frequently forgotten tests include pregnancy tests, blood tests indicated by medications (e.g., potassium in a patient on diuretics or drug levels), spirometry in the pulmonary patient, echocardiogram for evaluation for need for SBE prophylaxis.

Management

Commonly forgotten or inadequately done aspects of management in medical preoperative consultation include instructions to patients on discontinuation of habits affecting surgical risk (such as smoking) and medication administration immediately pre- and postoperatively (Tables 23.12, 23.13). Prophylaxis for sub-

---

Table 23.11. Commonly Forgotten or Underestimated Items of History-Physical-Lab In Medical Evaluation of the Ambulatory Surgical Patient[a]

1. One disease (review the problem list)
2. The generally sick patient
3. Medications (include ASA, birth control pills, over-the-counter drugs)
4. Inquiry about recent steroid use; evaluation of murmurs (? need for SBE prophylaxis)
5. Blood tests indicated by specific medical diseases or medications (e.g., drug levels, potassium for diuretics)
6. Pregnancy test (serum qualitative HCG)
7. Spirometry
8. Echocardiogram (evaluation of murmur regarding SBE prophylaxis)

---

[a] See also Table 23.4, p. 617.

Table 23.12. Commonly Forgotten Management Items in the Ambulatory Surgical Patient[a]

1. Tell patient to report to internist *and* surgeon even **minor intercurrent illnesses** (including minor "colds"), between physical and day of surgery. Also, postoperative problems of potential medical interest after surgery.
2. Order patient to stop **smoking, alcohol,** illicit **drugs, OTC medications** (no new OTC medications).
3. **Medication (preop) review**—what to do the a.m. of surgery regarding taking medicines when NPO. Discontinuing medications such as ASA, coumadin if indicated (and when to restart postoperatively).
4. **Corticosteroids**—administer or increase dose to cover stress (including patients who have recently been on but have discontinued steroids).
5. **SBE prophylaxis.**
6. **Teach patients** "what" to expect pre- and postoperatively.
7. Tell surgeon to **notify internist** if medical problems outside certain limits postoperatively (e.g., blood pressure over 180/100), in certain situations or diseases.
8. **Medications** (postop)—when to restart postoperatively and what to do if unexpected problems arise (i.e., call internist).

[a] See also Table 23.4, p. 617.

acute bacterial endocarditis must be considered in advance, as special arrangements are usually required for intravenous antibiotics, especially if a second, postoperative dose is needed. The patient

Table 23.13. Medical Consultation Report for Ambulatory Surgery: Additional Recommendations

Recommendations:
1. Patient instructed to take all medications a.m. of surgery with sip of H_2O, except Lasix. Aspirin discontinued 7 days preop.
2. Please notify me if any intercurrent illnesses before surgery (patient also instructed).
3. Please notify me of any perioperative medical complications; if blood pressure under 120/60 or over 180/100; check postop Chemstix and notify me if under 100 or over 300 mg%.
4. Please instruct patient if he can resume aspirin day after surgery.
5. Please notify me of any abnormal laboratory data preoperatively.

should be instructed to notify the *internist as well as surgeon* about even minor condition changes or intercurrent illnesses between examination and surgery. Reasonable postoperative expectations in terms of symptoms of medical diseases should be explained to the patient, as well as indications to call the internist because of change in condition or need for medical adjustment. The consultation report should contain guidelines for the surgeon on notification of the internist if certain limits are exceeded for select diseases (e.g., blood pressure), but gratuitous statements should be avoided.

Some patients will require temporary medication adjustment preoperatively, such as dosage adjustment of insulin or blood pressure medication. Both the surgeon and patient should be given guidelines on when to notify the internist for dose adjustment, such as an unexpectedly prolonged time NPO for a diabetic, or lower than usual blood pressure at time of recovery room discharge.

The aforementioned recommendations are summarized succinctly for the surgeon in the consultation report (Table 23.13). A straightforward explanation to the patient will usually suffice; supplementation by a simple written sheet of instructions similar to Table 23.13 will encourage patient understanding and compliance.

Remember, elective surgery is elective. If the internist feels further evaluation is needed, a new problem is uncovered, or a patient is unstable, elective surgery should be delayed until the diagnostic investigation or a period of observation is completed (see Chap. 3).

The brief time between examination and surgery may not allow for preparation of a typewritten consultation note. Brief letters or notes written on prescription pads are not adequate. A sample of a formatted report that can be completed quickly in handwriting, but is still complete and understandable is given in Table 23.14 (see also pp. 624–625).

Table 23.14. Structured Medical Evaluation Report for Preoperative Patient [a]

GREATER BALTIMORE MEDICAL CENTER
6701 North Charles Street, Towson, Maryland 21204
HISTORY AND PHYSICAL, PAT WITH NURSE PRACTITIONER

Sex M F	Exam. Date	Medical Dr.	Age

CC/PI:

Family History:			MGP/PGP	Mother	Father	Siblings	Offspring
CA	CVA	Anesthesia					
DM	Kidney dis.	rxn.					
HBP	Liver dis.	Bleeding					
Cardiac	Anemia	Txn. rxn.					

Meds:	Allergies:	Anesthesia Complications:
	Tobacco:	Transfusion Rx:
	ETOH:	Coag hx: Bleeding; Clotting Phlebitis
	DRUGS:	

MEDICAL HISTORY	**SURGICAL HISTORY**
	MAJOR INJURIES:
LAST PAP	

[a] Adapted and reproduced with permission of the Greater Baltimore Medical Center, Baltimore, Md., and P. Dunning, CANP.

REVIEW OF SYSTEMS

EYES:	Glaucoma	
ENT:	Sinusitis, tinnitus, hearing loss, epistaxis, frequent sore throats, hoarseness	
CNS:	Seizures, dizziness, syncope, weakness, numbness, headaches	
ENDOCRINE:	Thyroid disease, recent weight change, thirst, DM	
BREASTS:	Lumps, pain, discharge	
CARDIOVASCULAR:	Chest pain, palpitations, edema, claudication, phlebitis	
PULMONARY:	SOB, hemoptysis, productive cough, wheezing, asthma, pneumonia	
GI:	Recent change in bowel habits, ulcer, HH, GB disease, colitis, hemorrhoids, dysphagia, abdominal pain, jaundice, blood in stools, melena	
GU:	Frequent UTI's, renal stones, dysuria, hematuria, frequency, nocturia	

PHYSICAL EXAM

Pulse	Blood Pressure Lying Sitting	Respiration	Temperature	Height	Weight

Integument: Skin, hair, nails	
Head/Neck: Skull, thyroid, carotids	
Eyes: Pupils, conj., sclera	
ENT: Canals, TM's, mucosa	
Lymph Nodes: Cervical, supraclavicular, axillary, ing	
Breasts: Symmetry, palpation, nipples	
Lungs: Respirations, percussion, breath sounds	
Heart: PMI, rhythm, ectopics, murmur	
Peripheral Vascular: Femoral, dorsalis pedis, distal	
Abdomen: Tenderness, masses, scars, inspection	
Extremities: Edema, varicosities, color	
Neuro: Motor, sensory, orientation	

Other Pertinent Findings:

Impression:

Recommendations:

Signed: _____

SELECTING PREOPERATIVE TESTS: AN OVERVIEW

Recently, interest has developed in defining which preoperative laboratory tests should be routinely performed on all surgical patients. Most of the information accumulated has been on the cost-yield of a few selected tests; sparse data are available on many tests, and recommendations must be based on clinical experience, despite its limitations.

Below, considerations other than cost-benefit analysis will be reviewed; these considerations are crucial in understanding the recommendations that follow. The methodology for deciding on a "good" screening laboratory test will be outlined. The recommendations for individual tests are based on cost-yield studies from the literature, where available; expert consensus; and our own clinical experience. *The reader should understand that the available data are limited, and clinical circumstances vary widely as do local community practices. Thus, the general recommendations will have to be adapted to the physician's individual setting and patient.* Medicolegal considerations remain a concern. The recommendations for laboratory screening will be directed at screening adult, presumably healthy, patients for anesthesia; additional testing may be needed to evaluate any known medical disease, high-risk groups (e.g., Table 23.3), and the primary surgical disease in the individual patient. The recommendations in this section are for major surgery, requiring general or spinal anesthesia; modifications will need to be made for less extensive procedures (Table 23.3).

Most of the literature analyzes only one factor: the cost-benefit (or yield) of preoperative laboratory testing. Many other important factors affect the clinical decision to perform preoperative tests (Table 23.15). Clinically important factors not considered in the research literature are the nature of surgery (major vs. minor),

Table 23.15. Considerations in Selecting Preopeative Laboratory Screening Tests (Other than Yield of Abnormal Results and Estimation of Anesthetic-Surgical Risk)

1. Interval since and quality of last physical examination; extent of preoperative exam
2. Inability to evaluate by history-physical examination in an individual patient (e.g., poor historian; distant heart sounds due to COPD)
3. Efficient evaluation of patients with known medical disease
4. Evaluation of primary surgical problem
5. Nature of surgery (major/minor; inpatient/outpatient)
6. Type of anesthesia (local, regional, spinal, general)
7. Other need for information:
    a. Estimate operative risk
    b. Rare abnormality resulting in marked change in surgical plans (e.g. incidental lung cancer on chest x-ray)
    c. Rare, catastrophic abnormality
    d. Baseline for postoperative change/complication
    e. Determining drug levels; monitoring drug effects
    f. Medicolegal documentation
    g. Avoiding harm to others (e.g., tuberculosis)
8. Cost-saving of standardized test batteries

type of anesthesia, estimation of operative risk in the decision for surgery, baseline for postoperative changes and complications, and the rare but catastrophic abnormality in the surgical setting (e.g., thrombocytopenia in the craniotomy patient). The high cost of such rare catastrophies has not been considered in most cost-benefit studies. The inefficiencies of individualized testing include physician time in selecting tests based on historical information and the loss of the cost-savings of mass batteries (e.g., SMA-6) of tests run routinely. Certain high-risk groups may be underscreened in selected testing, such as the elderly or diabetics. The need for medicolegal documentation is a very real consideration in preanesthetic laboratory testing, aside from medical indications.

Most studies evaluating laboratory testing have assumed a highly complete history, physical examination, or retrospectively-sought clinical data knowing the patient outcome. Clinical information is often not this complete and laboratory testing serves a larger back-up function in actual practice. Complicating factors are the multiple indications for selected testing (e.g., 30 indications for a chest x-ray alone in one study [20]), and the needs of multiple physicians (anesthesiologist, surgeon, internist). The immense practical difficulty in considering all of these factors in an individual patient on a daily basis is obvious. While it is not difficult to look of 10 different indications for a chest x-ray in a study of selective use of x-rays preoperatively, the problem is magnified clinically by having to look for multiple indications for 15–20 tests from the perspective of three physicians. Practically, this would require a computerized system with its own cost and time requirement for input.

Although the preceding discussion has been limited to laboratory tests, the same type of analysis can be applied to parts of the history and physical examination.

Keep in mind that even cost-benefit data are limited by the small number and quality of studies available.

Standard criteria have been developed for selecting a good screening test (Table 23.16). Additional factors applicable to the preoperative patient include: (a) the disease should not be easily detectable by routine history-physical examination; (b) the test result should affect the surgical or anesthetic risk; and (c) early knowledge of the disease should affect perioperative management.

Screening tests can be further evaluated by obtaining the sensitivity, specificity, and predictive value of the test (Table 23.17). *Sensitivity* is the number of patients with a *positive test plus the disease* divided by the total number of patients with the disease (i.e., correctly identify patients with the disease). *Specificity* is the number of patients with a *negative test plus no disease* divided by the total

Table 23.16. Criteria for Screening Tests[a]

1. Treatable disease whose natural history is known
2. Important problem (high incidence/prevalence; clinically significant)
3. Screening test available (sensitivity, specificity, predictive value)
4. Arrangements for treatment and follow-up

[a]Modified from WHO criteria. World Health Organization: Mass health examination. PUBLIC Health Paper N. 45, Geneva, World Health Organization, 1971.

number of patients without the disease (i.e., correctly identify patients with *no* disease). *Predictive value* (of either a positive or negative test) is the probability of patient with a positive test having the disease (or negative test being disease-free); this is based on the sensitivity/spec-

Table 23.17. Evaluation of Screening Tests for Preoperative Evaluation

		DISEASE[a]	
		+	−
TEST[b]	+	True-positive (TP)	False-positive (FP)
	−	False-negative (FN)	True-negative (TN)

$$\text{Sensitivity} = \frac{TP}{TP + FN} \quad \text{(correctly identify patients } \textbf{with } \text{disease)}^{c}$$

$$\text{Specificity} = \frac{TN}{TN + FP} \quad \text{(correctly identify patients with } \textbf{no } \text{disease)}^{c}$$

Predictive value of **Positive** (+) test[c,d] $= \dfrac{TP}{TP + FP}$ (probability an individual patient with a positive test has the disease)

[a] + = disease present; − = disease absent in patients.
[b] + = test positive; − = test negative in patients.
[c]Sensitivity and specificity given overall accuracy for a large study population of patients; to obtain the value for an individual patient, the prevalence of the condition in the population must be calculated in (= predictive value). A simplified method of calculating predictive value is given.
[d]Predictive value of **Negative** test not shown in table $\left(= \dfrac{TN}{TN + FN} \right)$ (= probability individual patient with a negative test is disease-free).

ificity with a factor for the prevalence of the condition in the population calculated in (Bayes' theorem). Bayes' theorem states that the probability of a patient with a positive test having the disease is in part dependent on the prevalence of the disease in the population or patient group to which the patient belongs. The predictive value of a positive test is higher in patient populations where the prevalence of the disease is higher.

Other factors influencing the selection of screening tests include the selection of cut points for determining abnormal tests; the method used for the test, and the precision of the individual hospital laboratory.

SPECIFIC PREOPERATIVE TESTS: EVALUATION

History and Physical Examination (see also p. 115)

Little information is available on the yield of the total history and physical examination in preoperative evaluation; even less data are available on specific parts of the exam. Turnbull (8) found 104 "potentially important" abnormal laboratory screening tests in 1010 patients with normal clinical examinations in a chart review.

If the laboratory is used as the standard of accuracy (despite marked limitations in doing so and the laboratory's own inaccuracies), there is little and conflicting data on the accuracy of the history-physical examination in identifying abnormalities (Table 23.18). There seems to be reasonable sensitivity when the clinical evaluation is abnormal. Wide variation in results are obtained when the negative history-physical is examined for false-negative results, whether the laboratory criteria is any abnormal test or only clinically significant abnormal tests. The reasons for this variation in results is not clear, but may be due to different quality of clinical examinations, study criteria, and type of test considered. In most of the better studies, the clinical examination has identified a high percentage of significant diseases found by laboratory tests.

Studies have not looked at the yield of the individual portions of the history-physical examination (e.g., family history, neurologic exam).

Recommendations: guidelines for the

Table 23.18. Comparison History-Physical Examination to Laboratory in Preoperative Evaluation[a]

Study	Laboratory Test	% Abn. H&P + Abn. Lab (Sensitivity)	% N1. H&P + Abn. Lab (FN)	Significant False-Neg (FN)
Jakobsson (12)	EKG		8%	
Rucker (20)	CXR		0.3%	0%
Tornebrandt (21)	CXR		37%	37%
Boghosian (28)	CXR	62%	34%	34%
Haubek (3)	CXR		3%	0%
Thomsen (3)	CXR		7%	0.2%
Eisenberg (41)	PTT	18%	3%	0.2%
Kaplan (9)	Admission Lab Tests[b]		0.4%	0.2%
Turnbull (8)	Admission Lab Tests[b]		22%	10%
Median		40%	7%	0.2%

[a] Abbreviations: H&P, history and physical examination; U/A = urinalysis; CXR = chest x-ray; PTT = partial thromboplastin time; Abn., abnormal; N1., normal; Lab, laboratory test; TP, true-positives; FN, false-negatives (see Table 23.17).
[b] Admission lab tests included some combination of CBC, U/A, chemistry tests.

selection of the comprehensive versus limited history/physical examination are given in Tables 23.2, p. 616 (based on limited studies and clinical experience).

Admission Laboratory Tests

The overall yield of the traditional battery of admission laboratory tests (CBC, clotting studies, chemistries) has been low in most studies (Fig. 23.2) (8–9; 56–57). Individual components of these batteries are considered below.

ELECTROCARDIOGRAM (EKG)

The number of preoperative electrocardiograms found to be abnormal is significant, but the number unpredicted by history-physical examination is less (10%) (Table 23.19). Only a small number of unexpected EKGs result in changes in therapy or surgical plans.

The percentage of unexpected abnor-

mal EKGs in surgical patients rises with age, with few being found before age 35 (3, 12, 14).

Expert consensus (3, 11) indicates that routine EKGs in all patients are not indicated. Routine EKGs are indicated preoperatively in patients over ages 30–40. There is no agreement on the age cutoff, and it may be higher for women (ages 35–55).

Recommendations: Routine preoperative EKGs should be obtained in patients over ages 30–35; *an older* age group of 35–40 years may be optionally used for women (based on literature and expert consensus).

CHEST X-RAYS

The number of chest x-rays found to be abnormal in preoperative patients is high, but the number in patients without clinical indicators of chest disease is much

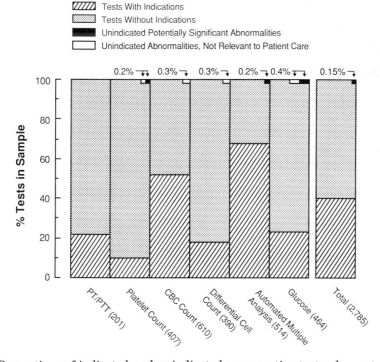

Figure 23.2. Proportions of indicated and unindicated preoperative tests, drawn to scale. Numbers in parentheses represent sample sizes used. PT/PTT indicates prothrombin time/partial thromboplastin time; CBC, complete blood cell. Automated multiple analysis is six factor. From: Kaplan EB, et al: The usefulness of preoperative laboratory screening. *JAMA* 253:3578, 1985, with permission. Copyright 1985, the American Medical Association.

Table 23.19.   Routine Preoperative EKGs: Yield

Study	No. of Patients	All Patients: Abnormals (%)	Normal Patients by H&P[a]	
			(%) Abnormals	% Abnormal *and* Change Management or Surgical Plans
Jakobsson (12)	731		8%	
Ferrer (14)	1,068	19%		
Paterson (15)	267	31%	16% (3% major abnormality)	2%
Rabkin (17)	812	21%		0%
Seymour (18)[b]	222	79%		
Turnbull (8)	1,010		10% (.4% major abnormality)	
Charpak (10)	1,610	38%		.3%
Bleary (56)	2,256	—	—	.3%
Catchleve (58)	60	20%	—	—
Median		26%	10% (2% major abnormality)	0.7%

[a] H&P, history and physical.
[b] Study restricted to patients over age 65.

smaller (Table 23.20). The number of chest x-ray findings that change medical or surgical management in patients with normal history-physical examinations is almost zero, except for one study of a small number of elderly patients. The overall yield of chest x-rays is small in healthy patients in available studies, but the total number of well-studied patients is small (Less than 2,000 in pooled studies). These numbers of patients may not be adequate to define risk and identify high-risk subgroups.

The percentage of abnormal x-ray findings increases with age in a general hospital population, from age 30 (2%) to over age 70 (45%) (3). Whether a baseline chest x-ray is helpful for comparison in the diagnosis of postoperative pulmonary complications cannot be decided on the basis of the one small study available (3).

Expert consensus (3, 19) has advised against routine chest x-rays solely because the patient is having surgery. Chest x-rays are indicated based on findings in the history-physical examination, and

possibly for the elderly because of the high incidence of concomitant disease, for cardiothoracic surgery, and surgery with a high risk of chest complications.

Recommendations: Routine chest x-rays need not be ordered solely because the patient is having surgery. Use of routine preoperative chest x-rays will depend on clinical judgment, with additional important factors being the patient's age, the type of anesthesia, and surgery. Factors indicating the need for a routine chest x-ray include, but are not limited to, elderly patients, general anesthesia, major surgery, surgery with a high risk of postoperative thoracic complications, and cardiothoracic surgery. Conversely, a patient under age 35 having regional or brief general anesthesia for a minor procedure does not necessarily need a routine chest x-ray. For the individual patient, clinical judgment based on these variables should supplement rigid guidelines based on studies, until more definitive studies (3) are available (based on literature, expert consensus, and clinical experience).

Table 23.20. Routine Preoperative Chest X-rays: Yield

Study	No. of Patients	All Patients: Abnormals (%)	Normal Patients by H&P[a]	
			(%) Abnormals	% Abnormal *and* Change Management or Surgical Plans
Haubek (3)[b]	204		3%	0%
Thomsen (3)[b]	1,227		6%	.2%
Rucker (20)[c]	368	13%	.3%	0%
Tape (24)	318	35%		0%
		(3–6% major abnormalites)		
Rees (26)	667	30%		
Charpak (10)	1,101	52%		
Turnbull (8)	1,010	4%		
Boghosian (28)	136		34%	
Tornebradt (21)[d]	100		37%	37%
Bleary (56)	2,765	—	—	.1%
Catchleve (58)	79	14%	—	—
Median		22%	6%	0%

[a] H&P, history and physical.
[b] Age > 40.
[c] Age > 59–60.
[d] Age > 70.

HEMATOLOGY

Few studies (3, 30–32) are available on the yield of the complete blood count and differential in routine perioperative assessment.

Preliminary, small studies have found a low incidence of abnormal hematocrits or hemoglobins in otherwise healthy surgical patients (Table 23.21). Small degrees of anemia may not increase surgical risk (30), as once thought. Expert consensus (1, 30) is generally that a hematocrit or hemoglobin test is indicated routinely because of the risk of anemia for anesthesia and the risk of further lowering of hematocrit by intraoperative bleeding, but dissenting views have been raised (3).

The yield of routine white blood cell counts in healthy preoperative patients has been 0.2%; 0% have changed medical or surgical management (8, 9). Expert consensus has not been reached for the routine white blood cell counts in surgical patients, again, based on inadequate data (3).

The yield of the routine differential white blood cell count in preoperative patients is low. In two studies of preoperative health patients and one study of a general hospital population (8, 31–32), no screening differential led to a significant new diagnosis or therapy. Expert consensus is that routine differential white blood cell counts are not needed in preoperative screening (3).

Recommendations: Routine hematocrit or hemoglobin counts should be obtained on preoperative patients, at least until adequate data on the safety of omitting this test in low risk subgroups are available (based on expert consensus, clinical experience). Routine white blood cell counts and differentials are not needed in preoperative patients (expert consensus).

CLOTTING STUDIES

Studies of common preoperative coagulation tests (partial thromboplastin time (PTT), prothrombin time (PT), platelet count, bleeding time) in otherwise low-risk patients (see p. 617) have found low

Table 23.21.   Routine Preoperative Hematocrit/Hemoglobin: Yield

Study	No. of Patients	All Patients: Abnormals (%)	Normal Patients by H&P[a]	
			(%) Abnormals	% Abnormal *and* Change Management or Surgical Plans
Kaplan (9)	610		.2%	0%
Turnbull (8)	1,010		.7%	.2%
Charpak (10)	3,004	4%		
Bleary (56)	1,728	—	—	1.6%
Median		4%	.5%	.6%

[a] H&P, history and physical.

yields of abnormal results and little effect on patient outcome (Table 23.22) (3, 37–39). The PTT has been best studied; inadequate numbers of patients have been studied for the PT and platelet count. Two studies found low yield to routine bleeding times in surgical patients (1.5% abnormal, 0 to 0.1% significantly abnormal) (38, 56). The bleeding history may not be as accurate as most clinicians assume (34–35). The low incidence of clotting disorders not identified by history, makes the best case theoretical predictive value of routine preoperative clotting studies very low, as has been demonstrated for the PTT (37).

Expert consensus is uniform in stating these tests are not routinely indicated in preoperative testing (3, 35, 37, 39, 42).

Recommendations: Routine hemostasis studies are not recommended in perioperative testing, except for high-risk surgery (neurosurgery), or where anticoagulation will be used intraoperatively (vascular and cardiac surgery) (based on literature and expert consensus).

SERUM GLUCOSE

Little data are available on the yield of routine serum glucoses screening for undiagnosed diabetes in surgical patients; what is known must be derived from yields of multi-test chemistry screening. The incidence of unexpected abnormal glucoses in routine preoperative testing was 1–2% (8, 9, 36); but may be as low as 0.3% (1). Changes in management occurred in 0.5% of patients screened (8–9, 56). The risks of occult adult-onset diabetes are probably less than juvenile diabetes in surgical patients. Expert consensus is not available for glucose screening. An alternative screening test is the urinalysis with testing for glycosuria, although this is less sensitive and specific than serum glucose; comparative figures are not available for surgical patients.

Recommendations: Urinalysis with a chemical test for glucose should be obtained in all surgical patients. Fasting serum glucose should be obtained in patients undergoing major surgical procedures or prolonged anesthesia (based on clinical experience).

TESTS OF RENAL FUNCTION (BUN, CREATININE, URINALYSIS)

Again, little information is available on routine preoperative testing of renal function. The yield of unexpected abnormalities of BUN and creatinine in otherwise healthy preoperative patients was 0.2% in limited studies (3, 8, 9, 56). The yield of preoperative urinalysis varies, depending on what is called abnormal; minor abnormalities such as a few white cells are common, but have little effect on physician management (43–44). Expert consensus is not available for renal function

Table 23.22.   Routine Tests of Hemostasis : Yield

Study	No. of Patients	All Patients: Abnormals (%)	Normal Patients by H&P[a]	
			(%) Abnormals	% Abnormal *and* Change Management or Surgical Plans
Partial thromboblastic time (PTT)				
Robbins (42)	1,000	14%		
Eisenberg (41)	750	4%	3%	0%
Suchman (39)			13%	[b]
Kaplan (9)	199	.5%	0%	0%
Trumbull (8)	210		3%	0%
Charpak (10)	952	8%	—	0%
Bleary (56)	2,914	—	—	0%
Rohrer (61)	282	5%	2.4%	
Median		4%	3%	0%
Prothrombin Time (PT)				
Kaplan (9)	201	1%	0%	0%
Trumbull (8)	213		0%	0%
Charpak (10)	935	8%		
Bleary (56)	2,931	—	—	0%
Rohrer (61)	2,825	.7%	.8%	—
Median		1%	0%	0%
Platelet Count				
Trumbull (8)	1,010		0%	0%
Bleary (56)	3,576			0.03%
Rohrer (61)	282	12%	8%	
Median		—	—	0%

[a] H&P, history and physical.
[b] No difference in bleeding complications between patients with and without elevated PTT.

tests. The recent availability of chemical tests for leukocyte esterase and totally automated urinalysis will probably require a reassessment of the cost-benefit of routine urinalysis.

Recommendations: A urinalysis is recommended for all surgical preoperative evaluations; dipstix evaluation using a dipstix, continuing tests for leukocyte esterase and nitrates, is adequate for screening (but not for surgical differential diagnosis). A creatinine should be obtained before major surgical procedures; a BUN is redundant, less accurate, and not needed unless for diagnostic purposes (based on clinical experience).

BASIC CHEMISTRY (ELECTROLYTES)

Routine preoperative electrolytes in normal patients yielded unexpected abnormalities in potassium in 0–1.5% of patients; of sodium in 0–0.5% of patients (3, 8–9, 56). Data are not available for abnormalities of chloride or carbon dioxide, but they would presumably be low. Expert consensus is not available.

Recommendations: Routine electrolytes do not need to be obtained for minor surgery. We prefer to obtain a potassium for general anesthesia, because of the risk, although the yield is low. A full set of electrolytes should be obtained for major procedures, until data are available on the safety of omitting this test (based on clinical experience).

LIVER ENZYMES

The yield of liver enzyme tests is not available for routine preoperative screening. Theoretical calculations indicate the yield would be low (1). The risk of occult hepatitis to the operating room team must be considered (1), but liver enzyme tests will have an uncertain effect on reducing this risk.

Recommendations: Routine testing of healthy preoperative patients for liver enzymes is not recommended. High-risk groups (Table 23.2) should be tested, including alcoholics, homosexuals, drug abusers, dialysis patients, and patients on drugs with a high risk of causing liver abnormalities (based on clinical experience).

MULTIPHASIC CHEMISTRY BATTERIES

Routine multiphasic 20-test chemistry panels have been investigated in general hospital populations and a small number of studies of surgical patients (3, 8–9, 45–52, 57). Data on yield in healthy surgical patients are difficult to extract from available publications. In general hospital populations, abnormal chemistry tests may be found in 10–40% of patients, but lead to a new diagnosis in only 0.2–10% of patients, and result in changes in management only in a small percentage. The number of false-positive tests is significant, since 20 tests are run, each with a false-positive rate of 2.5% in most laboratories (hence, the false-positive rate approaches the total gross yield of these tests); most of the other positive tests were accounted for by known diseases in the patients. Many of the unexpected abnormal results were ignored by the clinicians; no follow-up or action was taken.

Expert consensus generally recommends not obtaining routine multiple biochemical chemistry panels on healthy preoperative patients (3). These chemistry panels are frequently ordered in clinical practice.

Recommendations: Multiphasic chemistry 20-test batteries are not routinely indicated on healthy preoperative patients. A reasonable indication for such panels is the patient requiring multiple individual chemistry tests (as described above), where the battery would be less expensive (based on expert consensus, clinical experience).

NUTRITIONAL TESTING

This subject is discussed in Chapter 5, pp. 38–59.

PREGNANCY TESTING

Quantitative data are not available on the incidence of unsuspected pregnancy in surgical patients, but clinical experience suggests that it is low. Surgery during pregnancy carries some risk to the fetus (see p. 586). Expert consensus is not available on the indications for pregnancy testing in healthy preoperative patients.

Recommendations: A serum pregnancy test (qualitative HCG) should be obtained on women of childbearing age preoperatively, unless pregnancy is excluded for some other reason (sterilization, menses), based on the rare risk of harm to the fetus.

SEROLOGIC TESTING FOR SYPHILIS

Expert consensus is that routine testing for syphilis is no longer indicated, based on the low incidence of syphilis in most hospital populations.

Recommendations: Routine testing of all preoperative surgical patients for syphilis is not indicated (based on expert consensus).

HIV TESTING

Consideration of routine testing of surgical patients for human immunodeficiency virus (HIV) has been raised because of concerns for the safety of the operating team, and the effect of a fatal disease on surgical decision making, especially for elective surgery. The prevalence of undiagnosed HIV infection in surgical patients is not known and probably varies by hospital, depending on population. One inner city emergency room found a prevalence of 3% HIV seropositivity, many of which were not known to the care providers.

Routine HIV testing of surgical patients raises the ethical questions of high ratio of false-to true-positive tests in low-prevalence populations and of consent. Large logistical problems are raised, including the time required for testing, retesting of false-positive results (with resultant cancellation of surgery), and the required counseling of patients with positive results. The adverse effect of false-positive results on the patient must be considered.

Current expert recommendation is not to screen routinely for HIV in all healthy surgical patients (53–55), but the internist should keep abreast of recent developments in this controversial area.

Recommendations: Routine HIV testing of all healthy preoperative patients is not currently recommended at the time this book was written (based on expert consensus).

PULMONARY FUNCTION TESTS AND ARTERIAL BLOOD GASES

These are discussed in Chapter 6, p. 60.

NON-INVASIVE CARDIAC EVALUATION

This is discussed in Chapter 10, pp. 113–114.

READINGS

1. Robbins JA, Mushlin AI: Preoperative evaluation of the healthy patient. *Med Clin North Am* 63:1145–1156, 1979.
2. Gross RJ, Barker LR, Spees EK: Preoperative planning for the ambulatory patient. In Barker RL, et al (eds).: *Principles of Ambulatory Medicine*. Baltimore, Williams & Wilkins, 1986, pp 1235–1259, 1986.
3. Sox HC (ed): *Common Diagnostic Tests: Use and Interpretation*, Philadelphia, American College of Physicians, 1988.
4. Davis JE, Ugioka K: Selecting the patient for major ambulatory surgery: Surgical and anesthesiology evaluations. *Surg Clin North Am* 721–732, 1987.
5. Lagoe RJ, Milliren JW: A community-based analysis of ambulatory surgery utilization. *Amer J Public Health* 76:150–153, 1986.
6. Laffaye HA: The impact of an ambulatory surgical service in a community hospital. *Arch Surg* 124:601–603, 1989.
6a. Gold BS, Kitz, DS, Lecky JH, et al.: "Unanticipated admission to the hospital following ambulatory surgery." *JAMA* 262:3008–3010, 1989.
7. Lilienfield A, Lilienfield DE: *Foundations of Epidemiology* New York, Oxford University Press, 1980.
8. Turnbull JM, Buck C: The value of preoperative screening investigations in otherwise healthy individuals. *Arch Intern Med* 147:1101–1105, 1987.
9. Kaplan EB, Sheiner LB, Boeckmann AJ, et al.: The usefulness of preoperative laboratory screening. *JAMA* 253:3576–3581, 1985.
10. Charpak Y, Blery C, Chastang C, et al.: Usefulness of selectively ordered preoperative tests. *Med Care* 26:95–104, 1988.
11. Diagnostic and therapeutic technology assessment: Mandatory ECG before elective surgery. *JAMA* 250:540, 1983.
12. Jakobsson A, White T: Routine preoperative electrocardiograms. *Lancet* 1:972, 1984.
13. Goldberger AL, O'Konski M: Utility of the routine electrocardiogram before surgery and on general hospital admission. *Ann Intern Med* 105:552–557, 1986.
14. Ferrer MI: The value of obligatory preoperative electrocardiograms. *J Am Med Wom Assoc* 33:459–469, 1978.
15. Paterson KR, Caskie JP, Galloway DJ, et al.: The pre-operative electrocardiogram: An assessment. *Scott Med J* 28:116–118, 1983.
16. Rabkin SW, Horne JM: Preoperative electrocardiography: Its cost-effectiveness in detecting abnormalities when a previous tracing exists. *Can Med Assoc J* 121:301–306, 1979.
17. Rabkin SW, Horne JM: Preoperative electrocardiography: Effect of new abnormalities on clinical decisions. *Can Med Assoc J* 128:146–147, 1983.
18. Seymour DG, Pringle R, Maclennan WJ: The role of the routine pre-operative electrocardiogram in the elderly surgical patient. *Age and Ageing* 12:97–104, 1983.
19. National Center for Devices and Radiological Health: *The Selection of Patients for X-ray Examinations: Chest x ray Screening Examinations*. Rockville, Maryland: Food and Drug Administration, 1983. HHS public. no. (FDA) 83-8204.
20. Rucker L, Frye EB, Staten MA: Usefulness of screening chest roentgenograms in preoperative patients. *JAMA* 250:3209–3211, 1983.
21. Tornebrandt K, Fletcher R: Pre-operative chest x-rays in elderly patients. *Anaesthesia* 37:901–902, 1982.
22. Loder RE: Routine pre-operative chest radiography. *Anaesthesia* 33:972–974, 1978.
23. National Study by the Royal College of Radiologists: Preoperative chest radiology. *Lancet* II: 83–86, 1979.
24. Tape TG, Mushlin AI: How useful are routine chest x-rays of preoperative patients at risk for postoperative chest diseases? *J Gen Intern Med* 3:15–20, 1988.
25. Sagel SS, Evens RG, Forrest IV, et al.: Efficacy

of routine screening and lateral chest radiographs in a hospital-based population. *N Engl J Med* 291:1001–1004, 1974.

26. Rees AM, Roberts CJ, Bligh AS, et al.: Routine preoperative chest radiography in non-cardiopulmonary surgery. *Brit Med J* 1:1333–1335, 1976.

27. Hubbell FA, Greenfield S, Tyler JL, et al.: The impact of routine admission chest x-ray films on patient care. *New Engl J Med* 312:209–213, 1985.

28. Boghosian SG, Mooradian AD: Usefulness of routine preoperative chest roentgenograms in elderly patients. *J Amer Geriatr Soc* 35:142–146, 1987.

29. Tape TG, Mushlin AI: The utility of routine chest radiographs. *Ann Intern Med* 104:663–670, 1986.

30. Consensus Conference: Perioperative red blood cell transfusion. *JAMA* 260:2700–2703, 1988.

31. Connelly DP, McClain MP, Crowson TW, et al.: The use of the differential leukocyte count for inpatient casefinding. *Human Path* 13:294–300, 1982.

32. Shapiro MF, Hatch RL, Greenfield S: Cost containment and labor-intensive tests: The case of the leukocyte differential count. *JAMA* 252:231–234, 1984.

33. Shapiro MF, Greenfield S: The complete blood count and leukocyte differential count: An approach to their rational application. *Ann Intern Med* 106:65–74, 1987.

34. Borzotta AP, Keeling MM: Value of the preoperative history as an indicator of hemostatic disorders. *Ann Surg* 200:648–652, 1984.

35. Rapaport SI: Preoperative hemostatic evaluation: Which tests, if any? *Blood* 61:229–231, 1983.

36. Nye SW, Graham JB, Brinkhous KM: "The Partial Thromboplastin Time as a Screening Test for the Detection of Latent Bleeders." *Amer J Med Sci* 243:279–287, 1962.

37. Clarke JR, Eisenberg JM: A theoretical assessment of the value of the PTT as a preoperative screening test in adults. *Med Decision Making* 1:40–43, 1981.

38. Barber A, Green D, Galluzzo T, et al.: The bleeding time as a preoperative screening test. *Amer J Med* 78:761–764, 1985.

39. Suchman A, Mushlin AI: How well does the activated partial thromboplastin time predict postoperative hemorrhage? *JAMA* 256:750–753, 1986.

40. Suchman AL, Griner PF: Diagnostic uses of the activated partial thromboplastin time and prothrombin time. *Ann Intern Med* 104:810–816, 1986.

41. Eisenberg JM, Clarke JR, Sussman SA: Prothrombin and partial thromboplastin times as preoperative screening tests. *Arch Surg* 117:48–51, 1982.

42. Robbins JA, Rose SD: Partial thromboplastin time as a screening test. *Ann Intern Med* 90:796–797, 1979.

43. Kroenke K, Hanley JF, Copley JB, et al.: The admission urinalysis. *J Gen Intern Med* 1:238–242, 1986.

44. Lawrence VA, Kroenke K: The unproven utility of preoperative urinalysis. *Arch Intern Med* 148:1370–1373, 1988.

45. Bryan DJ, Wearne JL, Viau A, et al.: Profile of admission chemical data by multichannel automation: An evaluative experiment. *Clin Chem* 12:137–143, 1966.

46. Durbridge TC, Edwards F, Edwards RG, et al.: Evaluation of benefits of screening tests done immediately on admission to hospital. *Clin Chem* 22:968–971, 1976.

47. Belliveau RT, Fitzgerald JE, Nickerson DA: Evaluation of a routine profile chemistry screening of all patients admitted to a community hospital. *Amer J Clin Path* 53:447–451, 1970.

48. Whitehead TP, Woolton IDP: Biochemical profiles for hospital patients. *Lancet* II: 1439–1443, 1974.

49. Bradwell AR, Carmalt MHB, Whitehead TP: Explaining the unexpected abnormal results of biochemical profile investigations. *Lancet* II: 1071–1074, 1974.

50. Campbell IT, Gosling, P: Preoperative biochemical screening. *Brit Med J* 2:803–804, 1988.

51. Korvin CC, Pearce RH, Stanley J: Admissions screening: Clinical benefits. *Ann Intern Med* 83:197–203, 1975.

52. Cebul RD, Beck JR: Biochemical profiles: Applications in ambulatory screening and preadmission testing of adults. *Ann Intern Med* 106:403–413, 1987.

53. DeVita VT, Hellman S, Rosenberg SA: *AIDS: Etiology, Diagnosis, Treatment and Prevention.* Philadelphia, JB Lippincott, 1988.

54. Hagen MD, Meyer KB, Pauker SG: Routine preoperative screening for HIV: Does the risk to the surgeon outweigh the risk to the patient? *JAMA* 259:1357–1359, 1988.

55. Bayer R, Levine C, Wokf SM: HIV antibody screening: An ethical framework for evaluating proposed programs. *JAMA* 256:1768–1771, 1986.

56. Blery C, Szatan M, Fourgeaux B: Evaluation of a protocol for selective ordering of preoperative tests. *Lancet* I:139–141, 1986.

57. Durbridge TC, Edwards F, Edwards RG: An evaluation of multiphasic screening on admission to hospital. *Med J Aust* 1:703–705, 1976.

58. Catchlove BR, Wilson RM, Springs S, et al.: Routine investigations in elective surgical patients. *Med J Aust* 2:107–110, 1979.

59. Pineault R, Contandriopoulos AP, Valois M, et al.: Randomized clinical trial of one-day surgery. *Med Care* 23:171–182, 1985.

60. Mozes B, Lubin D, Modan B, et al.: Evaluation of an intervention aimed at reducing inappropriate use of preoperative blood coagulation tests. *Arch Intern Med* 149:1836–1838, 1989.

61. Rohrer MJ, Michelotti MC, Nahrwold DL: A prospective evaluation of the efficacy of preoperative coagulation testing. *Ann Surg* 208:554–557, 1988.

24

Useful Equations for the Consultant

William S. Kammerer

Our expanding ability to gather clinically relevant physiologic and pharmacokinetic data has led to a profusion of formulas, nomograms, and information on which to base diagnostic and therapeutic decisions. Memorization will suffice for those which we use frequently. However, memory cannot always be relied upon for the rest, or even for the original reference sources. Throughout this book, the authors have routinely included useful equations, rules of thumb, and clinical maxims appropriate to their subjects. This addendum is meant to serve as a partial catchall for additional information of use to the consulting internist. While information of this type is of great clinical usefulness, the "whole" patient and clinical situation is of equally great importance. Diagnosis and therapy "by the numbers" alone is not our intent.

The availability of portable programmable calculators will have a major impact on this aspect of medical practice, allowing us to have at our fingertips the ability to calculate drug dosage, cardiopulmonary performance, acid-base status, statistical significance, among others. The traditional bulging "peripheral brain" of most internists, consisting of innumerable pearls, cryptic notes, and references, may well be on the way to extinction, to be replaced by the silica-chip, microcircuited, programmable calculator.

General Information

Prefix	Multiplication Factor	Symbol
deca	10	da
hecto	10^2	h
kilo	10^3	k
mega	10^6	M
deci	10^{-1}	d
centi	10^{-2}	c
milli	10^{-3}	m
micro	10^{-6}	μ
nano	10^{-9}	n
pico	10^{-12}	p
femto	10^{-15}	f

Average Future Lifetime in U.S.*

Age Interval	Number Living†	Average Life Expectancy	White Male	White Female	All Others Male	All Others Female
0–1	100,000	72.4	69.3	77.0	63.6	72.5
1–5	98,387	72.6	69.4	77.0	64.2	73.1
5–10	98,104	68.6	65.6	73.2	60.5	69.3
10–15	97,930	63.9	60.8	68.3	55.6	64.5
15–20	97,747	59.0	55.9	63.4	50.8	59.5
20–25	97,251	54.3	51.3	58.6	46.2	54.7
25–30	96,572	49.7	46.8	53.7	42.0	50.0
30–35	95,902	45.0	42.1	48.9	37.8	45.3
35–40	95,186	40.3	37.5	44.1	33.7	40.7
40–45	94,164	35.7	32.9	39.3	29.7	36.3
45–50	92,643	31.3	28.4	34.7	25.9	32.0
50–55	90,335	27.0	24.2	30.2	22.3	27.9
55–60	86,855	23.0	20.3	25.9	19.0	24.1
60–65	81,778	19.3	16.7	21.8	16.1	20.7
65–70	74,502	15.9	13.6	18.0	13.6	17.5
70–75	65,367	12.7	10.8	14.3	11.2	14.3
75–80	58,151	10.1	8.5	11.1	9.6	12.5
80–85	38,694	7.9	6.6	8.5	8.5	11.0
85 and up	24,137	6.2	5.2	6.5	7.1	9.4

*Average number of years of life remaining at beginning of age interval.
Source: *World Almanac and Book of Facts, 1977.* Newspaper Enterprise Association, New York.
†Of 100,000 born alive, number living at beginning of age interval.

Metabolic-Physiologic

1. Correction of metabolic acidosis:
   HCO_3^- required = base deficit (meq/L) $\times$ 0.3 · (body weight in kg)
2. Correction of metabolic alkalosis:
   HCl (meq) required = base excess (meq/L) $\times$ 0.4 · (body weight in kg)
3. Correction of K^+ deficit:
   100–200 meq K^+ for each meq decrease in serum K^+ to 3.0 meq/L
   300–400 meq K^+ for each meq decrease in serum K^+ below 3.0 meq/L
   (In presence of alkalosis, serum K^+ first corrected by an increase of 0.7 meq for each 0.1-unit elevation of pH above 7.40)
4. Uric acid clearance (1):
   $$\frac{U \text{ uric} \cdot P\text{cr;}}{U \text{ cr.}} \quad \text{normal} = 0.4, \pm 0.1; >0.7 = \text{gout}$$
5. Correcting WBC count in traumatic spinal tap (2):
   $$\text{No. of WBCs introduced} = \frac{(\text{peripheral WBC}) \times (\text{RBC in CSF})}{\text{peripheral RBC count}}$$
6. CSF sugar values in patients with meningitis (3):
   Non-diabetic <½ blood glucose
   Diabetic <⅓ blood glucose

7. Drugs with a high sodium content:
   Carbenicillin (4.7 meq/gram)
   Penicillin G (1.7 meq/milion units)
   Ampicilin (3 meq/gram)
   Cephalothin (2.5 meq/gram)
   Kayexalate (65 meq/16 grams)
   Fleet's Phospho-soda (24 meq/5 ml)
8. Sodium, salt, milligrams, and milliequivalents:

Milliequivalents Na$^+$ (Approximate)	Milligrams Na$^+$	Grams Salt (NaCl) (Approximate)
11	250	0.6
22	500	1.3
43	1000	2.5
65	1500	3.8
87	2000	5.0
130	3000	7.6
174	4000	10.2

9. Relative corticosteroid potencies:

Agent	Glucocorticoid activity (cortisol = 1)	Mineralocorticoid activity (cortisol = 1)	Plasma Half-life (min)
Hydrocortisone (cortisol)	1	1	90
Cortisone	0.7	0.7	30
Prednisone	4	0.7	60
Prednisolone	4	0.7	200
Methylprednisolone	5	0.5	200
Triamcinolone	5	0	200
Dexamethasone	25	0–2	300
Betamethasone	30	0	300
Fludrocortisone	10	125	30
Aldosterone	0.1	400	
Corticosterone	0.35	2	70

Renal

1. Bedside estimate of creatinine clearance (4):

   a. For men $= \dfrac{\dfrac{98 - 16 \cdot (\text{Age} - 20)}{20}}{P_{cr}}$

   For women, use 90% of above value

   b. $\dfrac{\text{Ur. Cr. grams}}{\text{Serum Cr. mg \%}} - 70$

2. Urinary diagnostic indices (5)

	Prerenal Azotemia	Acute Oliguric Renal Failure	Acute Nonoliguric Renal Failure	Acute Obstructive Uropathy	Acute Glomerulonephriti
Urine osmolality, mOsm/kg H_2O	518 ± 35	369 ± 20	343 ± 17	393 ± 39	385 ± 61
Urine sodium, meq/L	18 ± 3	68 ± 5	50 ± 5	68 ± 10	22 ± 6
Urine/plasma urea nitrogen	18 ± 7	3 ± 0.5	7 ± 1	8 ± 4	11 ± 4
Urine/plasma creatinine	45 ± 6	17 ± 2	17 ± 2	16 ± 4	43 ± 7
Renail failure index ‡	0.6 ± 0.1	10 ± 2	4 ± 0.6	8 ± 3	$0.4 \pm 0.$
Fractional excretion of filtered sodium §	0.4 ± 0.1	7 ± 1.4	3 ± 0.5	6 ± 2	$0.6 \pm 0.$

$$‡ U_{Na} \Big/ \frac{U_{cr}}{P_{cr}}$$

$$§ U_{Na}/P_{Na} \Big/ U_{cr}/P_{cr}$$

Cardiovascular

Correlation of NYHA Functional Class with Cardiopulmonary Performance§

Functional class	1		2	3		4	
Ejection fraction	>0.55	0.50	0.40	0.30	0.20		0.1
End diastolic left ventricular pressure							
Rest	<12 mm Hg			>12 mm Hg			
After exercise	<12 mm Hg		>12 mm Hg				
Cardiac index (rest)	>2.5 L/min/M²			2.0		1.5	
Vital capacity				−30%		−35–50%	

§Adapted from Alderman (9), with permission

Normal values (6–8)
Cardiac index   3.5 L/min/M² ± 0.7
Stroke index   46 ml/min/M² ± 8.1
AVO_2 difference   4.1 vol % ± 0.6

	O_2 Saturation (%)
Right atrial pressure: mean <5 mm Hg	75
Pulmonary artery pressure: <32/13 mm Hg	75
Pulmonary artery wedge: mean < 13 mm Hg	97
End diastolic left ventricular pressure: <12 mm Hg	95

Calculation of Loading Doses for Phenobarbital and Hydantoin

$$L.D. = \frac{V \cdot (C_D - C_O)}{F}$$

C_D = Concentration desired
C_O = Concentration observed
F = Bioavailability

phenobarbital, hydantoin I.V.	= 1
phenobarbital p.o.	= 0.9
hydantoin p.o.	= 0.95

V = Volume of distribution:

phenobarbital	= 0.60L/Kg
hydantoin	= 0.65L/Kg

Aminoglycoside Dosing Guidelines

1. Calculate loading dose (LD) based on desired peak serum level

Gentamicin/Tobramycin		Amikacin	
LD	Peak level	LD	Peak level
1.5–2.0 mg/kg	4–6 mcg/ml	5.0 mg/kg	10–20 mcg/ml
2.0–2.5 mg/kg	6–8 mcg/ml	7.5 mg/kg	20–30 mcg/ml

2. Estimate patient's creatinine clearance (CrCl) from serum creatinine

$$\frac{CrCl}{\text{in ml/min}} = \frac{(140\text{-age})}{SCR \times 72} \times \text{wt. in kg} (\times 0.85 \text{ for females})$$

Minimum SCR
0.5 if <60 yrs.
1.0 if >60 yrs.

3. Determine maintenance dose (MD) and schedule using CrCl and LD according to the table below:

CrCl	MD = Percentage of LD	Dosing Interval
90	84%	q 8H
80	80%	q 8H
70	76%	q 8H
60	84%	q 12H
50	79%	q 12H
40	92%	q 24H
30	86%	q 24H
25	81%	q 24H
20	75%	q 24H

NOTE: These guidelines are not intended for use in patients with life threatening infections, changing renal function, marked obesity, CrCl <20ml/min, malnutrition, hemodialysis patients and in pediatric patients.

READINGS

1. Simkin PA, Hoover PL, Paxson CS, et al.: Uric acid excretion: Quantitative assessment from spot, midmorning serum and urine samples. *Ann Intern Med* 91:44–47, 1979.
2. Gottlieb AJ, Zamkoff KW, Jastremski MS, et al.: *The Whole Internist Catalog*, Philadelphia, WB Saunders, 1980.
3. Powers WJ: Cerebrospinal fluid to serum glucose ratios in diabetes mellitus and bacterial meningitis. *Am J Med* 71:217–220, 1981.
4. Jelliffe RW: Creatinine clearance: bedside estimate (letter to the editor). *Ann Intern Med* 79:604, 1979.
5. Miller TR, Anderson RJ, Linas SL, et al.: Urinary diagnostic indices in acute renal failure: A prospective study. *Ann Intern Med* 89:47–50, 1978.
6. Siber LM, Whitfield GF, Nagamatsu GR, et al.:

Surgical risk in a patient with recent myocardial infarction. *Hosp Physician* No. 6:31–36, 1979.

7. Anderson CC, Whitfield GF, Cohn J: Filling pressures and the critically ill patient: Part I. *Hosp Physician* No. 3:28–32, 1980.

8. Anderson CC, Cohn J, Whitfield GF: Filling pressures and the critically ill patient: Part II. *Hosp Physician* No. 5:39–46, 1980.

9. Alderman EL: Angiographic indicators of left ventricular function. *JAMA* 235:1055–1058, 1976.

GENERAL REFERENCES

10. Bennett WM, Muther RS, Parker RA, et al.: Drug therapy in renal failure: Dosing guidelines for adults. Part I: Antimicrobial agents, analgesics. *Ann Intern Med* 93:62–89, 1980.

11. Bennett WM, Muther RS, Parker RA, et al.: Drug therapy in renal failure: Dosing guidelines for adults. Part II: Sedatives, hypnotics, and tranquilizers; cardiovascular, antihypertensive, and diuretic agents; miscellaneous agents. *Ann Intern Med* 93:286–325, 1980.

12. Adverse interactions of drugs. *The Medical Letter* 23:17–28, 1981.

13. *Coronary Risk Handbook*. American Heart Association, New York, 1973.

Index

Page numbers in *italics* denote figures; those followed by "t" denote tables.